W9-ASP-269

Handbook of

DAIRY
FOODS AND
NUTRITION

Second Edition

CRC SERIES IN MODERN NUTRITION
Edited by Ira Wolinsky and James F. Hickson, Jr.

Edited by Ira Wolinsky

Forthcoming Titles Continued

Advanced Nutrition: Macronutrients, Second Edition, Carolyn D. Berdanier

Handbook of Nutrition for Vegetarians, Joan Sabate and Rosemary A. Ratzin-Tuner

Tryptophan: Biochemicals and Health Implications, Herschel Sidransky

Coenzyme Q: From Molecular Mechanisms to Nutrition and Health, Valerian E. Kagan and Peter J. Quinn

Nutraceuticals and Functional Foods, Robert E. C. Wildman

The Mediterranean Diet, Antonia L. Matalas, Antonios Zampelas, Vasilis Stavrinos, and Ira Wolinsky

Handbook of Nutrition and the Aged, Third Edition, Ronald R. Watson

Handbook of Nutraceuticals and Nutritional Supplements and Pharmaceuticals, Robert E. C. Wildman

Handbook of
DAIRY FOODS AND NUTRITION

Second Edition

Gregory D. Miller
Judith K. Jarvis
Lois D. McBean

 NATIONAL DAIRY COUNCIL

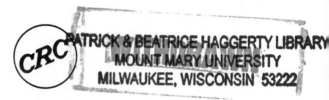

CRC Press
Boca Raton London New York Washington, D.C.

Library of Congress Cataloging-in-Publication Data

Miller, Gregory D.
    Handbook of dairy foods and nutrition/ Gregory D. Miller, Judith
K. Jarvis, Lois D. McBean. — 2nd ed.
        p.   cm. — (Modern nutrition)
    Includes bibliographical references and index.
    ISBN 0-8493-8731-0 (alk. paper)
    1. Dairy products in human nutrition Handbooks, manuals, etc.
I. Jarvis, Judith K.   II. McBean, Lois D.   III. Title.   IV. Series:
Modern nutrition (Boca Raton, Fla.)
QP144.M54M55 1999
613.2′6—dc21   99-32183
                                                                                        CIP

© 2000 by CRC Press LLC

No claim to original U.S. Government works
International Standard Book Number 0-8493-8731-0
Library of Congress Card Number 99-32183
Printed in the United States of America   2 3 4 5 6 7 8 9 0
Printed on acid-free paper

Series Preface

The CRC Series in Modern Nutrition is dedicated to providing the widest possible coverage of topics in nutrition. Nutrition is an interdisciplinary, interprofessional field par excellence. It is noted by its broad range and diversity. We trust the titles and authorship in this series will reflect that range and diversity.

Published for a broad audience, the volumes in the CRC Series in Modern Nutrition are designed to explain, review, and explore present knowledge and recent trends, developments, and advances in nutrition. As such, they will appeal to professionals as well as the educated layman. The format for the series will vary with the needs of the author and the topic, including, but not limited to, edited volumes, monographs, handbooks, and texts.

Contributors from any bona fide area of nutrition, including the controversial, are welcome.

I welcome the contribution of the book *Handbook of Dairy Foods and Nutrition, Second Edition* by my talented and energetic colleagues Gregory D. Miller, Ph.D., F.A.C.N., Judith K. Jarvis, M.S., R.D., L.D., Lois D. McBean, M.S., R.D. The first edition proved extremely useful and we have received lots of positive feedback. It serves as a resource for those interested in nutritional and clinical aspects of milk and milk products. The second edition is again timely, up-to-date, and covers an important subject area.

Ira Wolinsky, Ph.D.
University of Houston
Series Editor

Introduction

America's dairy farmers participate in a national check-off program that provides monies to promote the consumption of dairy foods. A large portion of these funds is used to support nutrition research, communication, and education. Since 1915, the National Dairy Council® has been committed to establishing programs and developing educational materials based on current scientific research, as well as providing sound scientific information in all of its communications.

This book is an update of the first edition of the *Handbook of Dairy Foods and Nutrition*. We have again attempted to review the most current scientific information available on the role and value of dairy foods in a healthful diet. It is a part of our ongoing effort to provide up-to-date information on foods and nutrition research to health professionals, educators, consumers, processors, and other interested groups. We hope this new edition will continue to be a useful resource on the role of dairy foods in health and nutrition.

The Authors

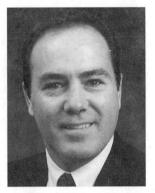

Gregory D. Miller, Ph.D., F.A.C.N., is vice president, nutrition research for National Dairy Council® (NDC), Rosemont, Illinois. Dr. Miller graduated in 1978 from Michigan State University with a B.S. degree in nutrition and in 1982 earned an M.S. degree in nutrition (toxicology) from The Pennsylvania State University. In 1986 he received a Ph.D. in Nutrition (toxicology) from The Pennsylvania State University.

He served as an undergraduate research assistant in nutrition-toxicology at Michigan State University in 1978 and was a graduate research assistant in the Center for Air Environment Studies and the Nutrition Department of The Pennsylvania State University from 1979 to 1986. Dr. Miller was a research scientist for Kraft, Inc., Glenview, Illinois from 1986 to 1989 and was a senior research scientist from 1989 to 1992.

Dr. Miller is a member of the American College of Nutrition, The American Society for Nutritional Sciences, The American Society for Clinical Nutrition, Institute of Food Technologists Nutrition Division, the American Dairy Science Association, and the International Society for the Study of Fatty Acids and Lipids. He was a scientific advisory panel member for the Office of Technology Assessment for the development of several reports to Congress on issues in the treatment and prevention of osteoporosis. He has chaired or co-chaired more than 20 workshops and symposia for national organizations including the American Society for Nutritional Sciences, American College of Nutrition, and the International Life Sciences Institute.

Dr. Miller is a member of the Editorial Board for the *Journal of the American College of Nutrition* and *Mature Medicine Canada*. He has served as a symposium editor for the *Journal of Nutrition* and the *Journal of the American College of Nutrition*. He is an editorial advisor for *Prepared Foods* and *Dairy Foods* magazines. He has served as a member of the board of directors and is secretary treasurer for the American College of Nutrition. He is currently a board member of the United States National Committee to the International Dairy Federation and is president of the International Dairy Federation's Commission on Science, Nutrition, and Education.

Among other awards, he has received the 1989 Kraft Basic Science Award and was listed in the 1992 *American Men and Women of Science* and the 1992 *Who's Who in Science*. In 1993, Dr. Miller was elected as a Fellow of the American College of Nutrition. He was selected as an outstanding alumnus by the Michigan State University in 1996, and received the Health and Human Development Alumni Recognition Award in 1996 from The Pennsylvania State University.

Dr. Miller has presented more than 65 invited lectures at national and international meetings and has published more than 85 research papers, reviews, articles, and abstracts. He has co-edited three books on diet, nutrition, and toxicology and contributed chapters to eight books. He is co-author of the *Handbook of Dairy Foods and Nutrition*.

Lois McBean, M.S., R.D., is a nutrition consultant for National Dairy Council. She is the author/editor of NDC's *Dairy Council Digest*, a bimonthly review of nutrition research for health professionals.

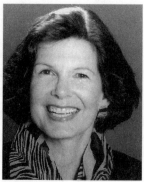

Lois McBean received a B.A. degree in 1966 from the University of Toronto, and obtained her M.S. degree in nutrition in 1968 from Cornell University. Lois is a registered dietitian and an active member of The American Dietetic Association, The American Society for Nutritional Sciences, and The Institute of Food Technology.

Prior to her career as a nutrition writer/editor and consultant, Lois McBean was a research nutritionist for the federal government in Washington, D.C., where she was involved in the establishment of zinc as an essential nutrient. Lois has written extensively on many diet and health issues, especially those related to the dairy industry. In addition to newsletters, she has authored numerous articles in peer-reviewed scientific journals, chapters in food and nutrition books, scientific backgrounders, fact sheets, educational materials (e.g., the *Calcium Counseling Resource*), speeches, video conference scripts, and press releases. The *Dairy Council Digest* and the *Calcium Counseling Resource* can be obtained by logging onto www.nationaldairycouncil.org.

Judith K. Jarvis, M.S., R.D., L.D., is manager of consumer and health professional information in the nutrition research department of the National Dairy Council. In this position, she writes scientific background papers, develops other educational pieces for health professionals, and manages quarterly mailings to the nutrition and health community. Judy monitors major medical/nutrition journals and writes or reviews summaries of current research for dissemination to local Dairy Councils and other dairy industry organizations. In addition, she reviews materials for technical accuracy from a variety of departments and develops corporate comments provided to regulatory agencies as

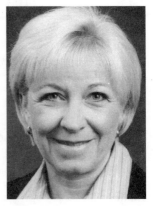

needed. Judy also answers technical inquiries related to dairy foods, nutrition, and health from local Dairy Councils, health professionals, the dairy and food industry, educators, government agencies, and consumers.

Judith Jarvis earned a bachelor of science degree in communications from the University of Illinois and a master of science degree in human nutrition and nutritional biology from the University of Chicago.

Prior to joining the National Dairy Council, she worked as a clinical dietitian, providing nutritional care and education to cardiac and renal patients. She is a member of The American Dietetic Association, the American College of Nutrition, and is current President of the Chicago Nutrition Association. She served as editor of the *American College of Nutrition* newsletter from 1995-1998 and has authored articles for scientific and nutrition journals.

Chapter Reviewers

Chapter 1
The Importance of Milk and Milk Products in the Diet
Robert G. Jensen, Ph.D.
Manfred Kroger, Ph.D.

Chapter 2
Dairy Foods and Cardiovascular Health
Ronald M. Krauss, M.D.
David Kritchevsky, Ph.D.

Chapter 3
Dairy Foods and Hypertension
David A. McCarron, M.D.
Michael Zemel, Ph.D.

Chapter 4
Dairy Foods and Colon Cancer
Martin Lipkin, M.D.
Michael J. Wargovich, Ph.D.

Chapter 5
Dairy Foods and Osteoporosis
Robert P. Heaney, M.D.
Connie M. Weaver, Ph.D.

Chapter 6
Bone Health and the Vegetarian
Robert P. Heaney, M.D.
Connie M. Weaver, Ph.D.

Chapter 7
Dairy Foods and Oral Health
William H. Bowen, D.D.S., Ph.D.
Dominick P. DePaola, D.D.S., Ph.D.

Chapter 8
Lactose Intolerance
Dennis A. Savaiano, Ph.D.
Michael Levitt, M.D.

Chapter 9
Contribution of Milk and Milk Products to Health throughout the Life Cycle
Connie M. Weaver, Ph.D.
Susan I. Barr, Ph.D., R.D.N.

Acknowledgments

We would like to thank and acknowledge the many people who have provided support in the development of this book. Special thanks are given to Laurel Fantis for help with preparation of manuscripts and obtaining permission for reproducing figures and tables; Nancy Warner for help in preparing tables and graphs and for word processing assistance; and Marya Spangler for help with literature searches and collecting data.

Two experts reviewed each chapter. A list of the chapters and reviewers is provided. We thank them for their helpful suggestions in the preparation of each chapter.

Contents

The Importance of Milk and Milk Products in the Diet

I. INTRODUCTION

Milk and other dairy foods were recognized as important foods as early as 4000 BC, evidenced by rock drawings from the Sahara depicting dairying. In Egyptian tombs dating back to 2300 BC remains of cheese were found.[1] About 3000 years ago milk and its products were familiar enough to be used as metaphors or analogues. An example is reference to the Promised Land as a land "flowing with milk and honey." During the Middle Ages, dairy products were important foods throughout Europe, although preferences for specific dairy foods varied geographically. In Greece and Rome, cheese, but not fresh milk or butter, was popular. In contrast, fresh milk and butter, but not cheese, were popular in northern Europe and Asia. Writings by Marco Polo who traveled to China between 1271 and 1295 describe the drying of milk and drinking of a fermented milk (probably koumiss) by nomadic tribes. From the Middle Ages through the eighteenth century, changes in the handling of milk came slowly and milking, churning, and cheese making were largely done by hand.[1]

In North America, milk and milk products were introduced with the arrival of the Europeans. In the early 1600s, the first dairy herd was established in the United States. With the Industrial Revolution, which brought railroads, steam engines, and refrigeration, fresh milk became available to a large population. Milking machines and automatic churners appeared in the 1830s followed by specialized cheese factories in the 1850s. As a result of continued advances and improvements in the dairy industry over the years, today a wide variety of milks and other dairy products is available.[2]

This chapter presents an overview of the nutritional contribution of milk and dairy products to our diets, including a discussion of specific nutrients such as energy, protein, carbohydrate, fat, vitamins, and minerals in these foods. Protecting the quality of milk and other dairy foods, trends in dairy food consumption, and the wide variety of dairy foods available, including chocolate milk, cheeses, cultured

1-8493-8731-0/00/$0.00+$.50

and culture-containing dairy foods, and whey products are discussed. For more in-depth information on this subject, readers are referred to several publications.[2-13]

II. RECOMMENDATIONS TO INCLUDE MILK AND MILK PRODUCTS IN THE DIET

A. Food Guide Recommendations

Official recommendations including the U.S. Department of Agriculture's (USDA) *Food Guide Pyramid*,[14] National Dairy Council's *Guide to Good Eating*,[15] and the USDA/Department of Health and Human Service's (DHHS) Dietary Guide-lines for Americans[16] all recognize milk and other milk products as one of the five major food groups. USDA's *Food Guide Pyramid* recommends 2 to 3 servings/day from the Milk, Yogurt, & Cheese Group.[14] National Dairy Council's *Guide to Good Eating* recommends 2 to 4 servings from the Milk Group.[15] Recognizing the higher calcium intakes recommended by the National Institutes of Health,[17] an American Academy of Pediatrics' publication includes a modified Food Guide Pyramid which advises adolescents to consume five daily servings/day from the Milk Group to meet calcium recommendations.[18]

Dairy foods are considered to be the preferred source of calcium.[17,19] Both an expert panel on "Optimal Calcium Intake" convened by the National Institutes of Health[17] and the American Medical Association[19] have recognized milk and other dairy foods as an important source of calcium for Americans. The 1995 Dietary Guidelines for Americans states that "many women and adolescent girls need to eat more calcium-rich foods to get the calcium needed for healthy bones throughout life. By selecting lowfat or fat-free milk products and other lowfat calcium sources, they can obtain adequate calcium and keep the fat from being too high."[16] The Dietary Guidelines advises Americans to eat two to three servings of dairy foods/day.[16]

B. Government Feeding Programs/Child Nutrition Programs

Milk and other dairy foods are an important component of the meals and snacks offered in the federal government's child nutrition programs.[2] In 1996, an estimated 4.8 billion half pints of fluid milk were served in child nutrition programs in schools: 3.7 billion half pints in the National School Lunch Program (NSLP), 945 million half pints in the School Breakfast Program (SBP), and 144 million half pints in the School Milk Program (SMP) (Table 1.1).[2] In addition to milk, other dairy foods such as cheese and yogurt are consumed as part of the child nutrition programs. USDA recently approved 4 ounces of yogurt as an acceptable alternate to one ounce of meat/meat alternate for breakfasts and lunches served under any of the child nutrition programs.[20]

Nationally representative evaluations of USDA's NSLP and SBP indicate that participation in these programs significantly increases children's intake of a range of nutrients, especially those such as calcium, phosphorus, riboflavin, and protein

Table 1.1 Milk Consumed Through Schools; 1989-1996

	School Lunch Program[1]	School Breakfast Program[2]	Special Milk Program[3]	Total Half-Pints Served	Total Gallons	% of U.S. Milk Production
	(half pints)	(half pints)	(half pints)			
1989	3,404,200,413	553,095,455	188,688,263	4,145,984,131	259,124,008	1.6
1990	3,407,714,459	594,321,133	181,248,099	4,183,283,691	261,455,231	1.5
1991	3,443,233,261	648,580,972	177,026,314	4,268,830,547	268,801,909	1.6
1992	3,486,635,622	716,148,024	174,431,839	4,377,213,484	273,575,843	1.6
1993	3,517,055,117	775,797,605	167,265,331	4,460,118,052	278,757,378	1.6
1994	3,571,489,027	841,380,973	158,845,879	4,571,715,679	285,732,230	1.6
1995*	3,615,393,894	906,288,934	151,353,428	4,673,036,256	292,064,766	1.6
1996	3,665,299,884	945,282,271	144,323,505	4,754,814,660	297,175,916	1.7

[1] Assumes that milk is served with 85% of lunches. [2] Assumes that milk is served with 84% of breakfasts.
[3] Special milk program available only at schools that do not participate in school lunch and breakfast programs. Percents of lunches and breakfasts served with milk based on "School Nutrition Dietary Study." * Revised.

Source: International Dairy Foods Association, Food Nutrition Service, Milk Facts 1997 Edition, Washington, D.C., Milk Industry Foundation, 1997. With permission.

found in milk and other dairy products.[21,22] Children who skip the SBP consume less daily energy, calcium, phosphorus, magnesium, and vitamins A and D than children who consume this meal.[23,24] Much of the beneficial effect of consuming NSLP and SBP meals is attributed to the increased intake of milk and milk products.[24,25] Children may not be able to make up for the nutrients such as calcium provided by these meals over the rest of the day.[24] Dairy foods such as milk and cheese are also an important component of other government feeding programs such as the Women, Infants, and Children (WIC) program.[26] This program provides specified amounts of milk, cheese, and other foods to eligible low-income, nutritionally at risk pregnant, breast feeding, and nonbreast feeding postpartum women and infants and children up to 5 years of age.

III. CONTRIBUTION OF MILK AND MILK PRODUCTS TO NUTRIENT INTAKE

A. Nutrient Contribution

Milk and other dairy products make a significant contribution to the nation's supply of nutrients (Table 1.2).[27] As estimated for 1994, dairy foods (excluding butter) contributed only 9% of the total calories available. Yet, these foods provided 73% of the calcium, 31% of the riboflavin, 33% of the phosphorus, 19% of the protein, 16% of the magnesium, 21% of the vitamin B_{12}, 17% of the vitamin A, 10% of the vitamin B_6, and 6% of the thiamin in addition to appreciable amounts of vitamin D and niacin equivalents available in the U.S. food supply.[27] While optional, nearly all milk sold in the United States today is fortified with vitamin D to obtain standardized amounts of 400 I.U. or 10 µg/quart.[28,29] Milk and other dairy foods are therefore nutrient dense foods, supplying a high concentration of many nutrients in relation to their energy (caloric) value.

B. Milk and Milk Products throughout Life

Intake of cow's milk and milk products contributes to health throughout life (see Chapter 9). According to the American Academy of Pediatrics,[30] the nutritional adequacy of diets for children should be achieved by consuming a wide variety of foods and children should be provided with sufficient energy to support their growth and development and to reach or maintain desirable body weight. Dairy foods are nutrient dense foods providing abundant amounts of protein, vitamins, and minerals necessary for growth and development. Studies indicate that intake of calcium-rich foods such as milk and other dairy foods during childhood and adolescence is an important determinant of peak bone mass and future risk of osteoporosis (see Chapter 5 on Dairy Foods and Osteoporosis). Unfortunately, the vast majority of children are not even consuming the two to three servings of dairy foods recommended by USDA's Food Guide Pyramid.[31,32] Researchers found that only slightly more than half (54%) of children ages 2 to 19 consumed 2 to 3 servings of dairy foods/day.[32]

Table 1.2   **Percent Nutrient Contribution of Dairy Foods, Excluding Butter, to the U.S. Per Capita Supply, 1994**

Nutrient	1994 %
Energy	9.3
Protein	19.3
Fat	12.3
Carbohydrate	5
Minerals	
Calcium	72.8
Phosphorus	32.8
Zinc	18.9
Magnesium	16.4
Iron	2.1
Vitamins	
Riboflavin	30.7
Vitamin B_{12}	21.0
Vitamin A	17.4
Vitamin B_6	9.7
Folate	7.3
Thiamin	6.2
Vitamin E	2.8
Ascorbic Acid	2.7
Niacin	1.4

Source: Gerrior, S., and Bente, L., *Nutrient Content of the U.S. Food Supply*, 1909-94. Home Economics Research Report No. 53, Washington, D.C.: U.S. Department of Agriculture, Center for Nutrition Policy and Promotion, 1997.

During adulthood, intake of dairy foods provides essential nutrients needed for body maintenance and protection against major chronic diseases. For example, milk and other dairy foods are an important source of calcium which reduces the risk of osteoporosis (see Chapter 5), hypertension (see Chapter 3), and colon cancer (see Chapter 4). For older adults in particular, milk and other dairy foods furnish a generous supply of nutrients in relation to calories. Adults, similar to children, are not consuming recommended servings of dairy foods.[33] A recent survey conducted by the USDA found that Americans are consuming an average of only 1.5 servings (1 serving from milk and $^1/_2$ serving from cheese) each day from the Milk Group or slightly more than half of the two to three servings/day recommended by USDA. Only 23% of those surveyed met the recommendations for dairy food intake. Even fewer adolescent girls (10%) and women 20 years and over (14%) consumed two to three servings/day from the Milk Group.[33]

C. Low Intake of Dairy Foods Compromises Nutrient Intake

Without consuming dairy foods, it is difficult to meet recommended intakes of calcium and vitamin D.[17,19] An investigation of approximately 800 high school students revealed that 79% of the students' calcium intake came from milk and other dairy foods.[34] In another study involving adolescents, calcium intake was positively associated with milk intake.[35] Similarly, adult women who met their calcium recommendations consumed significantly more servings of milk and milk products than women whose diets did not meet their calcium needs.[36]

Consuming milk and milk products improves the overall nutritional quality of the diet.[37-41] In an investigation in Oregon, adults who included more dairy foods in their diets for at least 12 weeks increased their intake of calcium as well as other nutrients such as magnesium, riboflavin, potassium, phosphorus, and vitamin D.[38] Other studies in adults[40] and children[39,41] indicate that intake of dairy foods improves the nutrient adequacy of the diet. Further, intake of dairy foods does not necessarily increase total calorie or fat intake, body weight, or percent body fat.[38-42]

IV. NUTRIENT COMPONENTS OF MILK AND MILK PRODUCTS

Although fluid whole cow's milk is a liquid food (88% water), it contains an average of 12% total solids and 8.6% solids-not-fat, an amount comparable to the solids content of many other foods. More than 100 different components have been identified in cow's milk. Important nutritional contributions of milk and milk products are protein, calcium, phosphorus, vitamin A, and several B-vitamins, especially riboflavin and vitamin B_{12} (Table 1.3).[6,7,43] Although this chapter focuses solely on cow's milk, readers may refer to Table 1.4 and Jensen[6] for information on the composition of milks from other animals.

A. Energy

The energy (calorie) content of milk and other dairy foods varies widely and depends mostly on the fat content of the milk but also on the addition of nonfat milk solids, sugars, and other energy-yielding components (Table 1.3). For example, whole milk (3.2% milk fat) provides 150 kcal per cup; reduced fat (2%) milk provides 121 kcal per cup; lowfat (1%) milk provides 104 kcal per cup; and nonfat (skim) milk provides 90 kcal per cup. As mentioned above, milk is considered to be a food of high nutrient density, providing a high concentration of nutrients in relation to its energy content. There is no scientific evidence that the intake of specific foods such as dairy foods contributes to overweight. Weight loss is achieved by reducing total caloric intake and/or increasing physical activity. For individuals concerned about reducing their body weight, there is a wide variety of dairy products of different energy content available. The Dietary Guidelines[16] cautions, however, that even people who consume lower fat foods can gain weight if they eat too much of foods high in starch, sugars, or protein.

B. Protein

Cow's milk is recognized as an excellent source of high quality protein.[6,8,44-46] In 1994, milk and other dairy foods (excluding butter) contributed 19% of the protein available in the nation's food supply.[27] Cow's milk contains about 3.5% protein by weight, accounts for about 38% of the total solids-not-fat content of milk, and

Table 1.3　Nutrient Content of Selected Dairy Foods

Nutrients	Units	Milk							Cheese					Cultured Dairy Foods		
		Whole 3.25% fat 1 cup	Reduced Fat 2% fat 1 cup	Lowfat 1% fat 1 cup	Nonfat 1 cup	Chocolate Whole 1 cup	Chocolate Reduced Fat 1 cup	Chocolate Lowfat 1 cup	Cheddar 1 oz.	Cream 1 oz.	Cottage 1 cup	Mozzarella Part Skim, Low Moisture 1 oz.	American Pasteurized Process 1 oz.	Yogurt Plain, Whole Milk 1 cup	Yogurt Plain, Nonfat Milk 1 cup	Buttermilk Lowfat 1 cup
Proximates																
Water	g	214.70	217.67	220.04	221.43	205.75	208.95	211.25	10.42	15.24	93.20	13.77	11.10	215.36	208.81	220.82
Energy	kcal	149.92	121.20	104.42	90.33	208.38	178.84	157.57	114.13	98.95	81.81	79.36	106.44	150.48	136.64	99.00
Energy	kj	627.08	507.52	436.53	377.30	872.50	747.50	660.00	477.41	413.91	342.39	331.98	445.38	629.65	570.85	414.05
Protein	g	8.03	8.13	8.53	8.75	7.93	8.03	8.10	7.06	2.14	14.00	7.79	6.28	8.50	14.04	8.11
Total lipid (fat)	g	8.15	4.69	2.38	0.61	8.48	5.00	2.50	9.40	9.89	1.15	4.85	8.86	7.96	0.44	2.16
Carbohydrate by difference	g	11.37	11.71	12.18	12.30	25.85	26.00	26.10	0.36	0.75	3.07	0.89	0.45	11.42	18.82	11.74
Fiber, total dietary	g	0.00	0.00	0.00	0.00	2.00	1.25	1.25	0.00	0.00	0.00	0.00	0.00	0.00	0.00	0.00
Ash	g	1.76	1.81	1.89	1.91	2.00	2.03	2.05	1.11	0.33	1.57	1.05	1.66	1.76	2.89	2.18
Minerals																
Calcium	mg	291.34	296.70	312.87	316.30	280.25	284.00	286.75	204.49	22.65	68.82	207.32	174.49	295.72	487.80	285.18
Iron	mg	0.12	0.12	0.12	0.12	0.60	0.60	0.60	0.19	0.34	0.16	0.07	0.11	0.12	0.22	0.12
Magnesium	mg	32.79	33.36	35.16	35.55	32.58	33.00	33.33	7.88	1.83	6.03	7.45	6.31	28.37	46.80	26.83
Phosphorus	mg	227.90	232.04	244.76	254.80	251.25	254.25	256.50	145.18	29.60	151.19	148.58	211.18	232.51	383.43	218.54
Potassium	mg	369.66	376.74	397.15	418.22	417.25	422.00	425.50	27.90	33.85	96.62	26.89	45.93	378.77	624.51	370.69
Sodium	mg	119.56	121.76	128.38	129.85	149.00	150.50	151.75	175.91	83.77	458.78	149.60	405.52	113.68	187.43	257.01
Zinc	mg	0.93	0.95	0.98	1.00	1.03	1.03	1.03	0.88	0.15	0.43	0.89	0.85	1.45	2.38	1.03
Copper	mg	0.02	0.02	0.03	0.03	0.16	0.16	0.16	0.01	0.01	0.03	0.01	0.01	0.02	0.04	0.03
Manganese	mg	0.10	0.01	0.01	0.01	0.19	0.19	0.19	0.00	0.00	0.00	0.00	0.00	0.01	0.01	0.01
Selenium	mcg	4.88	5.37	5.64	5.39	4.75	4.75	4.75	3.94	0.68	10.17	4.62	4.08	5.39	8.82	4.90

Table 1.3   Nutrient Content of Selected Dairy Foods (Continued)

Nutrients	Units	Milk							Cheese					Cultured Dairy Foods		
		Whole 3.25% fat 1 cup	Reduced Fat 2% 1 cup	Lowfat 1% fat 1 cup	Nonfat 1 cup	Chocolate Whole 1 cup	Chocolate Reduced Fat 1 cup	Chocolate Lowfat 1 cup	Cheddar 1 oz.	Cream 1 oz.	Cottage 1 cup	Mozzarella Part Skim, Low Moisture 1 oz.	American Pasteurized Process 1 oz.	Yogurt Plain, Whole Milk 1 cup	Yogurt Plain, Nonfat Milk 1 cup	Buttermilk Lowfat 1 cup
Vitamins																
Vitamin C ascorbic acid	mg	2.29	2.32	2.45	2.47	2.28	2.30	2.33	0.00	0.00	0.00	0.00	0.00	1.30	2.13	2.40
Thiamin	mg	0.09	0.10	0.10	0.10	0.09	0.09	0.10	0.01	0.01	0.02	0.01	0.01	0.07	0.12	0.08
Riboflavin	mg	0.40	0.40	0.42	0.43	0.41	0.41	0.42	0.11	0.06	0.19	0.10	0.10	0.35	0.57	0.38
Niacin	mg	0.21	0.21	0.22	0.22	0.31	0.32	0.32	0.02	0.03	0.15	0.03	0.02	0.18	0.30	0.14
Pantothenic acid	mg	0.77	0.78	0.82	0.83	0.74	0.75	0.76	0.12	0.08	0.24	0.03	0.14	0.95	1.57	0.67
Vitamin B6	mg	0.10	0.11	0.11	0.11	0.10	0.10	0.10	0.02	0.01	0.08	0.02	0.02	0.08	0.13	0.08
Folate	mcg	12.20	12.44	12.99	13.23	11.75	12.00	12.00	5.16	3.74	14.01	2.81	2.21	18.13	29.89	12.25
Vitamin B12	mcg	0.87	0.89	0.94	0.95	0.84	0.85	0.86	0.23	0.12	0.72	0.26	0.20	0.91	1.50	0.54
Vitamin A, IU	IU	307.44	500.20	499.80	499.80	302.50	500.00	500.00	300.23	404.56	41.81	199.30	342.92	301.35	17.15	80.85
Vitamin A, RE	mcg, RE	75.64	139.08	144.55	149.45	72.50	142.50	147.50	78.81	108.30	12.43	54.15	82.22	73.50	4.90	19.60
Vitamin E,	mg ATE	0.24	0.17	0.10	0.10	0.23	0.13	0.07	0.10	0.27	0.12	0.13	0.13	0.22	0.01	0.15
Lipids																
Fatty acids, saturated	g	5.07	2.92	1.48	0.40	5.26	3.10	1.54	5.98	6.23	0.73	3.08	5.58	5.14	0.28	1.34
4:0	g	0.26	0.15	0.08	0.03	0.25	0.14	0.06	0.30	0.28	0.04	0.16	0.30	0.24	0.01	0.07
6:0	g	0.16	0.09	0.05	0.01	0.15	0.08	0.04	0.15	0.08	0.01	0.03	0.10	0.16	0.01	0.04
8:0	g	0.09	0.05	0.03	0.01	0.09	0.05	0.02	0.08	0.10	0.01	0.04	0.11	0.10	0.01	0.03
10:0	g	0.21	0.12	0.06	0.01	0.20	0.11	0.05	0.17	0.19	0.02	0.08	0.18	0.23	0.01	0.05
12:0	g	0.23	0.13	0.07	0.01	0.22	0.12	0.05	0.15	0.13	0.02	0.05	0.14	0.27	0.02	0.06
14:0	g	0.82	0.47	0.24	0.06	0.79	0.44	0.19	0.94	1.02	0.12	0.49	0.91	0.84	0.05	0.22

	Unit															
16:0	g	2.15	1.23	0.63	0.18	2.22	1.31	0.65	2.78	2.99	0.35	1.48	2.58	2.17	0.12	0.57
18:0	g	0.99	0.57	0.29	0.06	1.17	0.74	0.44	1.14	1.15	0.13	0.59	1.08	0.78	0.04	0.26
Fatty acids, mono-unsaturated	g	2.36	1.35	0.69	0.16	2.48	1.47	0.75	2.66	2.79	0.33	1.38	2.54	2.19	0.12	0.62
16:1	g	0.18	0.11	0.05	0.02	0.18	0.10	0.05	0.29	0.28	0.04	0.13	0.29	0.17	0.01	0.05
18:1	g	2.05	1.18	0.60	0.13	2.18	1.31	0.68	2.24	2.38	0.30	1.18	2.13	1.82	0.10	0.54
20:1	g	0.00	0.00	0.00	0.00	0.00	0.00	0.00	0.00	0.00	0.00	0.00	0.00	0.00	0.00	0.00
22:1	g	0.00	0.00	0.00	0.00	0.00	0.00	0.00	0.00	0.00	0.00	0.00	0.00	0.00	0.00	0.00
Fatty acids, poly-unsaturated	g	0.30	0.17	0.09	0.02	0.31	0.18	0.09	0.27	0.36	0.04	0.14	0.28	0.23	0.01	0.08
18:2	g	0.18	0.11	0.05	0.02	0.20	0.12	0.06	0.16	0.22	0.03	0.10	0.17	0.16	0.01	0.05
18:3	g	0.12	0.07	0.03	0.01	0.12	0.07	0.03	0.10	0.14	0.01	0.04	0.11	0.07	0.00	0.03
18:4	g	0.00	0.00	0.00	0.00	0.00	0.00	0.00	0.00	0.00	0.00	0.00	0.00	0.00	0.00	0.00
20:4	g	0.00	0.00	0.00	0.00	0.00	0.00	0.00	0.00	0.00	0.00	0.00	0.00	0.00	0.00	0.00
20:5	g	0.00	0.00	0.00	0.00	0.00	0.00	0.00	0.00	0.00	0.00	0.00	0.00	0.00	0.00	0.00
22:5	g	0.00	0.00	0.00	0.00	0.00	0.00	0.00	0.00	0.00	0.00	0.00	0.00	0.00	0.00	0.00
22:6	g	0.00	0.00	0.00	0.00	0.00	0.00	0.00	0.00	0.00	0.00	0.00	0.00	0.00	0.00	0.00
Cholesterol	mg	33.18	18.30	9.80	4.90	30.50	17.00	7.25	29.74	31.10	4.97	15.31	26.76	31.12	4.41	8.58
Phytosterols	mg	0.00														
Amino Acids																
Tryptophan	g	0.11	0.12	0.12	0.12	0.11	0.11	0.12	0.09	0.02	0.16	0.11	0.09	0.05	0.08	0.09
Threonine	g	0.36	0.37	0.39	0.39	0.36	0.36	0.37	0.25	0.09	0.62	0.30	0.20	0.35	0.58	0.39
Isoleucine	g	0.49	0.49	0.52	0.53	0.48	0.49	0.49	0.44	0.11	0.82	0.37	0.29	0.46	0.77	0.50
Leucine	g	0.79	0.80	0.84	0.86	0.78	0.79	0.79	0.68	0.21	1.44	0.76	0.56	0.86	1.41	0.81
Lysine	g	0.64	0.64	0.68	0.69	0.63	0.64	0.64	0.59	0.19	1.13	0.79	0.62	0.76	1.26	0.68
Methionine	g	0.20	0.21	0.21	0.22	0.20	0.20	0.20	0.19	0.05	0.42	0.22	0.16	0.25	0.41	0.20
Cystine	g	0.07	0.08	0.08	0.08	0.07	0.08	0.08	0.04	0.02	0.13	0.05	0.04	0.08	0.13	0.08
Phenylalanine	g	0.39	0.39	0.41	0.42	0.38	0.39	0.39	0.37	0.12	0.76	0.41	0.32	0.46	0.77	0.43
Tyrosine	g	0.39	0.39	0.41	0.42	0.38	0.39	0.39	0.34	0.10	0.75	0.45	0.34	0.43	0.71	0.34
Valine	g	0.54	0.54	0.57	0.59	0.53	0.54	0.54	0.47	0.13	0.87	0.49	0.38	0.70	1.16	0.60

Table 1.3   Nutrient Content of Selected Dairy Foods (Continued)

| | | Milk | | | | | | | Cheese | | | | | Cultured Dairy Foods | | |
| | | Whole 3.25% fat | Reduced Fat 2% fat | Lowfat 1% fat | Nonfat | Chocolate Whole | Chocolate Reduced Fat | Chocolate Lowfat | Cheddar | Cream | Cottage | Mozzarella Part Skim, Low Moisture | American Pasteurized Process | Yogurt Plain, Whole Milk | Yogurt Plain, Nonfat Milk | Buttermilk Lowfat |
Nutrients	Units	1 cup	1 cup	1 cup	1 cup	1 cup	1 cup	1 cup	1 oz.	1 oz.	1 cup	1 oz.	1 oz.	1 cup	1 cup	1 cup
Arginine	g	0.29	0.30	0.31	0.32	0.29	0.29	0.29	0.27	0.08	0.64	0.34	0.26	0.26	0.42	0.31
Histidine	g	0.22	0.22	0.23	0.24	0.22	0.22	0.22	0.25	0.08	0.47	0.29	0.26	0.21	0.35	0.23
Alanine	g	0.28	0.28	0.29	0.30	0.27	0.28	0.28	0.20	0.07	0.73	0.24	0.16	0.36	0.60	0.29
Aspartic acid	g	0.61	0.62	0.65	0.66	0.60	0.61	0.62	0.45	0.15	0.95	0.56	0.37	0.67	1.11	0.65
Glutamic acid	g	1.68	1.70	1.79	1.83	1.66	1.68	1.70	1.73	0.49	3.03	1.82	1.30	1.66	2.75	1.58
Glycine	g	0.17	0.17	0.18	0.19	0.17	0.17	0.17	0.12	0.04	0.31	0.15	0.10	0.21	0.34	0.18
Proline	g	0.78	0.79	0.83	0.85	0.77	0.78	0.79	0.80	0.20	1.62	0.80	0.64	1.01	1.66	0.82
Serine	g	0.44	0.44	0.46	0.48	0.43	0.44	0.44	0.41	0.11	0.79	0.45	0.30	0.53	0.87	0.42
Other																
Caffeine	mg					5.00	5.00	5.00								
Theobromine	mg					57.50	57.50	57.50								

Source: USDA, ARS, USDA Nutrient Database for Standard, Reference Release 12, Nutrient Data Laboratory. www.nal.usda.gov/fnic/food comp, 1998.

Table 1.5 Protein Fractions Isolated from Cow's Milk and Some of their Properties

Protein and Protein Fraction	Approximate Percent of Skim Milk Protein	Isoelectric Point of pH (the pH at which the protein does not migrate in an electric field)	Molecular Weight	Distinctive Characteristics
I. Casein (precipitated from skim milk by acid at pH 4.6)	76–78		15,000–33,600	
α_{s1}-Casein	53–70	4.1	23,000–27,000	1% Phosphorus
α_{s2}-Casein	45–55	4.1	23,000	
β-Casein	25–35	4.5	24,000	0.6% Phosphorus
κ-Casein	8–15	4.1	19,000	
γ-Casein	3–7	5.8–6.0	21,000	0.1% Phosphorus
II. Non-Casein Proteins	14–24			
A. Lactalbumin (soluble in ½ saturated $(NH4)_2SO_4$ solution)				
β-Lactoglobulin	7–12	5.3	36,000	
α-Lactalbumin	2–5	4.2–4.5	14,440	7% Tryptophan
Blood Serum Albumin	0.7–1.3	4.7	69,000	Identical with bovine serum albumin
B. Lactoglobulin (insoluble in ½ saturated $(NH4)_2SO_4$ solution)				
Euglobulin	0.8–1.7	6.0	180,000–252,000	Contains antibodies
Pseudoglobulin	0.6–1.4	5.6	180,000–289,000	
IgG immunoglobulins				
IgG1	1–2		150,000	
IgG2	0.2–0.5		170,000	
IgM Immunoglobulin	0.1–0.2		900,000–1,000,000	
IgA Immunoglobulin	0.05–0.1		300,000–500,000	

Table 1.4   Nutrient Composition of Milks from Different [

Nutrient	Cow	Human	Buffalo		
Water, g	87.99	87.50	83.39		
Food energy, kcal	61	70	97		
kJ	257	291	404		
Protein (N x 6.38), g	3.29	1.03	3.75		
Fat, g	3.34	4.38	6.89		
Carbohydrate, total, g	4.66	6.89	5.18		
Fiber, g	0	0	0	0	
Ash, g	0.72	0.20	0.79	0.	
Minerals					
Calcium	119	32	169	134	
Iron, mg	0.05	0.03	0.12	0.05	
Magnesium, mg	13	3	31	14	
Phosphorus, mg	93	14	117	111	
Potassium, mg	152	51	178	204	
Sodium, mg	49	17	52	50	
Zinc, mg	0.38	0.17	0.22	0.30	
Vitamins					
Ascorbic Acid, mg	0.94	5.00	2.25	1.29	
Thiamin, mg	0.038	0.014	0.052	0.048	
Riboflavin, mg	0.162	0.036	0.135	0.138	
Niacin, mg	0.084	0.177	0.091	0.277	
Pantothenic Acid, mg	0.314	0.223	0.192	0.310	
Vitamin B_6, mg	0.042	0.011	0.023	0.046	
Folate, mcg	5	5	6	1	
Vitamin B_{12}, mcg	0.357	0.045	0.363	0.065	0.
Vitamin A, RE	31	64	53	56	42
IU	126	241	178	185	147
Cholesterol, mg	14	14	19	11	—

* Amount in 100 Grams Edible Portion

Dashes denote lack of reliable data for a constituent believed to be present in measurab[amounts.

Source: National Dairy Council, *Newer Knowledge of Milk and Other Fluid Dairy Products* 1993, p. 47. With permission.

contributes about 21% of the energy of whole milk.[6,12] As shown in Table 1.5, cow' milk protein is a heterogeneous mixture of proteins.[12] Milk also contains small amounts of various enzymes and traces of nonprotein nitrogenous materials.[6] Of the total protein in cow's milk, about 80% is casein and 20% is whey protein.[6] Casein, the dominant protein in cow's milk, can be fractionated electrophoretically into four major components: alpha-, beta-, gamma-, and kappa-casein. Casein is generally defined as the protein precipitated at pH 4.6, a property used in the manufacturing of cheese. Whey, which is more heterogeneous than casein, consists predominantly of beta-lactoglobulin and alpha-lactalbumin. Alpha-lactalbumin has a high content of the amino acid tryptophan, a precursor of niacin. Because of milk's tryptophan content, this food is an excellent source of niacin equivalents. One niacin equivalent is defined as one milligram of niacin or 60 mg of tryptophan. Other whey proteins present in smaller amounts are serum albumin, immunoglobulins (e.g., IgA, IgG,

Table 1.5 Protein Fractions Isolated from Cow's Milk and Some of their Properties

Protein and Protein Fraction	Approximate Percent of Skim Milk Protein	Isoelectric Point of pH (the pH at which the protein does not migrate in an electric field)	Molecular Weight	Distinctive Characteristics
C. Proteose–Peptone Fraction (not precipitated at pH 4.6 from skim milk previously heated to 95–100°C. 30 min.)	2–6	3.3–3.7	4,100–20,000	Not well defined Includes glycoproteins

Source: National Dairy Council, *Newer Knowledge of Milk and Other Fluid Dairy Products*, 1993, p. 19. With permission.

IgM), protease peptones, lactoferrin, and transferrin. Each of these proteins has unique characteristics. Whey protein concentrates and isolates are used as ingredients in a number of formulated food products.[47]

Nutritionally, cow's milk protein is considered to be high quality because it contains in varying amounts all of the essential amino acids that our bodies cannot synthesize and in proportions resembling amino acid requirements (Table 1.6).[8,44,45]

Table 1.6   Amino Acid Distribution in Milk

Amino Acids	Estimated Requirements of Adults[a] (Grams Per Day)	Milligrams Per Gram Milk Solids Not Fat[b]	Grams Per Cup (8 oz., 244 g) Whole Fluid Milk
Essential (Indispensable)			
Histidine	0.84	10.31	0.218
Isoleucine	0.70	22.98	0.486
Leucine	0.98	37.16	0.786
Lysine	0.84	30.12	0.637
Methionine	0.91[c]	9.50	0.201
Phenylalanine	0.98[d]	18.34	0.388
Threonine	0.49	17.12	0.362
Tryptophan	0.25	5.34	0.113
Valine	0.70	25.39	0.537
Non-essential (Dispensable)			
Alanine		13.10	0.277
Arginine		13.76	0.291
Aspartic Acid		28.79	0.609
Cystine		3.50	0.074
Glutamic Acid		79.48	1.681
Glycine		8.04	0.170
Proline		36.78	0.778
Serine		20.66	0.437
Tyrosine		18.34	0.388

[a] Values calculated for 70 kg adult male
[b] All values have been calculated based on 8.67 percent milk solids not fat for whole milk
[c] Value for total S-containing amino acids (methionine+cystine)
[d] Value for total aromatic amino acids (phenylalanine+tyrosine)

Source: National Dairy Council, *Newer Knowledge of Milk and Other Fluid Dairy Products*, 1993, p. 20. With permission

Only the sulfur amino acids (methionine plus cystine) in milk proteins are slightly limiting as compared with the adult's estimated requirement of essential amino acids. Because of its relative surplus of the amino acid lysine, cow's milk protein complements many plant proteins which normally are limited in lysine.[44] Also, because of its high quality, cow's milk protein is used as a standard reference protein to evaluate the nutritive value of food proteins.[45] The quality of a protein is determined by any one of the several parameters indicated in Table 1.7.

Individual milk proteins have been shown to exhibit a wide range of beneficial functions including enhancing calcium absorption and immune function, reducing blood pressure and the risk of cancer, and protecting against dental caries (see Chapter 7 on Dairy Foods and Oral Health).[45] A recent investigation demonstrates

Table 1.7   Average Measures of Protein Quality for Milk and Milk Proteins

	BV*	PD	NPU	PER	PDCAAS
Milk	91	95	86.45	3.1	1.21
Casein	77	100	76	2.9	1.23
Whey protein	104	100	92	3.6	1.15
Biological Value (BV)	=	Proportion of absorbed protein that is retained in the body for maintenance and/or growth.			
Protein Digestibility (PD)	=	Proportion of food protein absorbed			
Net Protein Utilization (NPU)	=	Proportion of protein intake that is retained (calculated as BV x PD)			
Protein Efficiency Ratio (PER)	=	Gain in body weight divided by weight of protein consumed			
Protein Digestibility Corrected Amino Acid Score (PDCAAS)	=	The amino acid score multiplied by a digestibility factor.			

* The BV of egg protein is defined as 100.

(Adapted from: *Nutritional Quality of Proteins*, European Dairy Association, 1997. With Permission.)

that peptides derived from bovine lactoferrin, a glycoprotein in milk and cheese, have antibacterial properties.[48] Limited evidence from *in vitro* and experimental animal studies indicates that milk proteins may protect against cancer.[49-51] McIntosh et al.[49] demonstrated that dairy protein-based diets reduced the development of cancer in Sprague-Dawley male rats which received a chemical carcinogen. As reviewed by Parodi,[51] whey proteins in particular appear to be anticarcinogenic. Whey proteins are rich in substrates (e.g., the sulfur amino acids, cysteine and methionine) for the synthesis of glutathione which has been demonstrated to prevent cancer under experimental conditions. The ability of whey proteins to enhance both humoral and cell-mediated immune responses in laboratory animals may also explain the anti-cancer activity of whey proteins. Alternatively, the presence of high-affinity binding proteins in the whey protein fraction may bind potential co-carcinogens, rendering them unavailable. Whey protein may also increase bone strength, according to a recent study of ovariectomized laboratory rats.[52] The researchers suggest that milk whey protein affects bone metabolism in these animals by increasing bone protein such as collagen and enhancing the bone breaking force.

A limited number of infants and young children exhibit allergic responses to cow's milk protein, primarily beta-lactoglobulin, casein, alpha-lactalbumin, and bovine serum albumin.[53,54] Estimates of the prevalence of cow's milk protein allergy or sensitivity (i.e., an abnormal immunological response to one or more of cow's milk proteins) vary between 0.3% and 7.5%.[55,56] Evidence also indicates that cow's milk sensitivity is often overdiagnosed and that, when strict diagnostic tests are used, only about 1 to 3% of infants and children during the first two years of life are sensitive to cow's milk protein.[54,56] The incidence is somewhat higher in infants who are fed cow's milk very early in life (i.e., before 3 to 4 months of age) and/or have a family history of allergies.[56] In the majority of cases, this condition is temporary and children often outgrow cow's milk protein allergy by 3 years of age.[53,54]

Although some researchers have suggested that milk proteins, particularly bovine serum albumin, trigger an autoimmune response that destroys pancreas beta cells in genetically susceptible children causing Type I or insulin-dependent diabetes (IDDM),[57-59] scientific evidence to date fails to support a causal association between cow's milk proteins and IDDM.[60-67] When the feeding practices of over 250 children with IDDM were compared to those of nondiabetic children, no association was found between early introduction of cow's milk during infancy and IDDM.[62] In another investigation involving 253 children (aged 9 months to 7 years) from 171 families of persons with IDDM, researchers found that children who developed B-cell autoimmunity (BCA), an early predictor of IDDM, were no more likely to have been exposed to cow's milk protein than children without BCA.[63] Blood levels of antibodies to bovine serum albumin (BSA) do not predict diabetes, according to several researchers.[60,64] An American Academy of Pediatrics (AAP) Work Group on Cow's Milk Protein and Diabetes Mellitus[68] encourages breast feeding for infants born into families with a history of IDDM, especially if a sibling already has the disease. Because there is no established association between intake of infant formulas containing cow's milk protein and diabetes, the AAP Work Group concluded that commercial infant formulas containing cow's milk protein are an acceptable alternative to breast milk for infants who are not breast fed. For infants at high risk of IDDM, the Work Group discourages the use of commercially available cow's milk and cow's milk protein during the first year of life. The AAP Work Group recommends that more research be conducted on cow's milk intake and IDDM in genetically susceptible infants.[68]

C. Carbohydrate

Lactose, the principal carbohydrate in milk, is synthesized in the mammary gland. Lactose accounts for about 54% of the total solids-not-fat content of milk and contributes about 30% of the energy (calories) of whole milk. Cow's milk contains about 4.8% lactose (12 to 12.5 g lactose/cup) compared with 7% (15 to 18 g lactose/cup) in human milk.[69,70] Refer to the table at the end of Chapter 8, "Lactose Content of Dairy Products."

In infants, some lactose enters the distal bowel (colon) where it promotes the growth of certain beneficial lactic-acid-producing bacteria which may help combat gastrointestinal disturbances resulting from undesirable putrefactive bacteria.[30] In addition, lactose favors the absorption of calcium and perhaps phosphorus in infants.[71] However, there is no scientific evidence that lactose improves calcium absorption in adults.[72]

Minor quantities of glucose, galactose, and oligosaccharides are also present in milk. Glucose and galactose are the products of lactose hydrolysis by the enzyme lactase.[6] Researchers speculate that galactose may have a unique role in the rapidly developing infant brain.[6] Some individuals have difficulty metabolizing lactose because of reduced lactase levels, a condition called lactase nonpersistence. However, recent research indicates that most persons with lactase nonpersistence are able to consume the amount of lactose in up to two cups of milk a day if taken with meals, one at breakfast and the other at dinner (see Chapter 8 on Lactose Intolerance).[73]

Other dairy foods such as aged cheeses and yogurts with live active cultures are also well tolerated.[73] In cheese making, lactose is converted to lactic acid by select microorganisms. A number of low-lactose and lactose-reduced milks and milk products are available. Commercial lactase hydrolyzes lactose in milk when added prior to processing. Lactose-reduced milk contains about 70% less lactose than regular milk. Lactose-free milk has about 99.9% of its lactose hydrolyzed.

D. Fat

Milk fat contributes unique characteristics to the appearance, texture, flavor, and satiability of dairy foods and is a source of energy, essential fatty acids, fat-soluble vitamins, and several other potential health-promoting components.[74]

Milk fat, the most complex of lipids, exists in microscopic globules in an oil-in-water emulsion in milk. Milk's lipids are mainly triglycerides or esters of fatty acids with glycerol (97-98%), 0.20 to 1.0% phospholipids, 0.22 to 0.41% free sterols (cholesterol, waxes, and squalene, an intermediate of cholesterol), traces of free fatty acids, and varying amounts of the fat-soluble vitamins A, D, E, and K (Table 1.8). The fat contributes about 48% of the energy of whole milk.

Table 1.8   Constituents of Milk Lipids

Class of Lipid	Per 100 Grams Whole Fluid Milk (3.34% Fat)	Per Cup (8 oz., 244g) Whole Fluid Milk
Vitamin A activity	126 IU (31 RE)	307 IU (76 RE)
Vitamin D	1.1356–2.8056 IU	2.771–6.846 IU
Vitamin E	0.080 mg	0.195 mg
Vitamin K	0.00334 mg	0.008 mg
Triglycerides	3.23–3.27 g	7.88–7.98 g
Diglycerides	0.01–0.02 g	0.02–0.05 g
Monoglycerides	0.53–1.27 mg	1.29–3.10 mg
Keto acid glycerides (total)	28.4–42.75 mg	69.3–104.3 mg
Ketonogenic glycerides	1.00–4.3 mg	2.44–10.5 mg
Hydroxy acid glycerides (total)	20.0–26.05 mg	48.8–63.56 mg
Lactonogenic glycerides	2.00 mg	4.88 mg
Neutral glyceryl ethers	0.53–0.67 mg	1.293–1.635 mg
Neutral plasmalogens	1.34 mg	3.270 mg
Free fatty acids	3.34–14.7 mg	8.15–35.87 mg
Phospholipids (total)	6.7–33.4 mg	16.30–81.50 mg
Sphingolipids (less sphingomyelin)	2.00 mg	4.88 mg
Free sterols	7.35–13.69 mg	17.93–33.40 mg
Cholesterol	14 mg	33 mg
Squalene	0.2338 mg	0.570 mg
Carotenoids	0.0233–0.0301 mg	0.057–0.073 mg

Adapted from National Dairy Council, *Newer Knowledge of Milk and Other Fluid Dairy Products*, 1993, p. 21. With permission.

Milk fat is not only characterized by a number of different fatty acids, but also by their chain lengths. More than 400 different fatty acids and fatty acid derivatives have been identified in milk fat, ranging from butyric acid with four carbon atoms to fatty acids with 26 carbon atoms.[6,74,75] Milk fat is unique among animal fats because it contains a relatively high proportion of short-chain and medium-chain saturated fatty acids (i.e., those with 4 to 14 carbons in length). The composition of milk fat varies somewhat according to the breed of the cow, stage of lactation, season, geographical location, and feed composition.[75] However, the fatty acids are approximately 62% saturated, 30% monounsaturated, 4% polyunsaturated, with the remaining 4% other minor types of fatty acids.[6,12] The saturated fatty acids present in the largest amount in milk fat are palmitic, stearic, and myristic acids. While saturated fatty acids generally contribute to an increase blood cholesterol levels, individual saturated fatty acids differ in their blood cholesterol-raising effects (see Chapter 2 on Dairy Foods and Cardiovascular Health). Long-chain saturated fatty acids such as lauric, myristic, and palmitic acids raise blood total and low density lipoprotein (LDL or the "bad") cholesterol levels, whereas stearic acid and short-chain saturated fatty acids such as butyric, caproic, caprylic, and capric acids have either a neutral effect or may lower blood cholesterol levels.[76,77] Milk fat contains about 50% long-chain saturated fatty acids and 10% short-chain fatty acids. The relative cholesterol-raising potential of lauric, myristic, and palmitic acids is controversial, although the differences appear to be modest.[76,78]

Oleic acid is the main monounsaturated fatty acid in milk fat.[6] Polyunsaturated fatty acids such as arachidonic acid are present in trace amounts. Arachidonic acid is required, but can be made from its precursor, linoleic acid, an essential fatty acid. Linoleic and linolenic acids are not synthesized in the human body or are synthesized at such a slow rate that they must be supplied by the diet. The essential polyunsaturated fatty acid linoleic acid is present in milk fat in a form which favors conversion to arachidonic acid. Omega-3-linoleic acid and its products, eicosapentaenoic acid (EPA) and docosahexaenoic acid (DHA), are also present in small but significant amounts. If linoleate and omega-3 linolenic acids are present in adequate quantities, arachidonic acid, EPA, and DHA are synthesized in sufficient amounts.

Average per capita consumption of trans fatty acids in the U.S. is about 8.1 to 12.8 g/day which represents about 4 to 12% of total dietary fat intake or 2 to 4% of total energy intake.[79] In bovine milk, trans fatty acids (particularly vaccenic acid) are present at a level of approximately 3% of total fat.[75] Dairy foods contribute less than 1 g/day of trans fatty acids — about 0.2 g/day of trans fatty acids/day from milk and 0.1 g/day from butter.[79] Trans fatty acids in milk fat result from the biohydrogenation of pasture and feed linoleic and linolenic acids by rumen microorganisms.[80] The main source of trans fatty acids in the U.S. diet is partially hydrogenated vegetable oils used in crackers and other baked goods, margarines, and fried snack foods. Not only are data on trans fatty acid intake in the U.S. limited, but research findings on the effect of trans fatty acids on risk of cardiovascular disease are inconsistent.[77,81] There is no scientific evidence that trans fatty acids in dairy foods are harmful to health. On the contrary, the predominant fatty acid in milk fat, trans-11-18:1, is converted to conjugated linoleic acid (CLA).[80] As discussed below, several potential health benefits of CLA have been identified.[82,83]

Information on the effect of individual fatty acids in milk fat on risk of coronary heart disease is limited and influenced greatly by genetics (see Chapter 2 on Dairy Foods and Cardiovascular Health). Findings to date do not support blanket recommendations to preferentially decrease intake of animal fats such as milk fat to reduce the risk of heart disease or other major chronic diseases. Rather moderation in total fat intake, from both animal and vegetable sources, is recommended.[16]

Cholesterol is a normal constituent in milk, although milk contains relatively little cholesterol (i.e., less than 0.5% of milk fat).[6] Because cholesterol occurs in the fat globule membrane, its concentration in dairy foods is related to the fat content (Table 1.3). A one-cup serving (8 fluid ounces) of whole, 2%, and nonfat (skim) milk contains 33 mg, 18 mg, and 4 mg cholesterol, respectively. Cholesterol in the body is the precursor of many important substances such as adrenocortical hormones, vitamin D, bile salts, and sex hormones. Milk and other dairy foods contributed about 16% of the cholesterol available in the food supply in 1994.[27] This share of cholesterol from dairy foods has remained about the same since the early 1900s, although the contribution of individual dairy foods to the availability of cholesterol has varied over the years. Today, more lowfat milks, yogurt, and cheese contribute to the availability of cholesterol than earlier in the century, whereas less cholesterol now comes from whole milk and cream than in the past. Not only do dairy foods make a relatively small contribution to total cholesterol intake, but dietary cholesterol, regardless of source, has a modest effect on blood cholesterol levels. Moreover, individuals vary widely in their blood cholesterol response to dietary cholesterol (see Chapter 2 on Dairy Foods and Cardiovascular Disease).

Milk fat, similar to other dietary fats, serves as a concentrated source of energy. Also, the fat of milk is highly emulsified, which facilitates its digestion. Fats must be liquid or emulsifed at body temperature to be digested and absorbed. The shorter the carbon chain or the degree of unsaturation, the lower the melting point of the fat. Since milk fat has a melting point lower than body temperature, it is efficiently utilized, particularly by the young and by older adults.

Emerging scientific findings indicate that milk fat contains several components such as conjugated linoleic acid (CLA), sphingomyelin, butyric acid, and myristic acid which may potentially protect against major chronic diseases (see Chapter 4 on Dairy Foods and Colon Cancer and Chapter 2 on Dairy Foods and Cardiovascular Health).[82] Milk fat is the richest natural dietary source of CLA, containing 2.4 to 28.1 mg/g.[83-85] The CLA content of most dairy products ranges from 2.5 to 9.1 mg/g fat. In cheeses, the CLA content is reported to range from 3.6 to 8 mg/g fat; in fluid milks from 3.3 to 6.4 mg/g fat; and in butter from 5.5 to 6.5 mg/g fat. Moreover, 90% of the CLA in dairy foods is in the cis-9, trans-11-18:2 isomeric form which is believed to be the biologically active CLA isomer.[80,82,84] This isomer has recently been given the trivial name, rumenic acid, by an ad hoc committee.[86] The CLA content of dairy foods is influenced primarily by the CLA content of the starting raw milk and the final fat content. In addition, the protein content, type of fermentation bacteria, and processing procedures such as agitation may make a small contribution to differences in the CLA content among and within dairy foods.[87] Pasteurization increases the CLA content of dairy foods and differences in protein content and the type of fermentation bacteria used in some dairy foods influence their CLA content.[85]

Physiological concentrations of CLA suppress cell growth in human malignant melanoma, colorectal, breast, lung, prostate, and ovarian cancer cell lines.[82,83] In experimental animal studies, CLA inhibits the growth of chemically induced epidermal, forestomach, colorectal, and mammary tumors.[83,88-90] Diets supplemented with 1% by weight or less of CLA inhibit mammary tumors in rats independent of the amount or type of dietary fat.[83] The CLA content of milk is believed to be one of milk's components (along with calcium and lactose) explaining the link between higher milk intake and decreased risk of breast cancer in a recent study which followed more than 4600 women for 25 years.[91] For a discussion of the potentially beneficial role of CLA against coronary heart disease, refer to Chapter 2. CLA may also play a beneficial role in bone formation and resorption,[92] enhance immune function,[93,94] and reduce body fat/increase lean body mass.[95,96] When experimental animals were fed CLA, food intake was transiently reduced, but the animals did not lose weight and even gained some weight.[95] Improved feed efficiency has been demonstrated in animals fed CLA, indicating that CLA affects body composition. When laboratory mice were fed CLA, whole body fat was reduced and body protein, water, and ash increased.[96]

Sphingomyelin, the most common sphingolipid, makes up about one-third of total milk phospholipids, although it can vary according to season and the cow's stage of lactation.[82] Sphingomyelin is present in cow's milk at a concentration of 0.1 mg/ml or about 0.2 to 1.0% of the total lipids of milk, or 1/4 to 1/3 of total milk phospholipids. Because sphingolipids are found mainly in the milk fat globule membrane, lowfat and nonfat as well as traditional dairy products are good sources of sphingolipids.[82] Dietary sphingolipids may have a protective role in cancer and possibly cardiovascular disease.[97]

A unique feature of milk fat is the presence of butyric acid which is found at a level of more than 3% of the major fatty acids in milk fat. No other common food contains this four-carbon short-chain fatty acid. Most butyric acid in the human body is derived from the fermentation of fiber in the digestive tract. Recent research findings indicate that butyric acid may protect against certain cancers.[82,98,99] In a variety of cancer cell lines (colon, leukemia, breast) butyrate inhibits the proliferation and induces differentiation and programmed cell death (i.e., apoptosis). At the molecular level, butyrate is associated with down-regulation or inactivation of the expression of cancer genes.[82,98] Butyrate may also inhibit tumor invasiveness and metastasis.[82,98]

Myristic acid, a saturated fatty acid that accounts for about 10% of milk fat,[6] may help the body fight infection. In laboratory mice, butter protects against the suppression in immune response induced by exposure to ultraviolet B radiation compared to margarine and linoleic acid-rich vegetable oils.[100] The researchers suggested that the fatty acid composition of the various fats may be responsible for their unique effect on immunity.[100] According to an experimental animal study, a specific protein involved in the activation of macrophages was increased when the animals were fed high levels of myristic acid.[101]

The question of whether or not milk fat favorably influences satiety is being entertained. Numerous studies under varying conditions have examined whether specific macronutrients such as fat, carbohydrate, and protein improve satiety or a feeling of fullness following intake. Compared to lowfat meals, a high fat meal empties more slowly from the stomach.[102] Little is known about the effect of specific fatty acids or different sources of fats such as milk fat on satiety. Research is needed to determine the satiety value of milk fat and certain fatty acids in milk fat. If milk fat per se, as compared to other sources of fat, is demonstrated to have a unique effect on satiety, this finding could support recommendations to include milk fat in the diet to help control hunger and food intake. A preliminary study involving healthy adults found that dairy fat affected satiety differently than nondairy fat.[103] Compared to nondairy fat, a meal consumed with dairy fat resulted in higher initial blood glucose levels and lower blood glucose levels four to six hours following the meal. The researchers acknowledge that the link between blood glucose and satiety is complex and recommend that additional research be conducted to determine the potential of dairy fat to influence satiety.[103] In a study of healthy men in France, a meal containing butter delayed the desire for the next meal.[104]

Milk fat may have a beneficial effect on bone health, according to experimental animal studies.[105,106] In a recent study in young chicks, intake of different dietary fats influenced changes in prostaglandin E_2 and other bone growth factors.[106] Saturated fat (butter or butterfat) lowered bone levels of the essential unsaturated fatty acid, arachidonic acid, which is a precursor of PGE_2, raised insulin-like growth factor (IGF-1), moderated PGE_2 production, and increased bone formation rate.[106] Also, in chicks fed saturated fat (butter), the higher bone formation rate was accompanied by an increase in blood levels of hexosamines, a component of bone matrix protein, reflective of increased bone turnover.[106] The chicks fed the saturated fat diet (butter) also maintained the highest blood levels of vitamin E. In a previous investigation, high blood levels of vitamin E were associated with increased bone formation rate.[107] A saturated fat diet increases the saturated/polyunsaturated fat ratio in bone and may spare vitamin E to enhance the formation of bone. These findings indicate that saturated fat (butter) may optimize bone formation by its effects on bone growth factors.

The potential to modify milk fat to provide a specific nutritional or health advantage is actively being investigated.[108] Manipulating the fatty acid content of milk fat by altering the feed of cows has been demonstrated to have a favorable effect on blood lipid levels in humans.[109] The monounsaturated fat content of milk can be increased by increasing the monounsaturated content of cows' feed.[110] According to a study involving 30 adults with Type IIa Hyperlipidemia, intake of butter and cheese that contained a higher content of monounsaturated fat content increased blood levels of high density lipoprotein (HDL) cholesterol, the "good" cholesterol.[111] The monounsaturated fat-rich dairy foods were produced by feeding cows full-fat soya beans. The cholesterol-raising properties of milk fat can be reduced by removing cholesterol, fractionating milk fat, or altering the fatty acid profile of milk fat by changing cows' feed. Manipulating the diets of dairy cows can also increase the CLA content of milk.[112]

E. Vitamins

All of the vitamins known to be essential to humans have been detected in milk. Vitamins A, D, E, and K are associated with the fat component of milk (Table 1.8). Vitamin A plays important roles in vision, cellular differentiation, growth, reproduction, and immunocompetence.[10] Both vitamin A and its precursors called carotenoids, principally B-carotene, are present in variable amounts in milk fat.[6] The carotenoids are the yellow pigments in milk fat responsible for the color of butter and along with the green riboflavin vitamin for milk's characteristic creamy color. About 11 to 50% of total vitamin A activity in milk is derived from carotenoids, the specific proportion depending on the breed and feed of the cow and season of year, among other factors.[10] Milk and milk products are an important source of vitamin A, providing about 17.4% of this vitamin in the U.S. food supply (Table 1.2).[27] Whole cow's milk (3.25% fat) provides about 307 IU (76 RE) of vitamin A per 8 ounce serving.[43] Three cups of whole milk, therefore, provide 23 to 28% of the Recommended Dietary Allowance (RDA) for vitamin A for adults.[43,113] Not only is cow's milk a good source of vitamin A, but B-lactoglobulin, the major protein component of bovine milk whey, may enhance vitamin A absorption.[114] Because vitamin A and carotene exist in the fat portion of milk, lower fat and fat free (skim) milks contain little of this vitamin. Consequently, fluid lower fat and fat free (skim) milks are required to be fortified with chemically derived vitamin A (retinol palmitate) to a level found in whole milk or 300 IU (6% DV) per 8-fluid-ounce serving. However, dairy processors are encouraged to continue to fortify lowfat milks to the current level of 500 IU of vitamin A per cup (10% DV), or 2,000 IU per quart.[115] If vitamin A is added to whole milk or other milks for which it is not required, the label must state this fact.[116]

Vitamin D, a fat-soluble vitamin which enhances the intestinal absorption of calcium and phosphorus, is essential for the maintenance of a healthy skeleton throughout life.[28] An inadequate intake of this vitamin results in inadequate mineralization of bone and leads to the development of rickets in children and osteomalacia in adults.[10] Also, vitamin D deficiency leads to secondary hyperparathyroidism which enhances mobilization of calcium from the skeleton, resulting in osteoporosis.[28] Vitamin D is present in low concentrations in unfortified milk (47 to 105 IU vitamin D per liter).[6,10] However, nearly all fluid milk, irrespective of its fat content, marketed in the U.S. is fortified to obtain the standardized amount of 400 IU (10 µg)/quart.[115] One cup (8 ounces) of vitamin D-fortified milk provides 25% of the Dietary Reference Intake [28] for this vitamin for most individuals. When a food is fortified with vitamin D, vitamin D must be listed on the nutrition label.[115] Vitamin D fortification of milk has been largely responsible for the virtual elimination of rickets in the United States.[117,118] Moreover, vitamin D fortification of fluid milks is supported by health professional organizations.[119,120] Consuming a sufficient intake of vitamin D fortified milk and milk products is especially important for individuals at risk of vitamin D deficiency such as those who have limited exposure to sunlight (e.g., housebound older adults).[28] To help ensure that milk contains the amount of vitamin D specified on the label, milk is monitored primarily by state governments in cooperation with the federal Food and Drug Administration (FDA).[121] The FDA recommends that the vitamin D content of milk be measured by a certified laboratory and determined to be acceptable by this regulatory agency.[121] According to good manufacturing practices (GMP), the acceptable range allowed for vitamin D fortification of milk is not less than 100% and not more than 150% of label claims (i.e., 400 to 600 IU vitamin D).[121] Milk remains an important and carefully monitored source of vitamin D in the diets of all who consume this food.

Vitamin E (mainly tocopherol) is an antioxidant, protecting cell membranes and lipoproteins from oxidative damage by free radicals.[10,122] This vitamin also helps to maintain cell membrane integrity and stimulate the immune response.[10] Some studies also support a protective role for vitamin E in certain cancers and cardiovascular disease.[122] Although widely available in the U.S. food supply, vitamin E is present in low concentrations in milk (0.1 mg alpha-tocopherol equivalents/100 g or 0.244 mg alpha-tocopherol equivalents per one cup). The RDA [113] for vitamin E ranges from three to 10 mg alpha-tocopherol equivalents. Vitamin K, which is necessary for blood clotting, is found in low concentrations in milk (0.4 to 1.8 μg/100 g).[6] Quantitative values for vitamin K in milk are few and variable. This vitamin may also have a protective role in bone health.[122]

In addition to the essential fat-soluble vitamins, milk and other dairy foods also contain all of the water-soluble vitamins in varying amounts required by man (Table 1.9). Significant amounts of thiamin (vitamin B_1), which acts as a coenzyme for many reactions in carbohydrate metabolism, are found in milk (0.04 mg/100g or 0.09 mg/cup). Three 8-ounce glasses of milk provide about 22% of the thiamin recommended for adults.[123] Pasteurization decreases thiamin in milk by about 10%.[6] Milk is also a good source of riboflavin or vitamin B_2. This vitamin functions as a precursor for certain essential coenzymes important in the oxidation of glucose, fatty acids, amino acids, and purines. The average riboflavin content of fluid whole milk is about 0.16 mg per 100 g. Three 8-ounce glasses of milk would supply 100 and 92%, respectively, of the 1.1 and 1.3 mg/day of riboflavin recommended for adults.[123] Niacin (nicotinic acid and nicotinamide) functions as part of a coenzyme in fat

Table 1.9   Water-Soluble Vitamins in Milk

Vitamin	Per 100 Grams Whole Fluid Milk	Per Cup (8 oz, 244g) Whole Fluid Milk
Ascorbic Acid, mg	0.94	2.29
Thiamin, mg	0.038	0.093
Riboflavin, mg	0.162	0.395
Niacin	0.084	0.205
Niacin Equivalents, mg*	0.856	2.088
Pantothenic acid, g	0.314	0.766
Vitamin B_6, mg	0.042	0.102
Folate, mcg	5	12
Vitamin B_{12}, mcg	0.357	0.871

* This value includes niacin equivalents from preformed niacin and from tryptophan. A dietary intake of 60 mg tryptophan is considered equivalent to 1 mg niacin. One "niacin equivalent" is equal to either of these amounts.

Adapted from: National Dairy Council, *Newer Knowledge of Milk and Other Fluid Dairy Products*, 1993, p. 28. With permission.

synthesis, tissue respiration, and utilization of carbohydrate. This vitamin promotes healthy skin, nerves, and digestive tract a well as aiding digestion and fostering a normal appetite. The average content of niacin in milk is 0.084 mg per 100 g. The presence of the amino acid tryptophan in milk protein can be used by the body for the synthesis of niacin. A dietary intake of 60 mg tryptophan is considered to be equivalent to one mg niacin in the body.[6] The niacin equivalents in three 8-ounce glasses of milk therefore equal 6.28 (0.630 mg preformed niacin plus 5.65 mg from tryptophan). This provides 45 to 42%, respectively, of the 14 and 15 mg of niacin per day recommended for adults.[123]

Milk is a good source of pantothenic acid, a component of coenzyme A which is involved in fatty acid metabolism. The average amount of pantothenic acid in milk is 0.31 mg per 100 g. Three glasses of milk provide 46% of the 5 mg of pantothenic acid per day recommended for adults.[123] Vitamin B_6 (pyridoxine, pyridoxal, pyridoxamine) functions as a coenzyme for more than 100 enzymes involved in protein metabolism. On the average, about 0.04 mg vitamin B_6 are found in 100 g milk. Three glasses of milk provide about 23 and 18%, respectively, of the 1.3 and 1.7 mg vitamin B_6 per day recommended for adults.[123] Folate (folic acid) is a growth factor and functions as a coenzyme in the transfer of one-carbon units in the de novo synthesis of nucleotides necessary for DNA synthesis.[123] Cow's milk contains a high-affinity folate binding protein (FBP), a minor whey protein, which promotes retention and increases the bioavailability of folate by slowing the rate of absorption.[124] The average level of folate in milk is 5 µg per 100 g. Three glasses of milk would supply 9% of the 400 mg folate/day recommended for nonpregnant, nonlactating adults.[123] Vitamin B_{12} is necessary for growth, maintenance of nerve tissues, and normal blood formation.[123] Milk is an excellent source of this vitamin, providing 0.36 µg per 100 g. Three glasses of milk would furnish all of the 2.4 µg vitamin B_{12} recommended for most adults. Milk is also a good source of biotin, a vitamin necessary for many carboxylation and decarboxylation reactions in carbohydrate, fatty acid, protein, and nucleic acid metabolism.[123] Milk contains about 3 ug biotin per 100 g. Three glasses of milk would provide about 73% of the 30 µg biotin/day recommended for adults.[123] Ascorbic acid (vitamin C), which forms cementing substance such as collagen in the body, is important in wound healing and increasing resistance to infections.[122] This vitamin also enhances the absorption of non-heme iron and may protect against some cancers and cardiovascular disease.[10] Milk contains only a small amount of ascorbic acid (0.94 mg per 100 g milk or 2.3 mg per 8-ounce cup). Processing or exposure to heat such as pasteurization reduces the vitamin C content of milk. The current RDA for vitamin C for most adults is 60 mg per day.[113]

F. Minerals

Milk and other dairy foods are important sources of major minerals particularly calcium, phosphorus, magnesium, potassium, and trace elements such as zinc (Tables 1.10 and 1.11). The mineral content of cow's milk is influenced by several factors including the stage of lactation, and environmental and genetic factors. For this reason, there may be wide variation in the content of specific minerals in milk.[10]

Table 1.10   Macrominerals in Milk

Macrominerals (mg)	Per 100 Grams Whole Fluid Milk	Per Cup (8 oz, 244 g) Whole Fluid Milk
Calcium	119	291
Chlorine	103	244
Magnesium	13	33
Phosphorus	93	228
Potassium	152	370
Sodium	49	120
Sulfur	25	61

Adapted from: National Dairy Council, *Newer Knowledge of Milk and Other Fluid Dairy Products*, 1993, p. 28. With permission.

Table 1.11   Trace Elements in Milk

Trace Elements	Per 100 Grams Whole Fluid Milk	Per Cup (8 oz, 244g) Whole Fluid Milk
Aluminum, mcg	46.0	112.24
Barium, mcg	—	—
Boron, mcg	27.0	65.88
Bromine, mcg	60.0	146.40
Bromine (coastal area), mcg	280.0	683.20
Chromium, mcg	1.5	3.66
Cobalt, mcg	0.06	0.15
Copper, mcg	13.0	31.72
Fluorine, mcg	15.0	36.60
Iodine, mcg	4.3	10.49
Iron, mg	0.0492	0.12
Lithium, mcg	—	—
Manganese, mcg	2.2	5.37
Molybdenum, mcg	7.3	17.81
Nickel, mcg	2.7	6.59
Rubidium, mcg	200.0	488.00
Selenium (nonseleniferous area), mcg	4.0	9.76
Selenium (seleniferous area), mcg	up to 127.00	up to 309.88
Silicon, mcg	143.0	348.92
Silver, mcg	4.7	11.47
Strontium, mcg	17.1	41.72
Tin, mcg	—	—
Titanium, mcg	—	—
Vanadium, mcg	0.0092	0.02
Zinc, mcg	0.03811	0.93

Adapted from: National Dairy Council, *Newer Knowledge of Milk and Other Fluid Dairy Products*, 1993, p. 29. With permission.

About 99% of the body's calcium is in bone and teeth with the remaining one percent in body fluids, nerves, heart, and muscle. Throughout life, calcium is continually being removed from bones and replaced with calcium. Consequently, the need for an adequate supply of dietary calcium is important throughout life, not only during the years of skeletal development. In addition to calcium's role in bone health, this mineral fulfills several other important physiological functions in human metabolism, as evidenced by its role in blood coagulation, myocardial function, muscle contractility, and integrity of intracellular cement substances and various membranes.[28]

Unfortunately, calcium is one nutrient for which dietary intake is likely to be below recommended levels.[125] Prolonged calcium deficiency is one of several factors contributing to osteoporosis, a disease characterized by low bone mass and increased risk of fractures (see Chapter 5 on Dairy Foods and Osteoporosis). An adequate intake of calcium protects against hypertension (see Chapter 3 on Dairy Foods and Hypertension) and possibly some cancers (see Chapter 4 on Dairy Foods and Colon Cancer). Calcium in milk may also reduce the risk of kidney stones.[126-129] In a four-year prospective study involving 45,000 male health professionals with no history of kidney stones, those who consumed a calcium-rich diet (1326 mg calcium) experienced a 44% lower risk of symptomatic kidney stones than men who consumed 516 mg calcium a day.[126] Calcium-rich foods such as nonfat and lowfat milk, cottage cheese, and ricotta cheese had the strongest association with decreased risk of kidney stones, whereas calcium supplements (above 500 mg a day) offered no protective effect.[126] Similar findings have been found in women with no history of kidney stones who were followed for 12 years.[127] The women who consumed more than 1119 mg calcium a day from foods such as dairy foods were 35% less likely to develop stones than those who consumed 430 mg calcium a day or less. In contrast to food sources of calcium, calcium supplements increased the risk of kidney stones.[127] In another prospective study involving women with no history of kidney stones, intake of nonfat milk was associated with decreased risk of kidney stones.[129] Researchers speculate that a diet high in calcium may reduce the risk of kidney stones by decreasing the intestinal absorption and excretion of oxalate, a substance found in many plants including spinach. A recent investigation involving 21 adults with a history of calcium oxalate kidney stones and normal urine calcium levels found that substituting 1 $\frac{1}{2}$ cups of fat free milk for apple juice increased urine calcium levels and decreased urine oxalate levels by an average of 18%.[128] The researchers recommend that milk be consumed simultaneously with oxalate-containing foods to bind the oxalate in the diet and reduce the risk of calcium oxalate kidney stones.

The National Academy of Sciences (NAS) has issued new calcium recommendations for the healthy U.S. population.[28] As shown in Table 1.12, three servings per day of Milk Group foods are needed to meet the calcium needs of children ages 1 to 8 years and adults 19 through 50 years. For older children (9 to 18 years) and adults (50 + years), four servings/day will meet their calcium recommendations. The absorption of calcium is facilitated by the presence of vitamin D. For this reason, vitamin D-fortified milk is an important source of dietary calcium.

Milk is also an important source of phosphorus, providing 228 mg per 8-ounce serving. This essential mineral plays a central role in metabolism and is a component of lipids, proteins, and carbohydrates.[10] Dietary recommendations for phosphorus are no longer tied to calcium.[28] Instead, phosphorus recommendations are now based on the amount of dietary phosphorus to maintain serum inorganic phosphate levels consistent with cellular and bone formation needs.[28] Three cups

Table 1.12 Number of Milk Group Servings to Meet Calcium Intake Recommendations

Age	Calcium Recommendation*	Number of Milk Group Servings**
Children 1–3	500 mg	3 servings**
Children 4–8	800 mg	3 servings
Children 9–18	1,300 mg	4 servings
Adults 19–50	1,000 mg	3 servings
Adults 50+	1,200 mg	4 servings

* Dietary Reference Intakes, 1997.
**A serving equals 8 oz. of milk, one cup of yogurt, $1\frac{1}{2}$ ounces of cheese
**Serving sizes for children ages 1-3 are 2/3 of adult size.

Source: Calcium Intake Recommendations. National Dairy Council internal communication, September 1997.

of milk will supply about 98% of the 700 mg phosphorus recommended per day for adults 19 years and older and 55% of the 1,250 mg phosphorus per day recommended for 9- to 18-year olds.

Magnesium, a required cofactor for over 300 enzyme systems in the body, is related to calcium and phosphorus in function. This mineral activates many of the body's enzymes, participates in the synthesis of protein from amino acids, and plays a role in the metabolism of carbohydrate and fat.[10,28] Because magnesium is widely distributed in foods, particularly those of vegetable origin, a deficiency of this nutrient is rare. The NAS recommends 420 and 320 mg magnesium per day for adult males and females 31 years and older, respectively.[28] Milk contains about 13 mg magnesium per 100 g.[43] Three 8-ounce glasses of milk will therefore provide 23.5% of the magnesium recommended for adult males and 31% for adult females.

Potassium contributes to the transmission of nerve impulses and helps to control skeletal muscle contraction. Accumulating scientific evidence supports a beneficial role for potassium in blood pressure control or prevention of hypertension (see Chapter 3 on Dairy Foods and Hypertension). Milk contains about 152 mg potassium per 100 g.[43] Three 8-ounce glasses of milk provide about 55% of the 2,000 mg potassium per day recommended for adults over 18 years of age.[113]

Milk and other dairy foods contain many trace elements or nutrients needed by the body at levels of only a few milligrams per day (Table 1.11). Of the more than 100 known trace elements, biological function has been demonstrated in seventeen and dietary recommendations have been established for iron, zinc, selenium, iodine, and fluoride.[28,113] Trace elements in cow's milk are highly variable and depend on the stage of lactation, season, milk yield, amount of the trace element in each cow's diet, post-pasteurization handling of milk, storage conditions, and accuracy of analysis.

Iron is found in low concentrations in milk providing 0.05 mg per 100 g. Increasing the iron intake of cows does not increase milk's iron content. In addition to its low iron content, the bioavailability of iron from cow's milk is low. To reduce the risk of iron deficiency anemia, cow's milk is not recommended for infants during the first year of life.[130] However, when cow's milk is fed as recommended (i.e., after 12 months of age), there is little risk of iron deficiency anemia.

Zinc is a constituent of over 200 enzymes involved in most major metabolic pathways such as the synthesis of ribonucleic acid, deoxyribonucleic acid, and protein.[6] This trace element is essential for growth and development, wound healing, immunity, and other physiological processes.[10] Zinc is also involved in gene expression and helps maintain the integrity of cell membranes.[6] Dairy foods such as milk, cheese, and yogurt are good sources of zinc.[10] Milk contains about 0.38 mg zinc per 100 g. The level of zinc in milk is mostly related to milk's protein content. Because only about 1 to 3% of zinc in cow's milk is in the lipid fraction, the zinc concentration of lowfat and fat free milk is virtually identical to that of whole milk. Three servings of milk provide about 19 and 23% of the zinc RDA[113] for adults (i.e., 15 mg per day for males, 12 mg per day for females). Milk and milk products provide 18.9% of the zinc available in the food supply.[27]

Selenium is an integral component of the enzyme glutathione peroxidase which helps to protect cell components from oxidative damage.[6,10,113] The selenium content of cow's milk varies widely depending on the selenium intake of the cow.[6] In geographical areas where plants are deficient in selenium, cow's milk contains 5 to 30 ng selenium/ml. In contrast, in areas such as South Dakota where plants are high in selenium, up to 1,300 ng/ml are found in cow's milk. Most of the selenium is found in the skim or serum portion of milk, with only 2 to 10% in the fat fraction.[6]

Iodine, which is naturally occurring in milk, is an essential component of the thyroid hormones, thyroxine and triiodothyronine, which regulate growth and metabolism.[10] The iodine content of cow's milk varies widely, depending on the geographical area and iodine intake of the cow. Low concentrations of iodine are used as a sanitizer in the dairy industry on equipment and to sanitize cows' udders prior to the milking process.[6] The iodine products used by the dairy industry are formulated with ingredients that have been approved by the FDA as safe to use in food. All sanitizers and their specific use are also approved by the FDA.[121] A survey of the iodine content of milks in 27 states revealed that this food does not contribute to excessive intakes of iodine.[131] The dairy industry makes special efforts to educate dairy farmers about the proper use of iodine as a sanitizer at the farm and in the plant.[131] Even at intakes 10 to 20 times the recommended intake of 150 µg iodine/day for most adults, there is little evidence of adverse health effects.[113] In general, iodine deficiency is a more likely occurrence than iodine toxicity. A deficiency of iodine can cause enlargement of the thyroid gland (goiter).[113]

Dietary intake recommendations for fluoride, which protects against dental caries, have recently been established.[28] Fluoride intake generally comes from fluoridated water and fluoridated dental products. Most foods, including dairy foods (0.25 mg/liter or kg), have low levels of this trace element. The content of other minerals in cow's milk and their physiological roles are reviewed by Fox.[10]

V. PROTECTING THE QUALITY OF MILK AND OTHER DAIRY FOODS

A. Who is Responsible for Milk's Quality?

Quality relates to the chemical, microbiological, physical, organoleptic, and safety properties of milk. Rigid sanitary conditions are employed to assure milk's quality or result in milk with a low bacterial count, good flavor and appearance, satisfactory keeping quality, high nutritive value, and freedom from disease-producing organisms and foreign constituents. Cow's milk is among the most perishable of all foods because of its excellent nutritive composition and fluid form. As it comes from the cow, milk provides a good medium for the growth of bacteria. Unless milk is constantly protected against contamination and adverse environmental conditions, it may also develop flavor changes. Milk is relied upon as an important source of many nutrients. For this reason, maximum retention of these nutrients must be assured at every stage of production, processing (e.g., pasteurization), and distribution of milk and milk products.

Protecting the quality of milk is everyone's responsibility — public health officials, the dairy and related industries, and consumers. Progress in dairy technology and public health has resulted in milk that can be depended upon as a safe, nutritious, pleasing food even though it may be produced hundreds or thousands of miles away from the point of consumption. Vigilance is continuously exercised in maintaining this quality as new challenges arise in the environment. Numerous controls and treatments are in place to ensure the quality of milk.

B. Pasteurized Milk Ordinance

The Pasteurized Milk Ordinance (PMO)[121] continues to be one of the most effective instruments for protecting the quality of the milk supply. It is a set of recommendations by the U. S. Public Health Service (USPHS)-FDA for voluntary adoption by states and other jurisdictions. Recognized by state and local milk regulatory agencies and the dairy industry, the PMO describes the steps necessary to protect the milk supply and the reasons for the procedures.[121] Although the PMO is a recommended standard for sanitary Grade A milk, legal responsibility for the provision of milk quality is exercised mostly by state and local governments whose requirements are in some instances more stringent than the PMO guidelines. To maintain or improve the quality of milk, the PMO is revised periodically as technological advances in processes, equipment, and research are made. The 1995 PMO represents the 29th revision since the first regulation in 1924.[121]

C. Unintentional Microconstituents

The dairy industry has stringent regulations and programs in place from the farm to the marketplace to ensure the public of safe and wholesome products. However, almost every food, including milk and dairy foods, may contain trace residues of contaminants, either naturally or from external sources. While it is impossible to completely eliminate these residues, risk of adverse health effects is minimal as a result of a strong regulatory system.[12]

Milk from cows given an antibiotic, primarily penicillin or tetracycline, to treat temporary bacterial infections such as mastitis, is withheld from the market until the milk is demonstrated to be free of the antibiotic or the level of the antibiotic is below an established safe level.[6,12] Milk is frequently tested for antibiotic residues to ensure that this requirement is observed.[121,132] There is little concern regarding antibiotic residues in food, particularly because the public is protected from these residues as a result of regulatory actions. Routine sampling and screening of milk for drug residues is conducted on a state-by-state basis following the procedures outlined in the PMO.[6,12]

Pesticide residues in most U.S. foods pose minimal, if any, health risk because of federal regulations which limit human exposure to these contaminants.[12] All pesticides sold in the United States must be approved for safety by the Environmental Protection Agency before they can be used. Tolerance or action levels for allowable pesticide residues in foods such as milk have been established by regulatory agencies.[12] The FDA, under its pesticide monitoring program and "Total Diet Study," collects and samples food nationwide for pesticide and other chemical contaminants.[132] This surveillance has demonstrated that pesticide contamination of foods in the U.S. is extremely low.[132] In 1996, 97.4% of 781 domestic samples of milk/dairy products/eggs analyzed had no residues detected and none contained residues in amounts over tolerance levels.[132]

Milk and other dairy products are also safe from radioactivity.[6] At present, the health risks from potentially dangerous radionuclides are minimal and do not warrant any changes in food technology or in individual food habits.[6] Milk has been used as an indicator for obtaining information on current radionuclide concentrations for forecasting trends because it is convenient to analyze and produced throughout the year. Officials have established standards or levels of radiation as guidelines at which remedial action and preventive measures would be taken to reduce the exposure if the need arose.

The dairy industry extensively tests any new procedures and technologies before widespread adoption to assure that they are safe for both cows and milk consumers. An example of such a relatively new technology is a milk production-enhancing hormone, bovine somatotropin (BST), which is approved by FDA for commercial use in the U.S.[133] This hormone increases milk output by up to 20% and improves milk production efficiency. Before its approval, BST and milk produced from BST-treated cows underwent extensive testing for its safety by the FDA, the National Institutes of Health, and numerous independent groups. Based on the scientific findings, regulatory agencies worldwide have independently concluded that milk produced by BST-treated cows is safe for human consumption and indistinguishable from milk produced by untreated cows.

D. Milk Treatments

Most market milk in the U.S. is homogenized, although this is an optional process. Homogenization results in milk or milk products in which the fat globules are reduced in size to such an extent that no visible cream separation occurs in the milk. This process basically results in milk of uniform composition or consistency and palatability without removing or adding any constituents. Homogenization increases the whiteness of milk because the greater number of fat globules scatters light more effectively. Homogenized milk is less susceptible to oxidized flavor and the softer curd formed aids digestion.[6,12]

Pasteurization is required by law for all fluid milk and milk products moved in interstate commerce for retail sale. Even under the best sanitary dairy practices, disease-producing organisms may enter raw milk accidentally from environmental and human sources. However, as a result of pasteurization and other safeguards, illness related to milk intake has decreased dramatically during the past six decades.[121] Today, milk and fluid milk products are associated with less than 1% of all disease outbreaks due to infected food and contaminated water compared to 25% in 1938.[121] The PMO outlines procedures for the proper pasteurization of milk and milk products. Basically, pasteurization is the heating of raw milk to 63°C for not less than 30 minutes or 72°C for 15 seconds, followed by rapid cooling to 7°C or less. Pasteurization destroys pathogenic bacteria, yeasts, molds, and most all other nonpathogenic bacteria. It also inactivates most enzymes that might cause spoilage through the development of off-flavors. Pasteurization makes milk bacteriologically safe and increases its shelf life to 10 to 14 days without significantly changing its nutritive value.[6]

Some milk and milk products undergo ultra-high-temperature (UHT) processing. This process, which involves thermal heating at or above 138°C for at least two seconds before or after packaging, results in a product with an extended shelf life under refrigerated conditions. UHT processing can extend the shelf life of fluid milk from 19 days to 90 days under refrigeration.[134] The levels of most nutrients in milk are not significantly affected by UHT processing and storage. With appropriate controls on the quality of milk, as well as on the processing and packaging, UHT milk tastes very much like conventionally pasteurized milk. When UHT milk is combined with aseptic packaging, the shelf life of milk can be extended from its typical refrigerated 19 days to six or more months without refrigeration.[134]

E. Storage and Handling

Proper handling of dairy products and open dating are designed to assure consumers of dairy products with a good shelf life, or the length of time after processing that the product will retain its quality. Open dating on milk and milk product containers indicates when the product should be withdrawn from retail sale. It is used by the dairy industry to reflect the age of individual packages, not the shelf life of products. Generally, depending upon storage conditions and care in the home, a product will remain fresh and usable for a few days beyond this "pull date" or "sell-by-date." Regulation of open dating varies among states and other municipalities.[12]

To preserve the quality of milk and dairy products, consumers are recommended to:

- use proper containers to protect milk from exposure to sunlight, bright daylight, and strong fluorescent light to prevent the development of off-flavor and a reduction in riboflavin, ascorbic acid, and vitamin B_6 content.
- store milk at refrigerated temperatures (7°C) or below as soon as possible after purchase.
- keep milk containers closed to prevent absorption of other food flavors in the refrigerator. An absorbed flavor alters the taste but the milk is still safe.
- use milk in the order purchased.
- serve milk cold.
- return milk containers to the refrigerator immediately to prevent bacterial growth. Never return unused milk to the original container.
- keep canned milk in a cool, dry place. Once opened, it should be transferred to a clean, opaque container and refrigerated.
- store dry milk in a cool, dry place and reseal the container after opening. Humidity causes dry milk to lump and may affect flavor and color changes. If such changes occur, the milk should not be consumed. Once reconstituted, dry milk should be treated like any other fluid milk (i.e., covered and stored in the refrigerator).
- serve UHT milk and other dairy products cold and store in the refrigerator after opening.

Freezing may be used to preserve some dairy foods. However, for milk and other fluid dairy products, freezing is not recommended. While freezing has little impact on the nutritional value of milk, it does decrease milk's quality and the delicate texture of most other dairy products. The dairy industry is aggressively investigating new technologies such as the use of carbon dioxide gas, bacteriocins (organic compounds such as lactate and acetate that inhibit the growth of spoilage microorganisms) produced by lactic acid bacteria, and irradiation to extend the shelf life of dairy foods.[134] For example, carbon dioxide gas is used in more than 15 commercial cottage cheese operations nationwide and the bacteriocin, nisin, has been approved by FDA for use in pasteurized cheese and processed cheese spreads to control the growth of pathogenic microorganisms.[134] However, gamma irradiation for liquid products is not feasible because of the off-flavors produced.

VI. KINDS OF MILK AND MILK PRODUCTS

A. Consumption Trends

Between 1960 and 1997, total milk production in the U.S. increased by 33 billion pounds (i.e., from 123 to 156 billion pounds).[2] Most of this milk is processed as fluid or beverage milk (Figure 1.1). Per capita consumption of total dairy products was 584 pounds in 1995, an increase of 20 pounds from 1970, but down 17 pounds from 1987.[135] In recent decades the consumption pattern of individual milks and milk products has changed dramatically.[11,135,136] Noteworthy trends include more use of lowfat milk, fluid cream products, yogurt, and cheese and less use of whole milk.[11,136] Consumption of lowfat milk has increased at the expense of whole milk (Figure 1.2). In 1995, reduced-fat and nonfat milks accounted for 64% of all beverage milks compared to 19% in 1970.[135] During this same time, use of whole milk dropped to 35.9% in 1995 compared to 81% in 1970. Among young children 5 years and under, fluid milk intake has decreased by 17% since the late 1970s, while consumption of carbonated soft drinks has increased by 18% and noncitrus juices, including grape-and apple-based mixtures, by 292%.[137]

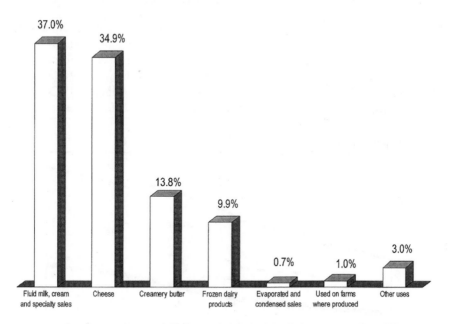

Figure 1.1   1996 U.S. milk supply utilization, by product. (From International Dairy Foods Association, Milk Facts 1997 Edition, Washington, D.C., 1997. With permission.)

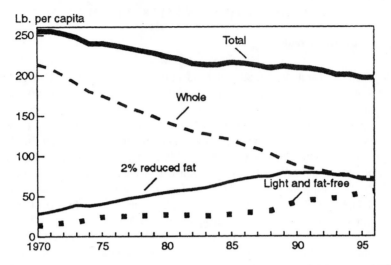

Figure 1.2 Per capita consumption of plain beverage milk declined 23% between 1970 and 1996. (From Putnam, J.J. and Allshouse, J.E., Food Consumption, Prices and Expenditures, 1970-95. USDA ERS Statistical Bulletin Number 939, 28.)

Although Americans are switching to lower fat milks, they are consuming more fluid cream products (e.g., half and half, light cream, eggnog), sour cream and cheese. From 1980 to 1995, per capita consumption of fluid cream products increased nearly 54%.[11] Average consumption of cheese more than doubled between 1970 and 1995 (i.e., from 11.4 pounds per capita to 27.3 pounds per capita) (Figure 1.3). Consumption of Cheddar cheese, Americans' favorite cheese, and Italian cheeses such as

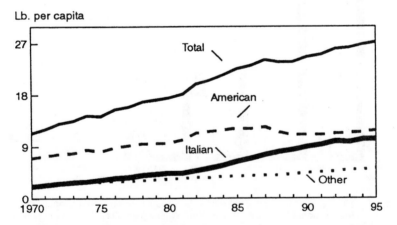

1/ Natural equivalent of cheese and cheese products. Excludes full-skim American and cottage-type cheeses.

Figure 1.3 Per capita consumption of cheese in 1995 was almost 2-1/2 times higher than in 1970. (From Putnam, J.J. and Allshouse, J.E., Food Consumption, Prices and Expenditures, 1970-95. USDA ERS Statistical Bulletin Number 939, 28.)

mozzarella, which are used in commercially manufactured foods and prepared foods (e.g., pizza, tacos), increased dramatically.[135] Between 1970 and 1996, per capita consumption of Cheddar cheese increased 59% and Italian cheeses more than quintupled.[136] In contrast, consumption of cottage cheese declined by one-half, or by 2.6 pounds.[136] Most of this decline in cottage cheese was in whole-milk cottage cheese. Despite numerous introductions of lower fat cheeses in the 1990s, these products account for only about a fifth of supermarket cheese sales and a much smaller proportion of total cheese used by food manufacturers and foodservice operators.[136] Similar to cheese, dramatic changes have occurred in the consumption of yogurt. Per capita consumption of yogurt increased six-and-a-half-fold between 1970 and 1995 (Figure 1.4).[135,136]

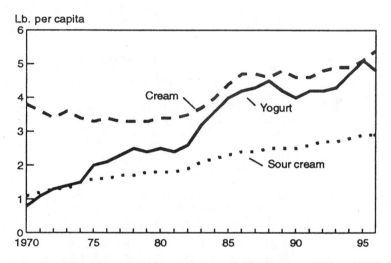

Figure 1.4   Per capita consumption of yogurt increased sixfold between 1970 and 1996. (From Putnam, J.J. and Allshouse, J.E., Food Consumption, Prices and Expenditures, 1970-95. USDA ERS Statistical Bulletin Number 939, 28.)

B. Wide Range of Milk and Milk Products

An ever-increasing variety of milk and other dairy products is available to meet the taste, nutrition, health, and convenience demands of consumers. For example, dairy products of varied fat content, of low or reduced lactose content, fortified with nutrients such as vitamins A, D, and calcium, and processed to improve keeping quality (e.g., ultrapasteurized) are available. These products include milks (unflavored, flavored, evaporated, condensed, sweetened condensed, dry, nonfat dry), cultured or culture-containing dairy foods (yogurt, kefir, acidophilus milk, cultured buttermilk, sour cream), creams (heavy, light, whipping, half-and-half), butter, ice cream, and cheeses, among other products. For a description of some of these dairy products refer to Table 1.13 and other publications.[2-4,12,13]

As a result of recent comprehensive food labeling regulations, consumers can now easily choose foods such as dairy foods that meet their specific needs.[116] All dairy products are required to carry a food label headed by the title, "Nutrition Facts"

Table 1.13   Definitions of Fluid Milks and Fluid Milk Products

Whole Milk – contains not less than 3.25% milk fat and 8.25% solids-not-fat. Addition of vitamins A and D is optional, but if added, vitamin A must be present at a level of not less than 2,000 International Units (IU) per quart; vitamin D is optional, but must be present at a level of 400 IU, if added. Characterizing flavor ingredients may also be added.

Lowfat Milk – contains 0.5, 1.5, or 2.0% milk fat and not less than 8.25% solids-not-fat. Lowfat milk must contain 2,000 IU vitamin A per quart. Addition of vitamin D is optional, but must be present at a level of 400 IU, if added. Characterizing flavoring ingredients may also be added.

Skim or Nonfat Milk – contains less than 0.5% milk fat and not less than 8.25% solids-not-fat. Skim or nonfat milk must contain 2,000 IU of vitamin A per quart. Addition of vitamin D is optional, but must be present at a level of 400 IU, if added. Characterizing flavoring ingredients may be added.

Cultured Milks – are produced by culturing any of the milks listed above with appropriate characterizing bacteria. The addition of certain characterizing ingredients and lactic-acid producing bacteria may permit, for example, the product to be labeled "cultured buttermilk," "cultured lowfat buttermilk," or "cultured skim milk (nonfat) buttermilk" depending upon the level of milk fat in the finished product.

Half-and-Half – consists of a mixture of milk and cream containing not less than 10.5% milk fat, but less than 18% milk fat.

Light Cream – contains not less than 18% milk fat, but less than 30%. Light cream may also be called "coffee cream" or "table cream."

Light Whipping Cream – contains not less than 30% milk fat, but less than 36% milk fat. Light whipping cream may also be called "whipping cream."

Heavy Cream – contains not less than 36% milk fat. Heavy cream may also be called "heavy whipping cream."

Sour Cream – is the product resulting from the addition of lactic acid-producing bacteria to pasteurized cream containing not less than 18% milk fat. Sour cream may also be called "cultured sour cream."

Sour Half-and-Half – is the product resulting from the addition of lactic acid-producing bacteria to half-and-half. Sour half-and-half contains not less than 18% milk fat. The product may or may not contain lactic acid-producing bacteria.

Dry Curd Cottage Cheese – is a soft, unripened cheese made from skim milk and/or reconstituted nonfat dry milk. The cheese curd is formed by the addition of either lactic acid-producing bacteria or acidifiers. The latter process is called direct acidification. Rennet and/or other suitable enzymes may be used to assist cured formation. Dry curd cottage cheese contains less than 0.5% milk fat and not more than 80% moisture. The product may also be called "cottage cheese dry curd."

Cottage Cheese – is the product resulting from the addition of a creaming mixture (dressing) to dry curd cottage cheese. Cottage cheese contains not less than 4% milk fat and not more than 80% moisture.

Lowfat Cottage Cheese – is the product resulting from the addition of a creaming mixture (dressing) to dry curd cottage cheese. Lowfat cottage cheese contains either 0.5, 1.0 , 1.5, or 2% milk fat and not more than 82.5% moisture.

Yogurt – is the product resulting from the culturing of a mixture of milk and cream products with the lactic acid-producing bacteria, *Lactobacillus bulgaricus* and *Streptococcus thermophilus*. Sweeteners, flavorings and other ingredients may also be added. Yogurt contains not less than 3.25% milk fat and 8.25% solids-not-fat.

Lowfat Yogurt – is similar in composition to yogurt except that it contains either 0.5, 1, 1.5 or 2% milk fat.

Nonfat Yogurt – is similar in composition to yogurt and lowfat yogurt except that it contains less than 0.5% milk fat.

Source: International Dairy Foods, *Milk Facts*, 1997 Edition, Washington, D.C., 1997. With permission.

Nutrition Facts

Serving Size 1 cup (244g)

Amount Per Serving

Calories 121   Calories from Fat 45

	% Daily Value*
Total Fat 5g	8%
Saturated Fat 3g	15%
Cholesterol 18mg	6%
Sodium 122mg	5%
Total Carbohydrate 12g	4%
Protein 8g	16%
Vitamin A	10%
Vitamin C	3%
Calcium	30%
Thiamin	6%
Riboflavin	24%

Not a significant source of iron and niacin.
Values are not available for fiber and sugars.

*Percent Daily Values are based on a
2,000 calorie diet.

Figure 1.5 Nutrition Facts label for 2% reduced fat milk. (From Label-Ease, National Dairy Council, 1997. With permission.)

which lists mandatory and optional dietary components per serving in a specified order (Figure 1.5). This label is required to include information on total calories and calories from fat and on amounts of total fat, saturated fat, cholesterol, sodium, total carbohydrate, dietary fiber, sugars, protein, vitamin A, vitamin C, calcium, and iron, in this order.[116] Other dietary components that may be listed voluntarily include: calories from saturated fat, amounts of polyunsaturated and monounsaturated fat, potassium, soluble and insoluble fiber, sugar alcohol, other carbohydrate, and other essential vitamins and minerals. If a claim is made about any of these components, or if a dairy food is fortified or enriched with any of them, listing of the optional component becomes mandatory. The quantitative amount per serving (e.g., grams, milligrams) of total fat, saturated fat, cholesterol, sodium, total carbohydrate, dietary fibers, sugars, and protein, is listed on the label. The amount of each of the above as well as of vitamins and minerals (e.g., vitamins A and C, calcium, iron) also is presented as a percentage of the Daily Value (% Daily Value). Daily Values are the label reference numbers based on current nutrition recommendations. Some labels list the Daily Values for a daily diet of 2000 and 2500 calories. Daily Values can help consumers determine how a food fits into an overall diet. These labeling regulations also provide consistent serving sizes and standard definitions for descriptive terms on food labels. Serving sizes, given in both household and metric measures (e.g., 1 cup [240 ml] for milk; 225 g [1 cup] yogurt), replace those previously set by manufacturers.

Uniform definitions for descriptive terms such as *free, low, high, good source, reduced, less, light, more*, and *% fat free* are now provided (Table 1.14). For example,

Table 1.14   Nutrient Content Descriptions for Dairy Products in the United States

1.	Free (without, no, zero)	• Based on value of nutrient per reference amount and per labeled serving size.
	Fat-free	• Less than 0.5 g fat
	Calorie-free	• Less than 5 calories
	Sodium-free	• Less than 5 mg sodium
	Cholesterol-free	• Less than 2 g saturated fat and 2 mg cholesterol
2.	Low (little, few, low source)	
	Low fat	• 3 g or less of fat per serving
	Low saturated fat	• 1 g or less of saturated fat per serving
	Low calorie	• 40 calories or less per serving
	Low sodium	• Less than 140 mg per serving
	Low cholesterol	• Less than 20 mg cholesterol and no more than 2 g saturated fat per serving
3.	High	• Food contains 20% or more of RDI of a nutrient per serving
4.	Good source	• Food contains 10-14% of RDI of a nutrient per serving
5.	Reduced	• Food contains 25% less of a nutrient or calories per serving than reference product. For cholesterol an additional requirement is maximum 2 g saturated fat per serving. The term reduced is used for nutritionally altered foods.
6.	Less (fewer)	• Food contains a minimum of 25% less of a nutrient or calories per serving. Additional requirement for cholesterol is maximum of 2 g saturated fat per serving. Food need not be nutritionally altered.
7.	Light (lite)	• If less than 50% of calories are from fat, calories should be reduced by 1/3 or fat content should be reduced by 50%.
		• If 50% or more of calories come from fat, reduction must be 50% of fat.
		• May also denote physical and organoleptic attributes, e.g., color.
8.	More	• Food, not necessarily nutritionally altered, contains at least 10% more of RDI of a nutrient.
9.	Percent fat free	• Food must be low-fat or fat-free. If a food contains 2 g fat per 50 g, it may be called 96% fat free.

Source: Kosikowski, F.V., and Mistry, V.V., *Cheese and Fermented Milk Foods*, 1997, p. 558. With permission.

free is defined as <5 calories; or <5 mg sodium; or <2 mg cholesterol; or <0.5 g saturated fat; or <2 mg cholesterol; or <0.5 g sugar.[116] The terms *light* and *reduced* (calorie, fat) are always used with a comparison to the reference food. The term *healthy* can be used on the label if the food is low in fat and saturated fat, has limited amounts of cholesterol and sodium, and contains at least 10% of the Daily Value for one or more of vitamins A or C, or iron, calcium, protein, or fiber.[138] Some dairy foods may also carry a health claim related to calcium and osteoporosis such as "Regular exercise and a healthy diet with enough calcium helps teen and young adult white and Asian women maintain good bone health and may reduce their high risk of osteoporosis later in life."[116] To carry a health claim, a food must contain no more than 20% of the Daily Value of fat (13 g), saturated fat (4 g), cholesterol (60 mg), and sodium (480 mg). For a calcium-osteoporosis claim, a food must also provide at least 20% of the reference daily intake of 1000 mg calcium (i.e., 200 mg calcium per serving). Also, for foods that might be fortified with large amounts of calcium, FDA requires a disclaimer indicating that a calcium intake of about 2000 mg per day is unlikely to provide any additional benefit.[116] Fat free (skim, nonfat), lowfat (1%), and reduced fat (2%) milk and milk products (e.g., lowfat/fat free yogurt) qualify for the calcium-osteoporosis health claim.[116]

A number of traditional foods, including whole milk, sour cream, cottage cheese, and yogurt have a standard of identity (i.e., the ingredients are fixed by law). Beginning January 1, 1998, the standards of identity for 12 lower fat dairy products, including lowfat milk, skim (nonfat) milk, lowfat cottage cheese, sweetened condensed skimmed milk, sour half-and-half, evaporated skimmed milk, low-fat dry milk, and the lower fat versions of all cultured dairy products, with the exception of yogurt, were eliminated.[139] These foods are now subject to the requirements of FDA's "general standard" which permits foods to be named by use of a defined nutrient content claim (e.g., *reduced fat* or *lowfat*) and a standardized term (e.g., "milk" or "cottage cheese"). This change was made to help consumers better understand the fat content of milk and other dairy foods. Under these rules, skim milk may now be called fat free or nonfat milk; 1% lowfat milk may be labeled "lowfat" or "light," and 2% lowfat milk is now called 2% reduced-fat milk. Labeling for whole milk (often referred to as vitamin D or homogenized milk) is unchanged (Table 1.15, Figure 1.6).[139] As a result of these labeling changes, consumers can expect to have many more choices of milk products, including *light* milk with at least 50% less fat than whole, or full-fat, milk and other reformulated milks with reduced fat contents with increased consumer appeal.[140] The American Heart Association acknowledges the value of milk and has awarded the "heart-check" seal to nonfat or fat free milk and 0.5% lowfat milk (Figure 1.6) indicating that these products meet the American Heart Association food criteria for saturated fat and cholesterol for healthy people over two years of age.

C. Chocolate Milk

Although a variety of flavored milks (e.g., strawberry, peanut butter, blueberry, root beer) are available locally and/or nationally, chocolate milk is by far the most popular flavored milk. Chocolate milk is milk to which chocolate or cocoa and

Table 1.15 Milk's Current Names

	(One Serving is 1 Cup or 8 Fluid Ounces)				
Past Name	Current Name (in Bold)	Calories	Fat (g)	Sat. Fat (g)	Calcium (mg)
Skim or Nonfat Milk	**Fat Free Milk** or Skim or Nonfat Milk	80	0	0	300 or 30% Daily Value
1% Lowfat Milk	1%* **Lowfat Milk**, or Light Milk	100	2.5	1.5	300 or 30% Daily Value
2% Lowfat Milk	2%* **Reduced Fat Milk**	120	5	3	300 or 30% Daily Value
Whole Milk	Whole Milk	150	8	5	300 or 30% Daily Value

* The milk fat percentages on labels are optional.

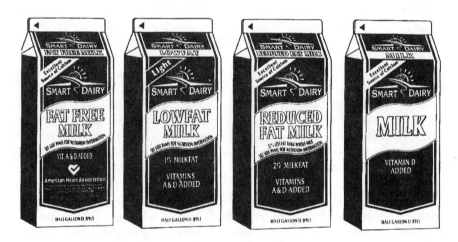

Figure 1.6   Current milk labels. (From MilkPEP, internal communication)

sweetener has been added. Similar to unflavored milks, chocolate milk has an excellent nutritional profile, providing significant amounts of high-quality protein, calcium, riboflavin, magnesium, phosphorus, niacin equivalents, vitamin B_{12}, vitamin A, and when added, vitamin D, as well as several other essential nutrients (Table 1.3).[43] Chocolate milk is a rich source of calcium. Each 8-ounce serving of chocolate milk provides 35% of the 800 mg recommended for this nutrient for children 4 through 8, 23% of the 1300 mg recommended for those 9 through 18 years, and 30% of the 1000 mg recommended for adults 19 through 50.[28,43] The nutrient content of chocolate milk, whole, 1% lowfat, 2% reduced fat, and fat free (skim or nonfat), is similar to that of the corresponding unflavored milk. The main exceptions are the higher contents of carbohydrate and calories in chocolate milk due to the addition of sucrose and other nutritive sweeteners.[43] In general, chocolate-flavored milks have about 60 calories more than their unflavored counterpart. An 8-ounce serving of chocolate lowfat (1%) milk contains 158 calories, 2% reduced fat chocolate milk contains 179 calories, and chocolate whole milk contains 208 calories (Table 1.3).

Chocolate milk is a highly nutritious, well-liked beverage. When children ages 8 through 13 were asked about their milk-drinking habits, 91% said that they liked chocolate milk.[141] When given a choice of milks, 57% of milk drinkers preferred chocolate milk over white milk.[141] One study demonstrated that offering chocolate milk at mealtime did not reduce preschoolers' intake of other foods.[142] Consuming chocolate milk as part of school lunch programs also can improve children's nutrient intake and reduce milk waste.[143,144] Providing 1% lowfat chocolate-flavored milk at school lunch increased children's intake of calcium, riboflavin, and phosphorus, according to a study by Garey et al.[144] When school food service directors in the southwest region of the U.S. were interviewed about the types of beverages offered in the school food service programs, approximately 78% supported serving chocolate milk.[145] Students' preference for chocolate milk and their increased milk (and calcium) intake were the two main reasons given by the directors for serving chocolate milk.[145] Findings of a recently reported study indicate that children who drank flavored milks had higher intakes of nutrients such as calcium and vitamin A than children who drank other beverages such as fruit drinks, soft drinks, or tea.[146] This study used data from the 1994-95 USDA Continuing Surveys of Food Intakes by Individuals to determine the daily intake of plain fluid milk, flavored milks, fruit juices, fruit drinks, soft drinks, and tea, and the contribution of these beverages to nutrient intake by children ages 1 to 5 and 6 to 11 years.[146]

There is no scientific evidence that chocolate milk, because of its sugar content, contributes to dental caries (see Chapter 7 on Dairy Foods and Oral Health). In fact, chocolate milk may contribute less to dental caries than other foods with similar sugar content. Because it is a liquid, chocolate milk is cleared from the mouth relatively quickly and therefore may be less cariogenic than many other foods such as raisins or candies that adhere to tooth surfaces. Moreover, several components in chocolate milk such as cocoa, milk fat, calcium, and phosphorus have been suggested to protect against dental caries. Likewise, there is no scientific evidence that sugar per se or in foods such as chocolate milk contributes to obesity or behavioral and learning disorders.[147,148] Chocolate milk contains a small amount (0.5 to 0.6%) of oxalic acid, a compound occurring naturally in cocoa beans and other plants. Although oxalic acid can combine with calcium to form an insoluble salt, there is no scientific evidence that oxalic acid in chocolate milk impairs calcium absorption.[149] The absorption of calcium from chocolate milk has been found to be similar to that of unflavored milk and other calcium-containing foods.[149]

D. Cheese

According to an ancient legend, cheese was discovered several thousand years before Christ by an Arabian merchant who placed milk in a pouch made from a sheep's stomach as he set out for a day's journey across the desert.[3] The rennet in the lining of the pouch, combined with the heat of the sun, caused the milk to separate into the curd of cheese and thin liquid now called whey. The art of cheese making is thought to have come to Europe from Asian travelers. During the Middle

Ages, cheese making flourished in countries such as Italy and France. In 1620 when the Pilgrims made their voyage to America, cheese was included in the Mayflower's supplies. In North America, cheese making remained a local farm industry until 1851 when the first cheese (Cheddar) factory opened in New York state. Shortly thereafter in 1868, a Limburger cheese factory was opened in Wisconsin.[3] Since these early years, the cheese industry has grown phenomenally both in total production and in the varieties of cheese products offered to consumers. Total natural cheese production in the U.S. grew from 418 million pounds in 1920 to 2.2 billion pounds in 1970 to 6 billion in the early 1990s to over 7.3 billion pounds in 1997.[3] Similarly, the production of processed cheese has increased over the years to more than two billion pounds a year in 1996.[3] Per capita consumption of natural cheese also has risen, specifically to 27.7 pounds in 1996, an increase of nearly a half pound from a year earlier (Figure 1.7). American varieties, which include Cheddar, Colby, and Monterey Jack, account for the largest percent followed by Italian varieties (e.g., mozzarella, ricotta, etc.). This increase in cheese consumption may be explained by cheese's pleasing taste, excellent nutritional value, versatility, economy, and more recently the introduction of innovative new products, a wider availability of specialty cheeses, more convenient packaging, and new ideas on how to use the product.

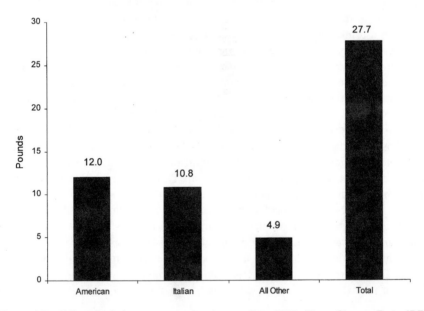

Figure 1.7   U.S. natural cheese per capita consumption, 1996. (From *Cheese Facts*, IDFA, 1997. With permission.)

Cheese is a concentrated dairy product made by draining off the whey after coagulation of casein, the major milk protein.[7,13] Casein is coagulated by acid produced by select microorganisms and/or by coagulating enzymes resulting in curd formation. Milk may also be acidified by adding food grade acidulants in the manufacture of certain varieties of cheese, such as cottage cheese. In fresh, unripened cheese (e.g., creamed cottage, cream cheese), the curd, separated from the whey, can be used immediately, whereas in matured or ripened cheeses (e.g., Cheddar, Swiss), the curd is treated further by the action of beneficial select strains of bacteria, mold, yeasts, or combinations of any of these ripening agents to produce a cheese of a specific flavor, texture, and appearance.[7] Natural cheese is produced directly from milk. Pasteurized blended cheese, process cheese, cheese foods, cheese spreads, and cold-pack cheeses are made by blending one or more different kinds of natural cheese with suitable emulsifying agents into a homogeneous mass. These cheeses are processed to produce uniform, safe, longer-keeping products.

Most cheeses produced in the U.S. have a standard of identity.[29] These federal standards define cheeses by specifying the ingredients used, the composition (maximum moisture content and minimum percentage of fat in the cheese solids or in the total mass of cheese), the requirements regarding pasteurization of the milk or an alternate minimum ripening period, production procedures, and any special requirements unique to a variety or class of cheese. However, manufacturers may list nutrient content claims on the labels of standardized foods (e.g., reduced fat cheese) if certain conditions are met.[116] The nutrient content claim (e.g., reduced fat) must meet FDA's definition which in the case of *reduced* fat is at least 25% less fat than in the standard product. Also, the modified food cannot be nutritionally inferior to the traditional standardized food. In addition, the new food must have performance characteristics similar to those of the standardized food. If not, the label must state the difference in performance. A modified food that uses a standardized term (e.g., Swiss cheese), but does not comply with the standard of identity, must be labeled either as an "imitation" if it is nutritionally inferior (e.g., imitation Swiss cheese), or as a "substitute," "alternative," or other appropriate term (e.g., Swiss cheese alternative) if it is not nutritionally inferior. The majority of imitation cheeses are imitation or alternate process cheeses. The dairy industry administers a program for identifying real dairy foods. The REAL Seal on a carton or package identifies cheese, milk, and other qualified dairy foods made from U.S. produced milk that meets federal and/or state standards.[7] This seal assures consumers that the food is not an imitation or substitute.

Cheese is a concentrated source of many of milk's nutrients.[7,27] About one-third of all the milk produced in the U.S. each year is used to make cheese (Figure 1.1).[3] About 10 pounds (five quarts) of milk are required to make one pound of Cheddar cheese and nine pounds of whey. During the typical cheese-making process, there is a significant partitioning of milk's nutrients with separation of the curds from the whey and changes in milk's nutrients during ripening of the cheese. The water-insoluble components of milk (casein, fat) primarily remain in the curd, whereas most of the water-soluble constituents (carbohydrates, salts, proteins smaller than casein) are in the whey (Table 1.16). The amount of various nutrients retained in the curd and whey largely depends on the type of cheese manufactured, the milk (whole, lowfat, reduced fat, nonfat), and manner of coagulation. During ripening, microorganisms and enzymes which transform the fresh curd into a cheese of specific flavor, texture, and appearance can also alter the nutrient content of the product.

Cheese makes an appreciable contribution to the amount of nutrients available in the U.S. food supply (Table 1.17). In 1994, cheese contributed 7.8% of the protein, 23% of the calcium, and nearly 5% of the riboflavin available. In addition, cheese

Table 1.16   Partition of Nutrients in Milk in Making Cheddar Cheese

Nutrient	Percentage in Curd[a]	Percentage in Whey[a]
Water	6	94
Total Solids	48	52
Casein	96	4
Soluble Proteins	4	96
Fat	94	6
Lactose	6	94
Calcium	62	38
Vitamin A	94	6
Thiamin	15	85
Riboflavin	26	74
Vitamin C	6	84

[a] Percentage of total in original milk at point of separation of curd and whey.

Note: The indicated loss of vitamin C, due to the destructive effect of light, is relatively unimportant because the milk itself is not a significant source of vitamin C, particularly pasteurized milk for cheese. Unaccountable losses usually are observed also with other vitamins, notably riboflavin, which also is affected by light. These losses are more noticeable in the whey than in the curd.

Source: National Dairy Council, *Newer Knowledge of Cheese and Other Cheese Products*, 1992, p. 25. With permission.

supplies many other nutrients in significant amounts. The protein of cheese is largely casein with small amounts of alpha-lactalbumin and beta-lactoglobulin. Together, these proteins in the curd amount to about four-fifths of the protein of the original milk. One fifth of milk's protein, mostly the soluble albumins and globulins, remain in the whey. The method of coagulation of milk as well as the degree of ripening (i.e., enzyme-coagulated or acid-coagulated) influence the protein content of cheese. In hard ripened cheeses, such as Cheddar and Swiss, relatively little hydrolysis of protein occurs, whereas in soft ripened cheeses, such as Camembert, protein is broken down to water-soluble compounds including peptides, amino acids, and ammonia. Cheese protein is classified as a high-quality protein because of its unique amino acid composition. Cheese contains all of the amino acids commonly found in food protein and in significant amounts. The relative surplus of one of the dietary essential amino acids, lysine, in cheese protein (as in the proteins of milk) makes cheese, as well as milk, valuable in supplementing vegetable proteins, especially those of grain products which are low in lysine.

The carbohydrate content, principally lactose, in ripened cheese is not nutritionally significant. Lactose is largely removed in the whey during cheese making.[7,13] The presence of small amounts (about 2%) of lactose in cheese depends on the quantity of entrapped whey in the curd. During ripening, this lactose is generally transformed to lactic acid and other products by bacteria, molds, yeasts, and enzymes that produce the characteristic flavor of specific cheeses. After 21 to 28 days of ripening, generally no lactose remains.[7] The legal addition of optional ingredients such as fat free milk and cheese whey during the manufacture of process cheese

Table 1.17   Percent Total Nutrients Contributed by Cheese to the U.S. Per Capita Food Supply, 1994

	Total Cheese %
Food Energy	3.1
Protein	7.8
Fat	5.6
Carbohydrate	0.2
Minerals	
Calcium	23.3
Iron	0.9
Magnesium	2.3
Phosphorus	9.5
Zinc	7.4
Potassium	0.9
Vitamins	
Ascorbic Acid	0.0
Thiamin	0.3
Riboflavin	4.6
Niacin	0.2
Folate	1.6
Vitamin B_6	1.2
Vitamin B_{12}	4.1
Vitamin A activity	5.8

Source: Gerrior S., and Bente, L., *Nutrient Content of the U.S. Food Supply,* 1909-94, Home Economic Research Report No. 53, Washington, D.C., USDA Center for Nutrition Policy and Promotion, 1997.

products may increase the carbohydrate content of these products. Because most varieties of cheese contain an insignificant amount of lactose, this food is well tolerated by consumers who are lactase nonpersistent (see Chapter 8 on Dairy Foods and Lactose Intolerance).

The milk fat content of cheese is mainly responsible for this food's satiety value, flavor, and texture. During curing or ripening, milk fat in cheese undergoes a certain amount of hydrolysis which results in the release of volatile fatty acids (e.g., butyric, caproic, and caprylic acids and higher carbon chain fatty acids) which in turn can contribute to the flavor of cheese. Cheeses vary widely in milk fat content, from almost 0% in plain cottage cheese dry curd (made with nonfat milk) to at least 33% in cream cheese made from whole cow's milk and cream. A higher fat cheese, such as cream cheese, is always enriched with cream and therefore contains a greater proportion of fat than protein. Cheeses such as Cheddar, Swiss, and Gouda generally have about the same amount of fat and protein. A reduced fat cheese has a higher protein-to-fat ratio. When fat is reduced, the taste and texture of cheese may be negatively altered. Numerous reduced fat cheeses have recently been introduced and efforts are being made to overcome some of these drawbacks.[7]

As mentioned above, the minimum milk fat (and maximum moisture) content of most cheeses is governed by federal and state regulations. Generally, natural cheeses such as Cheddar, Swiss, and Roquefort contain about 8 to 9 grams of fat per ounce. Processed cheeses have a fat content closely related to the cheese or mixtures of cheeses from which they are made. Generally, these processed cheeses contain about 7 to 9 grams of fat per ounce. Cheese foods and spreads have 6 to 7 grams of fat per ounce. Numerous processed cheeses with *reduced* or *less* fat or labeled *light* or *lite* are available on the market.[7] In addition, a fat free product called nonfat pasteurized process cheese product is available. Nutrient content descriptors are defined by law. The Nutrition Facts label on the cheese product indicates its fat and calorie content (Figure 1.8).

Although fat in cheese is similar to that of milk fat, the composition of fatty acids in cheese may differ from milk fat because of the ripening action in cheese. However, the fatty acid patterns for specific cheeses are not appreciably different from one another. A variety of cheeses, including Cheddar, are good sources of the anticancer agent, conjugated linoleic acid (CLA) (see Chapter 4 on Dairy Foods and Colon Cancer). CLA has been demonstrated to protect against both cancer and coronary heart disease in laboratory animals. In humans, intake of 112 g (or 4 ounces) of Cheddar cheese increased blood levels of CLA by 19 to 27%, according to a study of nine healthy men.[150] The cholesterol content of cheese varies with the fat content. Full-fat cheeses such as Cheddar cheese and cream cheese contain about 30 mg cholesterol per ounce. A one-third fat-reduced Cheddar cheese has approximately 21 mg of cholesterol per serving and fat-free cheeses contain about 5 mg cholesterol per serving.[7]

The vitamin content of cheese depends on the vitamins in the milk used, the manufacturing of the cheese, the cultures or microorganisms employed, and the conditions and length of the curing period. Wide variations in the vitamin content occur among individual samples of the same variety of cheese, as well as among different varieties. As most of the fat in milk is retained in the curd, cheese contains the fat-soluble vitamins of the milk used. Cheese such as Cheddar, which is made with whole milk, is a good source of vitamin A activity (298 RE or 1059 IU per 100 g), whereas, cheese made with 1% milk fat contains a relatively smaller amount of this vitamin (11 RE or 37 IU per 100 g). Water-soluble vitamins such as thiamin, riboflavin, niacin, vitamin B_6, pantothenic acid, biotin, and folacin remain in the whey. The more whey retained in the cheese, the greater the content of these vitamins in the cheese. Generally, any cheese variety high in one B vitamin is high in most of the other B vitamins. In surface-ripened cheeses such as Brie and Camembert and mold-ripened cheese varieties such as blue cheese or Gorgonzola, a higher concentration of B complex vitamins may occur on the outer layers of the cheese.

Cheese is a good source of minerals (Tables 1.3 and 1.17). However, similar to vitamins, the mineral content of cheese varies both within and among varieties. Cheeses contribute about 23% of the calcium available in the food supply in 1994.[27] The calcium content of cheese is largely influenced by the acidity at coagulation and by extent of expulsion of the whey from the curd. In ripened whole-milk cheeses made with a coagulating enzyme (e.g., Cheddar cheese), the calcium and phosphorus of milk remain for the most part in the curd. In contrast, cheese coagulated by lactic

Nutrition Facts

Serving Size 1 oz (28g) about 1 inch cube)
Servings Per Container Varied

Amount Per Serving

Calories 110   Calories from Fat 85

% Daily Value*

Total Fat 9g	**14%**
Saturated Fat 6g	**30%**
Cholesterol 30mg	**10%**
Sodium 180mg	**7%**
Total Carbohydrate 0g	**0%**
Dietary Fiber 0g	**0%**
Sugars 0g	
Protein 7g	

Vitamin A	6%
Vitamin C	0%
Calcium	20%
Iron	0%

*Percent Daily Values are based on a 2,000 calorie diet. Your daily values may be higher or lower depending on your calorie needs:

		Calories:	2,000	2,500
Total Fat	Less than		65g	80g
Sat Fat	Less than		20g	25g
Cholesterol	Less than		300mg	300mg
Sodium	Less than		2,400mg	2,400mg
Total Carbohydrate			300g	375g
Dietary Fiber			25g	30g

Calories per gram:
Fat 9 • Carbohydrate 4 • Protein 4

Figure 1.8 Sample label for Cheddar cheese. (From Kosikowski, F.V. and Mistry, V.V., Cheese and Fermented Milk Foods, Volume I: Origins and Principles, 3rd ed., 1997, 557. With permission.)

acid alone (e.g., cottage or cream cheese) contains less calcium and phosphorus because the calcium salts are removed from the casein as casein is precipitated.[7] Cheddar cheese contains 721 mg calcium per 100 g, whereas dry curd cottage cheese contains 32 mg calcium per 100 g. The calcium content of cottage cheese may be increased by adding calcium-containing creaming mixtures. Generally, cheeses that are high in calcium contain other minerals such as magnesium in appreciable amounts. Cheese contributes small, but variable, amounts of specific trace elements such as zinc to the diet.

The sodium content of cheese is variable because of the addition of sodium chloride (salt) as an optional ingredient during manufacturing. On average, one ounce of natural Cheddar cheese contributes only about 7% and a similar amount of natural Swiss cheese contributes about 3% of the daily sodium intake limit of 2400 mg/day.[113] Although Americans are advised to decrease their intake of sodium to reduce their risk of hypertension (see Chapter 3 on Dairy Foods and Hypertension), about two-thirds of adults are not susceptible to hypertension caused by salt sensitivity. Further, many experts question the benefit of low-salt diets for healthy people. Other factors such as excess body weight and reduced physical activity may play a more important role in the development of high blood pressure. However, for salt-sensitive individuals, sodium-free (5 mg or less per serving), low sodium (140 mg or less per serving), very low sodium (35 mg or less), reduced sodium (at least 25% less sodium), and *light* (reduced in sodium by 50% or more) cheeses are available.

Cheese is an important source of essential nutrients throughout life. As mentioned above, because of its low lactose content, cheese is an important source of many nutrients found in milk, particularly calcium, for individuals with lactose intolerance. Research also indicates that certain cheeses may protect against dental caries (see Chapter 7 on Dairy Foods and Oral Health). Studies in experimental animals and in humans demonstrate that intake of natural and processed cheeses reduces risk of tooth decay. Components in cheese such as calcium and possibly phosphorus may inhibit the demineralization and favor the remineralization of teeth.

Although concern has been expressed that intake of cheese contributes to constipation, there is no scientific evidence to support this belief.[151-153] In a study of older adults living in a retirement home, intake of cheese had no effect on intestinal transit time, fecal frequency, or fecal wet weight and consistency.[152] To prevent and treat constipation, individuals are advised to consume 20 to 35 grams of fiber a day from fresh produce and whole-grains, drink plenty of fluids, and exercise regularly.[153]

E. Cultured and Culture-Containing Dairy Foods

Cultured (fermented) dairy foods are milk products that result from the fermentation of milk or its products by starter cultures (selected specific microorganisms) that produce lactic acid under controlled conditions.[7,47] In culture-containing dairy products, concentrated cultures of bacteria such as *Lactobacillus acidophilus* or bifidobacteria are added to pasteurized and other types of heat-treated milk with no subsequent incubation or fermentation. In recent years, probiotic or health-promoting bacteria have been added to an array of dairy foods. There are a variety of cultured dairy foods differing in flavor and consistency such as acidophilus milk, Bulgarian buttermilk, cultured buttermilk, cultured or sour cream, kefir, koumiss, and yogurt.[7] All of these fermented milk products are characterized by the presence of lactic acid. Yogurt is made from milk fermented by a mixed culture of *Lactobacillus bulgaricus* and *Streptococcus thermophilus*. This dairy product may be plain, sweetened, flavored, or frozen. Culturing or fermenting dairy foods is a method of preserving these foods as well as improving taste, digestibility, and increasing the variety of dairy foods available.[47] In recent decades, cultured and culture-containing dairy foods have increased dramatically in part because of their healthy image, trendy flavors, and milder cultures.[154] Per capita sales of yogurt have increased from 1.5 pounds in 1974 to 4.8 pounds in 1996 (Figure 1.4).[2] As a result of the recent government ruling allowing yogurt to be used to meet all or part of the meat/meat alternate requirement for child and adult nutrition programs in the U.S.,[20] sales of yogurt may be expected to increase further in the near future.

Cultured and culture-containing dairy foods are important sources of many of milk's nutrients including protein, calcium, phosphorus, magnesium, riboflavin, vitamin B_{12}, and niacin equivalents (Table 1.3).[7,43] In general, the nutrient content of cultured and culture-containing foods is similar to that of the milk from which these products are made. However, factors such as the type and strain of bacteria, milk (whole, lowfat, nonfat) used, fermentation conditions, storage, and other treatments such as the addition of milk solids-not-fat, sweeteners, and fruits (e.g., in yogurts) can influence the nutrient composition of cultured and culture-containing dairy foods.[7] Some lactic acid-producing bacteria require vitamins for growth whereas others synthesize some vitamins. The mineral content of milk is relatively unchanged by fermentation. The fermentation of milk results in partial breakdown and better absorption of milk's protein, carbohydrate (lactose), and fat.[155] These changes are thought to result in a food of improved digestibility. Similar to their non-cultured counterparts, cultured dairy foods of varied fat and energy contents are available. For example, in the U.S. three categories of yogurt exist: yogurt (>3.25% fat, >8.25% milk solids-not-fat), lowfat yogurt (>0.5 to <2.0% fat, >8.25% milk solids-not-fat), and nonfat yogurt (<0.5% fat, >8.25% milk solids-not-fat).[29]

Since the early 1900s when Elias Metchnikoff, in his book, *The Prolongation of Life,* associated consumption of large quantities of Bulgarian fermented milk with a long life, numerous health benefits have been attributed to cultured dairy foods.[7] These include improved lactose utilization, control of intestinal infections, reduced blood cholesterol levels, and anticarcinogenic activity. Many cultured dairy foods are beneficial for individuals with lactose intolerance (see Chapter 8 on Lactose Intolerance). This beneficial effect is explained by the lower lactose content of some cultured dairy foods compared to milk and the ability of starter cultures used in the manufacture of yogurt with live, active cultures to produce the enzyme lactase which hydrolyzes lactose.[156] Although yogurt with active cultures is particularly advantageous for lactose intolerant individuals, unfermented or sweet acidophilus milk (i.e., pasteurized milk with *Lactobacillus acidophilus* added but not incubated), cultured buttermilk (i.e., pasteurized nonfat or lowfat milk cultured with *Streptococcus lactis* culture), and yogurt without live active cultures are tolerated about the same as milk. Yogurts with live active cultures can be identified by the National Yogurt Association's "Live and Active Culture" seal. Only yogurt products meeting specific requirements (i.e., at least 10 million organisms per gram at the time of purchase) may carry this seal.

Lactobacillus acidophilus bacteria may inhibit many common pathogenic and food spoilage organisms in the intestine which cause digestive problems such as diarrhea.[155] In addition, they may restore an appropriate balance of microorganisms in the intestinal tract following prolonged antibiotic therapy. A preliminary study found that consuming a cup of plain yogurt with *Lactobacillus acidophilus* each day for six months reduced vaginal yeast infections.[157] The *Lactobacillus* strain *GG* is particularly effective in treating and preventing antibiotic-associated diarrhea, traveler's diarrhea, and acute diarrhea in children.[158] In adults, *Lactobacillus GG* has been demonstrated to stimulate human bowel function by altering the microflora and suppressing fermentation in the intestine.[159] *Lactobacillus GG* may also improve tolerance to milk in infants[160] and adults[161] with cow's milk allergy.

In young children with persistent diarrhea, yogurt has been demonstrated to prevent further weight loss.[162] Also in an *in vitro* study, yogurt containing live active cultures and with a pH near 4.5 destroyed *Escherichia coli*, a bacterial species which causes diarrhea particularly among travelers to tropical areas.[163] Yogurt with a strain of bacteria known as *Lactobacillus gasseri* may be particularly advantageous for older adults with atrophic gastritis, a condition which predisposes individuals to intestinal infections and constipation.[164]

Certain cultured and culture-containing dairy foods may lower blood cholesterol levels (see Chapter 2 on Dairy Foods and Cardiovascular Health). Recent studies in laboratory animals have found that blood total and low density lipoprotein (LDL) cholesterol (the "bad" cholesterol) are reduced when the animals are fed whey from milk containing *Bifidobacterium longum* or *Lactobacillus acidophilus*,[165] yogurts with *Bifidobacteria*,[166] and yogurts made with *Streptococcus thermophilus* plus *Lactobacillus acidophilus*.[167]

Scientific findings indicate a potential protective role for lactic acid bacteria and cultured dairy foods against certain cancers such as colorectal cancer (see Chapter 4 on Dairy Foods and Colon Cancer) and breast cancer.[168,169] In an *in vitro* study of the effect of five different bacterial strains on the growth of a human breast cancer cell line, all five bacteria strains inhibited the growth of the breast cancer cell line, although *Bifidobacterium infantitis* and *Lactobacillus acidophilus* were the most effective.[169] The mechanism(s) for the cancer protective effect of specific cultures or culture-containing dairy foods is unknown. Lactic acid-producing cultures reduce fecal enzymes associated with the conversion of procarcinogens to carcinogens in some studies.[170] The tumor-suppressing effect of lactobacilli may also be explained by their effect on the host's immune system. When mice given a chemical carcinogen were fed yogurt, colorectal tumors and the inflammatory immune response were reduced compared to the control animals which were not given yogurt.[171] In another investigation in which mice were challenged with *Salmonella typhimurium*, the immune response was greater in animals fed yogurt than in those fed a milk-based diet.[172] In a study involving healthy young adults, consumption of two cups of yogurt with live active cultures each day for four months increased white blood cell levels of gamma-interferon which improves the immune defense.[173] Bacterial cultures in fermented dairy foods such as yogurt may reduce the risk of colon cancer by generating a variety of peptides from casein which influence colon cell division.[50]

Numerous nutritional and health benefits are attributed to bifidobacteria or dairy foods containing these bacteria.[174-176] Bifidobacteria synthesize several vitamins such as thiamin, riboflavin, vitamin B_6, and vitamin K in the large intestine.[174] Among their potential health benefits, bifidobacteria help maintain the normal intestinal microflora balance and inhibit pathogenic bacteria in the gut, especially in infants and the elderly; improve lactose and milk digestion in lactose intolerant individuals; prevent formation of carcinogens, possibly by removing procarcinogens or activating the body's immune system; and lower blood cholesterol levels. The addition of bifidobacteria and *S. thermophilus* to infant formulas has been demonstrated to reduce the risk of diarrhea in high-risk infants.[177] Despite the above promising findings of health benefits of cultured and culture-containing dairy foods, additional research is needed to confirm these benefits in humans.[7]

F. Whey Products

Whey is the portion of milk remaining after casein and fat are formed into cheese curd usually by acid, heat, or rennet.[7,13] Once regarded mainly as an animal feed product, today the uses of whey and whey products for human consumption have greatly expanded as a result of recognition of whey's excellent nutritional and functional properties. As used for human food, whey is concentrated by evaporation to condensed products or maximally concentrated by drying into dry products of milk. All whey for human use must be pasteurized. The food industry uses whey and its products in baked goods, beverages, flavorings (sauces, salad dressings), canned goods (fruits and vegetables), cheese products (dips, spreads, process cheese, confections), dry mixes, frozen foods, jams and jellies, fat substitutes, and meat, pasta, and milk products. Whey and modified whey products are an acceptable substitute for nonfat dry milk (NFDM) in some foods and may partially replace NFDM in frozen desserts. Whey cheese, such as ricotta cheese, is made by concentrating whey and coagulating the whey protein with heat and acid, with or without the addition of milk and milk fat.

Whey is recognized for its high nutritional quality. This by-product of the cheese industry contains the water-soluble nutrients of milk, specifically lactose, noncasein protein (albumins and globulins), and some minerals and vitamins (Table 1.16). There are two types of whey, sweet whey and acid whey. Sweet whey (pH greater than or equal to 5.6) is obtained from whole milk used in the manufacture of natural enzyme-produced cheeses such as Cheddar cheese. Acid whey (pH less than or equal to 5.1) is obtained from nonfat milk used in the manufacture of cottage or similar cheeses. An average composition of sweet and acid dry wheys is provided in Table 1.18. Wide ranges in the nutrient content of these wheys are recognized because of diverse manufacturing processes presently used for cheese from which sweet and acid whey products are obtained.

Fresh pasteurized liquid whey is rarely used as such for foods or feeds because of high transporting costs and susceptibility to deterioration during storage. Consequently, whey is processed to provide a wide range of products including condensed whey, dry whey, and modified whey products, each with unique functional characteristics (e.g., whipping/foaming, emulsification, high solubility, gelation, viscosity). These whey products contain a high concentration of whey solids that are easily transported, have enhanced storage stability, blend well with other foods, and are economical sources of milk solids.[7,13]

Condensed whey is the liquid food obtained by removing some of the moisture from whey. The whey may be condensed about tenfold, but all constituents other than moisture remain in the same relative proportions as in the original whey. Condensed whey may be directly added to processed cheese foods. Sweet condensed

Table 1.18   **Average Composition of Sweet and Acid Dry Wheys[a]**

Constituent	Sweet	Acid
Protein, Nx6.38 (%)	12.9	12.2
Fat (%)	1.1	0.5
Lactose (%)	74.5	63.0
Total ash (%)	8.3	10.7
Vitamins[b]		
Vitamin A (IU)	44	107
Vitamin C (mg)	1.5	0.3
Vitamin E (mg)	0.03	0.05
Thiamin (B1) (mg)	0.5	0.5
Riboflavin (B2) (mg)	2.2	11.8
Pyridoxine (B6) (mg)	0.6	0.6
Vitamin B12 (mcg)	2.4	2.5
Pantothenic Acid (mg)	5.6	1.8
Niacin (mg)	1.3	1.0
Folate (mcg)	11.6	0.03
Minerals		
Calcium (mg)	796	2279
Phosphorus (mg)	931.7	1516
Sodium (mg)	1079	1022
Potassium (mg)	2080	1885
Magnesium (mg)	176	247
Zinc (mg)	1.97	7.7
Iron (mg)	0.9	1.4
Copper (mg)	0.07	5.3
Selenium (mcg)	0.06	27.3

[a] Values per 100 g dry whey.

Source: USDA, ARS, USDA Nutrient Database for Standard Reference, Release 12, 1998, www.nal.usda.gov.fnic/foodcomp.

whey is used in candy formulas. Acid whey has a more limited use for humans. Dry whey, the most suitable form for use in foods or feeds, is the food obtained by removing about 95% of the moisture from whey but which contains all other constituents in the same relative proportions as in whey. This form of whey can be stored almost indefinitely under reasonable conditions without harm to its physical or nutritional properties. Modified whey products may be obtained by various processes and procedures such as ultrafiltration and reverse osmosis. Examples of modified whey products include partially delactosed whey, partially demineralized and demineralized whey, and whey protein concentrate. Partially delactosed whey contains no more than 60% lactose on a solids basis. Lactose (62 to 75% of dry whey) is removed by crystallization for use in many products such as a carrier or extender in pharmaceuticals. Partially demineralized whey contains a maximum of 7% mineral matter on a solids basis and demineralized whey contains a maximum of $1\frac{1}{2}$% on a solids basis. The minerals in whey (7 to 10% total in dry whey) are removed because they may contribute to an off-taste. Whey protein concentrate contains a minimum of 25% protein on a solids basis. In general, the protein level of whey protein concentrates ranges from 34 to 90%.[178] Whey protein concentrates may be added to coffee whiteners, soups, and infant formula because of their emulsification properties; to desserts and whipped toppings because of their ability to form foams; to meats and baked goods for texture and structure because of their gelling properties; and to lowfat cheeses because of their ability to soften cheese texture.[7] Whey protein edible coatings may be used to extend the shelf life of oxygen sensitive foods such as nuts, or fresh fruits and vegetables.

VII. SUMMARY

The nutritional and health benefits of milk and other dairy foods are well documented and sound scientific evidence supports their importance in the diet. In fact, these foods have a long history of contributing to health and well-being. Today, milk and other dairy foods are recognized as energy dense foods. Although they only contribute 9% of the total calories (energy) available in the U.S. food supply, these foods provide 73% of the calcium, 31% of the riboflavin, 33% of the phosphorus, 19% of the protein, 16% of the magnesium, 21% of the vitamin B_{12}, 17% of the vitamin A, 10% of the vitamin B_6, and 6% of the thiamin, in addition to appreciable amounts of vitamin D and niacin equivalents.[27] Dairy foods contribute to nutrient intake and health from childhood through older adult years. Unfortunately, many people fail to consume recommended servings of these foods which makes it difficult for them to meet nutrient recommendations. Consuming milk and other dairy foods improves the overall nutritional quality of the diet without necessarily increasing total energy or fat intake, body weight, or percent body fat.[37-42]

With respect to specific nutrients, cow's milk is an excellent source of high quality protein which contains in varying amounts all of the essential amino acids required for humans.[45] Because of its content of the amino acid tryptophan, milk is an excellent source of niacin equivalents. Experimental studies indicate that cow's milk protein may help to increase bone strength, enhance immune function, reduce blood pressure and risk of cancer, and protect against dental caries. The prevalence of cow's milk protein allergy or sensitivity is generally exaggerated and, if present in high risk children, is usually outgrown by three years of age.[53,54] Scientific findings fail to confirm the suggestion that cow's milk protein contributes to the development of Type I or insulin-dependent diabetes in genetically susceptible children.[60-68] Although the primary carbohydrate in cow's milk is lactose, its amount varies widely among different dairy foods. As discussed in Chapter 8, those who are lactase nonpersistent can comfortably consume the amount of lactose in up to two cups of milk/day when taken with meals. Fat in milk contributes to the appearance, texture, and flavor of dairy foods. Milk fat is also a source of energy, essential fatty acids, fat-soluble vitamins (A,D,E,K) and several health promoting components such as conjugated linoleic acid (CLA), sphingomyelin, butyric acid, and myristic acids.[6,82] For example, emerging scientific findings reveal that CLA may protect against certain cancers and cardiovascular disease, enhance immune function, and reduce body fatness/increase lean body tissue. Potentially beneficial roles of milk fat on satiety and bone health are being investigated.

Milk and other dairy foods are an important source of many vitamins and minerals. Vitamin A in whole milk, and added to fluid lower fat and fat free milks, plays a key role in vision, cellular differentiation, and immunity. Nearly all fluid milks in the U.S. are fortified with vitamin D. Vitamin D enhances the intestinal absorption of calcium and phosphorus and is essential for the maintenance of a healthy skeleton. In addition to these fat-soluble vitamins, milk and other dairy foods contribute appreciable amounts of water-soluble vitamins such as riboflavin, vitamin B_{12}, and vitamin B_6. Milk and milk products provide almost three-quarters of the calcium available in the nation's food supply. A sufficient intake of calcium reduces the risk of osteoporosis (see Chapter 5), hypertension (see Chapter 3), colon cancer (see Chapter 4), and some types of kidney stones. Three to four servings of milk and other dairy foods a day will meet the calcium recommendations for most people. In addition to calcium, these foods contribute other important minerals such as phosphorus, magnesium, potassium, and trace elements such as zinc.

The high nutritional value of milk, as well as its overall quality, are ensured by rigid sanitary conditions employed from farm to marketplace. Protecting the quality of milk is everyone's responsibility, from government health officials, to the dairy industry, to consumers. The Pasteurized Milk Ordinance[121] is an example of an effective instrument for protecting the quality of the nation's milk. To improve milk's quality, most milk is homogenized and pasteurized. Homogenization results in milk of uniform consistency which is less susceptible to off-flavors. Pasteurization is required by law for all fluid milk and milk products moved in interstate commerce for retail sale. As a result of pasteurization, milk and milk products are now associated with less than 1% of all disease outbreaks due to infected food and contaminated water compared to 25% in 1938.[121]

Today, consumers have a wide variety of dairy foods to choose from to meet their taste, nutrition, health, and convenience needs. Dairy foods of varied fat content, of low or reduced lactose content, fortified with nutrients such as vitamin A, vitamin D, and calcium, and processed to improve the keeping quality are readily available. These foods include milks (unflavored, flavored, evaporated, condensed, sweetened condensed, dry, nonfat dry), cultured and culture-containing dairy foods (yogurts, acidophilus milk, cultured buttermilk, sour cream), creams, butter, ice cream, and cheeses.[12,13] Over the years, consumption of individual milks and milk products has changed dramatically. Noteworthy trends include more use of reduced fat milks, yogurt, creams, and cheese, and less use of whole milk.[11,135] As a result of recent comprehensive food labeling regulations, consumers can now easily choose dairy foods that meet their specific needs by referring to the Nutrition Facts label on product packages.[116] To help consumers better understand the fat content of milk and other dairy foods, standards of identity for 12 lower fat dairy foods have been removed and new labels introduced. For example, skim (nonfat) milk can now be labeled *fat free* as well as nonfat and skim.[115]

The nutritional and health benefits of specific dairy foods such as chocolate milk, cheese, cultured and culture-containing dairy foods, and whey products are reviewed. Intake of chocolate milk, a highly nutritious, well-liked beverage, has been demonstrated to improve children's overall nutrient intake.[144-146] Cheese is a concentrated source of many of milk's nutrients.[13] Because of their insignificant amount of lactose, most cheeses are well tolerated by individuals with lactase nonpersistence (see Chapter 8). Cheeses are also a good source of CLA, and several varieties of cheese may protect against dental caries (see Chapter 7). Not only are cultured (fermented) and culture-containing dairy foods such as yogurt an excellent source of many of milk's nutrients, but they may offer health benefits including improved lactose digestion, control of intestinal infections, reduced blood cholesterol levels, and anticancer activity. These beneficial effects depend on the type and strain of bacteria, fermentation condition, type of milk, and other factors. Similar to cultured dairy foods, whey, a by-product of the cheese industry, is being recognized for its excellent nutritional and functional properties.[13] Clearly, consumers today are presented with an abundant array of safe, nutritious dairy foods tailored to meet their specific health and other needs.

REFERENCES

1. McGee, H., *On Food and Cooking: The Science and Lore of the Kitchen*, Macmillan, New York, 1984.
2. International Dairy Foods Association, *Milk Facts 1997 Edition,* Washington, D.C.: International Dairy Foods Association, September 1997.
3. International Dairy Foods Association, *Cheese Facts 1997 Edition,* Washington, D.C.: International Dairy Foods Association, 1997.
4. International Dairy Foods Association, *The Latest Scoop 1997 Edition.* Washington, D.C.: International Dairy Foods Association, 1997.
5. Wong, N. P., Jenness, R., Keeney, M., and Marth, E. H., Eds., *Fundamentals of Dairy Chemistry,* 3rd ed., Van Nostrand Reinhold, New York, 1988.
6. Jensen, R. G., Ed., *Handbook of Milk Composition*, Academic Press, New York, 1995.
7. Kosikowski, F. V. and Mistry, V. V., *Cheese and Fermented Milk Foods, Vol. 1. Origins and Principles, Vol. 11. Procedures and Analysis,* 3rd edition, F.V. Kosikowski and Associates, Brooktondale, NY, 1997.
8. Fox, P. F., Ed., *Advanced Dairy Chemistry, Vol. 1, Proteins*, Chapman and Hall, New York, 1992.
9. Fox, P. F., Ed., *Advanced Dairy Chemistry, Vol. 2, Lipids,* 2nd edition, Chapman and Hall, New York, 1995.
10. Fox, P. F., Ed., *Advanced Dairy Chemistry, Vol. 3, Lactose, Water, Salts, and Vitamins,* 2nd edition, Chapman and Hall, New York, 1997.
11. CAST (Council for Agricultural Science and Technology), *Contribution of Animal Products to Healthful Diets,* Task Force Report No. 131, Ames, Iowa: Council for Agricultural Science and Technology, October 1997.
12. National Dairy Council, *Newer Knowledge of Milk and Other Fluid Dairy Products*, National Dairy Council, Rosemont, IL, 1993.
13. National Dairy Council, *Newer Knowledge of Cheese and Other Cheese Products*, National Dairy Council, Rosemont, IL, 1992.
14. U.S. Department of Agriculture, Human Nutrition Information Service, *The Food Guide Pyramid*, Home and Garden Bulletin No. 252, Washington, D.C.: USDA/HNIS, 1992.
15. National Dairy Council, *Guide to Good Eating*, 6th ed., National Dairy Council, Rosemont, IL, 1994.

16. U.S. Department of Agriculture and U.S. Department of Health and Human Services, *Nutrition and Your Health: Dietary Guidelines for Americans,* 4th ed., Home and Garden Bulletin No. 232, Washington, D.C.: USDA/DHHS, 1995.

17. National Institutes of Health, *Optimal Calcium Intake,* NIH Consensus Statement 12, 4, NIH, Bethesda, MD, 1994.

18. Skiba, A., Loghmani, E., and Orr, D. P., Nutritional screening and guidance for adolescents, *Adolescent Health Update,* 9(2), 1, 1997.

19. American Medical Association, Council on Scientific Affairs, Intake of dietary calcium to reduce the incidence of osteoporosis, *Arch. Fam. Med.,* 6, 495, 1997.

20. U.S. Department of Agriculture, Food and Consumer Service, National School Lunch Program, School Breakfast Program, Summer Food Service Program for Children, and Child and Adult Care Food Program, Meat alternates used in the child nutrition programs, final rule, *Fed. Regist.,* 62(44), 10187, 1997.

21. Devaney, B., Gordon, A. R., and Burghardt, J. A., Dietary intakes of students, *Am. J. Clin. Nutr.,* 61(Suppl.), 205, 1995.

22. Hanes, S., Vermeersch, J., and Gale, S., The national evaluation of school nutrition programs: program impact on dietary intake, *Am. J. Clin. Nutr.,* 40, 390, 1984.

23. Sampson, A. E., Dixit, S., Meyers, A. F., and Houser, R., Jr., The nutritional impact of breakfast consumption on the diets of inner-city African-American elementary school children, *J. Natl. Med. Assoc.,* 87, 195, 1995.

24. Nicklas, T. A., Bao, W., Webber, L. S., and Berenson, G. S., Breakfast consumption affects adequacy of total daily intake in children, *J. Am. Diet. Assoc.,* 93, 886, 1993.

25. Mathematica Policy Research Inc., The School Nutrition Dietary Assessment Study, Food and Nutrition Service, U.S. Department of Agriculture, Princeton, N.J., 1993.

26. Food and Consumer Service, Public Affairs Staff, U.S. Department of Agriculture, Food and Nutrition Service, *Nutrition Program Facts and Preliminary Summary of Food Assistance Program Results for April 1998,* Alexandria, VA, 1998.

27. Gerrior, S. and Bente, L., *Nutrient Content of the U.S. Food Supply, 1909-94.* Home Economics Research Report No. 53, U.S. Department of Agriculture, Center for Nutrition Policy and Promotion, Washington, D.C., 1997.

28. Food and Nutrition Board, Institute of Medicine, Standing Committee on the Scientific Evaluation of Dietary Reference Intakes, *Dietary Reference Intakes for Calcium, Phosphorus, Magnesium, Vitamin D, and Fluoride,* National Academy Press, Washington, D.C., 1997.

29. U.S. Department of Health and Human Services, Food and Drug Administration, Code of Federal Regulations, Title 21, Part 131, Subpart B, Milk and cream, Part 133, Subpart B, Cheeses and Related Cheese Products, U.S. Government Printing Office, Washington, D.C., April 1998.

30. American Academy of Pediatrics, Committee on Nutrition, *Pediatric Nutrition Handbook,* 4th ed., American Academy of Pediatrics, Elk Grove Village, IL, 1998.

31. Munoz, K. A., Krebs-Smith, S. M., Ballard-Barbash, R., and Cleveland, L. E., Food intakes of U.S. children and adolescents compared with recommendations, *Pediatrics* 100 (3), 323, 1997.

32. Munoz, K. A., Krebs-Smith, S. M., Ballard-Barbash, R., and Cleveland, L. E., Errors in food intake article, *Pediatrics,* 101(Suppl.), 952, 1998.

33. U.S. Department of Agriculture, Agricultural Research Service, *Pyramid Servings Data, Results from USDA's 1995 and 1996 Continuing Survey of Food Intakes by Individuals,* Riverdale, MD: U.S. Department of Agriculture, December 1997, www.barc.usda.gov/bhnrc/foodsurvey/home.htm.

34. Barr, S. I., Associations of social and demographic variables with calcium intakes of high school students, *J. Am. Diet. Assoc.*, 94, 260, 269, 1994.
35. Albertson, A. M., Tobelmann, R. C., and Marquart, L., Estimated dietary calcium intake and food sources for adolescent females: 1980-92, *J. Adol. Health*, 20, 20, 1997.
36. Guthrie, J. E., Dietary patterns and personal characteristics of women consuming recommended amounts of calcium, *Family Economics and Nutrition Reviews,* 9, 33, 1996.
37. Barger-Lux, M. J., Heaney, R. P., Packard, P. T., Lappe, J. M., and Recker, R. R., Nutritional correlates of low calcium intake, *Clinics in Applied Nutr.*, 2(4), 39, 1992.
38. Karanja, N., Morris, C. D., Rufolo, P., Snyder, G., Illingworth, D. R., and McCarron, D. A., Impact of increasing calcium in the diet on nutrient consumption, plasma lipids, and lipoproteins in humans, *Am. J. Clin. Nutr.,* 59, 900, 1994.
39. Chan, G. M., Hoffman, K., and McMurray, M., Effects of dairy products on bone and body composition in pubertal girls, *J. Pediatr.*, 126, 551, 1995.
40. Devine, A., Prince, R. L., and Bell, R., Nutritional effect of calcium supplementation by skim milk powder or calcium tablets on total nutrient intake in postmenopausal women, *Am. J. Clin. Nutr.*, 64, 731, 1996.
41. Cadogan, J., Eastell, R., Jones, N., and Barker, M. E., Milk intake and bone mineral acquisition in adolescent girls: randomized, controlled intervention trial, *Br. Med. J.*, 315, 1255, 1997.
42. Badenhop, N. E., Ilich, J. Z., Skugor, M., Landoll, J. D., and Matkovic, V., Changes in body composition and serum leptin in young females with high vs. low dairy intake, *J. Bone Miner. Res.*, 12, 487s, 1997 (Abstr. # S537).
43. U.S. Department of Agriculture, Agricultural Research Service, *USDA Nutrient Database for Standard Reference, Release 12,* Nutrient Data Laboratory, www.nal.usda.gov/fnic/foodcomp, 1998.
44. Hagemeister, H., Sick, H., and Barth, C. A., Nitrogen balance in the human and effects of milk constituents, In: Role of Milk Protein in Human Nutrition, *Bull. Int. Dairy Federation*, 253, 3, 1990.
45. European Dairy Association, *Nutritional Quality of Proteins*, European Dairy Association, Brussels, Belgium, 1997.
46. International Dairy Federation, *Milk Protein Definition & Standardization*, International Dairy Federation, Brussels, Belgium, 1994.
47. Kurmann, J. A., Rasic, J. L., and Kroger, M., *Encyclopedia of Fermented Fresh Milk Products, An International Inventory of Fermented Milk, Cream, Buttermilk, Whey, and Related Products*, Van Nostrand Reinhold, New York, 1992.
48. Dionysius, D. A. and Milne, J. M., Antibacterial peptides of bovine lactoferrin: purification and characterization, *J. Dairy Sci.*, 80, 667, 1997.
49. McIntosh, G. H., Regester, G. O., LeLeu, R. K., Royle, P. J., and Smithers, G. W., Dairy proteins protect against dimethylhydrazine-induced intestinal cancers in rats, *J. Nutr.*, 125, 809, 1995.
50. MacDonald, R. S., Thornton, W. H., Jr., and Marshall, R. T., A cell culture model to identify biologically active peptides generated by bacterial hydrolysis of casein, *J. Dairy Sci.*, 77, 1167, 1994.
51. Parodi, P. W., A role for milk proteins in cancer prevention, *Austr. J. Dairy Technol.*, 53, 37, 1998.
52. Takada, Y., Matsuyama, H., Kato, K., Kobayashi, N., Yamamura, J.-I., Yahiro, M., and Aoe, S., Milk whey protein enhances the bone breaking force in ovariectomized rats, *Nutr. Res.*, 17, 1709, 1997.

53. Bock, S. A., Prospective appraisal of complaints of adverse reactions to foods in children during the first 3 years of life, *Pediatrics*, 79, 683, 1987.
54. Wharton, B., and Hide, D., Eds., The role of hypoallergenic formulae in cow's milk allergy and allergy prevention, *Eur. J. Clin. Nutr.*, 49(1), S1, 1995.
55. Jakobsson, I. and Lindberg, T., A prospective study of cow's milk protein intolerance in Swedish infants, *Acta Paediatr. Scand.*, 68, 853, 1979.
56. Foucard, T., Development of food allergies with special reference to cow's milk allergy, *Pediatrics*, 75 (Suppl.), 177, 1985.
57. Karjalainen, J., Martin, J. M., Knip, M., Ilonen, J., Robinson, B. H., Savilahti, E., Akerblom, H. K., and Dosch, H.-M., A bovine albumin peptide as a possible trigger of insulin-dependent diabetes mellitus, *N. Engl. J. Med.*, 327, 302, 1992.
58. Ahmed, T., Shibasaki, M., Kamota, T., Hirano, T., Sumazaki, R., and Takita, H., Circulating antibodies to common food antigens in Japanese children with IDDM, *Diabetes Care,* 20(1), 74, 1997.
59. Cavallo, M. G., Fava, D., Monetini, L., Barone, F., and Pozzilli, P., Cell-mediated immune response to B casein in recent-onset insulin-dependent diabetes: implications for disease pathogenesis, *Lancet*, 348, 926, 1996.
60. Atkinson, M. A. and Ellis, T. M., Infant diets and insulin-dependent diabetes: evaluating the "cows' milk hypothesis" and a role for anti-bovine serum albumin immunity, *J. Am. Coll. Nutr.*, 16, 334, 1997.
61. Paxson, J. A., Weber, J. G., and Kulczycki, A., Jr., Cow's milk-free diet does not prevent diabetes in NOD mice, *J. Am. Diabetes Assoc.*, 46(11), 1711, 1997.
62. Bodington, M. J., McNally, P. G., and Burden, A. C., Cow's milk and Type I childhood diabetes: no increase in risk, *Diabetic Med.*, 11, 663, 1994.
63. Norris, J. M., Beaty, B., Klingensmith, G., Yu, L., Hoffman, M., Chase, H. P., Erlich, H. A., Hamman, R. F., Eisenbarth, G. S., and Rewers, M., Lack of association between early exposure to cow's milk protein and B-cell immunity: Diabetes Autoimmunity Study in the Young (DAISY), *JAMA*, 276, 609, 1996.
64. Fuchtenbusch, M., Karges, W., Standl, E., Dosch, H.-M., and Ziegler, A.-G., Antibodies to bovine serum albumin (BSA) in type 1 diabetes and other autoimmune disorders, *Exp. Clin. Endocrinol. Diabetes*, 105, 86, 1997.
65. Schatz, D. A. and Maclaren, N. K., Cow's milk and insulin-dependent diabetes mellitus. Innocent until proven guilty, *JAMA*, 276, 647, 1996.
66. Scott, F. W., AAP recommendations on cow milk, soy, and early infant feeding, *Pediatrics*, 95, 515, 1995.
67. Ellis, T. M. and Atkinson, M. A., Early infant diets and insulin-dependent diabetes, *Lancet*, 347, 1464, 1996.
68. Work Group on Cow's Milk Protein and Diabetes Mellitus, American Academy of Pediatrics, Infant feeding practices and their possible relationship to the etiology of diabetes mellitus, *Pediatrics*, 94, 752, 1994.
69. Filer, L. J. and Reynolds, W. A., Lessons in comparative physiology: lactose intolerance, *Nutr. Today,* 32, 79, 1997.
70. Suarez, F. L. and Savaiano, D. A., Diet, genetics, and lactose intolerance, *Food Technol.* 51, 74, 1997.
71. Ziegler, E. E. and Fomon, S. J., Lactose enhances mineral absorption in infancy, *J. Pediatr. Gastroenterol. Nutr.*, 2, 288, 1983.
72. Nickel, K. P., Martin, B. R., Smith, D. L., Smith, J. B., Miller, G. D., and Weaver, C. M., Calcium bioavailability from bovine milk and dairy products in premenopausal women using intrinisic and extrinsic labeling techniques, *J. Nutr.*, 126, 1406, 1996.

73. McBean, L. D. and Miller, G. D., Allaying fears and fallacies about lactose intolerance, *J. Am. Diet. Assoc.,* 98, 671, 1998.
74. German, J. B. and Dillard, C. J., Fractionated milk fat: composition, structure, and functional properties, *Food Technol.,* 52, 33, 1998.
75. Jensen, R. G. and Lammi-Keefe, C. J., Current status of research on the composition of bovine and human milk lipids, in *Lipids in Infant Nutrition,* Huang, Y.S., and Sinclair, A.J., Eds., AOCS Press, Champaign, IL, 168-191, 1998.
76. Katan, M. B., Zock, P. L., and Mensink, R. P., Dietary oils, serum lipoproteins, and coronary heart disease, *Am. J. Clin. Nutr.,* 61(Suppl.), 1368s, 1995.
77. American Heart Association, Dietary guidelines for healthy Americans: a statement for health professionals by the Nutrition Committee, American Heart Association, *Circulation,* 94, 1795, 1996.
78. Temme, E. H. M., Mensink, R. P., and Hornstra, G., Comparison of the effects of diets enriched in lauric, palmitic, or oleic acids on serum lipids and lipoproteins in healthy women and men, *Am. J. Clin. Nutr.,* 63(6), 897, 1996.
79. ASCN/AIN Task Force on Trans Fatty Acids, Position paper on trans fatty acids, *Am. J. Clin. Nutr.,* 63, 663, 1996.
80. Parodi, P. W., Distribution of isomeric octadecenoic fatty acids in milk fat, *J. Dairy Sci.,* 59, 1870, 1976.
81. Lichtenstein, A. H., Trans fatty acids, plasma lipid levels, and risk of developing cardiovascular disease. A statement for healthcare professionals from the American Heart Association, *Circulation,* 95, 2588, 1997.
82. Parodi, P. W., Cows' milk fat components as potential anticarcinogenic agents, *J. Nutr.,* 127, 1055, 1997.
83. Parodi, P. W., Milk fat conjugated linoleic acid: can it help prevent breast cancer? *Proc. Nutr. Soc. N. Zealand,* 22, 137, 1997.
84. Chin, S. F., Liu, W., Storkson, J. M., Ha, Y. L., and Pariza, M. W., Dietary sources of conjugated dienoic isomers of linoleic acid, a newly recognized class of anticarcinogens, *J. Food Comp. Anal.,* 5, 185, 1992.
85. Lin, H., Boylston, T. D., Chang, M. J., Luedecke, L. O., and Shultz, T. D., Survey of the conjugated linoleic acid contents of dairy products, *J. Dairy Sci.,* 78, 2358, 1995.
86. Kramer, J. K. G., Parodi, P. W., Jensen, R. G., Mossoba, M. M., Yurawecz, M. D., and Adolf, R. O., Rumenic acid: a proposed common name for the major conjugated linoleic acid (CLA) isomer found in natural products, *Lipids,* 33, In press, 1998.
87. Shantha, N. C., Ram, L. N., O'Leary, J., Hicks, C. L., and Decker, E. A., Conjugated linoleic acid concentrations in dairy products as affected by processing and storage, *J. Food Sci.,* 60(4), 695, 720, 1995.
88. Thompson, H., Zhu, Z., Banni, S., Darcy, K., Loftus, T., and Ip, C., Morphological and biochemical status of the mammary gland as influenced by conjugated linoleic acid: implication for a reduction in mammary cancer risk, *Cancer Res.,* 57(22), 5067, 1997.
89. Ip, C. and Scimeca, J. A., Conjugated linoleic acid and linoleic acid are distinctive modulators of mammary carcinogenesis, *Nutr. Cancer,* 27(2), 131, 1997.
90. Visonneau, S., Cesano, A., Tepper, S. A., Scimeca, J. A., Santoli, D., and Kritchevsky, D., Conjugated linoleic acid suppresses the growth of human breast adenocarcinoma cells in SCID mice, *Anticancer Res.,* 17(2A), 969, 1997.
91. Jarvinen, R., Knekt, P., Seppanen, R., and Teppo, L., Diet and breast cancer risk in a cohort of Finnish women, *Cancer Lett.,* 114, 251, 1997.

92. Li, Y. and Watkins, B. A., Conjugated linoleic acids alter bone fatty acid composition and reduce ex vivo prostaglandin E_2 biosynthesis in rats fed n-6 or n-3 fatty acids, *Lipids*, 33(4), 417, 1998.

93. Chew, B. P., Wong, T. S., Shultz, T. D., and Magnuson, N. S., Effects of conjugated dienoic derivatives of linoleic acid and B-carotene in modulating lymphocyte and macrophage function, *Anticancer Res.*, 17, 1099, 1997.

94. Wong, M. W., Chew, B. P., Wong, T. S., Hosick, H. L., Boylston, T. D., and Shultz, T. D., Effects of dietary conjugated linoleic acid on lymphocyte function and growth of mammary tumors in mice, *Anticancer Res.*, 17, 987, 1997.

95. Chin, S. F., Storkson, J. M., Albright, K. J., Cook, M. E., and Pariza, M. W., Conjugated linoleic acid is a growth factor for rats as shown by enhanced weight gain and improved feed efficiency, *J. Nutr.*, 124, 2344, 1994.

96. Park, Y., Albright, K. J., Liu, W., Storkson, J. M., Cook, M. E., and Pariza, M. W., Effect of conjugated linoleic acid on body composition in mice, *Lipids*, 32, 853, 1997.

97. Merrill, A. H., Jr., Schmelz, E.-M., Wang, E., Dillehay, D. L., Rice, L. G., Meredith, F., and Riley, R. T., Importance of sphingolipids and inhibitors of sphingolipid metabolism as components of animal diets, *J. Nutr.*, 127, 830s, 1997.

98. Smith, J. G. and German, J. B., Molecular and genetic effects of dietary derived butyric acid, *Food Technol.*, 49, 87, 1995.

99. Aukema, H. M., Davidson, L. A., Pence, B. C., Jiang, Y.-H., Lupton, J. R., and Chapkin, R. S., Butyrate alters activity of specific CAMP-receptor proteins in a transgenic mouse colonic cell line, *J. Nutr.*, 127, 18, 1997.

100. Cope, R. B., Bosnie, M., Boehm-Wilcox, C., Mohr, D., and Reeve, V. E., Dietary butter protects against ultraviolet radiation-induced suppression of contact hypersensitivity in Skh:HR-1 hairless mice, *J. Nutr.*, 126, 681, 1996.

101. Hubbard, N. E., Socolich, R. J., and Erickson, K. L., Dietary myristic acid alters acylated proteins in activated murine macrophages, *J. Nutr.*, 126, 1563, 1996.

102. French, S. J., Murray, B., Rumsey, R. D. E., Sepple, C. P., and Read, N. W., Preliminary studies on the gastrointestinal responses to fatty meals in obese people, *Int. J. Obes.*, 17, 295, 1993.

103. Burton-Freeman, B., Davis, P. A., and Schneeman, B. O., Dairy products as dietary fat sources: effects on postprandial glucose and insulin, *FASEB J.*, Feb. 28, A372, (Abstr. 2157), 1997.

104. Himaya, A., Fantino, M., Antoine, J.-M., Brondel, L., and Louis-Sylvestre, J., Satiety power of dietary fat: a new appraisal, *Am. J. Clin. Nutr.*, 65, 1410, 1997.

105. Seifert, M. F. and Watkins, B. A., Role of dietary lipid and antioxidants in bone metabolism, *Nutr. Res.*, 17(7), 1209, 1997.

106. Watkins, B. A., Shen, C.-L., McMurtry, J. P., Xu, H., Bain, S. D., Allen, K. G. D., and Seifert, M. F., Dietary lipids modulate bone prostaglandin E_2 production, insulin-like growth factor-1 concentration and formation rate in chicks, *J. Nutr.*, 127, 1084, 1997.

107. Xu, H., Watkins, B. A., and Seifert, M. F., Vitamin E stimulates trabecular bone formation and alters epiphyseal cartilage morphometry, *Calcif. Tissue Int.*, 57, 293, 1995.

108. Kaylegian, K. E., Functional characteristics and nontraditional applications of milk lipid components in food and nonfood systems, *J. Dairy Sci.*, 78, 2524, 1995.

109. Noakes, M., Nestel, P. J., and Clifton, P. M., Modifying the fatty acid profile of dairy products through feedlot technology lowers plasma cholesterol of humans consuming the products, *Am. J. Clin. Nutr.*, 63, 42, 1996.

110. Lin, M.-P., Staples, C. R., Sims, C. A., and O'Keefe, S. F., Modification of fatty acids in milk by feeding calcium-protected high oleic sunflower oil, *J. Food Sci.,* 61(1), 24, 1996.

111. O'Callaghan, D., Stanton, A., Rafferty, S., Canton, M., Murphy, J., Harrington, D., Connolly, B., and Horgan, J., Are butter and cheese rich in monounsaturates beneficial in hyperlipidaemic patients? *J. Cardiovasc. Risk,* 3, 441, 1996.

112. Stanton, C., Lawless, F., Kjellmer, G., Harrington, D., Devery, R., Connolly, J.F., and Murphy, J., Dietary influences on bovine milk cis-9, trans-11-conjugated linoleic acid content, *J. Dairy Sci.,* 62(5), 1083, 1997.

113. Food and Nutrition Board, Commission on Life Sciences, National Research Council, *Recommended Dietary Allowances,* 10th Ed., National Academy Press, Washington, D.C., 1989.

114. Said, H. M., Ong, D. E., and Shingleton, J. L., Intestinal uptake of retinol: enhancement by bovine milk B-lactoglobulin, *Am. J. Clin. Nutr.,* 49, 690, 1989.

115. Food and Drug Administration, U.S. Department of Health and Human Services, Lowfat and skim milk products, lowfat and nonfat yogurt products, lowfat cottage cheese: revocation of standards of identity; food labeling; nutrient content claims for fat, fatty acids, and cholesterol content of food, *Fed. Regist.,* 61(225), 58991 (Nov. 20), 1996.

116. Food and Drug Administration, U.S. Department of Health and Human Services, Food labeling; general provisions; nutrition labeling; label format; nutrient content claims; health claims; ingredient labeling; state and local requirements; and exemptions; final rules, 21 CFR Parts 101 & 102, *Fed. Regist.* 58, 2065 (Jan. 6), 1993.

117. Anderson, J. J. B., and Toverud, S. U., Diet and vitamin D: a review with an emphasis on human function, *J. Nutr. Biochem.,* 5, 58, 1994.

118. American Medical Association, Council on Foods and Nutrition, Importance of vitamin D milk, *JAMA,* 159, 1018, 1955.

119. American Academy of Pediatrics, Committee on Nutrition, The relation between infantile hypercalcemia and vitamin D - public health implications in North America, *Pediatrics,* 40, 1050, 1967.

120. American Medical Association, The nutritive quality of processed foods: general policies for nutrient additives, *Nutr. Rev.,* 40, 93, 1982.

121. U.S. Department of Health and Human Services, Public Health Service, Food and Drug Administration, *Grade "A" Pasteurized Milk Ordinance, 1995 Revision,* PHS/FDA Pub. No. 229, Washington, D.C. USDHHS, PHS, FDA, 1995.

122. Ziegler, E. E. and Filer, L. J., Jr., Eds., *Present Knowledge in Nutrition,* 7th ed., Washington, D.C., ILSI Press, 1996.

123. Food and Nutrition Board, Institute of Medicine, Standing Committee on the Scientific Evaluation of Dietary Reference Intakes, *Dietary Reference Intakes for Thiamin, Riboflavin, Niacin, Vitamin B_6, Folate, Vitamin B_{12}, Pantothenic Acid, Biotin, and Choline,* National Academy Press, Washington, D.C., 1998.

124. Parodi, P. W., Cows' milk folate binding protein: its role in folate nutrition, *Austr. J. Dairy Technol.,* 52, 109, 1997.

125. U.S. Department of Agriculture, Agricultural Research Service, Data tables: results from USDA's 1994-96 Continuing Survey of Food Intakes by Individuals and 1994-96 Diet and Health Knowledge Survey. ARS Food Surveys Research Group, www.barc.usda.gov/bhnrc/foodsurvey/home.htm.

126. Curhan, G. C., Willett, W. C., Rumm, E. B., and Stampfer, M. J., A prospective study of dietary calcium and other nutrients and the risk of symptomatic kidney stones, *N. Engl. J. Med.,* 328, 833, 1993.

127. Curhan, G. C., Willett, W. C., Speizer, F. E., Spiegelman, D., and Stampfer, M. J., Comparison of dietary calcium with supplemental calcium and other nutrients as factors affecting the risk for kidney stones in women, *Ann. Intern. Med.,* 126, 497, 1997.

128. Massey, L. K. and Kynast-Gales, S. A., Substituting milk for apple juice does not increase kidney stone risk in most normocalciuric adults who form calcium oxalate stones, *J. Am. Diet. Assoc.,* 98, 303, 1998.

129. Curhan, G. C., Willett, W. C., Speizer, F. E., and Stampfer, M. J., Beverage use and risk for kidney stones in women, *Ann. Intern. Med.,* 128, 534, 1998.

130. American Academy of Pediatrics, Committee on Nutrition, The use of whole cow's milk in infancy, *Pediatrics,* 89, 1105, 1992.

131. Bruhn, J. C. and Franke, A. A., Iodine in cow's milk produced in the USA in 1980-1981, *J. Food Protection,* 48, 397, 1985.

132. Food and Drug Administration, *Food and Drug Administration Pesticide Program Residue Monitoring, 1996,* Food and Drug Administration, Washington, D.C., 1996.

133. Ropp, K. L., New animal drug increases milk production, *FDA Consumer,* 28(4), 24, 1994.

134. Dairy Management Inc., Extending shelf life in dairy foods, *Innovations in Dairy,* April 1998.

135. Putnam, J. J. and Allshouse, J. E., *Food Consumption, Prices, and Expenditures, 1970-95,* Food and Consumer Economics Division, Economic Research Service, U.S. Department of Agriculture, Statistical Bulletin No. 939, Washington, D.C., August 1997.

136. Putnam, J. and Gerrior, S., Americans consuming more grains and vegetables, less saturated fat, *Food Rev.,* 20(3), 2, 1997.

137. U.S. Department of Agriculture, Agricultural Research Center, *What We Eat In America 1994-96,* results from the 1994-95 Continuing Survey of Food Intakes by Individuals, Human Nutrition Research Center, Food Surveys Research Group, Beltsville, MD, April 1997.

138. Food and Drug Administration, Food labeling: nutrient content claims, definition of terms, healthy, Final rule, *Fed. Regist.,* 59, 24232 (May 10), 1994.

139. Food and Drug Administration, Lowfat and skim milk products, lowfat and nonfat yogurt products, lowfat cottage cheese: revocation of standards of identity; food labeling, nutrient content claims for fat, fatty acids, and cholesterol content of food, final rule, *Fed. Regist.,* 61, 58991 (Nov. 20), 1996.

140. Kurtzweil, P., Skimming the milk label, *FDA Consumer,* 32(1), 22, 1998.

141. National Dairy Council, Breakfast behavior among children age 8 to 13, Executive summary, April, 1995, Prepared by McDonald Research, Inc., Skokie, IL, 1995.

142. Wilson, J. E., Preschool children maintain intake of other foods at a meal including sugared chocolate milk, *Appetite,* 16, 61, 1991.

143. Bock, M. A., Cummings, M. N., Petersen, G., and Ortiz, M., Impact of having chocolate milk as a beverage alternative on milk waste in selected school lunch programs, *J. Am. Diet. Assoc.,* 89, A-25, 1989.

144. Garey, J. G., Chan, M. M., and Parlia, S. R., Effect of fat content and chocolate flavoring of milk on meal consumption and acceptability by schoolchildren, *J. Am. Diet. Assoc.,* 90, 719, 1990.

145. Kimbrough, J. R., Shanklin, C. W., and Gench, B. E., Beverage choices offered by school food service programs, *School Food Service Res. Rev.,* 24, 1990.

146. Grove, T. M., Heimbach, J. T., Douglass, J. S., Doyle, E., DiRienzo, D. B., and Miller, G. D., Nutritional contributions of flavored milks and alternative beverages in the diets of children, *FASEB J.,* 12(4), A 225, 1998.

147. Glinsmann, W. H., Irausquin, H., and Park, Y. K., Evaluation of health aspects of sugars contained in carbohydrate sweeteners, *J. Nutr.,* 116(Suppl.), 1, 1986.

148. White, J. W. and Wolraich, M., Effect of sugar on behavior and mental performance, *Am. J. Clin. Nutr.,* 62(Suppl.), 242, 1995.

149. Recker, R. R., Bammi, A., Barger-Lux, M. J., and Heaney, R. P., Calcium absorbability from milk products, an imitation milk, and calcium carbonate, *Am. J. Clin. Nutr.,* 47(1), 93, 1988.

150. Huang, Y.-C., Luedecke, L. O., and Shultz, T. D., Effect of cheddar cheese consumption on plasma conjugated linoleic acid concentrations in men, *Nutr. Res.,* 14(3), 373, 1994.

151. Sandler, R. S., Jordan, M. C., and Shelton, B. J., Demographic and dietary determinants of constipation in the U.S. population, *Am. J. Publ. Health,* 80, 185, 1990.

152. Mykkanen, H. M., Karhunen, L. J., Korpela, R., and Salminen, S., Effect of cheese on intestinal transit time and other indicators of bowel function in residents of a retirement home, *Scand. J. Gastroenterol.,* 29(1), 29, 1994.

153. National Institute of Diabetes and Digestive and Kidney Diseases, National Institutes of Health, *Constipation,* NIH Publ. No. 95-2754, National Digestive Diseases Information Clearinghouse, Bethesda, MD, July 1995.

154. Gorski, D., Cultured product trends, *Dairy Foods,* 98 (4), 33, 1997.

155. Hitchins, A. D. and McDonough, F. E., Prophylactic and therapeutic aspects of fermented milk, *Am. J. Clin. Nutr.,* 49, 675, 1989.

156. Kolars, J. C., Levitt, M. D., Aouji, M., and Savaiano, D. A., Yogurt – an autodigesting source of lactose, *N. Engl. J. Med.,* 310, 1, 1984.

157. Hilton, E., Isenberg, H. D., Alperstein, P., France, K., and Borenstein, M. T., Ingestion of yogurt containing *Lactobacillus acidophilus* as prophylaxis for Candidal Vaginitis, *Ann. Intern. Med.,* 116, 353, 1992.

158. Salminen, S., Functional dairy foods with *Lactobacillus* strain *GG, Nutr. Rev.,* 54(Suppl.), 99, 1996.

159. Benno, Y., He, F., Hosoda, M., Hashimoto, H., Kojima, T., Yamazaki, K., Lino, H., Mykkanen, H., and Salminen, S., Effects of *Lactobacillus GG* yogurt on human intestinal microecology in Japanese subjects, *Nutr. Today,* 31(Suppl.), 9, 1996.

160. Majamaa, H. and Isolauri, E., Probiotics: a novel approach in the management of food allergy, *J. Allergy Clin. Immunol.,* 99, 179, 1997.

161. Pelto, L., Salminen, S.J., and Isolauri, E., *Lactobacillus GG* modulates milk-induced immune inflammatory response in milk-hypersensitive adults, *Nutr. Today,* 31(Suppl.), 45s, 1996.

162. Boudraa, G., Touhami, M., Pochart, P., Soltana, R., Mary, J.-Y., and Desjeux, J.-F., Effect of feeding yogurt versus milk in children with persistent diarrhea, *J. Pediatr. Gastroenterol. Nutr.,* 11(4), 509, 1990.

163. Kotz, C. M., Peterson, L. R., Moody, J. A., Savaiano, D. A., and Levitt, M. D., *In vitro* antibacterial effect of yogurt on *Escherichia coli, Dig. Dis. & Sci.,* 35, 630, 1990.

164. Pedrosa, M. C., Golner, B. B., Goldin, B. R., Barakat, S., Dallal, G. E., and Russell, R. M., Survival of yogurt-containing organisms and *Lactobacillus gasseri (*ADH) and their effect on bacterial enzyme activity in the gastrointestinal tract of healthy and hypochlorhydric elderly subjects, *Am. J. Clin. Nutr.,* 61, 353, 1995.

165. Zommara, M., Tachibana, N., Sakono, M., Suzuki, Y., Oda, T., Hashiba, H., and Imaizumi, K., Whey from cultured skim milk decreases serum cholesterol and increases antioxidant enzymes in liver and red blood cells in rats, *Nutr. Res.*, 16(2), 293, 1996.

166. Beena, A. and Prasad, V., Effect of yogurt and bifidus yogurt fortified with skim milk powder, condensed whey and lactose-hydrolysed condensed whey on serum cholesterol and triacylglycerol levels in rats, *J. Dairy Sci.*, 64, 453, 1997.

167. Akalin, A. S., Gonc, S. and Duzel, S., Influence of yogurt and acidophilus yogurt on serum cholesterol levels in mice, *J. Dairy Sci.*, 80, 2721, 1997.

168. Van't Veer, P., Dekker, J. M., Lamars, J. W. J., Kok, F. J., and Schouten, E. G., Consumption of fermented milk products and breast cancer: a case-control study in the Netherlands, *Cancer Res.*, 49, 4020, 1989.

169. Biffi, A., Coradini, D., Larsen, R., Riva, L., and DiFronzo, G., Antiproliferative effect of fermented milk on the growth of a human breast cancer cell line, *Cancer*, 28(1), 93, 1997.

170. Ling, W. H., Korpela, R., Mykkanen, M., Salminen, S., and Hanninen, O., *Lactobacillus* strain *GG* supplementation decreases colonic hydrolytic and reductive enzyme activities in healthy female adults, *J. Nutr.*, 124, 18, 1994.

171. Perdigon, G., Valdez, J. C., and Rachid, M., Antitumor activity of yogurt: study of possible immune mechanisms, *J. Dairy Res.*, 65, 129, 1998.

172. Puri, P., Rattan, A., Bijlani, R. L., Mahapatra, S. C., and Nath, I., Splenic and intestinal lymphocyte proliferation response in mice fed milk or yogurt and challenged with *Salmonella typhimurium*, *Int. J. Food Sci. Nutr.*, 47, 391, 1996.

173. Halpern, G. M., Vruwink, K. G., Van de Water, J., Keen, C. L., and Gershwin, M. E., Influence of long-term yoghurt consumption in young adults, *Int. J. Immunotherapy*, 7(4), 205, 1991.

174. Hughes, D. B. and Hoover, D. G., Bifidobacteria: their potential for use in American dairy products, *Food Technol.*, 45, 74, 1991.

175. Hoover, D. G., Bifidobacteria: activity and potential benefits, *Food Technol.*, 47, 120, 1993.

176. Ishibashi, N. and Shimamura, S., Bifidobacteria: research and development in Japan, *Food Technol.*, 47, 126, 1993.

177. Saavedra, J. M., Bauman, N. A., Oung, I., Perman, J. A., and Yolken R. H., Feeding of *Bifidobacterium bifidum* and *Streptococcus thermophilus* to infants in hospitals for prevention of diarrhea and shedding of rotavirus, *Lancet*, 344, 1046, 1994.

178. Burrington, K. J., More than just milk, *Food Product Design*, 7, 91, 1998.

CHAPTER 2

Dairy Foods and Cardiovascular Health

I. INTRODUCTION

Coronary heart disease (CHD), the most common and serious form of cardio-vascular disease, is the leading cause of death in developed industrialized countries. Despite the dramatic decline in age-adjusted CHD mortality in the U.S. since 1950, CHD still accounts for more deaths than any other disease or groups of diseases.[1,2] In 1994, over 487,000 people died from heart-related diseases.[1] CHD cost the U.S. an estimated $95.6 billion in 1998 for medical treatment and lost productivity.[3] Considering the high incidence of CHD mortality and morbidity, as well as its economic toll, prevention or early management of risk factors for CHD is a major public health goal.[2,4,5]

Many risk factors, both genetic and environmental, contribute to the development of CHD.[1,6,7] The three most important modifiable risk factors for CHD are cigarette smoking, high blood pressure, and elevated blood cholesterol levels, particularly high low density lipoprotein cholesterol.[7] Other risk factors *likely* to contribute to CHD risk include diabetes mellitus, physical inactivity, low blood levels of high density lipoprotein cholesterol, elevated blood triglyceride levels, and obesity.[7] Factors that *may* increase CHD risk include psychosocial factors, lipoprotein(a), homocysteine, and oxidative stress. Advancing age, male gender, and a family history of early-onset CHD are CHD risk factors which cannot be modified.[7]

Not only is the multifactorial nature of CHD recognized by numerous federal government agencies and health professionals,[5-15] but a high blood cholesterol level has been regarded as one of the major modifiable risk factors. The National Cho-lesterol Education Program (NCEP)'s Adult Treatment Panel II [5] classifies desirable total blood cholesterol levels as levels below 200 mg/dl, borderline-high for values between 200 and 239 mg/dl, and high for total cholesterol levels 240 mg/dl and above.

The positive association between elevated blood cholesterol and CHD risk is supported by extensive epidemiological, laboratory, and clinical findings.[12,15] In recent years, blood lipid-protein agglomerates, collectively called lipoproteins, have been associated with CHD risk.[12,13] The four classes of lipoproteins, based on density as well as lipid and apolipoprotein (apo) composition, include chylomicrons, very low density lipoproteins (VLDL), low density lipoproteins (LDL), and high density lipoproteins (HDL). In addition, there are various subclasses of lipoproteins such as intermediate density lipoproteins (IDL), LDL subclass pattern B, and HDL_2 and HDL_3.

An elevated level of blood LDL cholesterol, the major cholesterol-carrying lipoprotein, is associated with increased risk of CHD.[12,13,16-18] In contrast, a low level of HDL cholesterol constitutes a major CHD risk factor. Lipoprotein subclasses are also predictive of CHD. [19] High blood concentrations of small, dense LDL (LDL subclass pattern B)[20] and Lp(a) lipoprotein are associated with increased risk of CHD.[7] Also, small HDL particles and large very low density lipoprotein (VLDL) particles may play a role in the development of CHD.[19] Routine lipid testing may therefore fail to accurately predict CHD risk. Whether or not a high blood triglyceride level is an independent risk factor for CHD is controversial.[17] Increased triglyceride levels in isolation are associated with elevated CHD risk, but in the presence of other risk factors triglyceride levels lose their predictive power.

Some studies indicate that lowering total and LDL cholesterol and increasing HDL cholesterol levels reduces risk of CHD, at least for individuals with high blood cholesterol levels.[15,21] Substantial evidence indicates a role for diet in influencing blood cholesterol and lipoprotein levels, although genetics also plays a major role.[6,12,14,22-26] Of all the dietary factors studied, fat intake has received the most attention. Extensive research accumulated over the past four decades has established that different types and amounts of dietary fats influence blood cholesterol levels. A high intake of total and saturated fat and, to a lesser extent, cholesterol are associated with elevated blood total and LDL cholesterol levels.[5,6,9-12,27-29] In contrast, diets high in carbohydrate have been associated with reduced levels of plasma total, LDL, and HDL cholesterol levels.[6,29]

Dietary recommendations for fat and cholesterol have been made to help Americans reduce their risk of CHD. These population-based guidelines issued by federal government agencies and nationally recognized health organizations recommend that all Americans two years of age and older consume a diet that provides no more than 30% of energy from fat, no more than 10% of energy from saturated fat, up to 10% of energy from polyunsaturated fat, and 300 mg or less of cholesterol a day.[5,6,8,10,11,30] These recommendations are for average intakes over several days. To help ensure that children readily meet their nutrient needs for growth and development, more flexible guidelines are recommended.[6,30-32] The American Heart Association,[6] the Dietary Guidelines for Americans,[30] and the American Academy of Pediatrics[31] all recommend that between the ages of two and five years, children should gradually adopt a diet that meets the above guidelines. Diets containing less than 30% of calories from fat are not recommended for children because of the difficulty in meeting sufficient calories and other nutrients for optimal growth and development.[31] A Working Group convened by Health Canada and the Canadian Paediatric Society recommends a gradual decrease in fat intake from the high fat diet of infancy to a diet that provides no more than 30% of energy from fat by the time linear growth (i.e., adolescence) is reached.[32]

Although daily intakes (percent of energy) of total fat, saturated fat, and choles-terol have decreased over the past decade, Americans' intakes generally exceed recommendations for these nutrients. As shown in Figure 2.1,[33] 30% of men and 39% of women meet the recommendations for total fat and 34% of men and 45% of women have saturated fat intakes at or below recommendations.[33] In contrast to total and saturated fat, more men (55%) and especially women (81%) are likely to meet the recommendation for cholesterol.[33] To help Americans meet dietary fat recommendations, the Department of Health and Human Services, Food and Drug Administration[34] has authorized the use of health claims relating to an association between dietary lipids, specifically fat and cholesterol, and CHD on the labels of certain foods. Such foods may bear the following health claim, "While many factors affect heart disease, diets low in saturated fat and cholesterol may reduce the risk of this disease."[34]

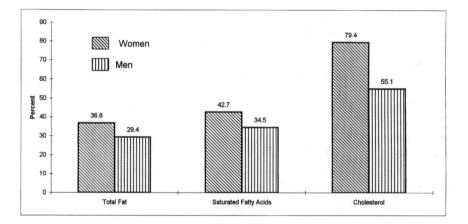

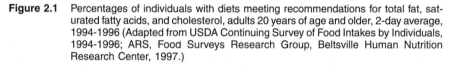

Figure 2.1   Percentages of individuals with diets meeting recommendations for total fat, sat-urated fatty acids, and cholesterol, adults 20 years of age and older, 2-day average, 1994-1996 (Adapted from USDA Continuing Survey of Food Intakes by Individuals, 1994-1996; ARS, Food Surveys Research Group, Beltsville Human Nutrition Research Center, 1997.)

To meet current dietary guidelines for fat and cholesterol, increased consumption of foods low in these nutrients is advised. With respect to dairy products, lower fat dairy foods often are recommended.[5,10,11,30] While the fat and cholesterol content of many dairy foods might be expected to increase blood cholesterol levels,[35-37] there is no direct evidence that consumption of whole fat dairy foods in moderation within the context of a total diet increases the risk of CHD.

II. CONTRIBUTION OF MILK AND MILK PRODUCTS TO FAT AND CHOLESTEROL INTAKE

The contribution of dairy foods to dietary intakes of fat and cholesterol can be found in Table 2.1.[38,39] According to the most recent USDA food disappearance data

Table 2.1   Dairy Product Contributions to Dietary Fat and Cholesterol in the United States

	Average Per Capita Contribution of Dairy Products to		
	Total Fat %	Saturated Fatty Acids %	Cholesterol %
USDA disappearance data, 1994			
Dairy products, excluding butter	12.3	23.6	16.1
Butter	3.0	5.8	3.2
Total	15.3	29.4	19.3
Food consumption data 1989–1991 CSFII	15.9	25.6	17.3

Adapted from Gerrior, S. and Bente, L., Nutrient Content of the U.S. Food Supply, 1909–94, U.S. Department of Agriculture, Center for Nutrition Policy and Promotion, Home Economics Research Report No. 53, 1997 and U.S. Department of Agriculture, ARS, Supplementary Table Set: Food and Nutrient Intakes by Individuals in the United States, 3 Days, 1989–91, Continuing Survey of Food Intakes by Individuals, 1989–91 (In photocopy form only), 1995.

and food intake data, dairy foods make a relatively small contribution to total fat and cholesterol intake. Dairy foods provide about one quarter of the saturated fat intake (Table 2.1, Figure 2.2).[38-40]

In 1994, dairy foods, excluding butter, contributed 12% of total dietary fat, 24% of saturated fat, and 16% of the cholesterol available in the U.S. food supply.[38] To put these data into perspective, the contribution of dairy foods to fat availability is far less than that provided by fats and oils (52%) or meat, poultry, and fish (25%).[38] Similarly, meat, poultry and fish contribute more to the saturated fat and cholesterol available in the U.S. food supply than do dairy foods (Figures 2.3 and 2.4).[38] Butter

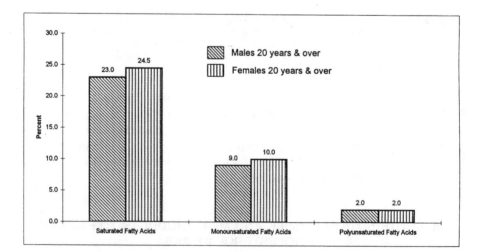

Figure 2.2   Contribution of dairy products to dietary fatty acid intake, 1994-96. (Adapted from U.S. Department of Agriculture, ARS, Data tables: Intakes of individual fatty acids: results from 1994-96 Continuing Survey of Food Intakes by Individuals, 1997.)

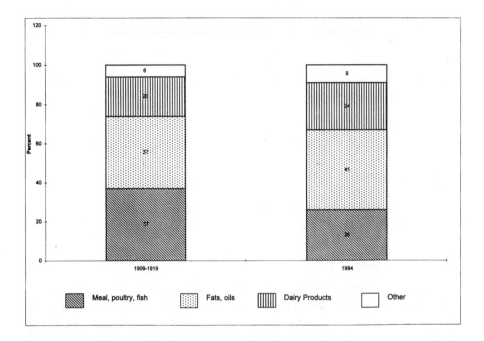

Figure 2.3 Sources of saturated fatty acids in the U.S. food supply. (Adapted from Gerrior, S. and Bente, L., Nutrient content of the U.S. food supply, 1909-1994. U.S. Department of Agriculture, Center for Nutrition Policy and Promotion, *Home Economics Research Report*, No. 53, 1997.)

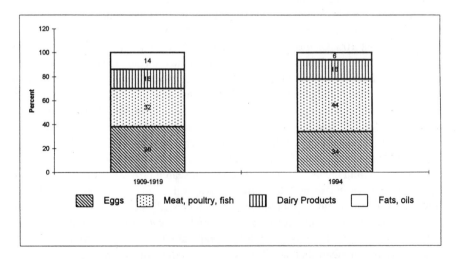

Figure 2.4 Sources of cholesterol in the U.S. food supply. (Adapted from Gerrior, S. and Bente, L., Nutrient content of the U.S. food supply, 1909-1994. U.S. Department of Agriculture, Center for Nutrition Policy and Promotion, Home Economics Research Report No. 53, 1997.)

contributed an estimated 3% of total fat, 6% of saturated fat, and 3% of the cholesterol available in the food supply in 1994.[38] In terms of actual intake, data from the 1989–91 Continuing Survey of Food Intakes by Individuals (CSFII) indicate that butter contributed 2.3% of total fat intake and 4.1% of saturated fat intake for adults.[41] For children 2 to 18 years of age, butter contributed 1.2% of total fat intake and 2% of saturated fat intake.[42]

III. DAIRY NUTRIENTS, DAIRY FOODS, AND CHD

A. Single Nutrients

Specific nutrients in dairy foods such as fat, protein, and vitamin D have been examined for their roles in influencing blood lipid and lipoprotein levels and CHD risk.

1. Dietary Fatty Acids

The quality (type) and quantity of dietary fatty acids affect blood total and lipoprotein cholesterol levels and CHD risk.[12,13,22-25] Both the degree of unsaturation and the chain length of a specific type of fatty acid influence blood total cholesterol and specific lipoprotein fractions. Fatty acids also may be classified as saturated fatty acids (SFA) (no double bonds), monounsaturated fatty acids (MUFA) (one double bond), or polyunsaturated fatty acids (PUFA) (2 or more double bonds). PUFAs are further subdivided according to the position of the first double bond as omega-6 PUFAs or omega-3 PUFAs.[12,13] When classified by length, fatty acids are short chain (<6 C), medium chain (6–10 C), or long-chain (12 or more C).

Milk fat has a unique fatty acid profile with approximately 62% SFAs, nearly 30% MUFAs, and 4% PUFAs, with the remaining 4% other types of lipids (Table 2.2).[12,43-45] With respect to chain length, short and medium chain SFAs generally constitute about 10% of the weight of total fatty acids, whereas long chain SFAs make up nearly 50% of the total weight of fatty acids.[44] Trans fatty acids, produced as a result of hydrogenation during digestion in the rumen, vary with concentrations estimated at 2.5 to 6.4% of milk fat.[44] Milk fat contains 360 mg cholesterol per 100 g fat. One 8 ounce serving of whole (3.5% fat) milk contains 34 mg cholesterol, whereas lowfat (1% lowfat or 2% reduced fat) milk and skim (nonfat or fat free) milk contain 18 and 14 mg cholesterol per 8 ounce serving, respectively.[45]

A considerable amount of research has focused on the influence of specific fatty acids on blood lipid levels.[13] Findings from this research provide information regarding the direction and differential effects of specific fatty acids on blood lipids. However, it is important to appreciate that dietary studies examining a single class of fatty acids often use liquid formula diets with high levels of either SFAs, MUFAs, or PUFAs. Consequently, it is difficult to extrapolate the findings from these studies to the typical American diet which contains a mixture of different types of fat in more moderate amounts from a variety of foods. Also, the unique physical forms of fats in foods, such as the milk fat globule, may impact the effects of fats on blood lipids.

Table 2.2 Fatty Acid Composition of Milk Fat

		Fatty Acids %	
		Fat	Milk Fat
Total SFA	C8:0	61.9	1.1
	C10:0		2.5
	C12:0		2.8
	C14:0		10.0
	C16:0		26.2
	C18:0		12.1
Total MUFA	C16:1	28.7	2.2
	C18:1		25.0
	C20:1		—
Total PUFA	C18:2	3.7	2.3
	C18:3		1.5
	Ratio[a]		
	P		0.06
	M		0.46
	S		1.0

[a] Ratios of polyunsaturated (P), monounsaturated (M) and saturated (S) fatty acids.

Adapted from McNamara, D.J., *J. Adv. Food Nutr. Res.*, 36, 253, 1992. With permission.

a. Saturated Fatty Acids (SFAs)

SFA intake is one of the strongest predictors of blood total, LDL, and HDL cholesterol levels.[6,12,13,22-25] Mathematical models predict that a 1% increase in energy as SFAs will raise blood cholesterol by 2 mg/dl.[23] This increase in total cholesterol induced by SFAs is attributed mainly to an increase in LDL cholesterol, although there also is an increase in HDL cholesterol.[12,13,23] It has long been appreciated that individual SFAs have different effects on blood cholesterol levels (Figure 2.5).[6,13,14,23,27,28,46] Specifically, palmitic (C16:0), myristic (C14:0), and lauric (C12:0) acids raise blood total and LDL cholesterol levels and have inconsistent effects on HDL levels, whereas stearic (C18:0) and medium chain SFAs have little or no effect on blood total, LDL, and HDL cholesterol levels.[6,13,14,23-28,46-48]

Although palmitic acid is the major SFA in the diet, findings regarding its hypercholesterolemic effect relative to lauric acid are inconsistent.[13,47-49] A recent review concludes that palmitic acid is hypercholesterolemic compared with lauric, stearic, and oleic fatty acids.[13] Well-controlled studies indicate that myristic acid is the most hypercholesterolemic saturated fatty acid,[13] although further studies are necessary to substantiate this conclusion. Given the relatively low intake of myristic acid, especially in comparison with palmitic acid, in the American diet, its potential contribution to high blood cholesterol is believed to be small.[12]

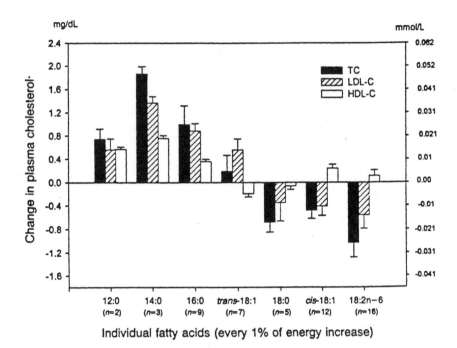

Figure 2.5   Effects of lauric (12:0), myristic (14:0), palmitic (16:0), elaidic (trans-18:1), stearic (18:0), oleic (cis-18:1), and linoleic (18:2n-6) acids compared with 18:1, TC, plasma total cholesterol. (From Kris-Etherton, P.M. and Yu, S., *Am. J. Clin. Nutr.*, 65[Suppl.], 1628, 1997. With permission.)

Stearic acid, compared with other long chain SFAs such as palmitic, myristic, and lauric acids, lowers blood total and LDL cholesterol levels when substituted for these SFAs.[13,47,50-53] In a metabolic ward study in which patients were fed formula liquid diets (40% of energy as fat) rich in either palmitic acid, stearic acid, or oleic acid (a MUFA), stearic and oleic acids had similar effects on blood cholesterol levels.[52] In an inpatient metabolic study in which 10 men, mean age 66, were fed liquid isocaloric diets differing in the type and amount of SFAs, lower concentrations of LDL cholesterol were observed when fats containing a high stearic acid content (e.g., beef tallow and cocoa butter) were fed.[53] In a strictly controlled metabolic study in Denmark involving healthy young men, a diet high in stearic acid (15% of total energy intake) favorably affected blood lipids compared with a diet high in palmitic acid or myristic and lauric acids (Figure 2.6).[47]

Short and medium chain SFAs are absorbed directly in the portal vein and not transported through the bloodstream to the liver by chylomicrons; consequently, these SFAs would be expected to have different effects on blood lipids than long chain fatty acids.[12] Despite limited data, the effects of medium-chain fatty acids on blood lipids are considered to be minimal.[12,13]

Although milk fat is an important source of SFAs, its content of stearic acid and short and medium chain fatty acids may minimize the expected increase in blood cholesterol compared to other "saturated" fats. In fact, preliminary findings of a study

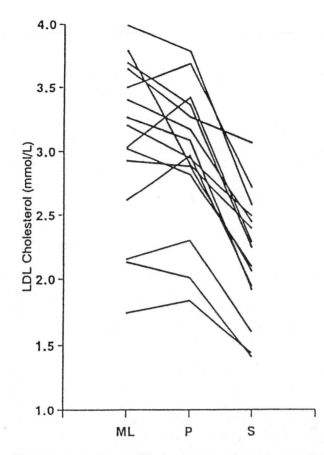

Figure 2.6   Plasma concentrations of LDL cholesterol in 15 subjects during three diets. ML is a diet high in myristic and lauric acids, P is a diet high in palmitic acid, and S is a diet high in stearic acid. Each point represents the mean of three determinations at the end of the 3-week diet intervention. To convert values for LDL cholesterol to milligrams per deciliter, multiply by 88.54. (From Tholstrup, T., et al., *Am. J. Clin. Nutr.*, 59, 371, 1994. With permission.)

involving healthy young men fed a 30% total fat, 9% SFA diet indicate that SFAs from dairy foods raise blood cholesterol less than from meat and coconut oil.[54] This finding is consistent with that of both Hegsted et al.[27] and Keys et al.[55] who, in the 1960s, reported that stearic acid did not fit into their respected predictive formulas.

b. Monounsaturated Fatty Acids (MUFAs)

MUFAs, particularly oleic acid (C18:1), are found in fats of both plant (olive oil) and animal (25 to 30% of the fatty acids in milk fat) origin. Olive oil, rapeseed oil (canola oil), cocoa butter, and beef are the major sources of MUFAs in the diet.[12]

MUFAs appear to have a neutral effect on blood cholesterol levels or to be mildly hypocholesterolemic.[6,13,28,29] As reviewed by Kris-Etherton and Yu,[13] oleic acid reduces total and LDL cholesterol levels when substituted for lauric, myristic, or palmitic saturated fatty acids. The effect of oleic acid on HDL cholesterol is less clear.[13] A recently reported meta-analysis of metabolic ward studies indicates that isocaloric replacement of carbohydrate with MUFAs increases HDL cholesterol levels.[25] Accumulating evidence indicates that when MUFAs are substituted for SFAs, their net effect on blood lipids and lipoproteins is similar to that of PUFAs without some of the disadvantages of a diet rich in PUFAs.[6] In addition to potentially maintaining or increasing HDL cholesterol levels, a MUFA-rich diet may be preferable to a PUFA-rich diet because it may slow the progression of atherosclerosis by generating LDL particles resistant to oxidation.[6] Also, MUFAs may not lower apo A-1, which is associated with HDL, as much as a PUFA rich diet.[56]

c. Polyunsaturated Fatty Acids (PUFAs)

There are two major classes of PUFAs: n-3 fatty acids found in fish oils and as minor constituents of some vegetable oils; and n-6 fatty acids including the essential fatty acid linoleic acid found in vegetable oils such as corn, cottonseed, and soybean oils. A number of studies indicate that substitution of n-6 PUFAs for SFAs in the diet lowers blood total and LDL cholesterol levels.[13,22-25,27] In contrast to studies indicating that MUFAs and PUFAs are equally effective in lowering blood cholesterol levels, Kris-Etherton et al.[57] observed that when whole food diets were used instead of formula diets, linoleic acid was more potent than oleic acid in lowering blood cholesterol levels and did not lower HDL cholesterol levels. In a recent review of the effects of individual fatty acids on plasma lipids in humans, Kris-Etherton and Yu[13] concluded that of all the fatty acids, PUFAs have the most potent hypocholesterolemic effect. Every 1% increase in PUFAs is predicted to lower total blood cholesterol levels by 0.9 mg/dL and LDL cholesterol levels by 0.5 mg/dL.[24] However, diets very high in linoleic acid reduce HDL as well as LDL cholesterol levels.

The American diet contains 5 to 7% of energy as PUFAs, an intake below the upper level of 10% of total energy recommended by federal government and other health professional organizations.[4,9-11] No data are available regarding the long-term effects of diets high in PUFAs.[14,23] However, high intakes of PUFAs have been implicated in the development of some cancers in laboratory animals and may increase the formation of gallstones in humans.[6,14]

Studies indicate that intake of n-3 fatty acids at levels achieved only by the use of supplements can reduce blood triglyceride levels (by 25 to 30%), decrease platelet aggregation and thrombogenicity, and elevate LDL cholesterol (by 5 to 10%) and HDL cholesterol (by 1 to 3%) levels, with relatively little effect on total cholesterol levels.[12,58,59] However, because the n-3 PUFA content of the U.S. diet is generally low, there is relatively little effect of these PUFAs on blood lipids. The American Heart Association[6] recommends that omega-3 fatty acids be obtained from intake of fish rather than from omega-3 fatty acid supplements.

d. Trans Fatty Acids

Trans fatty acids, generally isomers of cis MUFAs, are formed when liquid vegetable oils are partially hydrogenated to form margarine and shortening. Trans fatty acids occur naturally to some extent in dairy and meat products as a result of biohydrogenation of pasture and feed linoleic and linolenic acids by rumen micro-organisms in animals.[60,61] Cow's milk products contain an estimated 3 g of trans fatty acids per 100 g milk fat, whereas margarines can contain 10 times this amount.[62] It should be recognized that the biological effects of trans isomers found in milk fat may differ from artificially hydrogenated oils.[61] The predominant trans fatty acid in milk fat, trans-11-18.1, is converted to conjugated linoleic acid (CLA) which has several potential health benefits (see Chapter 1).[61]

Average availability of trans fatty acids in the typical American diet has been estimated to range from 2.6 g per day to 12.8 g per day.[60] Although intake of trans fatty acids is generally low, it has substantially increased over the past century.[63] Numerous investigations indicate that trans fatty acids have adverse effects on blood lipid and lipoprotein levels and/or are associated with increased risk of CHD when compared with their nonhydrogenated counterparts (i.e., cis-monounsaturated and cis-polyunsaturated fatty acids).[13,64-72]

In 1995, an expert panel assembled by the International Life Sciences Institute concluded, after an extensive review of the literature, that trans fatty acids raise blood cholesterol levels when substituted for PUFAs or cis-MUFAs.[67] In 1996, a joint task force of the American Society for Clinical Nutrition and the American Institute of Nutrition concluded that trans unsaturated fats adversely affect choles-terol profiles, but that these effects are less adverse than those for saturated fats.[66] According to the task force, trans unsaturated fats are reasonable substitutes for saturated, but not for polyunsaturated, fats. Other investigators disagree and consider trans unsaturated fatty acids to be just as adverse as saturated fatty acids with respect to CHD.[73,74] While the effect of trans unsaturated fats on total blood cholesterol levels may be intermediate between cis-MUFAs and saturates, trans fatty acids also have adverse effects on other CHD risk factors. Specifically, trans fatty acids increase blood total and LDL cholesterol levels, decrease HDL cholesterol levels, and raise lipoprotein (a) and triglyceride levels (Figure 2.7).[13,75]

Recent epidemiological studies implicate trans fatty acids as a potential risk factor for CHD.[65,68,69,71] The Health Professionals Follow-up study[69] and the Alpha-Tocopherol, Beta-Carotene Cancer Prevention Study[71] found a relative risk of CHD of 1.4 for men in the upper quintile of trans fatty acid intake. However, in the latter study, elaidic acid from vegetable trans fatty acids and not animal fatty acid intake was related to CHD risk. Also, only the highest quintile of trans fatty acid intake was significantly associated with increased risk of CHD.[71] No significant difference between trans fatty acid intake and CHD risk was found in the three intermediate quintiles of trans fatty acid intake from the lowest quintile.[71] According to the Framingham Study, for each additional teaspoon of margarine (a major dietary source of trans fatty acids) eaten per day, the relative risk of CHD in men was 1.1 at least in the second 11 years follow-up. [68] However, in the first 10 years of follow-up, no association was found between margarine intake and CHD.[68] New findings from the Nurses Health Study [65] reveal that women in the upper quintile of trans fat intake had a multivariate relative risk of CHD of 1.27. This 14-year follow-up study involving 80,082 women aged 34 to 59 years found that saturated and trans unsat-urated fats were associated with increased CHD risk, whereas total fat intake was

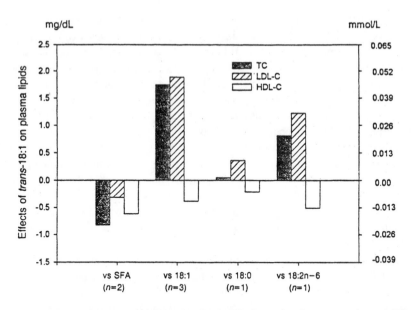

Figure 2.7　Trans-18:1 compared with other fatty acids (every ly. of energy exchange). Effects of trans fatty acids compared with saturated fatty acids (SFA), oleic acid (18:1), stearic acid (18:0), and linoleic acid (18:2). (From Kris-Etherton, P.M. and Yu, S., *Am. J. Clin. Nutr.*, 65[Suppl.], 1628, 1997. With permission.)

not significantly associated with risk of CHD.[65] Epidemiological studies, although suggestive, cannot demonstrate a causal relationship. The effect of trans fatty acids on human health can only be determined by randomized, controlled trials.[76]

A statement recently released by the Nutrition Committee of the American Heart Association concluded that trans fats should be replaced when possible by MUFAs or PUFAs in foods to reduce the risk of CHD.[60] This message should not be misinterpreted to mean that MUFAs and PUFAs can be consumed without limit or that there are "good" and "bad" foods based on their content of MUFAs, PUFAs, or trans fatty acids. Reducing total fat intake can lower both trans and saturated fat intake.

e. Conjugated Linoleic Acid and Sphingolipids

Other fatty acids present in dairy foods, such as conjugated linoleic acid, or CLA, and sphingolipids, may protect against CHD. CLA, a mixture of positional and geometric isomers of linoleic acid, is present in a number of foods and is especially rich in dairy foods. Although most of the research has focused on a potential anti-carcinogenic effect of CLA (see Chapter 4, Dairy Foods and Colon Cancer), experimental animal studies indicate that CLA may also reduce the risk of CHD.[77,78]

When rabbits received 0.5 g CLA per day in food, marked reductions were observed in plasma total and LDL cholesterol, the LDL/HDL cholesterol ratio, and triglyceride levels.[77] In addition, less atherosclerosis was detected in the aortas of CLA-fed rabbits. A more recent investigation by Nicolosi et al.[78] supports the above observations. In this study, hamsters were equally divided into five groups, a control group which received no CLA and either low (0.06% of energy), medium (0.11% of energy), or high (1.1% of energy) CLA or 1.1% of energy as linoleic acid for 11 weeks.[78] Compared to the control animals, the CLA-fed animals exhibited lower levels of plasma total cholesterol, non-HDL cholesterol (combined very low and LDL), and triglycerides. An antioxidant effect of CLA was suggested by determination of plasma tocopherol/total cholesterol ratios. In addition, measurement of the aortic fatty streak areas revealed less early atherosclerosis in the CLA-fed hamsters.[78] The findings led the researchers to conclude that CLA has the ability to reduce atherosclerosis risk factors and fatty streak formation which is an initial event in early atherosclerosis.[78]

Similar to CLA, most of the research on sphingolipids has focused on their potential anticarcinogenic properties (see Chapter 4, Dairy Foods and Colon Cancer). However, there is limited research from experimental animals indicating a potential role for sphingolipids in protecting against CHD.[79] Sphingolipids are an important type of fat found in milk and other dairy foods. Long-term feeding (two generations) of sphingolipids (1%) to laboratory rats significantly decreased total blood cholesterol levels by about 30%.[79] The potential protective roles of CLA and sphingolipids in cardiovascular health warrant additional study.

In summary, findings of the above studies of the effects of individual fatty acids on blood lipid levels indicate that many of the major fatty acids found in milk fat do not have a hypercholesterolemic effect.[72] These fatty acids include the long chain SFA, stearic acid; short chain SFAs; MUFAS; PUFAs, and possibly CLA and sphingolipids.

2. Dietary Fat Quantity

In addition to the type of dietary fat, the amount of dietary fat can influence blood lipid and lipoprotein levels.[12] According to equations developed by Hegsted et al.[27] and Keys et al.,[55] reducing total fat intake from 37% of energy to the recommended 30%, with equal proportions of SFAs, MUFAs, and PUFAs, would reduce blood total cholesterol by 14 mg/dl.

Variations in total fat intake, with or without changes in fat quality, can influence specific lipoproteins.[12,18] Drastic reductions in dietary fat calories (e.g., from 40% to less than 10% of energy) significantly lower blood LDL cholesterol, HDL cholesterol, and apo A-1 levels.[6,12,18,80] The extent of HDL lowering, however, is influenced by a number of factors including the type of carbohydrate (simple vs. complex) used to replace fat calories and the P to S ratio of the lowfat diet.[12] McNamara[12] estimates a 3 to 4 mg/dl decrease in blood HDL cholesterol levels for every 10% exchange of fat for carbohydrate calories.

Replacing fat intake with carbohydrate is predicted to have little effect on coronary risk because this diet decreases HDL cholesterol levels in addition to lowering LDL cholesterol levels.[18,81] Altering the quality or type of fat consumed (i.e., replacing SFA with USFAs) may be more effective in lowering the risk of CHD than previously appreciated.[18,65,82-84] Compared to a high carbohydrate, lowfat diet, a high fat diet low in SFAs but containing MUFAs increases HDL cholesterol levels and decreases triglyceride levels.[13] Because diets very low in fat (15% of calories) may induce adverse metabolic changes (i.e., reduce HDL cholesterol and increase triglyceride levels), and possibly lead to nutrient deficiencies in certain subgroups such as children, pregnant women, and older adults, the American Heart Association[6,85] does not recommend such diets for the general population.

3. Dietary Cholesterol

Within the range of dietary cholesterol usually consumed by most people, dietary cholesterol generally has a limited influence on blood cholesterol levels.[12,24,25,86] Dietary cholesterol has a much weaker influence than SFAs, specifically myristic, lauric, and palmitic acids, on blood total and LDL cholesterol levels.[6,24,25] During the past 30 years, 139 cholesterol feeding trials in 2,981 subjects have been carried out.[87] Findings from these trials are relatively consistent with a 100 mg change in dietary cholesterol resulting in a change in blood cholesterol levels of 2.5 mg/dl (Figure 2.8).[87]

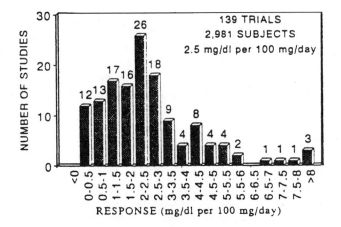

Figure 2.8   Histogram of the dose adjusted responses (change in plasma cholesterol [mg/dl] per 100 mg per day change in dietary cholesterol) for 139 published studies in 2,981 subjects testing dietary cholesterol as the single intervention variable. (From McNamara, D.J., *J. Am. Coll. Nutr.*, 16(6), 530, 1997. With permission.)

However, individuals vary in their blood cholesterol response to dietary cholesterol.[6,24,25,86-88] According to a review by McNamara,[87] 15 to 20% of the population is relatively sensitive to the effects of dietary cholesterol, whereas 80 to 85% are relatively insensitive. Reducing dietary cholesterol intake from 400 mg/day to 300 mg/day is estimated to lower plasma cholesterol levels by 3.2 mg/dl in cholesterol sensitive individuals (i.e., those who lack precise feedback control of endogenous cholesterol synthesis).[87] Cholesterol insensitive individuals compensate for decreases in dietary cholesterol by increasing endogenous cholesterol synthesis.[88] At present, there is no biological marker to identify individuals who are more or less sensitive to dietary cholesterol. Individuals with hyperlipidemia may be more sensitive to dietary cholesterol.[89] In a study involving 21 subjects, an acute load of cholesterol (700 mg) with a meal did not produce a more atherogenic profile except in subjects with hypertriglyceridemia.[89] The American Heart Association[6] summarizes the effects of dietary cholesterol on blood cholesterol levels as follows, "When compared with the effects of saturated fatty acids, the effects of dietary cholesterol on LDL cholesterol levels are weaker but can be substantial in some individuals. As with intake of saturated fatty acids, there is considerable interindividual variation in response to dietary cholesterol which should be considered when making individual dietary recommendations."

4. Protein (Casein)

Besides focusing on the fat content of milk and dairy foods, some investigators have reported that casein, the major protein in milk and dairy foods, is hypercholesterolemic when substituted for soy protein.[90-102] However, the effect of casein on blood cholesterol levels varies widely and appears to depend on experimental conditions including the amount of cholesterol in the diet, the percentage of protein and lipid in the diet, species, age and strain of the animal, duration of the study, the kind of casein, and the blood cholesterol level of the individual among other factors.[94-97]

Several studies indicate that a hypercholesterolemic effect of casein compared to soy protein is dependent on a cholesterol-rich diet.[90,91,93,101] In a cross-over study in which normolipidemic subjects consumed formula diets containing 500 mg cholesterol per day and 20% casein, blood LDL cholesterol levels increased by 10% and HDL cholesterol decreased by 10%.[93] When cholesterol intake was reduced to <100 mg/day, casein and soy protein had similar effects on blood lipoprotein levels. These findings support the suggestion that casein alters blood lipoprotein levels only in the presence of high dietary cholesterol.

In addition to dietary cholesterol, mineral intake may influence the hypercholesterolemic response to casein. In a study involving rabbits, a reduction in dietary minerals enhanced casein-induced hypercholesterolemia.[98] In rabbits, casein is hypercholesterolemic and atherogenic compared to soy. However, when the casein:soy ratio is 1:1, cholesterol levels and atherosclerosis are similar to those observed when 100% soy is fed.[99]

Most of the studies that have examined the effect of casein on blood cholesterol levels have been carried out in growing animals consuming a single source of protein.[98] Consequently, extrapolating the findings to adult humans consuming a mixed diet is questionable. Moreover, an individual's initial blood cholesterol level influences the response to proteins such as soybean.[95,96] Lowfat, low cholesterol diets containing isolated soybean protein (25 g/day or 50 g/day), as compared to casein, have been demonstrated to reduce blood cholesterol levels in men with elevated blood cholesterol, but not in those with lower initial blood cholesterol levels.[95,96] Also, the mechanism by which the type of protein influences blood cholesterol is unknown.[96] The suggestion that casein is hypercholesterolemic has not gained wide acceptance by the scientific community.[9]

5. Vitamin D

Some investigations indicate that vitamin D_3 (cholecalciferol), acting through its metabolite, 1,25 dihydroxyvitamin D_3 (calcitriol), plays an important role in modulating the function of the cardiovascular system.[103-107] Vitamin D is obtained by the action of sunlight on 7-dehydrocholesterol in the skin and from the diet. Because few foods contain vitamin D, almost all fluid milk in the U.S. is voluntarily fortified with vitamin D to obtain 400 IU per quart.[108] One 8-ounce serving of vitamin D fortified milk provides 25% of the amount of vitamin D recommended for everyone younger than 51 years of age (i.e., 5 μg/day or 200 IU/day) and 12.5% of the amount of vitamin D recommended for adults ages 51 through 70 years (i.e., 10 μg/day or 400 IU/day).[109]

Potential regulatory functions for calcitriol include enhancement of cardiac and vascular muscle contractility and changes in physical and morphological characteristics of the myocardium (e.g., heart weight to body weight ratio, myocardial collagen).[103,106,110] Depletion of vitamin D_3 in experimental animals has been demonstrated to increase the heart to body weight ratio.[106,110] When laboratory rats were fed a vitamin D_3 deficient diet for nine weeks, the heart to body ratio increased, cardiac myocytes were smaller but more numerous indicating hyperplasia, and c-myc protein levels in the rat hearts increased.[110] The authors suggest that vitamin D deficiency leads to a chronic increase in c-myc protein levels which in turn lead to myocyte hyperplasia and myocardial hypertrophy in the vitamin D_3-deficient heart [110] Maternal vitamin D deficiency has been demonstrated to slow metabolic and contractile development in neonatal rat hearts.[111] These findings indicate that vitamin D is associated with profound changes in physical and morphological properties of the heart and that this could have a significant effect on the contractile properties of the myocardium.

Other studies support a direct effect of calcitriol in cardiovascular function. When experimental animals were fed vitamin D deficient diets, both cardiac and vascular muscle contractile function increased.[104] To determine whether these changes were a direct response to calcitriol or an indirect result of the accompanying hypocalcemia, vitamin D deficient rats were fed a diet designed to maintain normal blood calcium and phosphorus levels.[105] The vitamin D endocrine system was found to be directly involved in maintaining normal contractile function.[105]

A specific receptor for calcitriol has been identified in cardiac myoblast cells.[112] Under normal physiological conditions, the vitamin D endocrine system may regulate myocardial metabolism.[102,107]

Some studies in humans support a potential beneficial role for vitamin D in cardiovascular health.[113-115] Low blood levels of 25-hydroxyvitamin D (25-OHD) and 1,25 dihydroxyvitamin D (1,25[OH]2D) were found in 17% and 26%, respectively, of patients with severe congestive heart failure.[113] In subjects at risk for CHD, serum 1,25 vitamin D levels were inversely associated with vascular calcification, a common feature of atherosclerosis. [114] Investigators in Norway attributed transitory congestive heart failure in an infant to severe vitamin D deficiency with hypocalcemia.[115]

These findings of involvement of the vitamin D endocrine system in cardiovascular function are preliminary. However, the possibility that vitamin D may contribute to a healthy cardiovascular system deserves further attention.

B. Genetics

Although efforts to prevent CHD have primarily focused on dietary and drug modifications of blood total cholesterol and lipoprotein cholesterol levels, accumulating findings indicate that genetics may have a more important effect on CHD risk than previously appreciated.[6,116-119] Blood lipid levels are shown to cluster in families, and studies of twins indicate significant genetic influences on lipid levels.[118] In fact, family history is considered to be a major risk factor for early onset CHD. [7]

Studies clearly indicate that individuals differ in their blood lipid responses to diet, notably with regard to dietary intake of fat and cholesterol.[88,120-126] A large variability in blood lipid responses among individuals following the National Cholesterol Education Program's (NCEP) Step 2 diet (i.e., 30% or less of calories from total fat, less than 7% of calories from saturated fat, and less than 200 mg cholesterol/day) has been reported (Figure 2.9).[123] Changes in blood LDL cholesterol levels ranged from +3% to –55% in men and +13% and –39% in women.[123] The range of individual responses to the same dietary intervention has been attributed to multiple genes, each with relatively small effect.[116,123] Moreover, this variability in response supports individualized dietary and lifestyle recommendations to prevent and treat CHD.[6] The identification of genes that influence an individual's risk for CHD ultimately may result in tests to identify individuals most likely to benefit from specific dietary or other lifestyle interventions and allow for individualized dietary recommendations.[6]

In recent years, considerable progress has been made in identifying genes influencing major risk factors for CHD such as total blood cholesterol, lipoproteins (HDL and LDL cholesterol), and apolipoproteins (apo B, A-I, A-II, A-IV, E).[116-118,123,126-132] Genetic defects in lipoprotein metabolism have increased our understanding of how specific lipoproteins influence premature CHD.[130,133-135] Several genes have been shown to affect blood HDL cholesterol levels and consequently CHD risk.[123] In many familial HDL cholesterol deficiency syndromes, abnormalities or deficiencies of apo A-I, the major protein in HDL cholesterol which protects against CHD, have been identified. Evidence from different strains of mice indicates that a unique genetic trait may influence HDL cholesterol and the atherosclerotic response to a high fat, high cholesterol diet. When mice genetically susceptible to diet-induced atherosclerosis received the human gene for apo A-I, HDL cholesterol levels were increased and fewer fatty lesions developed in the blood vessels than in control mice not receiving this gene.[131]

Genetics may have more influence on LDL than HDL cholesterol levels.[135] Levels of apo B, the protein in LDL, were more alike in identical than in fraternal twins, indicating that LDL levels are influenced by genes. Similarities were less apparent for apo A-I, implying that genetics may play a weaker role in HDL cholesterol levels.[135]

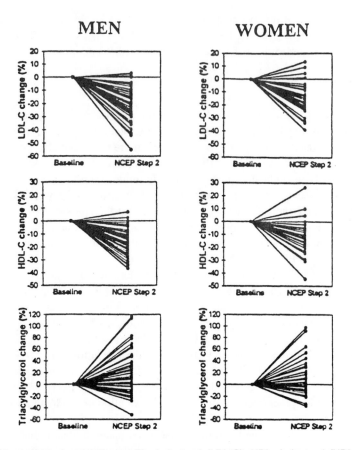

Figure 2.9   Individual variability in LDL-cholesterol (LDL-C), HDL-cholesterol (HDL-C), and triacyglycerol concentrations in response to a National Cholesterol Education Program (NCEP) Step 2 diet in men and women. (From Schaefer, E.J., et. al., *Am. J. Clin. Nutr.*, 65, 823, 1997. With permission.)

The influence of genetics on blood levels of LDL cholesterol and LDL subfraction patterns has been demonstrated in several investigations.[129,136,137] Familial forms of hypercholesterolemia, which are present in one in 500 persons in the general population, may result from deficient or defective LDL receptors.[138] A mutation in the gene coding for the LDL receptor prevents removal of LDL from the blood and results in a significant rise in LDL cholesterol and increased risk of CHD.[129,130,138] Genetic polymorphisms in apo E, which are important in the receptor-mediated uptake of small VLDL and intermediate density LDL, explain a small but significant proportion of the variation in LDL cholesterol.[119,123,128,139] Individuals with the E_4 allelic variant of apo E gene exhibit a greater reduction in LDL cholesterol on lowfat, low cholesterol diets than do individuals with other alleles.

Researchers have identified defects in genes controlling LDL subclasses which could explain much of the familial clustering of lipid and lipoprotein levels in certain families and their increased risk of premature CHD.[20,133,140-142] In a community-based study of 301 subjects from 61 nuclear families, two distinct LDL subclasses have been described.[20,133] Phenotype A is characterized by a predominance of large, buoyant LDL particles, whereas phenotype B consists mostly of small dense LDL particles.[20]

The phenotype B lipoprotein pattern is similar to that which has been described with increased CHD risk, specifically increased blood levels of triglyceride-rich lipoproteins and apo-B and low levels of HDL cholesterol.[134,136,140,143] As reviewed by Gardner et. al.,[26] data from the Stanford Five-City Project Study (1979-1992) involving over 248 adults and from the Physicians' Health Study of 14,916 men links small, dense LDLs with increased risk of CHD. Likewise in the Quebec Cardiovascular Study which followed 2443 men for 5 years, small dense LDLs increased CHD risk independent of other risk factors such as LDL cholesterol levels, body mass index, diabetes, blood pressure, age, alcohol intake, smoking, and a family history of heart disease.[144] LDL subclass pattern B has been associated with a threefold increase in risk of myocardial infarction.[136] The higher risk of atherosclerosis in individuals with phenotype B may be explained by the increased susceptibility to oxidation of the smaller, more dense LDL particles.[26,145,146] Also, compared to its larger counterparts, small dense LDL binds less well to LDL receptors, is cleared more slowly from circulation, and may enter the arterial wall at a faster rate.[147,148] Increased cholesterol deposition in the arterial wall increases the risk of atherosclerotic lesions.

Susceptibility to phenotype B appears to be inherited in most affected families as a single gene trait. Scientists have identified a possible genetic locus for this trait, designated ATHS (atherosclerosis susceptibility) on chromosome 19.[134] This and possibly other genes are responsible for the atherogenic lipoprotein phenotype (ALP), a common heritable trait shared by up to 30% of the population.[126] The trait is characterized by an atherogenic lipoprotein profile including LDL subclass pattern B. The effects of ATHS generally do not become apparent until after age 20 in men and after menopause in women.[136,143] The interaction of ATHS with other genetic or environmental factors such as diet may be responsible for a large proportion of the familial predisposition to CHD in the general population.[134]

The same genetic factors that determine an individual's plasma lipoprotein subclass profile and CHD risk also may affect the response to diet.[140-142] Adult males with LDL subclass pattern B have been found to differ from men with LDL subclass pattern A in their lipoprotein response to a lowfat diet.[140] In a randomized crossover investigation, 105 men consumed either a high fat (46% of calories from fat) or lowfat (24% of calories from fat) diet for six weeks. Following the lowfat diet, pattern B subjects exhibited twice the decrease in LDL cholesterol as pattern A subjects and plasma apo B levels decreased significantly, indicating a reduction in the total number of LDL particles (Figure 2.10). Thus, the genetically influenced LDL subclass pattern (A or B) is a significant factor contributing to the variation of LDL cholesterol response to a lowfat, high carbohydrate diet. The benefits of a reduced fat diet in terms of lipoprotein predictors of CHD risk, including LDL cholesterol, the ratio of LDL to HDL, and plasma apo B, were greatest in men who possessed LDL subclass pattern B.[140] This study also revealed that while the lowfat diet was especially beneficial for the pattern B men, it led to a more atherogenic lipoprotein response in some pattern A subjects.[140] Thus, a lowfat diet potentially

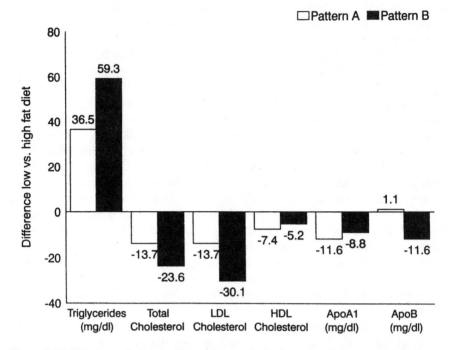

Figure 2.10 Differences between adults with genetically determined LDL subclass pattern A and B in their blood lipid, lipoprotein cholesterol, and apolipoprotein responses to a change from a high-to-low-fat diet. (Adapted from Dreon, D. M., et al., *FASEB J.*, 8, 121, 1994. With permission.)

may increase risk of CHD by switching some individuals' LDL subclass from A to a more atherogenic B subclass. Similar findings have been reported by a more recent investigation.[141] These observations illustrate the complex interaction between diet and genetics. Genetically determined LDL subclass pattern influences the blood lipid response to diet; conversely, diet influences changes in subclass pattern. Thus, both genetic and environmental factors, by influencing LDL subclass distributions, may contribute to differences in individuals' plasma lipoprotein response to a lowfat diet.[140,141]

A genetic predisposition to LDL pattern A or B may influence the blood lipid response to a reduced fat diet even if individuals themselves do not have this trait.[142] When 72 premenopausal women ages 25 through 44 years were switched from a 35% fat diet to a 20% fat diet for eight weeks, changes in LDL cholesterol levels were related to the number of parents expressing the pattern B phenotype. Specifically, LDL cholesterol reduction on a lowfat, high carbohydrate diet was greatest in daughters of two pattern B parents, intermediate in daughters with one pattern B parent, and least in daughters with no pattern B parents.[142] This genetic effect on the blood cholesterol response to diet was independent of the women's body weight, initial blood cholesterol levels, or their own LDL subclass pattern.[142]

Additional support for a diet-gene interaction is provided by Lopez-Miranda and colleagues.[149,150] When young men with a mutation in the gene responsible for apo

A-1 and previously normal cholesterol levels were fed a high fat diet (40% of calories) rich in monounsaturated fat, total and LDL blood cholesterol levels increased. These results were surprising given that the effect of monounsaturated fat on blood lipids generally is similar to that of a diet low in total and saturated fat. The authors conclude that for the 20% of the Caucasian population with this genetic mutation, reducing dietary fat successfully reduces plasma LDL cholesterol levels.[149] Genetic variations at the apo C_3 gene locus appear to influence the LDL cholesterol response to dietary monounsaturated fatty acids.[150] Based on these findings, an individual's genetic make-up not only influences the size and shape of LDL particles, but also may influence the metabolic response to dietary fat.

An understanding of how diet and genetics interact to influence CHD risk is becoming much greater. Identification of genetic polymorphisms that affect lipoproteins and CHD responses to specific dietary recommendations eventually will enable identification of individuals most likely to benefit from specific dietary modifications. It is clear that the same dietary pattern has unique effects in different individuals and that reduced fat diets may not be beneficial or equally beneficial for everyone.

Age and gender are other factors that can influence the extent to which individuals handle dietary fat, according to a recent investigation.[151] In this study, oxidation of the SFA, palmitic acid, in healthy children aged 5 to 10 years was almost twice that found in adults. Also, the metabolic disposal of palmitic acid was greater in men than in women.[151] These differences in handling of dietary fat between children and adults led the researchers to question the appropriateness of current recommendations for dietary fat, and particularly SFAs, for the population as a whole, including children from 5 years of age. [151]

The complicating factor of genetic diversity and differences among individuals in their ability to handle dietary fat because of age, gender, and possibly lifestyle factors supports dietary recommendations tailored to individuals. New dietary guidance issued by the American Heart Association[6] recognizes the importance of genetics in influencing individuals' response to diet. In the future, based on individual genetically based nutrition profiles, people may be able to map out a personal strategy of what to eat to minimize the risk of CHD. Greater individualization of dietary recommendations to reduce CHD, both for major subgroups of the population (e.g., children) and for individuals, is expected to improve the effectiveness of the intervention and reduce costs.[152]

C. Dairy Foods

Studies of the effects of single nutrients such as specific fats in dairy foods on blood lipid levels are important for identifying mechanisms underlying observed responses, but are of little practical relevance. In whole foods, complex interactions occur among nutrients which can modify the impact of a single nutrient on blood lipid levels. As reviewed below, studies employing dairy foods indicate that when these foods are consumed in usual amounts they do not appear to adversely affect blood lipid levels or increase risk of CHD. It is important to appreciate that the impact of a single food on risk of CHD also is influenced by the composition of the rest of the diet, as well as other lifestyle (e.g., physical activity, cigarette smoking) and genetic factors. Although there is a tendency to indict specific foods or food components, risk of CHD is associated with the total diet and other risk factors over time.

1. Milk and Culture-Containing Dairy Foods

Some researchers have hypothesized that certain dairy foods contain a blood cholesterol lowering "milk factor."[153-159] Interest in this possibility arose from the observation that Massai tribesmen of East Africa, who consume large quantities (4 to 5 liters per person per day) of fermented whole milk, have low blood cholesterol levels and a low incidence of CHD.[158]

Subsequent studies have examined the effect of a variety of dairy products on blood cholesterol levels. Several of these studies reveal that milk, yogurt, or *Lactobacillus acidophilus*-containing dairy foods are hypocholesterolemic in humans.[154,156,157,160,161] Howard and Marks[154] reported that humans exhibited a 5 to 15% decrease in blood cholesterol levels one week following intake of 2 quarts of whole and fat free milk a day, respectively. Likewise, Hepner et al.[157] found that supplementing ordinary diets with 3 cups of pasteurized and unpasteurized yogurt a day for one week reduced blood cholesterol levels by 5 to 10%. In another study, yogurt intake was found to be hypocholesterolemic in females.[160] Buonopane et al.[161] investigated the effect of consuming one quart of skim milk a day for eight weeks on blood cholesterol levels of 82 free-living adults. Blood cholesterol levels dropped 6.6% within 4 weeks in adults who consumed fat free milk and whose initial blood cholesterol levels were elevated (217 to 233 mg/dl). The hypocholesterolemic effect of fat free milk was greater in individuals with higher rather than lower baseline cholesterol levels.[161] A similar cholesterol-lowering effect of fat free milk (400 ml/day or about two glasses) was observed in postmenopausal Japanese women.[162] The reduction in blood cholesterol levels with fat free milk observed in these studies is in agreement with findings from other investigations.[163-165]

Experimental animal studies also indicate a hypocholesterolemic effect of several dairy products.[166-172] Kritchevsky et al.[167] showed that either whole or fat free milk fed to rats reduced blood cholesterol levels. When rabbits fed a high cholesterol diet received large amounts of yogurt, blood cholesterol levels decreased as compared to levels in rabbits on a similar diet without yogurt.[168] In weanling rats, blood cholesterol levels significantly decreased after four weeks as a result of intake of a commercial feed supplemented with *Lactobacillus acidophilus* fermented milk.[170] When the effects of yogurt and acidophilus yogurt on blood lipids were examined in mice, blood total and LDL cholesterol significantly decreased in the animals fed acidophilus yogurt.[172] In contrast, yogurt or acidophilus yogurt did not affect blood HDL cholesterol and triglyceride levels (Table 2.3).[172] In another study, total and LDL cholesterol levels decreased in laboratory rats fed yogurt containing either lactose hydrolyzed condensed whey or bifidobacteria, whereas whole milk and standard yogurt had no hypocholesterolemic effect.[173]

Zommara et al.[174] reported that whey from fat free milk fermented with bifidobacteria and lactic acid bacteria reduced blood total and LDL cholesterol levels, increased the activity of antioxidant enzymes, and increased the resistance of LDL

Table 2.3   Effect of Yogurt and Acidophilus Yogurt on Serum Lipids in Mice[1]

Dietary Treatment Group[3]	Cholesterol		HDL[2] Cholesterol		LDL Cholesterol		Triglycerides	
	d 28	d 56	d 28	d 56	d 28	d 56	d 28	d 56
				(mg/d)				
Control								
X̄	171.2[a,x]	168.1[a,x]	54.6	54.2	97.8[a,x]	96.6[a,x]	94.3	90.9
SD	3.0	3.9	3.1	3.1	3.6	2.4	5.8	5.9
Yogurt								
X̄	169.6[a,y]	157.7[b,x]	52.7	52.0	98.8[a,y]	88.3[b,x]	90.7	86.9
SD	5.0	6.8	3.0	3.8	5.4	4.3	6.7	5.3
Acidophilus yogurt								
X̄	139.9[b,x]	116.0[c,y]	51.0	51.3	70.4[b,x]	46.9[c,y]	92.6	88.7
SD	3.1	4.2	3.7	4.2	3.8	5.0	5.2	4.3

[a,b,c] Means within a column with no common superscript letters differ (P <0.01).

[x,y] Means within a row within a cholesterol group with no common superscript letters differ (P <0.01).

[1] Each value is a mean (±SD) of nine observations.

[2] HDL = High density lipoprotein; LDL = low density lipoprotein. The LDL cholesterol was calculated by the equation LDL cholesterol = serum cholesterol − HDL cholesterol − serum triglycerides.

[3] Mice were assigned to one of three dietary treatments for 56 d: 1) commercial rodent chow and water (control); 2) commercial rodent chow and yogurt made from milk inoculated with a 3% (vol/vol) liquid culture of *Streptococcus thermophilus* and *Lactobacillus delbrueckii* ssp. *bulgaricus* (yogurt), and 3) commercial rodent chow plus yogurt made from milk inoculated with a 0.01% (wt/vol) freeze-dried culture of *S. thermophilus* plus *Lactobacillus acidophilus* (acidophilus yogurt).

From Akalin, S., et al., *J. Dairy Sci.*, 80, 2721, 1997. With permission.

cholesterol to oxidation in laboratory rats. In this study, the non-fermented whey diet was less effective than wheys from cultured milk in reducing blood cholesterol and oxidative stress. [174] Mohan et al.[175] reported that blood cholesterol levels were significantly lower in probiotic-supplemented broiler chickens than in control animals. In another investigation, blood total and LDL cholesterol levels dropped when adult boars were fed diets high in cholesterol and acidophilus yogurt.[171] Keim et al.[166] found that rats fed a skim milk powder during the first week of weaning experienced an acceleration in the rate of blood cholesterol reduction that normally occurs during postweaning.

Additional studies in laboratory animals support a hypocholesterolemic effect of milk.[169] When experimental animals were fed diets containing whole milk or a casein-lactose mixture, blood cholesterol levels were lower in the animals receiving the whole milk. This finding led Schneeman et al.[169] to suggest that the blood lipid response to whole milk cannot be predicted simply from its fat content. This study also found that whole milk reduced blood triglyceride levels.[169] Although other investigators have reported that milk intake by animals or humans reduces blood triglyceride levels,[161,163] this finding is not consistently observed.[164,176] Moreover, the relationship between elevated blood triglyceride levels and CHD risk is inconclusive and considered to be less important than low levels of HDL cholesterols.[17]

The above studies indicate that milk consumption may lower blood cholesterol levels, with fat free milk eliciting the greatest response.[36] Further, the hypocholesterolemic effect of milk appears to be more pronounced in individuals with higher rather than lower blood cholesterol levels. Other factors such as minor components in milk produced in different regions also may explain differences in findings.

Although not all studies indicate a hypocholesterolemic effect of milk and milk products, intake of these foods has not been shown to *increase* blood lipid levels.[156,163,164,166,177-179] Thompson et al.[164] observed no significant change in blood cholesterol levels following intake of 1 liter supplements of various milk products fed daily for three weeks to human subjects. Likewise, McNamara et al.[177] found that 16 ounces of yogurt or a nonfermented dairy product (16 ounces lowfat milk, plus 10% milk solids) had no effect on plasma total, LDL, and HDL cholesterol levels when consumed by 18 normolipidemic males for four weeks. In a cross-sectional study involving over 300 adults and in which calcium intake was increased to 1500 mg/day using mostly dairy foods (milk, cheese, yogurt) for 12 weeks, there was no effect on blood lipid levels despite the increased consumption of dairy foods.[179]

Not only is evidence for a hypocholesterolemic effect of milk and some milk products inconsistent, but the identity of the "milk factor" is unknown. Possible candidates include hydroxymethylglutaryl-CoA reductase (a rate-limiting enzyme in cholesterol biosynthesis), lactose, and calcium.[153,155,164,180]

Several studies support a hypocholesterolemic effect of calcium.[157,179,181-187] These findings are of importance considering that dairy foods contribute 73% of the calcium available in the U.S. food supply.[38]

In a randomized single blind study, 13 men aged 38 to 49 years with moderate hypercholesterolemia were fed a metabolic diet approximating the typical American diet (i.e., 34% of calories from fat, 13% from SFAs, and 240 mg cholesterol a day) and either 400 mg or 2200 mg calcium (as calcium citrate malate)/day for ten days.[182] When compared to the low calcium diet, the high calcium diet lowered total cholesterol by 6%, LDL cholesterol by 11%, and apo B levels by 7% (Table 2.4). No significant differences in HDL cholesterol levels were observed.[182] The excretion of SFAs doubled during the high calcium diet, suggesting that calcium's beneficial effect may be explained by the formation of calcium-SFA complexes in the intestine. The findings of this study led the authors to conclude that increasing the calcium intake of a typical American diet "may be mildly effective in lowering total and LDL cholesterol concentrations, perhaps by its action on increasing saturated fatty acid excretion."[182] A complementary approach to the traditional recommendation to reduce SFA intake to lower risk of CHD might be to decrease the absorption of this lipid by increasing calcium intake. From the results of this study, it can be anticipated that the hypercholesterolemic effect of SFAs in a food such as whole milk may be ameliorated, at least in part, by the presence of calcium in the same food.

In a study involving 96 patients with mild to moderate hypercholesterolemia treated with a lowfat, low cholesterol diet, increasing calcium intake by 400 mg for 6 weeks reduced LDL cholesterol levels by 4.4% and increased HDL cholesterol

Table 2.4 Serum Lipid, Lipoprotein, and
Apolipoprotein Concentrations in Humans
Fed a Low or High Calcium Diet

Item	Low Ca		High Ca	
Cholesterol, mmol/L	5.99	± 0.62	5.66	± 0.57[a]
Triglycerides, mmol/L	1.74	± 0.82	1.89	± 0.90[2]
LDL cholesterol, mmol/L	4.13	± 0.54	3.67	± 0.49[a]
HDL cholesterol, mmol/L	1.06	± 0.23	1.11	± 0.34
Apolipoprotein B, g/L	10.4	± 1.7	9.7	± 1.5[a]
Apolipoprotein AI, g/L	12.1	± 1.8	12.3	± 1.7

[1] Values are means ± SD, $n = 3$. Samples from each subject
were assayed in triplicate.
[a] Indicates significantly different from low Ca diet at P <0.05.
[2] Mean of both periods assumes residual effect observed in
Period 1 attributed to baseline difference.

From Denke, M.A. et al., *J. Nutr.*, 123, 1047, 1993. With
permission.

Table 2.5 Changes in Lipid Levels After 6 Weeks of Treatment with Calcium Carbonate
or Placebo*

Type of Lipid	Diet Baseline	Placebo	Calcium Carbonate	% Change	P
Total cholesterol, mmol/L (mg/dL)	6.70 ± 0.86 (259.1 ± 33.2)	6.74 ± 0.83 (260.6 ± 32.0)	6.62 ± 0.89 (256 ± 34.4)	−1.7	NS
LDL cholesterol, mmol/L (mg/dL)	4.71 ± 0.77 (182.2 ± 29.7)	4.70 ± 0.74 (181.6 ± 28.5)	4.48 ± 0.76 (173.1 ± 29.3)	−4.4	0.001
HDL cholesterol, mmol/L (mg/dL)	1.34 ± 0.35 (51.7 ± 13.7)	1.36 ± 0.35 (52.5 ± 13.6)	1.40 ± 0.37 (54.3 ± 14.5)	4.1	0.031
Total cholesterol/ HDL ratio	5.3 ± 1.4	5.3 ± 1.3	5.0 ± 1.3	−4.5	0.012
LDL/HDL ratio	3.8 ± 1.2	3.7 ± 1.1	3.4 ± 1.1	−6.5	0.001
Lipoprotein Apo B, mmol/L (mg/dL)	2.07 ± 0.41 (80.0 ± 15.9)	2.21 ± 0.43 (85.3 ± 16.8)	2.15 ± 0.43 (83.3 ± 16.6)	−0.7	NS
Triglyceride, mmol/L (mg/dL)	1.41 ± 0.55 (124.7 ± 49.1)	1.50 ± 0.64 (133.1 ± 57.0)	1.61 ± 0.69 (143 ± 61.4)	9.6	NS

* LDL indicates low-density lipoprotein; HDL, high-density lipoprotein; and NS, nonsignificant.
From Bell, L., et al., *Arch. Intern. Med.*, 152, 2441, 1992. With permission.

by 4.1% (Table 2.5).[183] A blood cholesterol lowering effect of calcium has also been
demonstrated in experimental animals receiving a hypercholesterolemic diet.[187,188]

From these studies, it appears that the beneficial effect of calcium on blood lipid
levels is more pronounced in individuals with hypercholesterolemia than in those
with normal blood cholesterol levels. In addition to calcium's favorable effect on
blood lipids, this nutrient may protect against CHD by its effect on blood pressure
(see Chapter 3, Dairy Foods and Hypertension). Also, calcium, at least from milk,
has recently been linked to decreased risk of stroke.[189]

In a cohort of 3150 older, middle-aged (55 to 68 years) Japanese men enrolled in
the Honolulu Heart Program and followed for 22 years, intake of calcium from milk,
but not from nondairy sources, was associated with reduced risk of stroke.[189] Men who

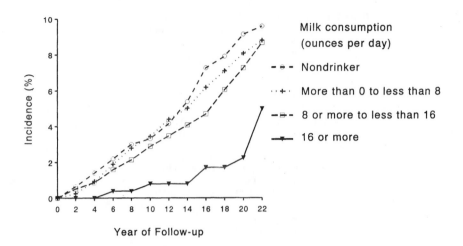

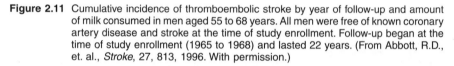

Year of Follow-up

Figure 2.11 Cumulative incidence of thromboembolic stroke by year of follow-up and amount of milk consumed in men aged 55 to 68 years. All men were free of known coronary artery disease and stroke at the time of study enrollment. Follow-up began at the time of study enrollment (1965 to 1968) and lasted 22 years. (From Abbott, R.D., et. al., *Stroke*, 27, 813, 1996. With permission.)

consumed 16 ounces per day or more of milk experienced half the rate of stroke (3.7 vs. 7.9 per 100, respectively) of men who did not drink milk (Figure 2.11). Although the rate of stroke decreased with increasing milk intake, the decline in stroke was modest for men who consumed less than 16 ounces per day. The finding that calcium intake from dairy sources, but not from nondairy sources, reduced risk of stroke indicates that other constituents in milk or concomitant health behaviors related to milk intake may be protective. The researchers concluded that, when combined with a balanced diet, weight control, and physical activity, drinking milk may help to decrease the risk of stroke.[189] Unlike some other investigations discussed above, dietary calcium or milk intake was not associated with reduced risk of CHD in this study.

2. Butter

Intake of butter generally causes blood total and LDL cholesterol levels to rise, more so when consumed by individuals with elevated blood cholesterol levels.[57,190,191] When moderately hypercholesterolemic subjects consumed a diet containing 36% of calories from fat, half of which was obtained from butter, blood total and LDL cholesterol levels increased.[190] Similarly, in an investigation in which normocholesterolemic young men were fed diets containing 37% of calories from fat, 81% of which was provided by cocoa butter, olive oil, soybean oil, or dairy butter, butter was hypercholesterolemic.[57] In contrast, Flynn et al.[192] reported that blood cholesterol levels did not significantly change in normocholesterolemic and hypercholesterolemic males consuming self-selected diets including two eggs/day with either butter or a high PUFA margarine for 12 weeks. However, individual responses in blood cholesterol levels were observed.[192]

Of interest are the findings of an investigation which examined the effects of five different fats, including butter, for six weeks on blood lipid and lipoprotein levels in 38 healthy, normolipidemic free-living men aged 30 to 60 years.[193] In this study, consuming butter at a level of about 19% of total calories (i.e., 60% of total fat intake or at least 20 times more than usually consumed) produced only a small (5%), although statistically significant, rise in total and LDL cholesterol levels.[193] Thus, under free-living conditions, as opposed to metabolic ward studies, intake of butter appears to have a relatively small influence on blood cholesterol levels.[193] No link between intake of butter and CHD was found in a prospective study examining the effect of margarine (a source of trans fatty acids) intake on the development of CHD among over 800 middle-aged men followed for 21 years.[68] The researchers caution, however, that conclusions may be premature because this study used a single 24-hour dietary recall which may not accurately reflect dietary intake.

IV. EFFICACY AND SAFETY OF LOWFAT DIETS

Various government and health professional organizations have provided similar guidelines regarding fat and cholesterol intake to lower the risk of CHD in the general population.[5,6,8,10,11,30] These organizations advise all healthy Americans two years of age and older to consume a diet that provides an average of no more than 30% of total calories as fat, less than 10% of total calories as SFAs, and less than 300 mg dietary cholesterol a day. For children, more flexible guidelines are recommended.[6,30-32] Specifically, between the ages of two and five years, children should gradually adopt a diet that meets the above guidelines.[6,30,31]

In recent years, a number of questions have arisen regarding the efficacy (i.e., in reducing CHD and improving life expectancy) and safety (i.e., nutritional adequacy) of following lowfat diets.[12,194-196] This is particularly true for very lowfat diets.[85] It is evident that the potential gain accrued by dietary interventions to reduce fat intake is unique to each individual. Consequently, future dietary guidelines may incorporate more individualized advice.[6]

A. Efficacy

Recent meta-analyses using data from both metabolic ward studies and studies in free-living populations indicate that lowering total dietary fat from 37% of calories and cholesterol from 385 mg/day to the NCEP Step 1 diet (i.e., 30% of calories as fat and 300 mg cholesterol/day) reduces blood total and LDL cholesterol by an average of 5%.[24,25] Also, a large degree of individual variability in response to this dietary intervention is reported. In a review of 16 published trials of six months or longer of the Step 1 diet, Ramsay et al.[197] found little effect on blood cholesterol levels in free-living individuals. However, in high risk subjects, reductions in blood cholesterol levels averaged about 2% over six months to six years, equivalent to an estimated reduction in coronary events of 3%.[197]

In the first study to evaluate the effectiveness of the NCEP's Step 2 diet (30% or less of total calories from fat, <7% of total calories from SFA, <200 mg cholesterol) on blood cholesterol levels in nearly 100 asymptomatic free-living adults with mild hypercholesterolemia, diet had only a small effect on blood cholesterol levels.[198] The lowfat diet reduced total and LDL blood cholesterol levels each by 5%, but was accompanied by a 5% decrease in HDL cholesterol. A low level of HDL cholesterol is an independent risk factor for premature CHD mortality and stroke.[199,200] The effect of the lowfat diet on blood cholesterol levels in this study was only one-third the level predicted by the NCEP Expert Panel. Although Schaefer et al.[123] reported more significant decreases in blood total and LDL cholesterol levels in 72 men and 48 women following the NCEP Step 2 diet, a wide variation in blood lipid responses was observed. Moreover, HDL cholesterol decreased and triglyceride levels rose.[123]

The total cholesterol/HDL ratio is a better predictor of CHD risk than either one alone.[201] A lowfat diet may result in no or even a slightly negative change in the total cholesterol/HDL ratio. Researchers have found that lowfat diets can lead to changes in lipoprotein metabolism associated with increased risk of CHD, such as a decrease in HDL cholesterol and increases in triglyceride and small dense LDL (subclass pattern B) levels.[25,81,119,140,142,202-205] Further, new research findings demonstrate that a lowfat diet increases blood Lp(a) levels and leads to detrimental changes in LDL particle size.[206,207] In a double-blind multicenter study called the Delta study, reducing total and SFA intake in healthy adults decreased blood total, LDL, and HDL cholesterol levels, and increased blood Lp(a) levels.[206] The researchers suggest that the potentially atherogenic changes (i.e., reduction in HDL cholesterol and increase in Lp(a) levels) in response to decreasing total and saturated fat intake must be weighed against the benefit of reducing LDL cholesterol levels.[206] In a recent cross-over diet study involving 103 healthy men, a lowfat diet (24% vs. 46% of calories as fat) was positively associated with increased levels of the more atherogenic small LDL particles.[207] This study found that an increase in SFAs, particularly myristic and palmitic acids, was positively associated with larger LDL particles and negatively associated with small LDL particles, whereas dietary stearic acid had no effect.[207] These findings indicate that SFAs may not be as detrimental to the lipoprotein profile as once believed.

Consuming a fat reduced diet appears to have an overall modest effect on blood cholesterol levels.[24,25] Moreover, only a proportion of the U.S. population responds to the fat content of the diet with a significant change in blood lipids.[140-142,151] In addition, very lowfat diets may have undesirable effects on blood lipids thereby potentially increasing some individuals' risk of developing CHD. For this reason, as well as the risk of nutrient deficiencies and unresolved questions regarding the effectiveness of very lowfat diets (i.e., no more than 15% of total calories from fat), the AHA does not recommend the use of these diets.[85] In particular, very lowfat diets could lead to health problems in young children, older adults, pregnant women, and individuals with hypertriglyceridemia or insulin-dependent diabetes mellitus.[85]

Several epidemiological and clinical trials of the impact of dietary (and drug) interventions on CHD and total mortality indicate little or no improvement in life expectancy or overall mortality.[208-217] Gains in life expectancy of only three to four months have been predicted for individuals who have reduced their dietary fat intake from 37 to 30%.[208,209] In general, the benefits of following a lowfat diet and lowering blood cholesterol levels on life expectancy are greater for people at higher risk of

CHD.[208,217] When the relationship between dietary variables and CHD mortality over 12 years was examined in 4546 adults participating in the Lipid Research Clinics Prevalence Follow-up Study, none of the dietary components examined (e.g., cholesterol, total fat, saturated fat) were linked to total deaths.[218] Although epidemiologic studies often demonstrate a beneficial effect of reducing dietary fat on CHD risk, findings from clinical studies are less impressive.[82] A review of six primary prevention trials in high risk, but otherwise healthy, people demonstrated no significant reduction in either CHD or all-cause mortality in most of the trials.[82] Similar findings were observed in the only two controlled secondary prevention trials in which diets low in saturated fat and cholesterol were fed to CHD patients.[82] In contrast, in five of six studies in which the type of fat fed was altered, a more beneficial effect on CHD mortality and, to a lesser extent, all-cause mortality was observed.[82] The author of this review concluded that diets high in polyunsaturated fat and low in saturated fat are preferable to diets low in total fat in reducing CHD risk. Similar findings are reported from the Nurses' Health Study.[83] In this prospective study of over 80,000 women, substituting MUFAs and PUFAs for SFAs and trans USFAs was more effective in preventing CHD than reducing total fat intake.[83]

The relationship between blood cholesterol levels and total mortality appears to be J-shaped, with increased mortality at both ends of the distribution.[219] At very low levels of blood cholesterol (<160 mg/dl) increased mortality due to some cancers, cerebral hemorrhage, respiratory disease, alcoholism, depression, suicide, and homicide has been reported.[220-227] Cowan et al.[228] reported that colon cancer risk was markedly elevated in men whose blood cholesterol level was below 187 mg/dl according to data from the Lipid Research Clinics Program mortality follow-up study. A 1990 National Heart, Lung and Blood Institute conference, which examined the findings from 19 international cohort studies involving nearly 300,000 adults, demonstrated that very low blood cholesterol levels were associated with four times the risk of death from noncardiovascular conditions.[222] Other more recent studies indicate a link between increased risk of death from noncardiovascular disease-related causes and low blood cholesterol levels.[226,227]

Several studies link suicidal behavior and depression with low blood cholesterol levels.[224,229-232] Findings from a 21-year study of over 50,000 adults in Sweden linked low blood cholesterol levels with an increased rate of suicide.[224] Likewise in the Paris Prospective Study involving over 6000 men, low blood cholesterol levels were associated with increased risk of suicide.[230] In a study of American males 70 years of age and older, depression was three times more common in those with low blood cholesterol levels than in men with higher blood cholesterol concentrations.[223] A study of 20 healthy postpartum women linked a decrease in blood cholesterol levels with an increased likelihood of depression.[229] Findings of an association between low blood cholesterol levels and depression is consistent with associations between low blood cholesterol and suicide and violent deaths. A recent meta-analysis of 32 studies conducted between 1965 and 1995 found a significant association between low blood cholesterol levels and increased violence.[232] A proposed mechanism for this association is low blood cholesterol's effect on decreasing brain levels of the neurotransmitter, serotonin.[233] However, more studies are needed to establish the relationship between blood cholesterol levels, mood, and suicide, and to identify an underlying mechanism(s).[234]

There is no scientific evidence that the association between low blood cholesterol levels and noncardiovascular disease mortality is causal, although this possibility cannot be ruled out.[212,215,217,222,226,235-237] Researchers have suggested that low blood cholesterol levels could be responsible for increased mortality (cause-effect), or that the higher mortality could be explained by another factor (preclinical disease) which would lower blood cholesterol levels (effect-cause).[236] Two recent studies involving data from the Framingham Study[237] and the Paris Prospective Study[226] support this latter explanation, specifically that low blood cholesterol levels are the result, rather than the cause, of diseases such as cancer. Another possibility is that a third factor (e.g., excess alcohol intake, cigarette smoking, untreated hypertension) could influence blood cholesterol levels and be a cause of death (confounding factor).[222,225,236,238]

Although blood cholesterol levels below 160 mg/dl are rare, evidence for greater overall health risk could have implications with respect to national cholesterol-lowering policies.[215,236] Increased effort should be directed toward identifying individuals most likely to benefit from dietary interventions to lower blood cholesterol levels.[215,236] Muldoon and colleagues[196] suggest that efforts to lower blood cholesterol levels "are best targeted towards those individuals with CHD or with multiple risk factors."

Although reducing dietary fat is a worthwhile goal for some individuals, it is not a "magic bullet" or simple solution to complex health problems such as CHD. Also, not everyone benefits or benefits equally from reducing dietary fat. In a recent investigation in the Netherlands involving 724 adults 85 years and older, high blood cholesterol levels were associated with reduced risk of death from all causes.[239] This study raises questions about the benefits of cholesterol lowering, at least in the "oldest old." Also in children, the few studies conducted in this population indicate that a fat-restricted diet has little or no effect on blood cholesterol levels.[32,240-242] Even in children with elevated blood cholesterol levels who received intensive dietary intervention and counseling (i.e., the Dietary Intervention Study in Children [DISC]), reducing dietary fat intake to 28% of calories combined with a family-oriented behavioral intervention over three years, resulted in only a small decrease in blood cholesterol levels (3.3 mg/dL or < 2%).[241] While children's growth and development were not adversely affected during the three years of this highly supervised intervention, children in the intervention group consumed approximately 150 fewer calories per day than those in the usual care group.[241] Children are at low risk of CHD and the scientific evidence is insufficient to conclude that childhood diets are related to CHD in adulthood.[32] According to a critical review, a lowfat diet has never been proven to be beneficial and may be potentially unsafe for children.[243] As discussed below, if carried too far or without care, attempts to reduce fat may compromise the health of both children and adults.

B. Safety

Not only may consumption of a lowfat diet be of limited or no benefit, particularly in terms of increasing life expectancy or delaying death, but it also may pose some potential risks. A reduction in dietary saturated fat and cholesterol may result in excessive intakes of PUFAs.[6,15] Safety concerns associated with PUFA-enriched diets include altered cell membrane fluidity which in turn could influence cell membrane function; increased formation of lipid hydroperoxides which could cause endothelial cell membrane injury; increased risk of certain cancers; elevated blood triglyceride levels; increased risk of gallstones; and reduced blood levels of protective HDL cholesterol.[6,9,15,81]

When women with apo E phenotype apo E 3/2 consumed a "therapeutic" diet with a high P:S ratio, "protective" HDL cholesterol levels decreased.[244] Because of unknown and potentially harmful effects of a high intake of PUFAs, the federal government and various health professional organizations recommend that intake of PUFAs not exceed 10% of energy intake.

The overall nutritional adequacy of the diet may be compromised by reducing fat intake to ≤30% kcal, according to several recent studies involving children and adults.[245-253] In a study in Bogalusa, Louisiana in which more than 800 children with an average age of 10 years were grouped according to fat intake, a higher percentage of children consuming a lowfat diet (<30% energy) failed to meet recommendations for vitamins B_6, B_{12}, E, thiamin, riboflavin, niacin, calcium, phosphorus, magnesium, and iron compared to those with a higher fat intake (30 to >40% of energy).[245] Further, children following self-selected lowfat diets consumed 20% more sugar, mainly in the form of candy, sweetened beverages, and desserts than children who consumed higher fat diets.[245]

When healthy predominately Hispanic preschool children in New York City reduced their fat intake to ≤30% kcal, their intakes of calcium and phosphorus were significantly reduced (Figure 2.12).[246] In another study using computer simulation dietary approaches to lower the fat intake of preschoolers, Sigman-Grant et al.[247] expressed concern that the nutritional intake of the children may be compromised. This study provided many options to reduce fat intake. However, the authors warned that utilization of more than one option to lower fat intake may result in insufficient energy and nutrient intake.[247] Although switching to skim (nonfat) milk was regarded as the "simplest" way to reduce the preschoolers' fat intake, actual acceptance of this food by the children was unknown.[247] Some children have demonstrated their dislike for skim (nonfat) milk.[254] If children drink less milk because they do not like the taste of lowfat milk, risk of calcium and other nutrient deficiencies increases.

Also, when fat free milk is substituted for higher fat versions to meet a child's recommended three cups a day, the diet may not provide sufficient energy. Fat restricted diets imposed by well-intentioned parents have led to growth failure in young children due to inadequate intake of energy, vitamins, and minerals.[254-256] When 663 children aged 8 to 10 years with elevated total and LDL cholesterol levels participated in the DISC study for three years, those who consumed a lowfat diet (28% of calories) had lower intakes of calcium, zinc, magnesium, phosphorus, vitamin B_{12}, thiamin, niacin, and riboflavin than children who consumed higher fat diets.[248] The researchers suggest that "adequate consumption of lean meats, fish, or poultry and non-fat dairy products when following a reduced fat diet will help ensure adequate intakes of zinc and calcium."[248]

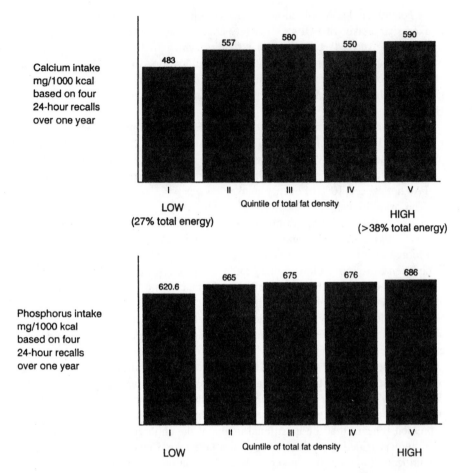

Figure 2.12 Intakes of calcium and phosphorus according to quintiles of total fat density in children. (Adapted from Shea, S., et al., *Pediatrics*, 92, 579, 1993. With permission.)

It is unnecessary to eliminate any food, including a specific dairy food, to meet dietary guidelines for fat intake. According to the American Academy of Pediatrics,[31] "if foods high in total fat, and cholesterol are eaten, they can be compensated for by eating less of these nutrients at other times. Because no single food item provides all the essential nutrients in the amounts needed, choosing a wide variety of food from all the food groups will ensure an adequate diet." This position is similar to that taken by the Joint Working Group of the Canadian Pediatric Society and Health Canada.[32] Following an extensive review of available scientific evidence, the Joint Working Group concluded that the dietary fat recommendations for adults are inappropriate for children until linear growth has stopped. Recognizing the need for flexibility in fat intake to meet children's energy needs for growth, development, and activity, the Joint Working Group did not specify a numerical target for total fat intake for children.[32] The 1995 Dietary Guidelines for Americans,[30] for the first time, recognized the unique nutritional needs of children. The Guidelines recommend that after the age of two years, children should "gradually adopt a diet that, by about five years of age, contains no more than 30% of calories from fat." The American Heart Association [6] and the American Academy of Pediatrics [31] also support this position. This advice encourages children to gradually transition to a lower fat diet between the ages of two and five years of age.

Adults who self-select lowfat (≤30% kcal) diets also may be at risk of deficiencies of nutrients, especially calcium, zinc, vitamin B_6, and magnesium.[249-253] According to an analysis of the 1987-88 Nationwide Food Consumption Survey, nutrient adequacy of the diet improves with increased fat intake.[250] In general, diets of adults participating in the survey did not simultaneously meet the goals of low energy from fat (30% kcal) and nutritional adequacy.[251] When the food group choices of young adults aged 18 to 24 years were examined, vitamin E, calcium, and zinc intakes were below two-thirds of recommended intakes in women whose diets contained 30% or less of energy from fat.[249] In contrast, women consuming higher fat diets (>30% of energy) had higher intakes of vitamins and minerals. In this study, men consuming lowfat diets had calcium intakes below recommended levels.[249] In a study of 107 women participating in a four-week hospital wellness program, women instructed to reduce fat (≤30% of energy) and cholesterol (<300 mg) intake tended to plan diets low in calcium and iron.[251]

According to a recent analysis of the diets of over 6,000 middle-aged men participating in the Multiple Risk Factor Intervention Trial (MRFIT), men at risk of CHD who switched to a lowfat diet often decreased their intakes of calcium, vitamin D, iron, and zinc.[252] Similar findings were reported in another investigation of the nutrient intakes of 409 adults following the NCEP Step I and II diets for six months.[253] Women who followed the lowfat diet advice significantly reduced their intakes of calcium and other nutrients such as vitamins D and E which were already low in their diets.[253] Men following these diets had low intakes of vitamin E and zinc. Women's low intakes of calcium and vitamin D were attributed to their low intake of milk. The findings of this study led the authors to recommend that "assessment and counseling for cholesterol-lowering diets should include attention to lowfat sources of calcium and zinc in women, and zinc in men."[253]

C. Dietary Compliance

A major problem with following lowfat (≤30% of energy) diets, especially among free-living populations, is long term adherence to such diets.[82,257-259] Prolonged compliance to diets reduced in fat and cholesterol is difficult even for individuals who receive intensive training and follow the diet initially.[257] In a 12-week study which followed over 100 patients with high blood cholesterol levels, compliance (as determined by changes in blood lipid and lipoprotein levels and from dietary records) to a lowfat (≤30% of energy), low cholesterol (≤300 mg/dl) diet was sustained in only 30% of the patients even after an initial three months of intensive diet training.[257] In another study, women participating in the Women's Health Trial were more likely to maintain a lowfat diet if they switched to lowfat versions of foods they normally consumed (except for cheese) and used lowfat cooking methods.[258] In contrast, compliance to a lowfat diet was more problematic if the women consistently avoided certain foods (e.g., meat, ice cream) and fats normally used as flavoring (e.g., butter).[258] Men participating in the MRFIT were more likely to adhere to a lowfat diet if they were older, did not drink alcohol or smoke, did not frequently eat away from home, had high blood cholesterol and blood pressure levels, and experienced fewer stressful life events.[260] A recent multicenter intervention trial involving 560 adults at risk of CHD who received either prepackaged foods or nutrition guidance on lowfat diets found that compliance was better in individuals receiving the pre-packaged foods (47%) than in those who self-selected lowfat diets (8%).[261] The adults receiving the prepackaged foods also consumed twice as much calcium and higher intakes of other nutrients than those who self-selected lowfat diets.[261] In general, the more restrictive the diet, the poorer the compliance.[82]

D. The Role of Various Dairy Foods in Meeting Dietary Guidelines for Fat Intake

The American Dietetic Association's 1997 Nutrition Trends Survey[262] found that 40% of consumers believed that they had to give up their favorite foods to have a healthful diet. Yet studies indicate that all foods can be included in a healthful diet. According to a computer analysis, individuals can choose from a variety of fat-reducing methods tailored to their tastes, lifestyles, and family's food choices.[263] This analysis indicates that individuals can meet recommended dietary goals for fat and cholesterol by making a variety of relatively simple dietary changes without reducing the amount of or eliminating foods such as whole milk or substituting lowfat for whole milk. Consequently, individuals who prefer the taste of whole milk over lower fat (2%, 1%, or fat free) milk can still meet their total fat goal by making other selections, for example, choosing only lean meats and reduced fat salad dressings.[263]

According to a recent analysis of the usage and impact of fat-modified products, adults who used two or three fat reduction strategies (e.g., fat free milk, lean meats, fat-modified products) achieved diets containing 30% or less of fat from calories, less than 10% of calories from saturated fat, reduced total calories, and high in vitamins and minerals.[264] The author states that energy and nutrient needs vary among individuals and that "all foods can fit into the boundaries of both micro- and macronutrient needs."[264] When eight healthy male volunteers aged 20 to 36 years consumed diets meeting the American Heart Association recommendations, plus one cup of whole or fat free milk per 1000 kcal of diet for six weeks, both of the milk diets provided a substantial reduction in fat intake compared to the subjects' usual diet.[156] Plasma total and LDL cholesterol levels were decreased on both milk diets compared with the baseline diet, although the reductions in blood total and LDL cholesterol were greater when the fat free milk was consumed.[156] Similar findings related to the inclusion of fast foods in a lowfat diet were reported by Davidson et al.[265] These investigators concluded that "familiar foods with a higher fat content in the context of a well-counseled balanced diet do not need to be sacrificed to comply with the goals of the NCEP."[265]

V. SUMMARY

Single nutrients have been demonstrated to have unique effects on blood lipid levels. Some dairy food nutrients (e.g., SFAs such as palmitic, myristic, and lauric acids, and cholesterol) are hypercholesterolemic, whereas others (e.g., MUFAs, PUFAs, the SFA stearic acid, medium chain SFAs) may have a modest hypocholesterolemic effect in comparison with longer chain SFAs. The effect of any single nutrient on blood lipid levels is highly individualized, in large part because of genetic variability. In addition, the effects of single nutrients may be different when delivered in the complex matrix of food and the overall diet.

There is little evidence from scientific studies which have examined foods, rather than specific nutrients, that dairy foods contribute to an atherogenic blood profile when consumed in recommended amounts. In studies in which various milks or culture-containing dairy products such as yogurt are consumed in moderate amounts, blood lipid levels generally do not increase.

To enhance the quality of life and reduce the risk of major chronic diseases including CHD, federal government agencies and nationally recognized health organizations recommend that the general healthy population two years of age and older consume a diet that provides no more than 30% of energy as fat, no more than 10% of energy as saturated fat, and 300 mg cholesterol or less a day. Research indicates that not everyone will receive the predicted CHD benefit from following these dietary recommendations. In fact, the Joint Working Group of the Canadian Pediatric Society and Health Canada, following an extensive review of scientific evidence concluded that a numerical target for total fat intake for children is inappropriate, and dietary fat recommendations for adults should not apply to children until after linear growth has stopped. The 1995 Dietary Guidelines for Americans, the American Heart Association, and the American Academy of Pediatrics each recommend that children between the ages of two and five years gradually adopt a diet that contains no more than 30% of energy as fat.

Some studies report that lowfat diets are ineffective in reducing CHD and improving life expectancy, and lead to potential health risks (e.g., nutritional inadequacies). In addition, only a proportion of the U.S. population responds to the fat content of the diets with a significant change in blood lipids and an even smaller portion is responsive to the cholesterol content of their diets. Scientists are identifying genes that influence blood lipid and lipoprotein levels and individuals' responses to specific dietary interventions. This genetic information one day may allow identification of individuals most likely to benefit from consuming a lowfat diet (or other intervention). These considerations, along with the difficulty experienced by many in adhering to fat-restricted diets, are resulting in increased emphasis on an individualized approach to identifying and treating CHD.

Improved identification of individuals at high risk of CHD and of those who will benefit most from specific interventions can be expected to improve health, reduce mortality, and decrease healthcare costs. Individuals who need to follow a lowfat diet can choose from a variety of fat-reducing strategies which can include all dairy foods. There are no "good" foods or "bad" foods relative to blood cholesterol levels or CHD risk. If an individual consumes favorite foods (e.g., whole milk, ice cream) in moderation and reduces fat intake by making other personal food choices (e.g., choosing lowfat salad dressings, fewer snack foods such as potato chips), compliance to a fat reduced diet can improve.

For a healthy vigorous existence for as long as possible, it is important to consume a variety of foods from each of the major food groups in moderation. Also important in the prevention and treatment of CHD is consideration of the individual's total risk profile (i.e., body weight, physical activity, cigarette smoking, etc.). Recognition of the variety of genetic and environmental (dietary and nondietary) factors involved in the development of CHD is leading health professionals to move away from "one-size-fits-all" dietary recommendations to more individualized guidance. As stated by Kritchevsky,[266] "the cause of heart disease, particularly CHD, is not as cut and dried as it may have appeared to be only a few short years ago." Better targeting of dietary interventions to reduce CHD can improve their effectiveness and lower costs. A narrow focus on a single food, food group, or diet can be counterproductive and may, in fact, be deleterious to health.

REFERENCES

1. American Heart Association, *1997 Heart and Stroke Statistical Update,* American Heart Association, Dallas, TX,1997.
2. U.S. Department of Health and Human Services, Public Health Service, Centers for Disease Control, National Center for Health Statistics, *Healthy People 2000 Review 1995-96*, DHHS Pub. No. (PHS) 96-1256, Hyattsville, MD, November 1996.
3. American Heart Association, Economic cost of cardiovascular diseases, www.americanheart.org/Scientific/HSstats98/10econom.htm1, 1998.
4. Department of Health and Human Services, Public Health Service, *Healthy People 2000: National Health Promotion and Disease Prevention Objectives,* Full Report, with commentary, U.S. Government Printing Office,Washington, D.C., 1990.
5. National Cholesterol Education Program (NCEP), Summary of the Second Report of the National Cholesterol Education Program (NCEP) Expert Panel on Detection, Evaluation, and Treatment of High Blood Cholesterol in Adults (Adult Treatment Panel 11), *JAMA*, 269, 3015, 1993.
6. American Heart Association, Nutrition Committee, Dietary guidelines for healthy American adults, *Circulation*, 94, 1795, 1996.
7. Pasternak, R. C., Grundy, S. M., Levy, D., and Thompson, P. D., Spectrum of risk factors for coronary heart disease, *J. Am. Coll. Cardiol.,* 27, 978, 1996.
8. *Surgeon General's Report on Nutrition and Health*, DHHS (PHS) Publ. No. 88-50210, U.S. Government Printing Office, Washington, D.C., 1988.
9. Committee on Diet and Health, Food and Nutrition Board, Commission on Life Sciences, National Research Council, *Diet and Health: Implications for Reducing Chronic Disease Risk,* National Academy Press, Washington, D.C., 1989.
10. National Cholesterol Education Program (NCEP), Report of the National Cholesterol Education Program (NCEP) Expert Panel on Population Strategies for Blood Cholesterol Reduction, Bethesda, MD, U.S. Department of Health and Human Services, Public Health Service, National Institutes of Health, National Heart, Lung and Blood Institute, February 1990.

11. National Cholesterol Education Program (NCEP), Report of the National Cholesterol Education Program (NCEP) Expert Panel on Blood Cholesterol Levels In Children And Adolescents, Bethesda, MD, U.S. Department of Health and Human Services, Public Health Service, National Institutes of Health, National Heart, Lung, and Blood Institute, April 1991.

12. McNamara, D. J., Dietary fatty acids, lipoproteins, and cardiovascular disease, *Advances in Food and Nutrition Res.*, 36, 253, 1992.

13. Kris-Etherton, P. M. and Yu, S., Individual fatty acid effects on plasma lipids and lipoproteins: human studies, *Am. J. Clin. Nutr.*, 65(Suppl.), 1628s, 1997.

14. Grundy, S. M., What is the desirable ratio of saturated, polyunsaturated, and monoun-saturated fatty acids in the diet? *Am. J. Clin. Nutr.*, 66(Suppl.), 988s, 1997.

15. FASEB and LSRO, Evaluation of publicly available scientific evidence regarding certain nutrient-disease relationships, 9. Lipids and cardiovascular disease, November 1991.

16. Stamler, J., Wentforth, D., and Neaton, J. D., Is relationship between serum cholesterol and risk of premature death from coronary heart disease continuous and graded? Findings in 356,222 primary screenees of the Multiple Risk Factor Intervention Trial (MRFIT), *JAMA*, 256, 2823, 1986.

17. NIH Consensus Development Panel on Triglyceride, High-Density Lipoprotein, and Coronary Heart Disease, Triglyceride, high-density lipoprotein, and coronary heart disease, *JAMA*, 269, 505, 1993.

18. Katan, M. B., High-oil compared with low-fat, high-carbohydrate diets in the prevention of ischemic heart disease, *Am. J. Clin. Nutr.*, 66(Suppl.), 974s, 1997.

19. Freedman, D. S., Otvos, J. D., Jeyarajah, E. J., Barboriak, J. J., Anderson, A. J., and Walker, J. A., Relation of lipoprotein subclasses as measured by proton nuclear magnetic resonance spectroscopy to coronary artery disease, *Arterioscler. Thromb. Vasc. Biol.*, 18, 1046, 1998.

20. Austin, M. A., Breslow, J. L., Hennekens, C. H., Buring, J. E., Willett, W. C., and Krauss, R. M., Low-density lipoprotein subclass patterns and risk of myocardial infarction, *JAMA*, 260, 1917, 1988.

21. Lipid Research Clinics Program, The Lipid Research Clinics coronary primary prevention study II., The relationship of reduction in incidence of coronary heart disease to cholesterol lowering, *JAMA*, 251, 365, 1984.

22. Grundy, S. M. and Denke, M. A., Dietary influences on serum lipids and lipoproteins, *J. Lipid Res.*, 31, 1149, 1990.

23. Hegsted, D. M., Ausman, L. M., Johnson, J. A., and Dallal, G. E., Dietary fat and serum lipids: an evaluation of the experimental data, *Am. J. Clin. Nutr.*, 57, 875, 1993.

24. Howell, W. H., McNamara, D. J., Tosca, M. A., Smith, B. T., and Gaines, J. A., Plasma lipid and lipoprotein responses to dietary fat and cholesterol: a meta-analysis, *Am. J. Clin. Nutr.*, 65, 1747, 1997.

25. Clarke, R., Frost, C., Collins, R., Appleby, P., and Peto, R., Dietary lipids and blood cholesterol: quantitative meta-analysis of metabolic ward studies, *Br. Med. J.*, 314, 112, 1997.

26. Gardner, C. D., Fortmann, S. P., and Krauss, R. M., Association of small low-density lipoprotein particles with the incidence of coronary artery disease in men and women, *JAMA*, 276, 875, 1996.

27. Hegsted, D. M., McGandy, R. B., Myers, M. L., and Stare, F. J., Quantitative effects of dietary fat on serum cholesterol in man, *Am. J. Clin. Nutr.*, 17, 281, 1965.

28. Yu, S., Derr, J., Etherton, T. D., and Kris-Etherton, P. M., Plasma cholesterol predictive equations demonstrate that stearic acid is neutral and monounsaturated fatty acids are hypocholesterolemic, *Am. J. Clin. Nutr.,* 61, 1129, 1995.

29. Mensink, R. P. and Katan, M. B., Effect of dietary fatty acids on serum lipids and lipoproteins in a meta-analysis of 27 trials, *Arterioscler. Thromb.,* 12, 911, 1992.

30. U.S. Department of Agriculture and U.S. Department of Health and Human Services, *Nutrition and Your Health: Dietary Guidelines for Americans,* 4th Ed., Home and Garden Bulletin No. 232, Washington, D.C., USDA/DHHS, 1995.

31. American Academy of Pediatrics, Committee on Nutrition, Cholesterol in children, *Pediatrics,* 101, 141, 1998.

32. Zlotkin, S. H., A review of the Canadian "Nutrition Recommendations Update: Dietary Fat and Children," *J. Nutr.,* 126, 1022s, 1996.

33. U.S. Department of Agriculture, Agricultural Research Service, Data tables: results from USDA's 1996 Continuing Survey of Food Intakes by Individuals and 1996 Diet and Health Knowledge Survey, ARS Food Surveys Research Group, www.barc.usda.gov/bhnrc/foodsurvey/home.htm.

34. Department of Health and Human Services, Food and Drug Administration, Food Labeling: health claims and label statements; dietary saturated fat and cholesterol and coronary heart disease, *Fed. Register,* 58(3), 2739, 1993 (Jan. 6).

35. Segall, J. J., Is milk a coronary health hazard?, *Br. J. Prev. Soc. Med.,* 31, 81, 1971.

36. Ney, D. M., Symposium: the role of the nutritional and health benefits in the marketing of dairy products. Potential for enhancing the nutritional properties of milk fat, *J. Dairy Sci.,* 74, 4002, 1991.

37. Nagaya, T., Yoshida, H., Hayashi, T., Takahashi, H., Kawai, M., and Matsuda, Y., Serum lipid profile in relation to milk consumption in a Japanese population, *J. Am. Coll. Nutr.,* 15(6), 625, 1996.

38. Gerrior, S. and Bente, L., Nutrient content of the U.S. food supply, 1909-94, U.S. Department of Agriculture, Center for Nutrition Policy and Promotion, Home Economics Research Report No. 53, 1997.

39. U.S. Department of Agriculture, Agricultural Research Service, Supplementary table set: food and nutrient intakes by individuals in the United States, 3 days, 1989-91, Continuing Survey of Food Intakes by Individuals, 1989-91 (in photocopy form only), 1995.

40. U.S. Department of Agriculture, Agricultural Research Service, Data tables: intakes of 19 individual fatty acids: results from 1994-96 Continuing Survey of Food Intakes by Individuals, ARS food surveys research group, www.barc.usda.gov/bhnrc/foodsurvey/home.htm.

41. Subar, A. F., Krebs-Smith, S. M., Cook, A., and Kahle, L. L., Dietary sources of nutrients among U.S. adults, 1989 to 1991, *J. Am. Diet. Assoc.,* 98, 537, 1998.

42. Subar, A. F., Krebs-Smith, S. M., Cook, A., and Kahle, L. L., Dietary sources of nutrients among US children, 1989-1991, *Pediatrics,* 102, 913, 1998.

43. Ney, D. M., Lai, H.-C., Lasekan, J. B., and Lefevre, M., Interrelationship of plasma triglycerides and HDL size and composition in rats fed different dietary saturated fats, *J. Nutr.,* 121, 1311, 1991.

44. CAST (Council for Agricultural Science and Technology), *Food Fats and Health,* Task Force Report No. 118., Council for Agricultural Science and Technology, Ames, Iowa, December 1991.

45. U.S. Department of Agriculture, Agricultural Research Service, USDA Nutrient Data-base for Standard Reference, Release 12, Nutrient Data Laboratory, www.nal.usda.gov/fnic/foodcomp, 1998.

46. Mensink, R. P., Effects of the individual saturated fatty acids on serum lipids and lipoprotein concentrations, *Am. J. Clin. Nutr.*, 57(Suppl.), 711, 1993.

47. Tholstrup, T., Marckmann, P., Jespersen, J., and Sandstrom, B., Fat high in stearic acid favorably affects blood lipids and factor VII coagulant activity in comparison with fats high in palmitic acid or high in myristic and lauric acids, *Am. J. Clin. Nutr.*, 59, 371, 1994.

48. Denke, M. A. and Grundy, S. M., Comparison of effects of lauric and palmitic acid on plasma lipids and lipoproteins, *Am. J. Clin. Nutr.*, 56, 895, 1992.

49. Temme, E. H., Mensink, R. P., and Hornstra, G., Comparison of the effects of diets enriched in lauric, palmitic, or oleic acids on serum lipids and lipoproteins in healthy women and men, *Am. J. Clin. Nutr.*, 63, 897, 1996.

50. Grundy, S. M., Influence of stearic acid on cholesterol metabolism relative to other long-chain fatty acids, *Am. J. Clin. Nutr.*, 60(Suppl.), 986, 1994.

51. Kritchevsky, D., Stearic acid metabolism and atherogenesis: history, *Am. J. Clin. Nutr.*, 60(Suppl.), 997, 1994.

52. Bonanome, A. and Grundy, S. M., Effect of dietary stearic acid on plasma cholesterol and lipoprotein levels, *N. Engl. J. Med.*, 318, 1244, 1988.

53. Denke, M. A. and Grundy, S. M., Effects of fats high in stearic acid on lipid and lipoprotein concentrations in men, *Am. J. Clin. Nutr.*, 54, 1036, 1991.

54. Ginsberg, H. N., Barr, S., Johnson, C., Karmally, W., Holleran, S., and Ramakrishnan, R., Comparison of the effects of AHA Step 1 diets enriched in dairy, meat, or coconut oil products on plasma lipids and lipoproteins in normal men, *Circulation*, 86(4), I-404 (Abstr.), 1992.

55. Keys, A., Anderson, J. T., and Grande, F., Serum cholesterol response to changes in the diet, IV, Particular saturated fatty acids in the diet, *Metab. Clin. Exp.*, 14, 776, 1965.

56. Wahrburg, U., Martin, H., Sandkamp, M., Schulte, H., and Assmann, G., Comparative effects of a recommended lipid-lowering diet vs a diet rich in monounsaturated fatty acids on serum lipid profiles in healthy young adults, *Am. J. Clin. Nutr.*, 56, 678, 1992.

57. Kris-Etherton, P. M., Derr, J., Mitchell, D. C., Mustad, V. A., Russell, M. E., McDon-nell, E. T., Salabsky, D., and Pearson, T. A., The role of fatty acid saturation on plasma lipids, lipoproteins, and apolipoproteins. I. Effects of whole food diets high in cocoa butter, olive oil, soybean oil, dairy butter, and milk chocolate on the plasma lipids of young men, *Metabolism*, 42(1), 121, 1993.

58. Harris, W. C., N-3 fatty acids and lipoproteins: comparisons of results from human and animal studies, *Lipids*, 31, 243, 1996.

59. Harris, W. S., N-3 fatty acids and serum lipoproteins: human studies, *Am. J. Clin. Nutr.*, 65(Suppl.), 1645, 1997.

60. Lichtenstein, A. H., Trans fatty acids, plasma lipid levels, and risk of developing cardiovascular disease, A statement for healthcare professionals from the American Heart Association, *Circulation*, 95, 2588, 1997.

61. Parodi, P. W., Distribution of isomeric octadecenoic fatty acids in milk fat, *J.Dairy Sci.*, 59, 1870, 1976.

62. Hunter, J. E. and Applewhite, T. H., Reassessment of trans fatty acid availability in the U.S. diet, *Am. J. Clin. Nutr.*, 54, 363, 1991.

63. Willett, W. C. and Asherio, A., Trans fatty acids: are the effects only marginal? *Am. J. Public Health*, 84, 722, 1994.

64. Zock, P. L. and Katan, M. B., Butter, margarine, and serum lipoprotein, *Atherosclerosis*, 13, 7, 1997.

65. Hu, F. B., Stampfer, M. J., Manson, J. E., Rimm, E., Colditz, G. A., Rosner, B. A., Hennekens, C. H., and Willett, W. C., Dietary fat intake and the risk of coronary heart disease in women, *N. Engl. J. Med.*, 337, 1491, 1997.

66. Feldman, E. B., Kris-Etherton, P. M., Kritchevsky, D., and Lichtenstein, A., for the ASCN/AIN Task Force on Trans Fatty Acids of the American Society for Clinical Nutrition and American Institute of Nutrition, Position paper on trans fatty acids, *Am. J. Clin. Nutr.*, 63, 663, 1996.

67. Report of the Expert Panel on Trans Fatty Acids and Coronary Heart Disease, Trans fatty acids and coronary heart disease risk, *Am. J. Clin. Nutr.*, 62(Suppl.), 655s, 1995.

68. Gillman, M. W., Cupples, L. A., Gagnon, D., Millen, B. E., Ellison, R. C., and Castelli, W. P., Margarine intake and subsequent coronary heart disease in men, *Epidemiology* 8, 144, 1997.

69. Ascherio, A., Rimm, E. B., Giovannucci, E. L., Spiegelman, D., Stampfer, M., and Willett, W. C., Dietary fat and risk of coronary heart disease in men: cohort follow up study in the United States, *Br. Med. J.*, 313, 84, 1996.

70. Aro, A., Jauhiainen, M., Partanen, R., Salminen, I., and Mutanen, M., Stearic acid, trans fatty acids, and dairy fat: effects on serum and lipoprotein lipids, apolipoproteins, lipoprotein (a), and lipid transfer proteins in healthy subjects, *Am. J. Clin. Nutr.*, 65, 1419, 1997.

71. Pietinen, P., Ascherio, A., Korhonen, P., Hartman, A. M., Willett, W. C., Albanes, D., and Virtamo, J., Intake of fatty acids and risk of coronary heart disease in a cohort of Finnish men: the Alpha Tocopherol, Beta-Carotene Cancer Prevention Study, *Am. J. Epidemiol.*, 145, 876, 1997.

72. Bernier, L. A., Roundtable discussion on milk fat, dairy foods, and coronary heart disease risk, *J. Nutr.*, 123, 1175, 1993.

73. Mensink, R. P. and Katan, M. B., Effect of dietary trans fatty acids on high-density and low-density lipoprotein cholesterol levels in healthy subjects, *N. Engl. J. Med.*, 323, 439, 1990.

74. Katan, M. B., Commentary on the supplement, Trans fatty acids and coronary heart disease risk, *Am. J. Clin. Nutr.*, 62, 518, 1995.

75. Sundram, K., Ismail, A., Hayes, K. C., Jeyamalar, R., and Pathmanathan R., Trans (elaidic) fatty acids adversely affect the lipoprotein profile relative to specific saturated fatty acids in humans, *J. Nutr.*, 127, 514s, 1997.

76. Shapiro, S., Do trans fatty acids increase the risk of coronary artery disease? A critique of the epidemiologic evidence, *Am. J. Clin. Nutr.*, 66(Suppl.), 1011s, 1997.

77. Lee, K. N., Kritchevsky, D., and Pariza, M. W., Conjugated linoleic acid and atherosclerosis in rabbits, *Atherosclerosis*, 108, 19, 1994.

78. Nicolosi, R. J., Rogers, E. J., Kritchevsky, D., Scimeca, J. A., and Huth, P. J., Dietary conjugated linoleic acid reduces plasma lipoproteins and early aortic atherosclerosis in hypercholesterolemic hamsters, *Artery,* 22(5), 266, 1997.

79. Kobayaski, T., Shimizugawa, T., Osakabe, T., Watanabe, S., and Okuyama, H., A long-term feeding of sphingolipids affected the levels of plasma cholesterol and hepatic tricyglycerol but not tissue phospholipids and sphingolipids, *Nutr. Res.*, 17(1), 111, 1997.

80. Schaefer, E. J., Lichtenstein, A. H., Lamon-Fava, S., McNamara, J. R., Schaefer, M. M., Rasmussen, H., and Ordovas M., Body weight and low-density lipoprotein cholesterol changes after consumption of a low-fat ad libitum diet, *JAMA*, 274, 1450, 1995.

81. Katan, M. B., Effect of low-fat diets on plasma high-density lipoprotein concentrations, *Am. J. Clin. Nutr.*, 67(Suppl.), 573s, 1998.

82. Oliver, M. F., It is more important to increase the intake of unsaturated fats than to decrease the intake of saturated fats: evidence from clinical trials relating to ischemic heart disease, *Am. J. Clin. Nutr.*, 66(Suppl.), 980s, 1997.

83. Hu, F. B., Stampfer, M. J., Manson, J. E., Rimm, E., Colditz, G. A., Rosner, B. A., Hennekens, C. H., and Willett, W. C., Dietary fat intake and the risk of coronary heart disease in women, *N. Engl. J. Med.*, 337, 1491, 1997.

84. Morgan, S. A., O'Dea, K., and Sinclair, A. J., A low-fat diet supplemented with monounsaturated fat results in less HDL-C lowering than a very-low-fat diet, *J. Am. Diet. Assoc.*, 97, 151, 1997.

85. Lichtenstein, A. H. and Van Horn, L., for the Nutrition Committee, Very lowfat diets, *Circulation*, 98, 935, 1998.

86. Ginsberg, H. N., Karmally, W., Siddiqui, M., Holleran, S., Tall, A. R., Blaner, W. S., and Ramakrishnan, R., Increases in dietary cholesterol are associated with modest increases in both LDL and HDL cholesterol in healthy young women, *Arterioscler. Thromb. Vasc. Biol.*, 15, 169, 1995.

87. McNamara, D. J., Cholesterol intake and plasma cholesterol: an update, *J. Am. Coll. Nutr.*, 16(6), 530, 1997.

88. McNamara, D. J., Kolb, R., Parker, T. S., Batwin, H., Samuel, P., Brown, C. D., and Ahrens, E. H., Jr., Heterogeneity of cholesterol homeostasis in man: Response to changes in dietary fat quality and cholesterol quantity, *J. Clin. Invest.*, 79, 1729, 1987.

89. Clifton, P. M. and Nestel, P. J., Effect of dietary cholesterol on postprandial lipoproteins in three phenotypic groups, *Am. J. Clin. Nutr.*, 64, 361, 1996.

90. Lovati, M. R., West, C. E., Sirtori, C. R., and Beynen, A. C., Dietary animal proteins and cholesterol metabolism in rabbits, *Br. J. Nutr.*, 64, 473, 1990.

91. Anonymous, Casein versus soy protein: further elucidation of their differential effect on serum cholesterol in rabbits, *Nutr. Rev.*, 49, 121, 1991.

92. Terpstra, A. H. M., Holmes, J. C., and Nicolosi, R. J., The hypocholesterolemic effect of dietary soybean protein vs. casein in hamsters fed cholesterol-free or cholesterol-enriched semipurified diets, *J. Nutr.*, 121, 944, 1991.

93. Meinertz, H., Nilausen, K., and Faergeman, O., Soy protein and casein in cholesterol-enriched diets: effects on plasma lipoproteins in normolipidemic subjects, *Am. J. Clin. Nutr.*, 50, 786, 1989.

94. Forsythe, W. A., Green, M. S., and Anderson, J. J. B., Dietary protein effects on cholesterol and lipoprotein concentrations: a review, *J. Am. Coll. Nutr.*, 5, 533, 1986.

95. Potter, S. M., Bakhit, R., Essex-Sorlie, D., Weingartner, K., Chapman, K., Winter, L., Nelson, A., Nelson, R., Ham, J., Savage, W., Prabhudesai, M., and Erdman, J. W., Jr., Depression of plasma cholesterol in men by consumption of baked products containing soy protein, *Am. J. Clin. Nutr.*, 58, 501, 1993.

96. Bakhit, R. M., Klein, B. P., Essex-Sorlie, D., Ham, J. O., Erdman, J. W., Jr., and Potter, S. M., Intake of 25 g of soybean protein with or without soybean fiber alters plasma lipids in men with elevated cholesterol concentrations, *J. Nutr.*, 124, 213, 1994.

97. Guermani, L., Villaume, C., Bau, H.-M., Mejean, L., and Nicolas, J. P. Effect of different kinds of dietary casein on blood cholesterol and triglycerides in pair fed rats, *Nutrition*, 8, 101, 1992.

98. Samman, S., Khosla, P., and Carroll, K. K., Influence of dietary minerals on apolipoprotein B metabolism in rabbits fed semipurified diets containing casein, *Atherosclerosis*, 82, 69, 1990.

99. Kritchevsky, D., Tepper, S. A., Czarnecki, S. K., Klurfeld, D. M., and Story, J. A., Experimental atherosclerosis in rabbits fed cholesterol-free diets. 9. Beef protein and textured vegetable protein, *Atherosclerosis*, 39, 169, 1981.

100. Beynen, A. C. and Sugano, M., Dietary protein as a regulator of lipid metabolism: State of the art and new perspectives, *J. Nutr. Sci. Vitaminol.*, 36(Suppl.), 1, 185, 1990.

101. Sakono, M., Fukuyama, T., Ni, W. H., Nagao, K., Ju, H. R., Sato, M., Sakata, N., Iwamoto, H., and Imaizumi, K., Comparison between dietary soybean protein and casein of the inhibitory effect on atherogenesis in the thoracic aorta of hypercholesterolemic (ExHc) rats treated with experimental hypervitamin D, *Biosci. Biotechnol. Biochem.*, (Japan), 61, 514, 1997.

102. Messina, M. and Erdman, J. W., Jr. Eds., First international symposium on the role of soy in preventing and treating chronic disease, *J. Nutr.*, 125(Suppl.), 567s, 1995.

103. Weishaar, R. E. and Simpson, R. U., The involvement of the endocrine system in regulating cardiovascular function: emphasis on vitamin D_3, *Endocrine Rev.*, 10, 351, 1989.

104. Weishaar, R. E. and Simpson, R. U., Vitamin D_3 and cardiovascular function in rats, *J. Clin. Invest.*, 79, 1706, 1987.

105. Weishaar, R. E. and Simpson, R. U., Vitamin D_3 and cardiovascular function, II., Direct and indirect effects, *Am. J. Physiol.*, 253, E675, 1987.

106. Weishaar, R. E., Kim, S.-N., Saunders, D. E., and Simpson, R. U., Involvement of vitamin D_3 with cardiovascular function, III., Effects on physical and morphological properties, *Am. J. Physiol.*, 258, E134, 1990.

107. Simpson, R. U. and Weishaar, R. E., Involvement of 1,25 dihydroxyvitamin D_3 in regulating myocardial calcium metabolism: Physiological and pathological actions, *Cell Calcium*, 9, 285, 1988.

108. Food and Drug Administration, Department of Health, Education, and Welfare, Milk and cream, Title 21, Part 18., *Fed. Regist.*, 38, 27924, 1973.

109. IOM (Institute of Medicine), *Dietary Reference Intakes for Calcium, Phosphorus, Magnesium, Vitamin D, and Fluoride,* Standing Committee on the Scientific Evaluation of Dietary Reference Intakes, Food and Nutrition Board, National Academy Press, Washington, D.C., 1997.

110. O'Connell, T. D., and Simpson, R. U., 1,25-dihydroxyvitamin D_3 regulation of myocardial growth and c-myc levels in the rat heart, *Biochem. Biophys. Res. Commun.*, 213, 59, 1995.

111. Morris, G. S., Zhou, Q., Hegsted, M., and Keenan, M. J., Maternal consumption of a low vitamin D diet retards metabolic and contractile development in the neonatal rat heart, *J. Mol. Cell. Cardiol.*, 27, 1245, 1995.

112. Simpson, R. U., Thomas, G. A., and Arnold, A. J., Identification of 1,25-dihydroxy vitamin D_3 receptors and activities in muscle, *J. Biol. Chem.*, 260, 8882, 1985.

113. Shane, E., Mancini, D., Aaronson, K., Silverberg, S. J., Seibel, M. J., Addesso, V., and McMahon, D. J., Bone mass, vitamin D deficiency, and hyperparathyroidism in congestive heart failure, *Am. J. Med.*, 103, 197, 1997.

114. Watson, K. E., Abrolat, M. L., Malone, L. L., Hoeg, J. M., Doherty, T., Detrano, R., and Demer, L.L., Active serum vitamin D levels are inversely correlated with coronary calcification, *Circulation*, 96, 1755, 1997.

115. Brunvand, L., Haga, P., Tangsrud, S. E., and Haug, E., Congestive heart failure caused by vitamin D deficiency? *Acta Pediatr.*, 84, 106, 1995.

116. Krauss, R. M., Genetic influences on lipoprotein response to dietary fat and cholesterol: an overview, *Am. J. Clin. Nutr.*, 62, 457s, 1995.

117. Berdanier, C. D., Ed., *Nutrients and Gene Expression*, CRC Press, Boca Raton, FL, 1996.

118. Simopoulos, A. P., *Genetic Variation and Dietary Response*, Karger, New York, 1997.

119. Dreon, D. M. and Krauss, R. M., Diet-gene interactions in human lipoprotein metabolism, *J. Am. Coll. Nutr.*, 16, 313, 1997.

120. Hopkins, P. N., Effects of dietary cholesterol on serum cholesterol: a metaanalysis and review, *Am. J. Clin. Nutr.*, 55, 1060, 1992.

121. Katan, M. B., Beynen, A. C., and de Vries, J. H. M., Existence of consistent hypo- and hyperresponders to dietary cholesterol in man, *Am. J. Epidemiol.*, 123, 221, 1986.

122. Quivers, E. S., Driscoll, D. J., Garvey, C. D., Harris, A. M., Harrison, J., Huse, D. M., Martaugh, P., and Weidman, W. H., Variability in response to a low-fat, low-cholesterol diet in children with elevated low-density lipoprotein cholesterol levels, *Pediatrics*, 89, 925, 1992.

123. Schaefer, E. J., Lamon-Fava, S., Ausman, L. M., Ordovas, J. M., Clevidence, B. A., Judd, J. T., Goldin, B. R., Woods, M., Gorbach, S., and Lichtenstein, A. H., Individual variability in lipoprotein cholesterol response to National Cholesterol Education Program Step 2 diets, *Am. J. Clin. Nutr.*, 65, 823, 1997.

124. Denke, M. A. and Grundy, S. M., Individual responses to a cholesterol-lowering diet in 50 men with moderate hypercholesterolemia, *Arch. Intern. Med.*, 154(3), 317, 1994.

125. Denke, M. A., Review of human studies evaluating individual dietary responsiveness in patients with hypercholesterolemia, *Am. J. Clin. Nutr.*, 62(Suppl.), 471s, 1995.

126. Carmena-Ramon, R., Ascaso, J. F., Real, J. T., Ordovas, J. M., and Carmena, R., Genetic variation at the ApoA-IV gene locus and response to diet in familial hypercholesterolemia, *Artherioscler. Thromb. Vasc. Biol.*, 18, 1266, 1998.

127. Ordovas, J. M., Lopez-Miranda, J., Mata, P., Perez-Jimenez, F., Lichtenstein, A. H., and Schaefer, E. J., Gene-diet interaction in determining plasma lipid response to dietary intervention, *Atherosclerosis*, 118(Suppl.), 11s, 1995.

128. Gylling, H., Konula, K., Koivisto, U. M., Mittinen, H. E., and Miettinen, T. A., Polymorphisms of the genes encoding apoproteins A-1, B, C-III, and E and LDL receptor, and cholesterol and LDL metabolism during increased cholesterol intake. Common alleles of the apoprotein E gene show the greatest regulatory impact, *Arterioscler. Thromb. Vasc. Biol.*, 17, 38, 1997.

129. Breslow, J. L., Deeb, S., Lalouel, J. M., LeBoeuf, R., Schaefer, E. J., Tyrder, H. A., Wilson, P., and Young, S., Genetic susceptibility to atherosclerosis, *Circulation*, 80, 724, 1989.

130. Mahley, R. W., Weisgraber, K. H., Innerarity, T. L., and Rall, S. C., Jr., Genetic defects in lipoprotein metabolism, *JAMA*, 265, 78, 1991.

131. Rubin, E. M., Krauss, R. M., Spangler, E. A., Verstuyft, J. G., and Clift, S. M., Inhibition of early atherogenesis in transgenic mice by human apolipoprotein AI, *Nature*, 353, 265, 1991.

132. Boomsma, D. I., Kaptein, A., Kempen, H. J. M., Leuven, J. A. G., and Princen, H. M. G., Lipoprotein (a): relation to other risk factors and genetic heritability, Results from a Dutch parent-twin study, *Atherosclerosis*, 99, 23, 1993.

133. Austin, M. A., King, K. M., Vranizan, K. M., and Krauss, R. M. Atherogenic lipoprotein phenotype: a proposed genetic marker for coronary heart disease risk, *Circulation*, 82, 495, 1990.

134. Nishina, P. M., Johnson, J. P., Naggert, J. K., and Krauss, R. M., Linkage of atherogenic lipoprotein phenotype to the low density lipoprotein receptor locus on the short arm of chromosome 19, *Proc. Natl. Acad. Sci. USA*, 89, 708, 1992.

135. Lamon-Fava, S., Jimenez, D., Christian, J. C., Fabsitz, R. R., Reed, T., Carmelli, D., Gastelli, W. P., Ordovas, J. M., Wilson, P. W. F., and Schaefer, E. J., The NHLBI twin study: heritability of apolipoprotein A-1, B, and low density lipoprotein subclasses and concordance for lipoprotein (a), *Atherosclerosis*, 91, 97, 1991.

136. Austin, M. A., King, M.-C., Vranizan, K. M., Newman, B., and Krauss, R. M., Inheritance of low-density lipoprotein subclass patterns: results of complex segregation analysis, *Am. J. Hum. Genet.*, 43, 838, 1988.

137. De Graaf, J., Swinkels, D. W., de Haan, A. F. J., Demacker, P. N. M., and Stalenhoef, A. F. H., Both inherited susceptibility and environmental exposure determine the low-density lipoprotein-subfraction pattern distribution in healthy Dutch families, *Am. J. Hum. Genet.*, 51, 1295, 1992.

138. Brown, M. S. and Goldstein, J. L., Teaching old dogmas new tricks, *Nature*, 330, 113, 1987.

139. Reilly, S. L., Ferrell, R. E., Kottke, B. A., and Sing, C. F., The gender-specific apolipoprotein E genotype influence on the distribution of plasma lipids and apolipoproteins in the population of Rochester, Minnesota, II., Regression relationships with concomitants, *Am. J. Hum. Genet.*, 51, 1311, 1992.

140. Dreon, D. M., Fernstrom, H. A., Miller, B., and Krauss, R. M., Low-density lipoprotein subclass patterns and lipoprotein response to a reduced fat diet in men, *FASEB J.*, 8, 121, 1994.

141. Krauss, R. M. and Dreon, D. M., Low-density-lipoprotein subclasses and response to a low-fat diet in healthy men, *Am. J. Clin. Nutr.*, 62, 478s, 1995.

142. Dreon, D. M., Fernstrom, H. H., Williams, P. T., and Krauss, R. M., LDL subclass patterns and lipoprotein response to a low-fat, high-carbohydrate diet in women, *Arterioscler. Thromb. Vasc. Biol.*, 17, 707, 1997.

143. La Belle, M., Austin, M. A., Rubin, E., Krauss, R. M., Linkage analysis of low-density lipoprotein subclass phenotypes and the apolipoprotein B gene, *Genetic Epidemiol.*, 8, 269, 1991.

144. Lamarche, B., Tchernof, A., Moorjani, S., Cantin, B., Dagenais, G. R., Lupien, P. J., and Despres, J.-P., Small, dense low-density lipoprotein particles as a predictor of the risk of ischemic heart disease in men, *Circulation*, 95, 69, 1997.

145. De Graaf, J., Hak-Lemmers, H. L. M., Hectors, M. P. C., Demacker, P. N. M., Hendriks, J. C. M., and Stalenhoef, A. F. H., Enhanced susceptibility to in vitro oxidation of the dense low density lipoprotein subfraction in healthy subjects, *Atherosclerosis*, 11(2), 298, 1991.

146. Tribble, D. L., Holl, L. G., Wood, P. D., and Krauss, R. M., Variations in oxidative susceptibility among six low density lipoprotein subfactions of differing density and particle size, *Atherosclerosis*, 93, 189, 1992.

147. Packard, C. J. and Shepard, J., Lipoprotein heterogeneity and apolipoprotein B metabolism, *Arterioscler. Thromb. Vasc. Biol.*, 17, 3542, 1997.

148. Bjornheden, T., Babyi, A., Bondjers, G., and Wiklund, O., Accumulation of lipoprotein fractions and subfractions in the arterial wall, determined in an in vitro perfusion system, *Atherosclerosis*, 123, 43, 1996.

149. Lopez-Miranda, J., Ordovas, J. M., Espino, A., Marin, C., Salas, J., Lopez-Segura, F., Jimenez-Perepera, J., and Perez-Jimenez, F., Influence of mutation in human apolipoprotein A-1 gene promoter on plasma LDL cholesterol response to dietary fat, *Lancet*, 343, 1246, 1994.

150. Lopez-Miranda, J., Jansen, S., and Ordovas, J. M., Influence of the Sst1 polymorphism at the apolipoprotein C-III gene locus on the plasma low-density-lipoprotein-cholesterol response to dietary monounsaturated fat, *Am. J. Clin. Nutr.*, 66, 97, 1997.

151. Jones, A. E., Murphy, J. L., Stolinski, M., and Wootton, S. A., The effect of age and gender on the metabolic disposal of [1-^{13}C] palmitic acid, *Europ. J. Clin. Nutr.*, 52, 22, 1998.

152. Callaway, C. W., Dietary guidelines for Americans, *J. Am. Coll. Nutr.*, 16(6), 510, 1997.

153. Richardson, T., The hypocholestermic effect of milk – a review, *J. Food Protect.*, 41, 226, 1978.

154. Howard, N. A. and Marks, J., Hypocholesterolemic effect of milk, *Lancet*, 2, 255, 1977.

155. Hitchins, A. D. and McDonough, F. E., Prophylactic and therapeutic aspects of fermented milk, *Am. J. Clin. Nutr.*, 49, 675, 1989.

156. Steinmetz, K. A., Childs, M. T., Stimson, C., Kushi, L. H., McGovern, P. G., Potter, J. D., and Yamanaka, W. K., Effect of consumption of whole milk and skim milk on blood lipid profiles in healthy men, *Am. J. Clin. Nutr.*, 59, 612, 1994.

157. Hepner, G., Fried, R., St. Jeor, S., Fusetti, L., and Morin, R., Hypocholesterolemic effect of yogurt and milk, *Am. J. Clin. Nutr.*, 32, 19, 1979.

158. Mann, G. V. and Spoerry, A., Studies of a surfactant and cholesteremia in the Masai, *Am. J. Clin. Nutr.*, 27, 464, 1974.

159. Mann, G. V., A factor in yogurt which lowers cholesteremia in man, *Atherosclerosis*, 26, 335, 1977.

160. Bazzare, T. L., Wu, S. L., and Yuhas, J. A., Total and HDL-cholesterol concentrations following yogurt and calcium supplementation, *Nutr. Rep. Int.*, 28, 1225, 1983.

161. Buonopane, G. J., Kilara, A., Smith, J. S., and McCarthy, R. D., Effect of skim milk supplementation on blood cholesterol concentration, blood pressure, and triglycerides in a free-living human population, *J. Am. Coll. Nutr.*, 11(1), 56, 1992.

162. Maruyama, C., Nakamura, M., Ito, M., and Ezawa, I., The effect of milk and skim milk intake on serum lipids and apoproteins in postmenopausal females, *J. Nutr. Sci. Vitaminol.*, 38, 203, 1992.

163. Rossouw, J. E., Burger, E.-M., van der Vyver, P., and Ferreira, J. J., The effect of skim milk, yogurt, and full cream milk on human serum lipids, *Am. J. Clin. Nutr.*, 34, 351, 1982.

164. Thompson, L. U., Jenkins, D. J. A., Amer, M. A. V., Reichert, R., Jenkins, A., and Kamulsky, J., The effect of fermented and unfermented milks on serum cholesterol, *Am. J. Clin. Nutr.*, 36, 1106, 1982.

165. Bierenbaum, M. L., Wolf, E., Raff, M., Maginnis, W. P., Amer, M. A., Kleyn, D., and Bisgeier, G., The effect of dietary calcium supplementation on blood pressure and sodium lipid levels: preliminary report, *Nutr. Rep. Int.*, 36, 1147, 1987.

166. Keim, N. L., Marlett, J. A., Amundson, C. H., and Hagenmann, L. D., Variability in cholesterolemic response of rats consuming skim milk, *J. Food Prot.*, 45, 541, 1982.

167. Kritchevsky, D., Tepper, S. A., Morrissey, R. B., Czarnecki, S. K., and Klurfeld, D. M., Influence of whole or skim milk on cholesterol metabolism in rats, *Am. J. Clin. Nutr.*, 32, 597, 1979.

168. Thakur, C. P. and Jha, A. N., Influence of milk, yoghurt and calcium on cholesterol-induced atherosclerosis in rabbits, *Atherosclerosis*, 39, 211, 1981.

169. Schneeman, B. O., Rice, R., and Richter, B. D., Reduction of plasma and hepatic triacylglycerides with whole milk-containing diets in rats, *J. Nutr.*, 119, 965, 1989.

170. Grunewald, K. K., Serum cholesterol levels in rats fed skim milk fermented by *Lactobacillus acidophilus*, *J. Food Sci.*, 47, 2078, 1982.

171. Danielson, A. D., Peo, E. R., Jr., Shahani, K. M., Lewis, A. J., Whalen, P. J., and Amer, M. A., Anticholesteremic property of *Lactobacillus acidophilus* yogurt fed to mature boars, *J. Anim. Sci.*, 67, 966, 1989.

172. Akalin, A. S., Gonc, S., and Duzel, S., Influence of yogurt and acidophilus yogurt on serum cholesterol levels in mice, *J. Dairy Sci.*, 80, 2721, 1997.

173. Beena, A. and Prasad, V., Effect of yogurt and bifidus yogurt fortified with skim milk powder, condensed whey and lactose-hydrolysed condensed whey on serum cholesterol and triacylglycerol levels in rats, *J. Dairy Sci.*, 64, 453, 1997.

174. Zommara, M., Tachibana, N., Sakono, M., Suzuki, Y., Oda, T., Hashiba, H., and Imaizumi, K., Whey from cultured skim milk decreases serum cholesterol and increases antioxidant enzymes in liver and red blood cells in rats, *Nutr. Res.*, 16(2), 293, 1996.

175. Mohan, B., Kadirvel, R., Natarajan, A., and Bhaskaran, M., Effect of probiotic supplementation on growth, nitrogen utilization, and serum cholesterol in broilers, *Br. Poult. Sci.*, 37, 395, 1996.

176. Naito, C., The effect of milk intake on serum cholesterol in healthy young females: randomized controlled studies, *Ann. NY Acad. Sci.*, 598, 482, 1990.

177. McNamara, D. J., Lowell, A. E., and Sabb, J. E., Effect of yogurt intake on plasma lipid and lipoprotein levels in normolipidemic males, *Atherosclerosis*, 79, 167, 1989.

178. Maruyama, C. and Ezawa, I., The effect of milk and skim milk intake on serum lipids and apoproteins in young females, *J. Nutr. Sci. Vitaminol.*, 37, 53, 1991.

179. Karanja, N., Morris, C. D., Rufolo, P., Snyder, G., Illingworth, D. R., and McCarron, D. A., Impact of increasing calcium in the diet on nutrient consumption, plasma lipids, and lipoproteins in humans, *Am. J. Clin. Nutr.*, 59, 900, 1994.

180. Hitchins, A. D., Wong, N. P., and McDonough, F. E., Effects of dietary lactose on serum cholesterol, triglycerol and calcium levels on selected serum and digestive enzyme activities in the rat, *Nutr. Rep. Int.*, 36, 773, 1987.

181. Karanja, N., Morris, C. D., Illingsworth, D. R., and McCarron, D. A., Plasma lipids and hypertension: response to calcium supplementation, *Am. J. Clin. Nutr.*, 45, 60, 1987.

182. Denke, M. A., Fox, M. M., and Schulte, M. C., Short-term dietary calcium fortification increases fecal saturated fat content and reduces serum lipids in men, *J. Nutr.*, 123, 1047, 1993.

183. Bell, L., Halstenson, C. E., Halstenson, C. J., Macres, M., and Keane, W. F., Cholesterol-lowering effects of calcium carbonate in patients with mild to moderate hypercholesterolemia, *Arch. Intern. Med.*, 152, 2441, 1992.

184. Groot, P. H. E., Grose, W. F. A., Dijkhuis-Stoffelsma, R., Fernandes, J., and Ambagtsheet, J. J., The effect of oral calcium carbonate administration on serum lipoproteins of children with familial hypercholesterolemia (type II-A), *Eur. J. Pediatr.*, 135, 81, 1980.

185. Bhattacharyya, A. K., Thera, C., Anderson, J. T., Grande, F., and Keyes, A., Dietary calcium and fat: effect on serum lipids and fecal excretion of cholesterol and its degradation in products in man, *Am. J. Clin. Nutr.*, 22, 1161, 1969.

186. Mitchell, W. D., Fyfe, T., and Smith, D. A., The effect of oral calcium on cholesterol metabolism, *J. Atheroscler. Res.*, 8, 913, 1968.

187. De Rodas, B. Z., Gilliland, S. E., and Maxwell, C.V., Hypocholesterolemic action of *Lactobacillus acidophilus* ATCC 43121 and calcium in swine with hypercholesterolemia induced by diet, *J. Dairy Sci.*, 79, 2121, 1996.

188. Jacques, H., Lavigne, C., Desrosiers, T., Giroux, I., and Hurley, C., The hypercholesterolemic effect of cod protein is reduced in the presence of high dietary calcium, *Can. J. Physiol. Pharmacol.*, 73, 465, 1995.

189. Abbott, R. D., Curb, J. D., Rodriguez, B. L., Sharp, D. S., Burchfiel, C. M., and Yano, K., Effect of dietary calcium and milk consumption on risk of thromboembolic stroke in older middle-aged men. The Honolulu Heart Program, *Stroke*, 27, 813, 1996.

190. Cox, C., Mann, J., Sutherland, W., Chisholm, A., and Skeaff, M., Effects of coconut oil, butter and safflower oil on lipids and lipoproteins in persons with moderately elevated cholesterol levels, *J. Lipid Res.*, 36, 1787, 1995.

191. Chisholm, A., Mann, J., Sutherland, W., Duncan, A., Skeaff, M., and Frampton, C., Effect on lipoprotein profile of replacing butter with margarine in a lowfat diet: randomised crossover study with hypercholesterolemic subjects, *Br. Med. J.*, 312, 931, 1996.

192. Flynn, M. A., Nolph, G. B., Sun, G. Y., Navidi, M., and Krause, G., Effects of cholesterol and fat modification of self-selected diets on serum lipids and their specific fatty acids on normocholesterolemic and hypercholesterolemic humans, *J. Am. Coll. Nutr.*, 10(2), 93, 1991.

193. Wood, R., Kubena, K., O'Brien, B., Tseng, S., and Martin, G., Effect of butter, mono- and polyunsaturated fatty acid-enriched butter, trans fatty acid margarine, and zero trans fatty acid margarine on serum lipids and lipoproteins in healthy men, *J. Lipid Res.*, 34(1),1, 1993.

194. Reaven, G. M., Looking at the world through LDL-cholesterol-colored glasses, *J. Nutr.*, 116, 1143, 1986.

195. Ockene, I. S. and Ma, Y., Low serum cholesterol: good or bad? *Med. Exerc. Nutr. Health*, 3, 63, 1994.

196. Muldoon, M. F., Bonci, L. J., Rodriguez, V., Kaplan, J. R., and Manuck, S. B., Health effects of serum cholesterol reduction: the potential for good and the potential for harm. *Med. Exerc. Nutr. Health*, 3, 74, 1994.

197. Ramsay, L. E., Yeo, W. W., and Jackson, P. R., Dietary reduction of serum cholesterol: time to think again, *Br. Med. J.*, 303, 953, 1991.

198. Hunninghake, D. B., Stein, E. A., Dujovne, C. A., Harris, W. S., Feldman, E. B., Miller, V. T., Tobert, J. A., Laskarzewski, P. M., Quiter, E., Held, J., Taylor, A. M., Hopper, S., Leonard, S. B., and Brewer, B. K., The efficacy of intensive dietary therapy alone or combined with Lovastatin in outpatients with hypercholesterolemia, *N. Engl. J. Med.*, 328, 1213, 1993.

199. Goldbourt, U., Yaari, S., and Medalie, J. H., Isolated low HDL cholesterol as a risk factor for coronary heart disease mortality. A 21-year follow-up of 8000 men, *Arterioscler. Thromb. Vasc. Biol.*, 17, 107, 1997.

200. Tanne, D., Yaari, S., and Goldbourt, U., High-density lipoprotein cholesterol and risk of ischemic stroke mortality. A 21-year follow-up of 8586 men from the Israeli Ischemic Heart Disease Study, *Stroke*, 28, 83, 1997.

201. Kinosian, B., Glick, H., and Garland, G., Cholesterol and coronary heart disease: predicting risks by levels and ratios, *Ann. Intern. Med.*, 121, 641, 1996.

202. Knopp, R. H., Walden, C. E., Retzlaff, B. M., McCann, B. S., Dowdy, A. A., Albers, J. J., Gey, G. O., and Cooper, M. N., Long-term cholesterol-lowering effects of 4 fat-restricted diets in hypercholesterolemic and combined hyperlipidemic men, *JAMA*, 278, 1509, 1997.

203. Jeppersen, J., Schaaf, P., Jones, C., Zhou, M.-Y., Chen, Y.-D. I., and Reaven, G. M., Effects of low-fat, high-carbohydrate diets on risk factors for ischaemic heart disease in postmenopausal women, *Am. J. Clin. Nutr.*, 65, 1027, 1997.

204. Walden, C. E., Retzlaff, B. M., Buck, B. L., McCann, B. S., and Knopp, R. H., Lipoprotein lipid response to the National Cholesterol Education Program Step II diet by hypercholesterolemic and combined hyperlipidemic women and men, *Arterioscler. Thromb. Vasc. Biol.*, 17, 375, 1997.

205. Cheung, M. C., Lichtenstein, A. H., and Schaefer, E. J., Effects of a diet restricted in saturated fatty acids and cholesterol on the composition of apolipoprotein A-1-containing lipoprotein particles in the fasting and fed states, *Am. J. Clin. Nutr.*, 60, 911, 1994.

206. Ginsberg, H. N., Kris-Etherton, P., Dennis, B., Elmer, P. J., Ershow, A., Lefevre, M., Pearson, T., Roheim, P., Ramakrishnan, R., Reed, R., Stewart, K., Stewart P., Phillips, K., and Anderson, N., for the DELTA Research Group, Effects of reducing dietary saturated fatty acids on plasma lipids and lipoproteins in healthy subjects, The Delta Study, Protocol 1, *Arterioscler. Thromb. Vasc. Biol.*, 18, 441, 1998.

207. Dreon, D. M., Fernstrom, H. A., Campos, H., Blanche, P., Williams, P. T., and Krauss, R. M., Change in dietary saturated fat intake is associated with change in mass of large low-density-lipoprotein particles in men, *Am. J. Clin. Nutr.*, 67, 828, 1998.

208. Tsevat, J., Weinstein, M. C., Williams, L. W., Tosteson, A. N. A., and Goldman, L., Expected gains in life expectancy from various coronary heart disease risk modifications, *Circulation*, 83, 1194, 1991.

209. Browner, W. S., Westenhouse, J., and Tice, J. A., What if Americans ate less fat? A quantitative estimate of the effect on mortality, *JAMA*, 265, 3285, 1991.

210. Holme, I., An analysis of randomized trials evaluating the effect of cholesterol reduction on total mortality and coronary heart disease incidence, *Circulation*, 82, 1916, 1990.

211. Roussouw, J. E. and Rifkind, B. M., Does lowering serum cholesterol levels lower coronary heart disease risk?, *Endocrinol. Metab. Clin. N. Am.*, 19, 279, 1990.

212. Kritchevsky, S. B. and Kritchevsky, D., Serum cholesterol and cancer risk: an epidemiologic perspective, *Annual Reviews Nutrition*, 12, 391, 1992.

213. Kritchevsky, S. B., Dietary lipids and the low blood cholesterol-cancer association, *Am. J. Epidemiol.*, 135, 509, 1992.

214. Kaplan, N. M., Lipid intervention trials in primary prevention: a critical review, *Clin. & Exptl. Hyptens. – Theory & Practice*, A14 (1&2), 109, 1992.

215. Jacobs, D. R., Jr. and Blackburn, H., Models of effects of low blood cholesterol on the public health, Implications for practice and policy, *Circulation*, 87, 1033, 1993.

216. Manolio, T. A., Ettinger, W. H., Tracy, R. P., Kuller, L. H., Borhani, N. O., Lynch, J. C., and Fried, L. P., for the CHS Collaborative Research Group: Epidemiology of low cholesterol levels in older adults: The Cardiovascular Health Study, *Circulation*, 87, 728, 1993.

217. Smith, G. D., Song, F., and Sheldon, T. A., Cholesterol lowering and mortality: the importance of considering initial level of risk, *Br. Med. J.*, 306, 1367, 1993.

218. Esrey, K. L., Joseph, L., and Grover, S. A., Relationship between dietary intake and coronary heart disease mortality: Lipid Research Clinics Prevalence Follow-up Study, *J. Clin. Epidemiol.,* 49, 211, 1996.

219. Martin, M. J., Hulley, S. B., Browner, W. S., Kuller, L. H., and Wentworth, D., Serum cholesterol, blood pressure, and mortality: Implications from a cohort of 361,662 men, *Lancet,* 2, 933, 1986.

220. Pekkanen, J., Nissinen, A., Vartiainen, E., Salonen, J. T., Punsar, S., and Karvonen, M., Changes in serum cholesterol level and mortality: a 30-year follow-up, *Am. J. Epidemiol.,* 139, 155, 1994.

221. Multiple Risk Factor Intervention Trial Research Group, Serum cholesterol level and mortality, *Arch. Intern. Med.,* 152, 1490, 1992.

222. Jacobs, D., Blackburn, H., Higgins, M., Reed, D., Iso, H., McMillan, G., Neaton, J., Nelson, J., Potter, J., Rifkind, B., Rossouw, J., Shekelle, R., and Yusuf, S., Report of the conference on low blood cholesterol: Mortality associations, *Circulation,* 86, 1046, 1992.

223. Morgan, R. E., Palinkas, L. A., Barrett-Connor, E. L., and Wingard, D. L., Plasma cholesterol and depressive symptoms in older men, *Lancet,* 341, 75, 1993.

224. Lindberg, G., Rastam, L., Gullberg, B., and Eklund, G. A., Low serum cholesterol concentration and short term mortality from injuries in men and women, *Br. Med. J.,* 305, 277, 1992.

225. D'Agostino, R. B., Belanger, A. J., Kannel, W. B., and Higgins, M., Role of smoking in the U-shaped relation of cholesterol to mortality in men. The Framingham Study, *Am. J. Epidemiol.,* 141, 822, 1995.

226. Zureik, M., Courbon, D., and Ducimetiere, P., Decline in serum total cholesterol and the risk of death from cancer, *Epidemiology,* 8, 137, 1997.

227. Raiha, I., Marniemi, P., Puukka, P., Toikka, T., Ehnolm, C., and Sourander, L., Effect of serum lipids, lipoproteins, and apolipoproteins on vascular and nonvascular mortality in the elderly, *Arterioscler. Thromb. Vasc. Biol.,* 17, 1224, 1997.

228. Cowan, L. D., O'Connell, D. L., Criqui, M. H., Barrett-Connor, E., Bush, T. L., and Wallace, R. B., Cancer mortality and lipid and lipoprotein levels: the Lipid Research Clinics Program Mortality Follow-up Study, *Am. J. Epidemiol.,* 131, 468, 1990.

229. Ploeckinger, B., Dantendorfer, K., Ulm, M., Baischer, W., Derfler, K., Musalek, M., and Dadak, C., Rapid decrease of serum cholesterol concentration and postpartum depression, *Br. Med. J.,* 313, 664, 1996.

230. Zureik, M., Courbon, D., and Ducimetiere, P., Serum cholesterol concentration and death from suicide in men: Paris Prospective Study, *Br. Med. J.,* 313, 649, 1996.

231. Gallerani, M., Manfredini, R., Caracciolo, S., Scapoli, C., Molinari, S., and Fersini, C., Serum cholesterol concentrations in parasuicide, *Br. Med. J.,* 310, 1632, 1995.

232. Golumb, B. A., Cholesterol and violence: is there a connection?, *Ann. Intern. Med.,* 128, 478, 1998.

233. Steegmans, P. H. A., Fekkes, D., Hoes, A. W., Bak, A. A. A., van der Does, E., and Grobbee, D. E., Low serum cholesterol concentration and serotonin metabolism in men, *Br. Med. J.,* 312, 221, 1996.

234. Brown, S. L., Lowered serum cholesterol and low mood: the link remains unproved, *Br. Med. J.,* 313, 637, 1996.

235. Smith, G. D., Shipley, M. J., Marmot, M. G., and Rose, G., Plasma cholesterol concentration and mortality, The Whitehall study, *JAMA,* 267, 70, 1992.

236. Hulley, S. B., Walsh, J. M. B., and Newman, T. B., Health policy on blood cholesterol, time to change directions, *Circulation,* 86, 1026, 1992.

237. Sharp, S. J. and Pocock, S. J., Time trends in serum cholesterol before cancer death, *Epidemiology*, 8, 132, 1997.

238. Iribarren, C., Reed, D. M., Burchfiel, C. M., and Dwyer, J. H., Serum total cholesterol and mortality, *JAMA*, 273, 1926, 1995.

239. Weverling-Rijnsburger, A. W. E., Blauw, G. J., Lagaay, A. M., Knook, D. L., Meinders, A. E., and Westendorp, R. G. J., Total cholesterol and risk of mortality in the oldest old, *Lancet*, 350, 1119, 1997.

240. Olson, R. E., The folly of restricting fat in the diet of children, *Nutrition Today*, 30(6), 1995.

241. The Writing Group for the DISC Collaborative Research Group, Efficacy and safety of lowering dietary intake of fat and cholesterol in children with elevated low-density lipoprotein cholesterol. The Dietary Intervention Study in Children (DISC), *JAMA*, 273, 1429, 1995.

242. Newman, T. B., Garber, A. M., Holtzman, N. A., and Hulley, S. B., Problems with the report of the expert panel on blood cholesterol levels in children and adolescents, *Arch. Pediatr. Adolesc. Med.*, 149, 241, 1995.

243. Gaull, G. E., Giombetti, T., and Woo, R. W. Y., Pediatric dietary lipid guidelines: a policy analysis, *J. Am. Coll. Nutr.*, 14(5), 411, 1995.

244. Cobb, M. M., Teitlebaum, H., Risch, N., Jekel, J., and Ostfeld, A., Influence of dietary fat, apolipoprotein E phenotype, and sex on plasma lipoprotein levels, *Circulation*, 86, 849, 1992.

245. Nicklas, T. A., Webber, L. S., Koschak, M. L., and Berenson, G. S., Nutrient adequacy of lowfat intakes for children: The Bogalusa Heart Study, *Pediatrics*, 89, 221, 1992.

246. Shea, S., Basch, C. E., Stein, A. D., Contento, I. R., Irigoyen, M., and Zybert, P., Is there a relationship between dietary fat and stature or growth in children three to five years of age?, *Pediatrics*, 92, 579, 1993.

247. Sigman-Grant, M., Zimmerman, S., and Kris-Etherton, P. M., Dietary approaches for reducing fat intake of preschool-age children, *Pediatrics*, 91, 955, 1993.

248. Obarzanek, E., Hunsberger, S. A., Van Horn, L., Hartmuller, V. V., Barton, B. A., Stevens, V. J., Kwiterovich, P. O., Franklin, F. A., Kimm, S. Y. S., Lasser, N. L., Simons-Mortor, D. G., and Lauer, R. M., Safety of a fat-reduced diet: The Dietary Intervention Study in Children (DISC), *Pediatrics*, 100, 51, 1997.

249. Hampl, J. S. and Betts, N. M., Comparisons of dietary intake and sources of fat in low- and high-fat diets of 18- to 24-year-olds, *J. Am. Diet. Assoc.*, 95, 893, 1995.

250. Murphy, S. P., Rose, D., Hudes, M., and Viteri, F. E., Demographic and economic factors associated with dietary quality for adults in the 1987-88 Nationwide Food Consumption Survey, *J. Am. Diet. Assoc.*, 92, 1352, 1992.

251. Sowada, B. J., Kendall, P. A., and Jansen, G. R., Effect of behavioral style on using a nutrient approach in diet planning, *J. Nutr. Education*, 25, 5, 1993.

252. Dolecek, T. A., Johnson, R. L., Grandits, G. A., Farrand-Zukel, M., and Caggiula, A. W., Nutritional adequacy of diets reported at baseline and during trial years 1-6 by the special intervention and usual care groups in the Multiple Risk Factor Intervention Trial, *Am. J. Clin. Nutr.*, 65(1), 305s, 1997.

253. Retzlaff, B. M., Walden, C. E., McNeney, W. B., Buck, B. L., McCann, B. S., and Knopp, R. H., Nutritional intake of women and men on the NCEP Step I and Step II diets, *J. Am. Coll. Nutr.*, 16(1), 52, 1997.

254. Smith, M. M. and Lifshitz, F., Excess fruit juice consumption as a contributing factor in nonorganic failure to thrive, *Pediatrics*, 93, 438, 1994.

255. Pugliese, M. Y., Weyman-Daum, M., Moses, N., and Lifshitz, F., Parental health beliefs as a cause of nonorganic failure to thrive, *Pediatrics*, 80, 175, 1987.

256. Lifshitz, F. and N. Moses, Growth failure: a complication of dietary treatment of hypercholesterolemia, *Am. J. Dis. Child.*, 143, 537, 1989.

257. Henkin, Y., Garber, D. W., Osterlund, L. C., and Darnell, B. E., Saturated fats, cholesterol, and dietary compliance, *Arch. Intern. Med.*, 152, 1167, 1992.

258. Kristal, A. R., White, E., Shattuck, A. L., Curry, S., Anderson, G. L., Fowler, A., and Urban, N., Long-term maintenance of a low-fat diet: durability of fat-related dietary habits in the Women's Health Trial, *J. Am. Diet. Assoc.*, 92, 553, 1992.

259. Kris-Etherton, P., and Burns, J. H., *Cardiovascular Nutrition*, Chicago, IL., The American Dietetic Association, 1998.

260. Van Horn, L. V., Dolecek, T. A., Grandits, G. A., and Skweres, L., Adherence to dietary recommendations in the special intervention group in the Multiple Risk Factor Intervention Trial, *Am. J. Clin. Nutr.*, 65(1), 289s, 1997.

261. McCarron, D. A., Oparil, S., Chait, A., Haynes, R. B., Kris-Etherton, P., Stern, J. S., Resnick, L. M., Clark, S., Morris, C. D., Hatton, D. C., Metz, J. A., McMahon, M., Holcomb, S., Snyder, G. W., and Pi-Sunjer, F. X., Nutritional management of cardiovascular risk factors, *Arch. Intern. Med.*, 157, 169, 1997.

262. The American Dietetic Association, *Nutrition Trends Survey 1997*, Executive Summary, Chicago, IL., The American Dietetic Association, 1997.

263. Smith-Schneider, L. M., Sigman-Grant, M. J., and Kris-Etherton, P. M., Dietary fat reduction strategies, *J. Am. Diet. Assoc.*, 92, 34, 1992.

264. Sigman-Grant, M., Can you have your low-fat cake and eat it too? The role of fat-modified products, *J. Am. Diet. Assoc.*, 97(Suppl.), 76s, 1997.

265. Davidson, M. H., Kong, J.C., Drennan, K. B., Story, K., and Anderson, G. H., Efficacy of the National Cholesterol Education Program Step 1 Diet, *Arch. Intern. Med.*, 156, 305, 1996.

266. Kritchevsky, D., History of recommendations to the public about dietary fat, *J. Nutr. Suppl.*, 28, 449s, 1998.

CHAPTER 3

Dairy Foods and Hypertension

I. INTRODUCTION

Hypertension, defined as a blood pressure equal to or greater than 140 mm Hg systolic (contracting) and/or 90 mm Hg diastolic (resting), affects up to 50 million or one in every four American adults.[1,2] The prevalence of this common chronic disease increases with age and is higher for African Americans than for Hispanic and non-Hispanic whites (Table 3.1).[1-4] At younger ages, men are at greater risk of high blood pressure than women, whereas in later years the prevalence is higher among women.[2] Hypertension can also result as a complication of pregnancy.[2]

Table 3.1   Hypertension* Prevalence by Age in Civilian, Noninstitutionalized Population, 1988 through 1991

Age, Y	% Hypertensive
18–29	4
30–39	11
40–49	21
50–59	44
60–69	54
70–79	64
80+	65

* Defined as the average of three blood pressure measurements of 140/90 mm Hg or more on a single occasion or reported taking of antihypertensive medication.

From National High Blood Pressure Education Program Working Group, *Arch. Intern. Med.*, 153, 186, 1993. With permission.

Uncontrolled high blood pressure increases the risk for coronary heart disease, stroke, cardiac failure, and kidney disease.[1,5] Compared to people with normal blood pressure, those with high blood pressure are at three to four times the risk of

1-8493-8731-0/00/$0.00+$.50
© 2000 by CRC Press LLC

developing coronary heart disease and seven times as likely to experience a stroke.[4] Control of blood pressure can reduce morbidity and mortality from coronary heart disease, stroke, and renal failure.[4] Morbidity and mortality from diseases attributable to hypertension have declined in the past 20 years as a result of better detection and treatment of hypertension.[1] However, more than a quarter of all people with high blood pressure are unaware of their condition.[1] For 1998, the cost of hypertension is estimated at nearly $32 billion in direct medical (e.g., cost of physicians, medications) and indirect (e.g., lost wages, lowered productivity) expenditures.[6]

Given the high prevalence, serious health consequences, and staggering economic burden of hypertension, the U.S. Department of Health and Human Services' National Health Promotion and Disease Prevention Objectives for the year 2000[4] call for reducing uncontrolled high blood pressure. A specific goal is to double blood pressure control (i.e., from an estimated 24% to at least 50%) in people with high blood pressure. Relatively small reductions in blood pressure can have a major positive impact on health.[7,8]

Both genetic and environmental factors influence blood pressure.[1,9] To date, no one factor has been identified as the cause of hypertension. Because of the high cost of and potential adverse side effects associated with pharmacological therapy for this disease, individuals are encouraged to adopt lifestyle modifications to treat or reduce their risk of high blood pressure (Table 3.2).[1] These lifestyle modifications include weight reduction if overweight, increased aerobic physical activity, moderation in dietary sodium and alcohol intake, and adequate consumption of calcium, potassium, and magnesium.[1]

Table 3.2   Lifestyle Modifications for Hypertension Prevention & Management

- Lose weight if overweight.
- Limit alcohol intake to no more than 1 oz (30 mL) ethanol (e.g., 24 oz [720 mL] beer, 10 oz [300mL] wine, or 2 oz [60 mL] 100-proof whiskey) per day or 0.5 oz (15 mL) ethanol per day for women and lighter weight people.
- Increase aerobic physical activity (30 to 45 minutes most days of the week).
- Reduce sodium intake to no more than 100 mmol per day (2.4 g sodium or 6 g sodium chloride).
- Maintain adequate intake of dietary potassium (approximately 90 mmol per day).
- Maintain adequate intake of dietary calcium and magnesium for general health.
- Stop smoking and reduce intake of dietary saturated fat and cholesterol for overall cardiovascular health.

From 6th Report of the Joint National Committee on Prevention, Detection, Evaluation, and Treatment of High Blood Pressure, NIH Publ. No. 98-4080, November 1997.

Excess body weight, especially central or abdominal obesity, increases risk of hypertension, and weight reduction in individuals who are at least 10% above ideal weight may reduce blood pressure.[1,8,10-14] As little as 5 to10 pounds weight loss reduces blood pressure in many overweight hypertensive patients.[1] Weight loss also may reduce or eliminate the need for antihypertensive medication.[1,10] Regular aerobic physical activity, such as 30 to 45 minutes of brisk walking most days of the week, also can lower blood pressure in many previously sedentary hypertensive patients.[1]

Because Americans generally consume an excess of 150 mmol of sodium a day, lowering sodium intake to less than 100 mmol a day (less than 6 g of sodium chloride or less than 2.4 g sodium a day) is recommended depending on the individual.[1,15] However, reducing sodium intake is not uniformly effective for everyone.[16,17] The blood pressure response to changes in dietary sodium chloride is variable and depends in part on whether an individual is normotensive or hypertensive or salt sensitive or salt resistant. A recent meta-analysis found that reducing sodium intake lowered blood pressure more in hypertensive adults than in normotensive adults.[18] In salt sensitive individuals, blood pressure increases with salt loading and decreases with salt restriction. In salt resistant individuals, blood pressure does not change with salt intake.[17] Certain population groups including hypertensive individuals, African Americans, obese persons, patients with kidney disease, individuals with a family history of hypertension, adults aged 65 years and older, and people with low plasma renin levels are more likely to be salt sensitive than others.[17] Genetics may be a major determinant of salt sensitivity and ongoing studies are attempting to identify specific genes, as well as nongenetic factors, that contribute to this trait. At present, there is no genetic or biochemical test to identify salt sensitive from salt resistant individuals. Interactions among dietary components such as chloride, calcium, potassium, and magnesium may also contribute to variability in the blood pressure response to dietary sodium.[17] To help consumers meet dietary recommendations for sodium, the Food and Drug Administration, in addition to requiring mandatory sodium labeling, allows health claims relating to an association between dietary sodium and high blood pressure on food labels.[16] Diets reduced in sodium are potentially low in several essential nutrients such as calcium, potassium, and magnesium which have been demonstrated to be beneficial in blood pressure regulation.[17,19,20] Also, low sodium diets have recently been associated with premature death.[21] Moderation in sodium intake (i.e., 2.4 g a day) is therefore recommended.[1,15]

According to the *Sixth Report on Prevention, Detection, Evaluation, and Treatment of High Blood Pressure*,[1] consuming an adequate intake of calcium, potassium, and magnesium lowers blood pressure. Dairy foods (e.g., fluid milk, yogurt) are the best food source for providing all three nutrients simultaneously in meaningful amounts.[22] In 1994, dairy foods contributed 73% of the calcium, 18.5% of the potassium, and 16% of the magnesium available in the nation's food supply.[22] As indicated in Table 3.3, dairy foods provide an appreciable percentage of the recommendations for calcium, potassium, and magnesium.[23-25]

This chapter reviews the mounting evidence supporting the beneficial role of these three nutrients, both individually and in combination (as in dairy foods), and of a dietary pattern including dairy foods in the control of blood pressure. It is important to recognize that nutrients are not consumed in isolation, but as interactive components of the total diet.[17,26] The high degree of interactions of nutrients may account for some of the heterogeneity in blood pressure response to variations in intake of individual nutrients.[26] Moreover, findings from a single intervention (i.e., a specific nutrient) may underestimate the effects achieved with combined interventions. Recent studies indicate that dietary patterns of nutrients as they occur together in foods significantly lower blood pressure.[27,28]

Table 3.3   Calcium, Potassium, and Magnesium Content of Selected Dairy Foods

Dairy Product	Calcium		Potassium		Magnesium	
	mg	(% AI)[1]	mg	(% RDA)[2]	mg	(% RDA)[3]
Whole Milk, 1 cup	291	(29)	370	(19)	33	(10)
Lowfat Milk, 2%, 1 cup	297	(30)	377	(19)	33	(10)
Skim Milk, 1 cup	302	(30)	406	(20)	28	(9)
Lowfat (1%) Chocolate Milk, 1 cup	287	(29)	426	(21)	33	(10)
Buttermilk, Cultured, 1 cup	285	(29)	371	(19)	27	(8)
Yogurt, Plain Lowfat, 8 fl. ounces	415	(42)	531	(27)	40	(13)
Yogurt, Plain Skim Milk, 8 fl. ounces	452	(45)	579	(29)	43	(13)

[1] 1000 mg calcium; [2] 2,000 mg potassium; [3] 320 mg magnesium. From Institute of Medicine 1997; Food and Nutrition Board, 1989.

II. CALCIUM, DAIRY FOODS, AND BLOOD PRESSURE

Since the early 1980s, a considerable body of evidence has accumulated from investigations in experimental animals, epidemiological studies, and clinical intervention trials in humans to support a beneficial role for calcium or calcium-rich foods such as milk and other dairy foods in blood pressure control.[26,29,30]

A. Experimental Animal Studies

A blood pressure-lowering effect of calcium has been demonstrated in several models of genetically hypertensive rats, including spontaneous hypertensive rats (SHR), salt-sensitive Dahl rats, DOC-salt rats, and Lyon genetically hypertensive rats,[26,29,31-35] as well as in normotensive Wistar-Kyoto (WKY) rats.[36] A low calcium intake increases the hypertensive effect of a high-sodium chloride diet while a high calcium intake lowers sodium chloride-induced blood pressure or attenuates the development of hypertension in these animals. More calcium is needed to reduce blood pressure in genetic hypertensive rats than in normotensive animals.[37] An inverse relationship between calcium and blood pressure also has been shown in pregnant and nonpregnant rats[38] and in insulin resistant (diabetic) Zucker obese rats.[39]

Abnormalities in calcium metabolism (e.g., reduced serum ionized calcium, increased parathyroid hormone, enhanced urinary calcium excretion) have been described in several animal models of hypertension.[35,40-46] Blakeborough et al.[46] reported that less calcium is absorbed in SHR rats than in normotensive WKY rats.

Several studies demonstrate that the hypotensive effect of calcium in experimental animals requires a normal or high normal intake of sodium chloride.[40,41,44,47-49] Oshima et al.[47] found that a high calcium diet lowered blood pressure in SHR rats only when intake of sodium chloride was high. These findings indicate that increased calcium helps to prevent dietary sodium chloride-induced hypertension. Oparil et al.[44] observed that dietary calcium supplementation prevented salt-sensitive hypertension in SHR rats by increasing diuretic and natriuretic responses to acute volume loading and by activating central nervous system pathways (i.e., neuronal mechanisms). Wyss et al.[48] likewise concluded that neuronal mechanisms underlie the blood pressure-lowering effect of dietary calcium in salt-sensitive SHR rats. Specifically, the addition of calcium to a high sodium chloride diet may prevent a rise in blood pressure by preventing the sodium chloride-induced decrease in anterior hypothalamic norepinephrine.[48]

In DOC-salt rats (a low renin model of experimental hypertension which is particularly sensitive to the hypotensive effects of calcium) a high calcium diet was demonstrated to attenuate the rise in renal vascular resistance which accompanies DOC-salt hypertension.[41,50] DiPette et al.[50] reported that this effect of calcium was associated with a suppression of 1,25-dihydroxyvitamin D_3. Calcium regulatory hormones, namely parathyroid hormone and 1,25-dihydroxyvitamin D_3, have been demonstrated to have properties that can increase peripheral vascular resistance.[51-53] Enhanced vascular relaxation may be a mechanism whereby calcium supplementation reduced blood pressure in sodium-volume-dependent hypertension.[41]

Increased dietary calcium has been reported to reduce smooth muscle reactivity in SHR rats. Porsti et al.[54] investigated the effects of oral calcium supplementation on blood pressure and intracellular free calcium concentration in SHR (hypertensive) and WKY (normotensive) rats. They also measured associated changes in vascular smooth muscle reactions. Calcium supplementation altered vascular smooth muscle responses and significantly attenuated the rise in systolic blood pressure and reduced intracellular free calcium in the hypertensive, but not normotensive, animals (Figure 3.1).

Experimental animal studies have demonstrated that increased calcium intake not only protects against salt-induced increases in blood pressure, but also modifies the effects of specific fats on blood pressure. Karanja et al.[55] observed that supplemental calcium reduced the severity of hypertension associated with a corn oil-rich diet in SHR rats. Further, a high calcium/butter fat diet was as effective as fish oil in lowering blood pressure (Figure 3.2).

B. Epidemiological Studies

Numerous epidemiological studies support an inverse relationship between dietary calcium and blood pressure, with the strongest association between low intakes of calcium and higher blood pressure (Figure 3.3).[26,29,30,37,56-64] These studies demonstrate that the calcium intake of hypertensive individuals is lower than that of normotensive individuals. McCarron and Morris,[56] for example, reported that hypertensive women consumed 21% less calcium than their normotensive controls. Karanja et al.,[65] in a cross-sectional study of 326 hypertensive and normotensive subjects, found that hypertensives consumed significantly lower amounts of calcium, magnesium, and potassium (i.e., nutrients found in substantial quantities in dairy foods) than normotensive subjects. They also demonstrated that intake of these minerals could be restored to recommended levels with dairy foods and without impacting blood lipid levels.[65]

Epidemiological studies have demonstrated an inverse association between calcium intake and hypertensive disorders of pregnancy (gestational hypertension and

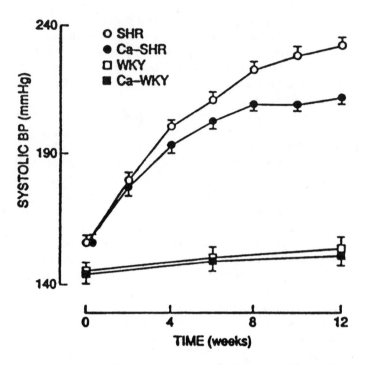

Figure 3.1 Line graphs show effect of high calcium (Ca) diet on systolic blood pressure (BP) in the spontaneously hypertensive rats (SHR) and Wistar-Kyoto rats (WKY) during the 12-week study, Development of hypertension was attenuated in the Ca-SHR group (p<0.0001) (n = 16 for SHR and Ca-SHR, and n = 9 for WKY and Ca-WKY groups), (From Porsti, I., Arvola, P., Wuorela, H., and Vapaatalo, H., *Hypertension*, 19, 85, 1992. With permission.)

preeclampsia).[30] Similarly, an inverse association between calcium intake and blood pressure has been observed in children.[66,67] According to a study involving 80 preschoolers, systolic blood pressure dropped by 2.0 mmHg for each 100 mg calcium per 1000 Kcal/day consumed.[66] Simons-Morton et al.[67] reported an inverse association between calcium intake and diastolic blood pressure based on data analyzed from 662 children participating in the Dietary Intervention Study in Children (DISC). This three year study, which provided dietary advice to lower fat intake by eight-year-old children with elevated low density lipoprotein cholesterol levels, also found that higher intakes of magnesium, potassium, protein, and carbohydrate were associated with lower blood pressure.[67] This blood pressure lowering effect of calcium in children is supported by an intervention trial.[68] In a study involving 101 school-aged children (11 years at baseline), increasing calcium intake by 600 mg a day for 12 weeks lowered systolic blood pressure, especially in children whose calcium intake was initially low. [68] Ensuring adequate calcium intake during childhood may be one way to lower the risk of developing hypertension later in life. There is some evidence supporting the concept that essential hypertension has its roots in childhood and high blood pressure represents a significant clinical problem.[69] Approximately one-half of children with high blood

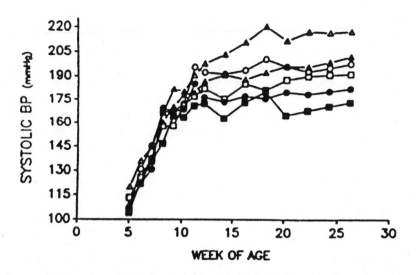

Figure 3.2   Line graph showing time course of blood pressure (BP) development for each of the six diets, △, CO/0.25% Ca²⁺; ○, BF/0.25% Ca²⁺; □, FO/0.25% Ca²⁺; ▲, CO/2.0% Ca²⁺; ●, BF/2.0% Ca²⁺; ■, FO/2.0% Ca²⁺., CO, corn oil; BF, butterfat; FO, fish oil. (From Karanja, N., Phanouvong, T., and McCarron, D. A., *Hypertension*, 14, 674, 1989. With permission.)

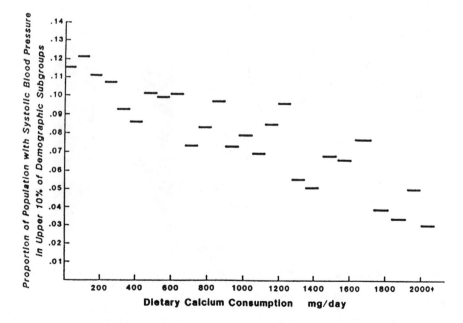

Figure 3.3   Percentage of individuals at risk of developing or having hypertension on the basis of daily calcium intake as reported in the National Health and Nutrition Examination Survey (NHANES) I. (From McCarron, D. A., et al., *Am. J. Clin. Nutr.*, 54, 215s, 1991. With permission.)

pressure have hypertension as adults, according to the Bogalusa Heart Study which followed 1505 children for 15 years.[70]

Several prospective studies support a blood pressure-lowering effect of calcium. Findings from the first four years of follow-up of the Nurses Health Study involving nearly 60,000 females in the U.S. demonstrated a 23% reduction in the relative risk for developing hypertension with a dietary calcium intake of at least 800 mg/day compared with an intake of less than 400 mg/day (Figure 3.4).[59] The lower risk of hypertension was independently associated with calcium from both dairy and non-dairy sources. Calcium intake has also been demonstrated to have a strong independent inverse association with risk of hypertension in men, according to a four year prospective study which examined the relationship between various nutritional factors and blood pressure in 30,681 predominantly white U.S. male health professionals, 40 to 75 years of age, without diagnosed hypertension.[71] High blood pressure was associated with calcium intakes below 500 mg/day. In a 10 year epidemiological follow-up study of the First National Health and Nutrition Examination Survey (NHANES I) involving over 6600 adults, those who reported higher calcium intakes were less likely to develop hypertension ten years later than subjects who reported lower calcium intakes.[62]

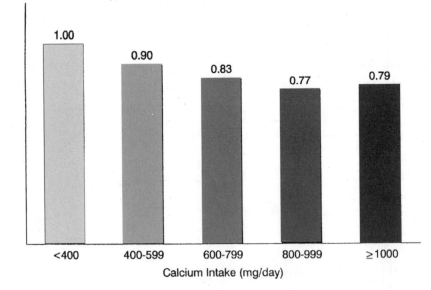

Relative Risk of Hypertension

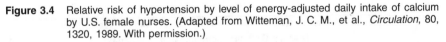

Calcium Intake (mg/day)

Figure 3.4   Relative risk of hypertension by level of energy-adjusted daily intake of calcium by U.S. female nurses. (Adapted from Witteman, J. C. M., et al., *Circulation*, 80, 1320, 1989. With permission.)

In 1995, Cappuccio et al.[72] conducted a meta-analysis of 23 published epidemiological studies that examined the relation between dietary calcium intake and blood pressure. A modest but statistically significant inverse association was found between dietary calcium intake and blood pressure.[72] However, Birkett[63] identified various problems with the data used in this meta-analysis and subsequently re-analyzed the data correcting for various shortcomings. The re-analyzed meta-analysis revealed a stronger inverse association between dietary calcium and blood pressure than originally reported.[63] Birkett[63] pointed out the difficulties in carrying out and interpreting meta-analyses and cautioned that failure to consider confounding factors such as age, body mass index, alcohol intake, and other nutrients can influence the results of meta-analyses.

Calcium from dairy foods specifically has been associated with a decrease in blood pressure in numerous epidemiological studies. In a cross-sectional survey of 5000 predominantly white adults from southern California, Ackley et al.[73] found that male hypertensives reported a lower intake of whole milk than male normotensives. In an analysis of a smaller subset, both total calcium intake and calcium from milk were lower in untreated hypertensives than in normotensives. No differences in nonliquid dairy products were found between normotensives and hypertensives. In the partial correlation analysis, whole milk calcium intake was more strongly inversely related to systolic blood pressure than total calcium intake, while the reverse was found for diastolic blood pressure.

Similarly, Garcia-Palmieri et al.,[74] in a report from the Puerto Rico Heart Study, found that milk intake was inversely associated with both systolic and diastolic blood pressure in men and that this correlation was independent of coffee and alcohol intake, weight, education, cigarette smoking, and other dietary variables. Systolic blood pressure was reduced by 2 mmHg for every two cups of milk (730 mg calcium) consumed per day. No association was observed between non-dairy calcium intake and blood pressure. Reed et al.,[75] in a study of diet and blood pressure among 800 Japanese men in Hawaii, observed that calcium from dairy foods, but not from nondairy foods, was inversely associated with blood pressure. The authors attributed this finding to the fact that dairy foods contain not only calcium but other nutrients (e.g., potassium) that influence blood pressure.

In a cross-sectional study of calcium intake and blood pressure of 1790 adults in Erie County, New York, Freudenheim et al.[76] found that the calcium intake of normotensives tended to be higher than that of hypertensives, and that calcium from milk and yogurt (but not cheese) was inversely associated with diastolic blood pressure in Caucasian females. These findings are in agreement with those of a previous study which found that milk, but not cheese, protected against hypertension.[77]

A study reported by Iso et al.[60] involving over 1900 Japanese men ages 40 to 69 years found that systolic blood pressure was higher among men whose daily calcium intake, particularly from dairy foods, was low (i.e., 449 to 695 mg). The authors suggest that increasing total calcium intake by 300 mg (i.e., the amount in an 8 ounce glass of milk) corresponds to a 1.6 mmHg decrease in systolic blood pressure. Recognizing that dairy calcium intake typically is low among the Japanese, Iso and coworkers[60] recommend that this population group increase their calcium intake, primarily by consuming more milk and milk products.

A high calcium intake (1575 mg/day) from dairy products during the first 20 weeks of pregnancy was associated with a low risk of gestational hypertension in a case-control study in Quebec, Canada.[78] The association was independent of body mass index, exercise, maternal age, education, and cigarette smoking. In a study of pregnant women from the Child Health and Development Study, women who drank two glasses of milk a day were at the lowest risk for preeclampsia.[79]

With few exceptions, epidemiological findings support a beneficial role for calcium, particularly from dairy foods such as milk, in blood pressure control.[63] As discussed below, a number of dietary and nondietary confounding variables influences the relationship between calcium intake and blood pressure. Recognition of these variables does not undermine the beneficial role of calcium in blood pressure control, but rather helps to identify those individuals who will benefit most from an increase in dietary calcium and supports the importance of food sources of calcium.

C. Clinical Studies

Clinical intervention trials using different biochemical indices and sources of calcium (i.e., supplements or calcium from foods such as dairy products) indicate a beneficial, although variable, blood pressure-lowering effect of calcium.[26,29,30,56,61,80-83]

When McCarron and Morris[56] compared the blood pressure response of 48 hypertensive and 32 normotensive individuals to 1000 mg of calcium salt (as the carbonate or citrate) per day for eight weeks, the blood pressure response of the hypertensive patients was greater than that of the normotensives. However, there was considerable individual variation for both groups. In the hypertensive patients, increased calcium intake significantly lowered systolic and diastolic blood pressures by 3.8 mm Hg and 2.3 mmHg, respectively.[56] Likewise, a meta-analysis of 22 randomized clinical trials of the effect of calcium supplementation (1000 mg a day) on blood pressure in 1231 persons revealed that calcium lowered systolic blood pressure more in hypertensive persons (−1.68 mmHg) than in normotensive persons (−0.53 mm Hg).[81] Calcium supplementation was associated with a statistically significant decrease in systolic blood pressure of 1 to 2 mm Hg both in the overall sample and in hypertensive individuals. In this meta-analysis, calcium significantly reduced systolic blood pressure, but not diastolic blood pressure.[81] Calcium supplementation also had the largest blood pressure lowering effect in older persons and women.

Boucher et al.[84] suggest that the findings reported above[81] indicating that calcium's hypotensive effect is greater in hypertensive than in normotensive individuals may be explained by the cut-off used to define normotensive and hypertensive individuals and/or failure to do a regression analysis on the effect of increased calcium based on baseline blood pressure levels. In their meta-analysis of 33 randomized controlled studies involving 2412 individuals, both normotensive and hypertensive, Boucher et al.[82] examined the relation between baseline blood pressure and calcium supplementation by using regression analysis. In this meta-analysis, increasing calcium intake by 1000 mg to 2000 mg a day was associated with a small, but statistically significant reduction in systolic blood pressure (−1.27 mmHg), but not diastolic blood pressure (−0.24 mm Hg) for the study group as a whole.

In essential hypertensive patients, Resnick et al.[85] observed that patients with a serum profile of lower renin, lower ionized calcium, and elevated 1,25-dihydroxyvitamin D levels experienced a significantly greater reduction in blood pressure in response to calcium supplementation (2 g/day) than hypertensive patients with the opposite profile. Similarly, Grobbee and Hofman[86] observed that calcium supplementation (1 g/day) lowered diastolic blood pressure in mildly hypertensive adults aged 16 to 29 years, especially in subjects with high plasma parathyroid hormone levels and/or low serum total calcium. Strazzullo et al.,[87] in a long-term (15 week) double-blind trial of calcium supplementation (1 g/day) in patients with mild hypertension, also found that hypertensive patients with abnormal calcium metabolism (e.g., hypercalciuria) were most likely to respond to increased calcium with a reduction in blood pressure.

Additional findings by Resnick et al.,[88] similar to those from experimental animal studies (see above), indicated that calcium supplementation was effective in offsetting the pressure-elevating effect of salt in salt sensitive individuals. Zemel et al.,[89] on the basis of their studies in salt sensitive African Americans, also concluded that salt sensitive hypertensives are more likely to demonstrate blood pressure reductions in response to calcium supplementation than individuals who are not salt sensitive. Vaughan et al.[90] found that systolic and diastolic blood pressure decreased (9% and 8%, respectively) in mildly hypertensive men who consumed a high calcium (1400 mg/day), moderate sodium (3300 mg/day) diet for six weeks compared to men who consumed a low calcium (400 mg/day), moderate sodium diet. Sodium excretion increased 13 to 21% in the men who consumed the high calcium diet.[90]

Increasing calcium also helps to maintain normal blood pressure during pregnancy and reduce the risk of preeclampsia.[29,83,91-95] Pregnancy-induced hypertension occurs in 10 to 20% of all pregnancies. Women pregnant for the first time or pregnant with twins or triplets are at highest risk of pregnancy-induced hypertension. Preeclampsia, a severe complication of pregnancy that develops in previously normotensive women, is characterized by hypertension, retention of fluid, and proteinuria. It usually presents between the 20th week of gestation and term. The condition occurs in 2 to 8% of all pregnancies or a higher percentage in high-risk pregnancies and can endanger the health of both the mother and child.[83]

Belizan et al.[93] in a multicenter, double-blind, randomized clinical trial involving 1194 Argentinean women in their first pregnancies, found that risk of hypertensive disorders of pregnancy was significantly lower in women who received 2000 mg of elemental calcium (as the carbonate) than in those who received a placebo (9.8 vs. 14.8%). The protective effect of calcium was more evident after the 28th week of pregnancy than at earlier stages (Figure 3.5). Low calcium levels and low plasma renin identified individuals most likely to benefit from calcium.[93] A beneficial effect of increased calcium during pregnancy was also demonstrated in teenagers enrolled in the Johns Hopkins Hospital Adolescent Pregnancy Program.[95] The teens who received an additional 2000 mg of calcium a day not only had lower blood pressures but also were less likely to deliver premature infants than the teens who were not supplemented with calcium.[95] Knight and Keith[94] reported that calcium supplementation (1 g/day for 20 weeks) significantly lowered diastolic blood pressure in hypertensive, but not normotensive, pregnant women.

A recent meta-analysis of fourteen randomized trials involving 2459 pregnant women found that increasing calcium intake by 1500 to 2000 mg a day during pregnancy lowered systolic and diastolic blood pressure by 5.40 mmHg and

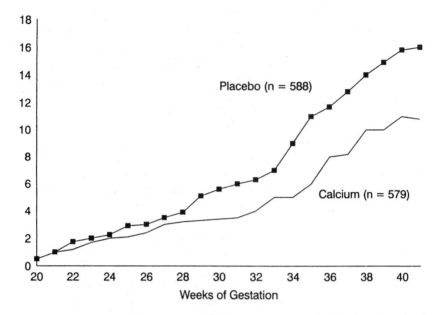

Figure 3.5   Percentage of women in the calcium and placebo groups in whom hypertensive disorders of pregnancy (gestational hypertension and preeclampsia) developed according to the week of gestation. (From Belizan, J. M. J., et al., *N. Engl. J. Med.*, 325, 1402, 1991. With permission.)

3.44 mmHg, respectively (Figure 3.6).[83] This meta-analysis also found that increasing calcium intake reduced the incidence of pregnancy-induced hypertension by 70% and preeclampsia by 62%.[83] It is estimated that several billion dollars a year in health care costs related to hypertensive disorders of pregnancy could be saved by increasing dietary calcium intake to recommended levels during pregnancy.[96]

In contrast to these positive results, the Calcium for Preeclampsia Prevention (CPEP) trial, conducted among over 4500 healthy pregnant women at five U.S. medical centers, found only a slight, but nonsignificant beneficial effect of 2000 mg of supplemental calcium on risk of preeclampsia, pregnancy-associated hypertension, or other adverse outcomes of pregnancy.[97] The failure to find a significant beneficial effect of calcium on pregnancy outcome in this study may be explained by the women's already relatively high calcium intake of 1100 mg a day and low risk status as measured by factors such as education level. Also, this study did not evaluate the effect of a dairy source of calcium. Because calcium-rich foods such as dairy foods contain other nutrients including potassium and magnesium which are associated with lowering blood pressure, the benefits could be even greater if calcium were obtained from foods rather than supplements.[83] Despite the findings of the CPEP trial, an adequate or increased level of intake of calcium is recommended during pregnancy.[23,29,98] Meeting calcium needs during pregnancy may lower the risk of hypertensive disorders during pregnancy and its adverse

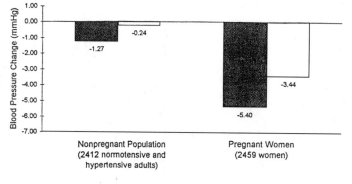

Figure 3.6 Blood pressure lowering effect of calcium in a nonpregnant population and in pregnant women, according to meta-analyses. (Adapted from Bucher, H.C., et al., *JAMA*, 275, April 10, 1016, 1996, Copyright 1996, American Medical Association. With permission)

outcomes, as well as have a beneficial effect on the blood pressure of the off-spring.[99,100] An inverse association has been reported between maternal calcium intake and the blood pressure of breast fed infants at 1, 6, and 12 months of age.[100] In a follow-up study, systolic blood pressure was significantly lower in seven-year-old children whose mothers received 2000 mg of supplemental calcium during pregnancy than in children whose mothers did not receive extra calcium.[99] The researchers speculate that high calcium intake during pregnancy may influence or program mechanisms in the fetus to regulate blood pressure.[99]

Clinical trials utilizing dairy foods as a source of calcium have shown a hypotensive effect.[101-103] A small hypotensive effect of milk intake was related to its mineral content in a six week double-blind trial examining regular milk versus a "mineral-poor" milk (Figure 3.7).[102] In this study of young normotensive women, the decrease in systolic blood pressure was significantly greater in the group supplemented with the regular milk (–4.1%) than in the women given the mineral-poor milk (–1.3%). No effect on diastolic blood pressure was observed. When the researchers compared their findings with those of trials of calcium supplements alone, they found that the effect of milk on blood pressure was greater and more rapid than that of calcium alone.[102] Thus, the combination and/or interaction of nutrients in milk may be more hypotensive than the blood pressure lowering effect of individual nutrients. Another study in normotensive subjects reported by Bierenbaum et al.[101] found that dairy products as a source of calcium (1150 mg/day) significantly reduced systolic blood pressure by an average of 5 mm Hg. A hypotensive effect of yogurt intake has been demonstrated. Zemel et al.[103] reported that calcium (600 mg/day) in the form of yogurt was more effective than calcium carbonate supplements in reducing systolic blood pressure and intracellular calcium in black non-insulin dependent diabetic hypertensives.

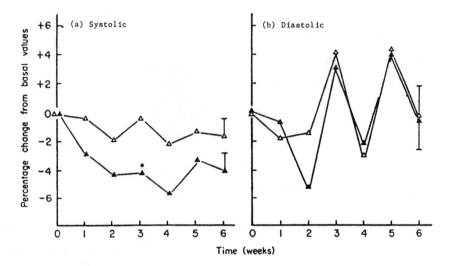

Figure 3.7   Mean percentage changes in systolic and diastolic blood pressure from basal values vs. time. Bar represents 1 SEM. (▲) = normal milk group; (△) = 'mineral-poor' milk group. Significance level between groups: *P<0.05. (From Van Beresteijn, E. C. H., Van Schaik, M., and Schaafsma, G., *J. Intern. Med.*, 228, 477, 1990. With permission.)

Findings from these clinical intervention studies using different indices suggest that increased calcium intake is most effective in lowering blood pressure in the face of a calcium deficit as can be found in pregnancy, in older age, among African American and diabetic subjects, and in individuals with lower renin activity, lower circulating calcium levels, higher urinary calcium excretion, secondary hyperparathyroidism, and elevated vitamin D hormone. It therefore is understandable that reviews of clinical trials of calcium on blood pressure may indicate variable findings and that pooled analyses may point to modest effects.[3,61,81,82] As discussed below, the hypotensive effect of calcium is influenced by a variety of factors.

D. Determinants of a Hypotensive Response to Calcium

Heterogeneity in the blood pressure response to calcium is not surprising given interactions among nutrients in the diet and food and the fact that hypertension is the expression of a variety of disorders with different mechanisms which singly or in combination result in increased vascular tone and total peripheral resistance.[26,29,30,64] A number of factors related to the study design, the individual, and the composition of the diet influence the effect of calcium on blood pressure.

1. Study Design

The duration of the intervention and the dose of calcium can influence blood pressure response.[30] According to McCarron and Morris,[56] at least eight weeks of intervention is necessary for the antihypertensive effect of calcium to be expressed.

Thus, the failure of some calcium intervention trials to find an effect, such as those reported by van Berestyne et al.[104] and Kynast-Gales and Massey,[105] may be explained in part by their short duration (<8 weeks).

"Negative" findings for a hypotensive role of calcium also may be due to an insufficient amount of supplemental calcium or to a high level of calcium intake prior to supplementation. Inaccurate determination of blood pressure and dietary calcium intake, inconsistent screening of subjects for factors such as salt intake, and a small sample size also may contribute to the failure of some studies to demonstrate an inverse association between calcium and blood pressure.[30]

2. Individual Characteristics

In general, older persons appear to be particularly responsive to the blood pressure-lowering effect of increased calcium intake.[81,106-108] This may be explained by the lower initial calcium intake and reduced ability to absorb calcium in older adults. Studies indicate that individuals with low initial calcium intakes (e.g., African Americans, elderly) are more responsive to the blood pressure-lowering effects of calcium than are calcium-replete individuals.[43,53,60,106,109] That is, an antihypertensive effect from calcium cannot be expected from a population whose calcium intake already meets or exceeds recommended intakes. The failure of some studies to demonstrate a significant blood pressure lowering effect of calcium may be explained by the participants' already high calcium intake.[97,109,110]

The concept of a threshold of calcium above which there is an attenuated relationship between calcium intake and blood pressure has been recognized by several investigators.[29,37,53,82,96,109,111] According to McCarron et al.,[37] the "set point" of this threshold is 700-800 mg calcium per day (i.e., risk of hypertension increases at calcium intakes below this level), although many factors such as other dietary components and genetics can influence this "set point."

An individual's initial blood pressure status also may influence the blood pressure response to calcium supplementation. Individuals with a higher initial blood pressure may be more likely to respond to increased calcium intake with a reduction in blood pressure than individuals with a lower initial blood pressure.[56,61,80-82] However, whether or not hypertensives are more responsive to a hypotensive effect of calcium than are normotensives remains to be conclusively established.[84] Systolic blood pressure also appears to be affected more often than diastolic pressure by increased calcium intake.[43,56,60,61,80-82,102]

Body weight may influence the hypotensive effect of calcium, although this is controversial. There is a strong and consistent relationship between body weight and blood pressure. Overweight increases risk of hypertension while weight loss reduces blood pressure.[3,8-14] Failure of increased calcium to lower blood pressure in some overweight individuals may be explained by the overriding influence of excess weight compared to a low calcium intake.[59,71]

"Salt sensitivity" is a potential predictor of blood pressure response to calcium.[29,43,51-53,85,86,92,112-114] Salt sensitive, low renin individuals exhibit disturbances in calcium metabolism such as low serum ionized calcium, increased calciuresis, and elevated levels of calcium regulatory hormones (i.e., parathyroid hormone and 1,25 dihydroxyvitamin D) (Figure 3.8). Individuals with characteristics of salt sensitivity have been observed to be more likely to respond to dietary calcium with a decrease in blood pressure, at least when sodium intake is not restricted, than non-salt sensitive individuals. The protective effect of calcium in salt sensitive individuals appears to be most pronounced in the presence of a high sodium intake.[52,113,115-117] A low salt intake may preclude a blood pressure lowering response to calcium supplementation as calcium serves to attenuate the hypertensive response to high salt diets. Zemel et al.[113] found that hypertensive salt sensitive African American adults consuming a high sodium (4000 mg) low calcium (356 mg) diet exhibited a decrease in blood pressure in response to increased calcium intake (956 mg/day), whereas adding calcium to a low sodium (1000 mg) diet was without effect on blood pressure.

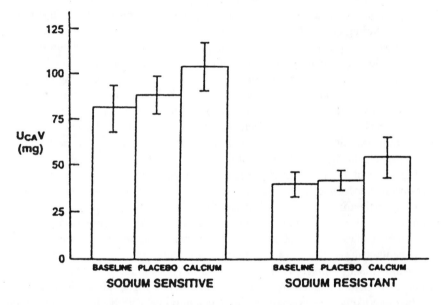

Figure 3.8   Mean ± standard deviation for urinary calcium excretion in sodium sensitive (left panel) and sodium resistant (right panel) subjects at baseline, during placebo, and during calcium supplementation. Sodium sensitive subjects had significantly (P<.001) greater calcium excretion during all three periods. (From Weinberger, M. H., Wagner, U. L., and Fineberg, N. S., *Am. J. Hypertens.*, 6, 799, 1993. With permission.)

Although there is no uniformly agreed upon protocol to identify salt sensitive individuals, an estimated 30 to 60% of hypertensives and 25 to 40% of normotensive individuals are considered to be salt sensitive, especially African Americans and the elderly.[118] One study reported alterations in calcium metabolism (e.g., increased parathyroid hormone and urinary calcium excretion and low serum calcium) in normotensive children of hypertensive parents, but not in children of normotensive parents.[119] If these findings are confirmed, changes in calcium metabolism may one day be used to predict hypertension.

3. Other Dietary Components

Interactions among calcium and other nutrients or dietary components may contribute to inconsistent effects of calcium on blood pressure.[17,26,64] As studies indicate, calcium's effect on blood pressure is influenced by salt intake. Other dietary components such as potassium, magnesium, and alcohol intake also may influence the antihypertensive effect of calcium.[17,26,29,37,59,62,64,75,108,115,120,121] The protective effect of calcium on blood pressure has been shown to be diminished in the presence of high intakes of alcohol.[59,121] This means that calcium in amounts higher than recommended intakes may be necessary to reduce elevated blood pressure in individuals who consume high alcohol intakes (>20 g/day or more than two drinks/day). Hamet et al.[115] suggest that high intakes of calcium (800 mg/1000 kcal) may help protect against sodium-induced as well as alcohol-induced hypertension. In contrast, less calcium may be needed to lower blood pressure in individuals consuming a high intake of potassium.[121] The effect of any single nutrient on blood pressure may be too small to detect, whereas several antihypertensive nutrients consumed together in a diet such as the "Dietary Approaches to Stop Hypertension" or DASH diet appear to have a more significant effect.[27,106] Clearly, nutrients interact in their effect on blood pressure regulation.[26]

4. Who is Most Likely to Respond?

There is no absolute predictor of the blood pressure response to increased calcium intake. However, the following groups indicated in Table 3.4 are considered to be the most likely to respond to increased calcium intake with a decrease in blood pressure.[37,53,122] Also specific clinical characteristics described in Table 3.4 predict individuals likely to have a blood pressure reduction in response to increased calcium intake.[53]

Table 3.4   Groups and Clinical Characteristics Associated with an Antihypertensive Effect on Calcium

Groups	Clinical Characteristics
Blacks	Salt sensitive
Southeast Asians (Japanese)	Elevated parathyroid hormone
Alcoholics	Elevated 1,25-dihydroxyvitamin D
Diabetics	Low ionized calcium
Salt Sensitive Subjects	Hypercalciuria
Pregnant Women	Low renin activity
Elderly People	
Individuals consuming low calcium diets	

Adapted from McCarron et al., *Am. J. Clin. Nutr.*, 54(Suppl. 1), 215s, 1991, and Sowers, J. R., et al., *Am. J. Hypertens.*, 4, 557, 1991.

III. POTASSIUM AND BLOOD PRESSURE

Experimental animal studies, epidemiological investigations, and clinical trials in humans indicate that an adequate potassium intake may protect against hypertension.[26,58,123-126] Overall findings also indicate that dietary potassium (e.g., in foods such as fruits, vegetables, and dairy foods) may have a major role as a non-pharmacological agent in the control of high blood pressure.[1] Not only may potassium protect against hypertension and its associated vascular diseases including stroke, but it also may reduce the need for antihypertensive medication.[26]

A. Experimental Animal Studies

In several animal models of hypertension, high potassium intake reduces blood pressure, often by attenuating a salt-induced rise in blood pressure.[26,124,125,127-129] In a study involving Dahl salt-sensitive and salt-resistant rats, low potassium intake not only was associated with increased blood pressure in both strains but it also increased the hypertensive effects of a high salt diet, even in previously salt-resistant rats.[128] In another experiment involving hypertensive rats, a high potassium diet markedly influenced salt sensitivity, evidenced by the reduction in blood pressure and mortality in the rats fed a high potassium, high sodium diet compared to those fed a normal potassium, high sodium diet.[125] Animal studies also indicate that increased dietary potassium may protect against vascular damage or stroke.[129]

B. Epidemiological Studies

Epidemiological investigations indicate an inverse association between potassium intake and blood pressure, although the findings are not entirely consistent. Higher intake of potassium was associated with lower mean systolic blood pressure and lower risk of hypertension in a study of 10,372 individuals, 18 to 74 years, who participated in the first Health and Nutrition Examination Survey (NHANES I).[58] In the INTERSALT study (i.e., a study investigating the relationships between electrolytes and blood pressure in over 10,000 adults in 52 population centers around the world) potassium intake or serum, urine, or total body potassium was inversely associated with blood pressure.[130,131] According to analyses of INTERSALT data, an increase in urinary potassium excretion of 60 mmol/day is associated with a 2.7 mmHg reduction in systolic blood pressure.[130] The INTERSALT data also suggest a drop in systolic blood pressure by 3.4 mmHg with a decrease in the 24-hour urinary sodium-potassium ratio from 3.1 (170 mmol of sodium/55 mmol potassium) to 1.0 (70 mmol of sodium /70 mmol potassium).[131]

When the relationship between electrolytes (sodium, potassium, calcium, and magnesium) and blood pressure was investigated in over 400 Yi farmers in the People's Republic of China, dietary, serum, and urinary potassium levels were inversely associated with systolic and diastolic blood pressures.[120] An increase in potassium intake of 100 mmol/day (7.5 g) corresponded to a decrease of 8.3 mm Hg and 5.7 mmHg in systolic and diastolic blood pressures, respectively.[120]

In 615 older men of Japanese ancestry participating in the Honolulu Heart Study, total potassium intake (i.e., from food and supplements) was significantly and inversely associated with both systolic and diastolic blood pressures.[132] Potassium from food was associated with both systolic and diastolic blood pressures, while supplemental potassium was associated only with diastolic blood pressure. Moreover, when potassium intake from dairy and non dairy sources was examined, dairy potassium was inversely associated with systolic and diastolic blood pressures, while nondairy potassium showed only a borderline inverse association with systolic blood pressure.[132] This epidemiological study indicates that potassium from dairy foods has a stronger relationship to blood pressure than potassium from nondairy foods.

Prospective studies support a beneficial role for dietary potassium in blood pressure regulation.[8,12,71,133] When 30,681 predominantly white American male health professionals aged 40 to 75 years without diagnosed hypertension increased their dietary potassium intake, risk of hypertension was significantly lower after adjusting for age, relative weight, as well as alcohol and energy intake (Figure 3.9).[71] In men participating in the Multiple Risk Factor Intervention Trial (MRFIT), dietary potassium intake was inversely associated with both systolic and diastolic blood pressure.[8] During the six years of the trial, potassium had a greater blood pressure lowering effect on systolic than diastolic blood pressure. In the Nurses Health Study II, an epidemiological cohort study of 300 women with normal blood pressure and habitually low intakes of potassium, increasing potassium intake to 102 mmol/day for 16 weeks significantly lowered systolic and diastolic blood pressures by 2.0 and 1.7 mmHg, respectively.[126]

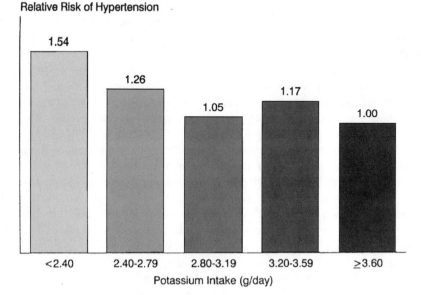

Relative Risk of Hypertension

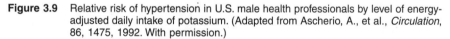

Figure 3.9   Relative risk of hypertension in U.S. male health professionals by level of energy-adjusted daily intake of potassium. (Adapted from Ascherio, A., et al., *Circulation*, 86, 1475, 1992. With permission.)

Findings of a longitudinal study in the Netherlands involving 233 children aged 5 to 17 years suggest that a sufficient intake of potassium (especially from food) or a reduction in the dietary sodium to potassium ratio may be beneficial in the early prevention of hypertension.[133] Children with a high dietary intake of potassium had a smaller yearly increase in systolic blood pressure than children with a low potassium intake. The sodium to potassium ratio also had an inverse relationship with blood pressure, although there was no clear effect for sodium alone. These findings indicate that in the early stages of hypertension (i.e., rise in blood pressure in childhood), blood pressure is raised more by a deficiency of potassium than by an excess of sodium. According to a three-year study of potassium supplementation (or sodium reduction), increased dietary potassium reduced blood pressure within the first two decades of life in adolescent girls.[134]

Similar to findings from experimental animal studies, some epidemiological studies in humans suggest that potassium's effect on the development of arterial disease may be independent of changes in blood pressure.[135,136] In a 12-year prospective study, a high intake of potassium from food sources reduced risk of stroke without a marked lowering of blood pressure.[135] When the relationship between urinary cations obtained from the INTERSALT study and cerebrovascular mortality was examined, 24-hour urinary potassium excretion was inversely associated with cerebrovascular disease mortality in women with no change in systolic and diastolic blood pressures.[136]

C. Clinical Studies

Clinical trials in normotensive and, in particular hypertensive, individuals point to a blood pressure-lowering effect of increased potassium intake.[137-139] In a recent randomized, cross-over trial in the United Kingdom, systolic blood pressure decreased by an average of 15 points in eight hypertensive patients over 68 years old who increased their intake of potassium by 60 mmol a day for one month and 48 mmol for four additional months.[139] In an investigation of African Americans who consumed a low potassium diet (32 to 35 mmol/day), those receiving a potassium supplement (80 mmol/day) for three weeks experienced a decrease in systolic and diastolic blood pressure of 6.9 and 2.5 mmHg, respectively.[138]

Further support for the concept that potassium intake may reduce the risk of developing hypertension comes from a recent meta-analysis of 33 randomized, controlled clinical trials involving over 2600 participants (age range 18 to 79 years).[137] Potassium supplementation significantly reduced systolic and diastolic blood pressure by 3.11 and 1.97 mmHg, respectively (Figure 3.10). Greater reductions were observed in the hypertensive group which exhibited decreases in systolic and diastolic blood pressures of 7.2 and 2.8 mmHg, respectively.[137] Also, the blood pressure-lowering effect of potassium appeared to be more pronounced in subjects consuming a high sodium intake. These findings led the authors of the meta-analysis to suggest that increasing potassium intake may be beneficial for the prevention and treatment of hypertension, especially in individuals who have difficulty lowering their sodium intake.[137]

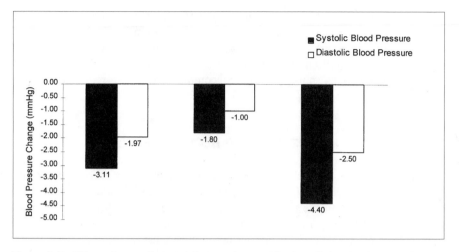

Figure 3.10 Effect of potassium supplementation on blood pressure in normotensive and hypertensive subjects. (Adapted from Whelton, P.K., et al. *JAMA*, 277, May 28, 1624, 1997. Copyright 1997, American Medical Association. With permission.)

Increasing dietary potassium intake from foods (e.g., fruits, vegetables, milk) appears to be as beneficial as potassium supplements in lowering blood pressure.[140] This was demonstrated in a study in which 28 hypertensive patients undergoing drug (antihypertensive) therapy increased their dietary potassium intake by an average of 50% (from 2.76 to 4.35 g/day), while another 26 participants maintained their usual diets.[140] The participants consuming the high potassium diets needed less medication (i.e., 36% reduction in drug use) than the control group to keep their blood pressure under 165/95 mmHg.

In general, the hypotensive effect of potassium is more pronounced in hypertensive than in normotensive individuals.[137] African Americans and others whose potassium intake is habitually low appear to benefit more from increased potassium intake than do whites or other groups consuming higher amounts of potassium.[138,141] African Americans usually consume and excrete less potassium and their blood pressure tends to be higher than Caucasians.[141] African Americans also have lower plasma renin sensitivity than Caucasians. A 10-week trial of the effect of a 80 mEq potassium chloride supplement a day on blood pressure showed that plasma renin activity in African Americans increased to the same level as Caucasians after potassium supplementation.[141] This finding suggests that the low plasma renin activity in African Americans is due in part to their low potassium intake. Thus, increasing dietary intake of food sources of potassium may be particularly beneficial for African Americans and others whose prevalence or risk of hypertension is high.

The effects of potassium on blood pressure also are influenced by other nutrients such as sodium, calcium, and magnesium.[142-144] Most studies that have demonstrated an antihypertensive effect of potassium have involved subjects consuming a high sodium (salt) rather than a low sodium diet.[137,142] A major mechanism by which increased potassium intake lowers blood pressure appears to be related to natriuresis (sodium excretion). Thus, individuals on high sodium diets need to maintain an adequate potassium intake to reduce their risk for hypertension. Increased potassium intake also reduces urinary losses of calcium and magnesium, nutrients demonstrated to have a protective effect on blood pressure.[26] Ensuring an adequate intake of potassium (i.e., 50 to 90 mmol/day), preferentially from foods such as vegetables, fruits, and dairy foods (milk, yogurt) is recommended to help reduce the risk of hypertension.[1,15]

IV. MAGNESIUM AND BLOOD PRESSURE

Magnesium has been observed to directly and indirectly affect cardiac and vascular smooth muscle.[145] Because magnesium promotes vascular smooth muscle relaxation, it is reasonable to suggest that this mineral may play a role in blood pressure regulation. Experimental animal, human epidemiological and clinical studies support a protective role for magnesium in hypertension, although the evidence is less conclusive than that for calcium or potassium.[26,145]

A. Experimental Animal Studies

Lower levels of magnesium in the plasma, kidney, heart, lung, and tibia and lower erythrocyte intracellular free magnesium have been found in the SHR (hypertensive) strain of rat compared to normotensive WKY rats.[146-148] In several different experimental rat models of hypertension, alterations in urinary magnesium excretion are reported.[145] Also diets that increase or decrease intracellular free magnesium lower or raise blood pressure, respectively.[145] Experimental animals fed a magnesium-deficient diet have been shown to exhibit an increase in blood pressure, and high magnesium diets attenuate the development of hypertension.[149-151] When the effect of dietary magnesium supplementation (10 g/kg diet) on blood pressure of Sprague-Dawley normotensive and mineralocorticoid-salt (DOCA-salt) hypertensive rats was investigated, magnesium supplementation significantly reduced blood pressure in the hypertensive, but not normotensive, rats.[152]

B. Epidemiological Studies

In a review of epidemiological studies of magnesium and blood pressure (mostly cross-sectional), Whelton and Klag[153] reported inconsistent findings. According to these authors, methodological shortcomings in the studies, including their brief duration, use of a single 24-hour dietary recall to measure magnesium intake, and the complicating presence of antihypertensive medication, preclude definitive conclusions regarding the effects of magnesium on blood pressure. Interactions among nutrients also influence the findings.[37,75] Reed and colleagues,[75] in their analysis of data from the Honolulu Heart Project, were unable to isolate the beneficial effects of magnesium from those of potassium and calcium.

Three studies reviewed by Whelton and Klag,[153] however, deserve mention, the first two because of their strong designs and the third because of a possible added explanation for the inconsistent findings. Magnesium was examined in a cross-sectional study of 61 dietary variables and blood pressure in 615 men participating in the Honolulu Heart Study, a community-based study of coronary heart disease and stroke in a cohort of elderly Japanese men living in Oahua, Hawaii. Magnesium intake had the strongest inverse association with both systolic and diastolic blood pressures (Figure 3.11).[132] Systolic and diastolic blood pressures were found to be 6.4 and 3.1 mm Hg lower, respectively, in the highest vs. the lowest quintile of magnesium intake.[132] In a hospital-based study in Detroit, dietary magnesium (determined by 4-day food records) was higher in Caucasian normotensive subjects than in either African American normotensives or Caucasian or African American hypertensives.[113] When serum magnesium levels and blood pressure were examined, Resnick et al.[154] found no difference in serum magnesium levels between hypertensive and control patients. However, when these investigators separated the hypertensive patients according to their renin status, those with high renin hypertension had the lowest serum magnesium levels.[154] These studies provide some evidence for a role for magnesium in regulating blood pressure.

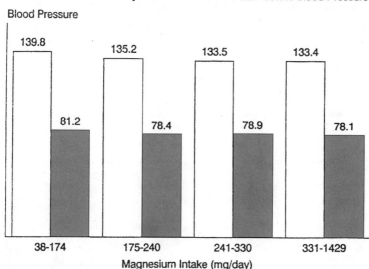

Figure 3.11 Inverse association between total magnesium intake and systolic and diastolic blood pressure in Japanese men. (Adapted from Jeffres, M. R., et al., *Am. J. Clin. Nutr.*, 45, 469, 1987. With permission.)

Prospective studies support a protective role for magnesium in the regulation of blood pressure.[12,59,71] Dietary magnesium had an independent and significant inverse association with hypertension in the first four years of follow-up (1980 to 1984) of the Nurses Health Study.[59] This prospective study examined the relationship of various nutritional factors to hypertension in over 58,000 predominantly Caucasian U.S. female registered nurses, aged 34 to 59 years.[59] The nurses who consumed at least 280 mg of magnesium a day had a one-third less chance of developing hypertension than those who consumed lower intakes of magnesium (i.e., <200 mg/day). The main contributors to magnesium intake in this study were fruits and vegetables (27%), cereals (17%), and dairy products (13%). The nurses who consumed at least recommended intakes for magnesium and calcium experienced a 35% reduction in risk of developing hypertension. In contrast, those who consumed intakes of these nutrients below recommended levels experienced a 23% lower risk of developing hypertension.[59] In the second four years of follow-up (i.e., 1984 to 1988) of 41,541 U.S. females participating in the Nurses Health Study,[12] magnesium intake was inversely associated with systolic and diastolic blood pressures, but not with the incidence of hypertension.

A beneficial role for magnesium in blood pressure regulation has also been reported in a prospective study involving nearly 31,000 predominantly Caucasian U.S. male health professionals, after adjusting for age, relative weight, and alcohol and energy intake (Figure 3.12).[71] Another study of over 15,000 subjects found an inverse association between dietary and blood levels of magnesium with systolic and diastolic blood pressures.[155] In older adults participating in a study in the Netherlands, increasing magnesium intake by 100 mg a day from foods was associated with a decrease in systolic and diastolic blood pressure of 1.2 and 1.1 mmHg, respectively.[144] In this study, the blood pressure lowering effect of magnesium was greater in men than in women.

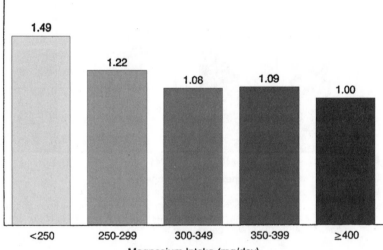

Figure 3.12 Relative risk of hypertension by level of energy-adjusted daily intake of magnesium in U.S. male health professionals. (Adapted from Ascherio, A., et al., *Circulation*, 86, 1475, 1992. With permission.)

C. Clinical Studies

Clinical studies of the influence of magnesium on blood pressure have yielded inconsistent findings, thus neither proving nor refuting an antihypertensive effect of this mineral. In phase I of the Trials of Hypertension Prevention,[110] no difference in blood pressure was observed between 227 subjects who received magnesium supplements (360 mg/day) for six months vs. 234 who received a placebo. However, the possibility of low magnesium absorption and low compliance, as well as the decrease in blood pressure in the placebo group, may have contributed to the lack of a blood pressure-lowering effect of magnesium in this trial. The hypotensive effect of magnesium may be restricted to magnesium-deficient individuals.[156] According to a three-month study of 13 patients with mild hypertension, oral supplements of magnesium lowered blood pressure only in patients identified as magnesium deficient based on blood magnesium levels.[156] However, in the Nurses Health Study II, increasing magnesium intake to 585 mg/day for 16 weeks in normotensive women whose usual dietary intake of magnesium was low had no effect on blood pressure.[126] Other methodological variables such as the use of antihypertensive medication and the length of follow-up may contribute to the inconsistent findings. In the Multiple Risk Factor Intervention Trial, dietary magnesium was inversely related to systolic and diastolic blood pressures with the greater effect for men not receiving antihypertensive medication.[8] Also, in a double-blind, placebo-controlled study involving 91 women with mild to moderate hypertension, increasing magnesium intake by 485 mg (20 mm) a day had no significant effect on blood pressure after three months of magnesium supplementation.[157] However, after six months, magnesium modestly, but significantly, reduced diastolic blood pressure (3.4 mm Hg). The decrease in systolic blood pressure (2.7 mmHg) was not significant.[157] Possible interactions of magnesium with other nutrients also may explain the inconsistent effects of magnesium on blood pressure.[145] Vigorous testing using long-term studies is needed to determine the effectiveness of dietary magnesium in reducing the risk of high blood pressure.[145,158]

V. DIETARY PATTERNS INCLUDING DAIRY FOODS AND BLOOD PRESSURE

Clearly, the impact of individual nutrients on blood pressure is complicated by the complexity of dietary interactions. To gain increased understanding of the combined effects of nutrients that occur together in foods, the National Institutes of Health sponsored a multicenter feeding trial to examine the effects of dietary patterns on blood pressure.[27] This landmark study, called the Dietary Approaches to Stop Hypertension (DASH) study, found that a diet high in lowfat dairy foods, fruits, and vegetables reduced saturated and total fat significantly and quickly (within two weeks) lowered blood pressure in subjects with high normal hypertension. This study is unique in that it examines the effect of dietary patterns of nutrients as in foods on blood pressure, as opposed to individual nutrients.[27]

More than 450 adults with systolic blood pressures of less than 160 mmHg and diastolic pressures of 80 to 95 mmHg were enrolled in the study.[27] About half of the participants were women and nearly 60% were African Americans. For eight weeks, participants were fed one of three diets: a "control diet" similar to what many Americans consume (i.e., low in fruits, vegetables, and dairy products and containing 36% of calories from fat); a "fruits and vegetables" diet (i.e., higher in fiber, potassium, and magnesium than in the control diet, but similar in fat); or a "combination" diet high in lowfat dairy foods, fruits, and vegetables and reduced in total fat (26% of calories), saturated fat, and cholesterol (i.e., higher in fiber, protein, potassium, magnesium, and calcium than the control diet). All three diets were equal in salt content (i.e., 3 g sodium/day) and all participants maintained body weight.

At the end of the eight weeks, the combination diet, the reduced fat diet that added lowfat dairy foods along with fruits and vegetables, produced the largest reductions in blood pressures (Figure 3.13).[27] Overall, this diet reduced systolic

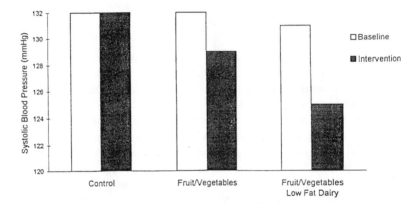

Figure 3.13 The effect of dietary patterns on systolic blood pressure in a cohort of 459 adults with high normal hypertension. (Adapted from Appel, L.J., et al., *N. Engl. J. Med.*, 336, 1117, 1997.)

blood pressure by 5.5 mmHg and diastolic blood pressure by 3.0 mmHg compared to the control diet. For participants with hypertension, the blood pressure lowering effect of the combination diet was even more impressive, with an average reduction of 11.4 mmHg for systolic and 5.5 mmHg for diastolic blood pressures.[27] These declines not only were apparent within two weeks, but they also rivaled those produced by antihypertensive medications.[106] Also, this diet did not produce gastrointestinal symptoms and the blood pressure-lowering effect was independent of body weight, sodium intake, or alcohol intake.[27] The fruits and vegetables diet reduced systolic and diastolic blood pressures by 2.8 mmHg and 1.1 mmHg, respectively, compared with the control diet.

Participants following the combination diet consumed almost three servings of dairy foods (two low in fat and one traditional product) a day (i.e., a mean of 1260 mg calcium a day). They also consumed 8 to 10 servings a day of fruits and vegetables. Because the study population was reflective of the general U.S. population and because all responded, the researchers suggest that the study results are generalizable to the entire U.S. population.[27] Consuming a diet similar to the combination diet and following other lifestyle recommendations to lower blood pressure could help prevent hypertension and, for some hypertensives, may reduce or eliminate the need for blood pressure medication.[27] This position is supported by other investigators.[28,106] A beneficial effect on blood pressure was demonstrated in another study in which the composition of the total diet was manipulated.[28] This study involved 560 adults with hypertension, dyslipidemia, or diabetes at 10 medical centers in the U.S. The participants were randomized to receive either prepackaged meals meeting individual nutrient requirements or they self-selected an American Heart Association Step 1 or Step 2 diet under a nutritionist's guidance for 10 weeks. Although blood pressure improved on both nutrition plans, the prepackaged meal plan resulted in a greater decrease in blood pressures (i.e., 6.4 and 4.2 mmHg for systolic and diastolic blood pressures, respectively) than the self-selected diets (i.e., 4.6 and 3.0 mmHg for systolic and diastolic blood pressures, respectively).[28] The beneficial effects on blood pressure with the prepackaged meal plan were accompanied by improvements in dietary levels of calcium, potassium, and magnesium approximating intakes achieved in the DASH study. The authors conclude that consuming nutritionally balanced meals that meet the recommendations of national health organizations can improve cardiovascular risk factors such as blood pressure.[28]

The findings of these studies[27,28] are important considering that small decreases in blood pressure have favorable effects on risk of cardiovascular disease, stroke, coronary heart disease, and all-cause mortality in adults.[7,8]

VI. SUMMARY

Accumulating scientific evidence indicates that an adequate intake of calcium, potassium, and magnesium, three nutrients found simultaneously in meaningful amounts in dairy foods, has a positive effect on blood pressure and helps to reduce the risk of hypertension. This disease affects one in every four American adults and is a major risk factor for coronary heart disease, stroke, and renal failure.

While much remains to be learned about the relationship between calcium and blood pressure, most investigators recommend that individuals consume current recommended intakes of this mineral to treat or reduce risk of hypertension.[1,3,37,53,114] Calcium supplements are not advised to reduce blood pressure.[1,29] Rather, food sources of calcium such as dairy foods are recommended because, in addition to calcium, they provide other nutrients such as potassium and magnesium which may protect against hypertension.[65,105] Milk and other dairy foods make a significant contribution to the nation's supply of nutrients.[22] Diets low in dairy foods compromise the nutritional quality of the diet.[65,159-162] Studies in both adults[65,159] and children[161,162] indicate that consumption of dairy foods improves the overall nutrient adequacy of the diet. Moreover, increasing calcium intake to 1500 to 1600 mg/day (i.e., an amount greater than the 1000 to 1300 mg currently recommended for adults[23]) from dairy foods (e.g., yogurt, skim and low fat milk) does not raise plasma lipids, lipoproteins, or body weight (i.e., other risk factors for coronary heart disease),[65] a finding supported by other investigators.[159,161-163] In addition, consuming calcium-rich foods such as dairy products is likely to be associated with fewer compliance problems than associated with salt-restricted diets.[53] Consuming calcium-rich foods such as dairy foods is also advantageous considering that salt-restricted diets are often limited in other essential nutrients such as calcium, iron, magnesium, and vitamin B_6.[19]

The minimum requirement for potassium is approximately 1600 to 2000 mg a day.[24] Given the high cost (>$200 a year) and potential health hazards associated with potassium supplements, especially for patients at risk of high blood potassium levels, diet is the preferred means to meet potassium needs.[140,143,164] Dairy foods, because of their potassium content, may be especially beneficial for African Americans, the elderly, and others at high risk for hypertension; for hypertensives on drugs (i.e., dairy foods may reduce their need for medication); and for young people to lower their later risk of this disease.

Rigorous testing in long-term studies is needed to determine the effectiveness of dietary magnesium as an approach to blood pressure control.[158] In the meantime, foods rich in magnesium such as vegetables, whole grains, fruits, and dairy foods are recommended to protect against hypertension,[53,132] especially for individuals whose intake of magnesium is low such as women, African Americans, and alcoholics.

Considering that the costs associated with hypertension are estimated at nearly $32 billion a year,[6] and that the U.S. government is committed to cutting health care costs, prevention of hypertension by consuming a nutritionally adequate diet containing recommended servings of dairy foods is essential. The National Heart, Lung and Blood Institute (NHLBI), in its new guidelines to prevent and treat high blood pressure,[1] recommends that people consume adequate intakes of calcium, potassium, and magnesium from food sources. Support for the importance of food sources of nutrients comes from a recent multicenter study called the Dietary Approaches to Stop Hypertension (i.e., DASH).[27] This study found that a dietary pattern consisting of three servings a day of lowfat dairy foods and eight to ten servings a day of fruits and vegetables, a pattern that provides calcium, potassium, and magnesium at the 75th percentile of Americans' intake, effectively lowers blood pressure in both normotensive and hypertensive individuals.[27] The DASH diet has been adopted as the official diet of the NHLBI's most recent recommendations to prevent hypertension.[1]

REFERENCES

1. Joint National Committee on Prevention, Detection, Evaluation, and Treatment of High Blood Pressure, The Sixth Report of the Joint National Committee on Prevention, Detection, Evaluation, and Treatment of High Blood Pressure, *Arch. Intern. Med.*, 157, 2413, 1997.

2. Federation of American Societies for Experimental Biology, Life Sciences Research Office, Prepared for the Interagency Board for Nutrition Monitoring and Related Research, Third Report on Nutrition Monitoring in the United States, Volume 1, U.S. Government Printing Office, 1995.

3. National High Blood Pressure Education Program Working Group, National High Blood Pressure Education Program Working Group Report on Primary Prevention of Hypertension, *Arch. Intern. Med.*, 153, 186, 1993.

4. U. S. Department of Health and Human Services, Public Health Service, Healthy People 2000, National Health Promotion and Disease Prevention Objectives, DHHS Pub. No. (PHS) 91-50212, U.S. Government Printing Office, Washington, D.C., September 1990.

5. Kannel, W. B., Blood pressure as a cardiovascular risk factor, *JAMA*, 275, 1571, 1996.

6. American Heart Association, Economic cost of cardiovascular diseases, www.amer-icanheart.org/Scientific/HSstats98/10econom. html.

7. Cook, N. R., Cohen, J., Herbert, P. R., Taylor, J. O., and Hennekens, C. H., Implications of small reductions in diastolic blood pressure for primary prevention, *Arch. Intern. Med.*, 155, 701, 1995.

8. Stamler, J., Caggiula, A. W., and Grandits, G. A., Relation of body mass and alcohol, nutrient, fiber, and caffeine intakes to blood pressure in the special intervention and usual care groups in the Multiple Risk Factor Intervention Trial, *Am. J. Clin. Nutr.*, 65(Suppl.), 338s, 1997.

9. Preuss, H. G., Diet, genetics, and hypertension, *J. Am. Coll. Nutr.*, 16, 296, 1997.

10. McCarron, D. A. and Reusser, M. E., Body weight and blood pressure regulation, *Am. J. Clin. Nutr.*, 63(Suppl.), 423s, 1996.

11. Pickering, T. G., Lessons from the Trials of Hypertension Prevention, Phase II, Energy intake is more important than dietary sodium in the prevention of hypertension, *Arch. Intern. Med.*, 157, 596, 1997.

12. Ascherio, A., Hennekens, C., Willett, W. C., Sacks, F., Rosner, B., Manson, J., Witteman, J., and Stampfer, M. J., Prospective study of nutritional factors, blood pressure, and hypertension among U.S. women, *Hypertension*, 27, 1065, 1996.

13. The Trials of Hypertension Prevention Collaborative Research Group, Effects of weight loss and sodium reduction intervention on blood pressure and hypertension incidence in overweight people with high-normal blood pressure. Results of the Trials of Hypertension Prevention, phase II, *Arch. Intern. Med.*, 157, 657, 1997.

14. Whelton, P. K., Kumanyika, S. K., Cook, N. R., Cutler, J. A., Borhani, N. O., Hennekens, C. H., Kuller, L. H., Langford, H., Jones, D. W., Satterfield, S., Lasser, N. L., and Cohen, J. D. for the Trials of Hypertension Prevention Collaborative Research Group, Efficacy of nonpharmacologic interventions in adults with high-normal blood pressure: results from phase I of the Trials of Hypertension Prevention, *Am. J. Clin. Nutr.*, 65(Suppl.), 652s, 1997.

15. U.S. Department of Agriculture, U.S. Department of Health and Human Services, Nutrition and Your Health: Dietary Guidelines for Americans, Fourth Edition, Home and Garden Bulletin No. 232, December 1995.

16. Food and Drug Administration, U.S. Department of Health and Human Services, Food labeling: health claims and label statements; sodium and hypertension, *Fed. Register*, 58(Jan. 6), 2820, 1993.

17. Oparil, S. Ed., Conference on dietary sodium and health, *Am. J. Clin. Nutr.*, 65(Suppl. 2), 583s, 1997.

18. Graudal, N. A., Galloe, A. M., and Garred, P., Effects of sodium restriction on blood pressure, renin, aldosterone, catecholamines, cholesterols, and triglyceride. A meta-analysis, *JAMA*, 279, 1383, 1998.

19. Morris, C. D., Effect of dietary sodium restriction on overall nutrient intake, *Am. J. Clin. Nutr.*, 65(Suppl.), 687s, 1997.

20. McCarron, D. A., Weder, A. B., Egan, B. M., Krishna, G. G., Morris, C. D., Cohen, M., and Oparil, S., Blood pressure and metabolic responses to moderate sodium restriction in Isradipine-treated hypertensive patients, *Am. J. Hypertens.*, 10, 68, 1997.

21. Alderman, M. H., Cohen, H., and Madhavan, S., Dietary sodium intake and mortality: The National Health and Nutrition Examination Survey (NHANES I), *Lancet*, 351, 781, 1998.

22. Gerrior, S. and Bente, L., Nutrient Content of the U.S. Food Supply, 1909-94, U.S. Department of Agriculture, Center for Nutrition Policy and Promotion, Home Economics Research Report No. 53, 1997.

23. IOM (Institute of Medicine), Dietary Reference Intakes for Calcium, Phosphorus, Magnesium, Vitamin D, and Fluoride, Standing Committee on the Scientific Evaluation of Dietary Reference Intakes, Food and Nutrition Board, National Academy Press, Washington, D.C., 1997.

24. Food and Nutrition Board, Subcommittee on the Tenth Edition of the RDAs, Recommended Dietary Allowances, 10th Edition, National Academy Press, Washington, D.C., 1989.

25. U.S. Department of Agriculture, Agricultural Research Service, USDA Nutrient Database for Standard Reference, Release 12, Nutrient Data Laboratory, www.nal.usda.gov/fnic/foodcomp, 1998.

26. Reusser, M. E. and McCarron, D. A., Micronutrient effects on blood pressure regulation, *Nutr. Rev.*, 52, 367, 1994.

27. Appel, L. J., Moore, T. J., Obarzanek, E., Vollmer, W. M., Svetkey, L. P., Sacks, F. M., Bray, G. A., Vogt, T. M., Cutler, J. A., Windhauser, M. M., Lin, P.-H., and Karanja, N., for the DASH Collaborative Research Group, A clinical trial of the effects of dietary patterns on blood pressure, *N. Engl. J. Med.*, 336, 1117, 1997.

28. McCarron, D. A., Oparil, S., Chait, A., Haynes, R. B., Kris-Etherton, P., Stern, J. S., Resnick, L. M., Clark, S., Morris, C. D., Hatton, D. C., Metz, J. A., McMahon, M., Holcomb, S., Snyder, G. W., and Pi-Sunyer, F. X., Nutritional management of cardiovascular risk factors, *Arch. Intern. Med.*, 157, 169, 1997.

29. Hamet, P., The evaluation of the scientific evidence for a relationship between calcium and hypertension, *J. Nutr.*, 125(Suppl.), 311s, 1995.

30. Osborne, C. G., McTyre, R. B., Dudek, J., Roche, K. E., Scheuplein, R., Silverstein, B., Weinberg, M. S., and Salkeld, A. A., Evidence for the relationship of calcium to blood pressure, *Nutr. Rev.*, 54, 365, 1996.

31. Hatton, D. C. and McCarron, D. A., Dietary calcium and blood pressure in experimental models of hypertension. A review, *Hypertension*, 23(4), 513, 1994.

32. McCarron, D. A., Lucas, P. A., Shneidman, R. J., LaCour, B., and Drueke, T., Blood pressure development of the spontaneously hypertensive rat after concurrent manipulations of dietary Ca2+ and Na+: Relation to intestinal Ca2+ fluxes, *J. Clin. Invest.*, 76, 1147, 1985.

33. Ayachi, S., Increased dietary calcium lowers blood pressure in the spontaneously hypertensive rat, *Metabolism*, 28, 1234, 1979.

34. Pernot, F., Schleiffer, R., Bergmann, C., Vincent, M., Sassard, J., and Gairard, A., Dietary calcium, vascular reactivity, and genetic hypertension in the Lyon rat strain, *Am. J. Hypertens.*, 3, 846, 1990.

35. Schleiffer, R. and Gairard, A., Blood pressure effects of calcium intake in experimental models of hypertension, *Semin. Nephrol.*, 15, 526, 1995.

36. McCarron, D. A., Blood pressure and calcium balance in the Wistar-Kyoto rat, *Life Sci.*, 30, 683, 1982.

37. McCarron, D. A., Morris, C. D., Young, E., Roullet, C., and Drueke, T., Dietary calcium and blood pressure: modifying factors in specific populations, *Am. J. Clin. Nutr.*, 54(Suppl. I), 215s, 1991.

38. Belizan, J. M., Pineda, O., Sainz, E., Menendez, L. A., and Villar, J., Rise of blood pressure in calcium-deprived pregnant rats, *Am. J. Obstet. Gynecol.*, 141, 163, 1981.

39. Ambrozy, S. L., Shehin, S. E., Chiou, C.-Y., Sowers, J. R., and Zemel, M. B., Effects of dietary calcium on blood pressure, vascular reactivity and vascular smooth muscle calcium efflux rate in Zucker rats., *Am. J. Hypertens.*, 4, 592, 1991.

40. Porsti, I. and Makynen, H., Dietary calcium intake: effects on central blood pressure control, *Semin. Nephrol.*, 15, 550, 1995.

41. Makynen, H., Kahonen, M., Wu, X., Arvola, P., and Porsti, I., Endothelial function in deoxycorticosterone-NaCl hypertension. Effect of calcium supplementation, *Circulation*, 93, 1000, 1996.

42. Hamet, P., Skuherska, R., Cherkaoui, L., Pang, S. C., Amer, V., and Tremblay, J., Calcium levels and platelet responsiveness in spontaneously hypertensive rats on high calcium diet (Abst.), *J. Hypertens.*, 4(Suppl. 6), 716s, 1986.

43. Sowers, J. R., Zemel, M. B., Standley, P. R., and Zemel, P. C., Calcium and hypertension, *J. Lab. Clin. Med.*, 114, 338, 1989.

44. Oparil, S., Chen, Y.-F., Jin, H., Yang, R.-H., and Wyss, J. M., Dietary Ca2+ prevents NaCl-sensitive hypertension in spontaneously hypertensive rats via sympatholytic and renal effects, *Am. J. Clin. Nutr.*, 54(Suppl.), 227s, 1991.

45. Young, E. W., Bukoski, R. D., and McCarron, D. A., Calcium metabolism in experimental hypertension, *Proc. Soc. Exp. Biol. Med.*, 187, 123, 1988.

46. Blakeborough, P., Neville, S. G., and Rolls, B. A., The effect of diets adequate and deficient in calcium on blood pressures and the activities of intestinal and kidney plasma membrane enzymes in normotensive and spontaneously hypertensive rats, *Br. J. Nutr.*, 63, 65, 1990.

47. Oshima, T., Young, E. W., Hermsmeyer, K., and McCarron, D. A., Modification of platelet and lymphocyte calcium handling and blood pressure by dietary sodium and calcium in genetically hypertensive rats, *J. Lab. Clin. Med.*, 119, 151, 1992.

48. Wyss, J. M., Chen, Y. F., Meng, Q., Jin, H., Jirikulsomchok, S., and Oparil, S., Dietary Ca2+ prevents NaCl-induced exacerbation of hypertension and increases hypothalamic norepinephrine turnover in spontaneously hypertensive rats, *J. Hypertens.*, 7, 711, 1989.

49. Wuorela, H., The effect of high calcium intake on intracellular free [Ca2+] and Na+ –H+ exchange in DOC-NaCl-hypertensive rats, *Pharmacol. & Toxicol.*, 71, 376, 1992.

50. DiPette, D. J., Greilich, P. E., Nickols, G. A., Graham, G. A., Green, A., Cooper, C. W., and Holland, O. B., Effect of dietary calcium supplementation on blood pressure and calcitropic hormones in mineralocorticoid-salt hypertension, *J. Hypertens.*, 8, 515, 1990.

51. Resnick, L. M., Calcium calcitropic hormones in human and experimental hypertension, In: Laragh, J. H., Brenner, B., and Kaplan, N. M., Eds., *Endocrine Metabolism in Hypertension*, Raven Press, New York, 265, 1989.

52. Resnick, L. M., Muller, F. B., and Laragh. J. H., Calcium regulating hormones in essential hypertension, relation to plasma renin activity and sodium metabolism, *Ann. Intern. Med.*, 105, 649, 1986.

53. Sowers, J. R., Zemel, M. B., Zemel, P. C., and Standley, P. R., Calcium metabolism and dietary calcium in salt sensitive hypertension, *Am. J. Hypertens.*, 4, 557, 1991.

54. Porsti, I., Arvda, P., Wuorela, H., and Vapaatalo, H., High calcium diet augments vascular potassium relaxation in hypertensive rats, *Hypertension*, 19, 85, 1992.

55. Karanja, N., Phanouvong, T., and McCarron, D. A., Blood pressure in spontaneously hypertensive rats fed butterfat, corn oil, or fish oil, *Hypertension*, 14, 674, 1989.

56. McCarron, D. A. and Morris, C. D., Blood pressure response to oral calcium in persons with mild to moderate hypertension, *Ann. Intern. Med.*, 103, 825, 1985.

57. McCarron, D. A., Calcium metabolism and hypertension, *Kidney Int.*, 35, 717, 1989.

58. McCarron, D. A., Morris, C. D., Henry, H. J., and Stanton, J. L., Blood pressure and nutrient intake in the United States, *Science*, 224, 1392, 1984.

59. Witteman, J. C. M., Willett, W. C., Stampfer, M. J., Colditz, G. A., Sacks, F. M., Speizer, F. E., Rosner, B., and Hennekens, C. H., A prospective study of nutritional factors and hypertension among U.S. women, *Circulation*, 80, 1320, 1989.

60. Iso, H., Terao, A., Kitamura, A., Sato, S., Naito, Y., Kiyama, M., Tanigaki, M., Iida, M., Konishi, M., Shimamoto, T., and Komachi, Y., Calcium intake and blood pressure in seven Japanese populations, *Am. J. Epidemiol.*, 133, 776, 1991.

61. Grobbee, D. E. and Waal-Manning, H. J., The role of calcium supplementation in the treatment of hypertension, current evidence, *Drugs*, 39(1), 7, 1990.

62. Dwyer, J. H., Li, L., Dwyer, K. M., Curtin, L. R., and Feinleib, M., Dietary calcium, alcohol, and incidence of treated hypertension in the NHANES I epidemiologic follow-up study, *Am. J. Epidemiol.*, 144, 828, 1996.

63. Birkett, N. J., Comments on a meta-analysis on the relationship between dietary calcium intake and blood pressure, *Am. J. Epidemiol.*, 148, 223, 1998.

64. Morris, C. D. and Reusser, M. E., Calcium intake and blood pressure: epidemiology revisited, *Sem. Nephrol.*, 15, 490, 1995.

65. Karanja, N., Morris, C. D., Rufolo, P., Snyder, G., Illingworth, D. R., and McCarron, D. A., Impact of increasing calcium in the diet on nutrient consumption, plasma lipids, and lipoproteins in humans, *Am. J. Clin. Nutr.*, 59, 900, 1994.

66. Gillman, M. W., Oliveria, S. A., Moore, L. L., and Ellison, R. C., Inverse association of dietary calcium with systolic blood pressure in young children, *JAMA*, 267, 2340, 1992.

67. Simons-Morton, D. G., Hunsberger, S. A., Van Horn, L., Barton, B. A., Robson, A. M., McMahon, R. P., Muhonen, L. E., Kwiterovich, P. O., Lasser, N. L., Kimm, S. Y. S., and Greenlick, M. R., Nutrient intake and blood pressure in the Dietary Intervention Study in Children, *Hypertension*, 29, 930, 1997.

68. Gillman, M. W., Hood, M. Y., Moore, L. L., Nguyen, U.-S. D. T., Singer, M. R., and Andon, M. B., Effect of calcium supplementation on blood pressure in children, *J. Pediatr.*, 127, 186, 1995.

69. Task Force Update on the Report (1987) on Blood Pressure in Children and Adolescents, A Working Group Report from the National High Blood Pressure Education Program, NIH Publ., No. 96-3790, September 1996.

70. Bao, W., Threefoot, S. A., Srinivasan, S. R., and Berenson, G. S., Essential hypertension predicted by tracking of elevated blood pressure from childhood to adulthood: The Bogalusa Heart Study, *Am. J. Hypertens.*, 8, 657, 1995.

71. Ascherio, A., Rimm, E. B., Giovannucci, E. L., Colditz, G. A., Rosner, B., Willett, W. C., Sacks, F., and Stampfer, M. J., A prospective study of nutritional factors and hypertension among U.S. men, *Circulation*, 86, 1475, 1992.

72. Cappuccio, F. P., Elliott, P., Allender, P. S., Pryer, J., Follman, D. A., and Cutler, J. A., Epidemiologic association between dietary calcium intake and blood pressure: a meta-analysis of published data, *Am. J. Epidemiol.*, 142, 935, 1995.

73. Ackley, S., Barrett-Connor, E., and Suarez, L., Dairy products, calcium, and blood pressure., *Am. J. Clin. Nutr.*, 38, 457, 1983.

74. Garcia-Palmieri, M. R., Costas, R. Jr., Cruz-Vidal, M., Sorlie, P. D., Tillotson, J., and Havlik, R. J., Milk consumption, calcium intake, and decreased hypertension in Puerto Rico: Puerto Rico Heart Health Program Study, *Hypertension*, 6, 322, 1984.

75. Reed, D., McGee, D., Yano, K., and Hankin, J., Diet, blood pressure, and multicollinearity, *Hypertension*, 7, 405, 1985.

76. Freudenheim, J. L., Russell, M., Trevisan, M., and Doemland, M., Calcium intake and blood pressure in blacks and whites, *Ethnicity Dis.*, 1, 114, 1991.

77. Trevisan, M., Krogh, V., Farinaro, E., Panico, S., and Mancini, M., Calcium-rich foods and blood pressure: findings from the Italian National Research Council Study (The Nine Communities Study), *Am. J. Epidemiol.*, 127, 1155, 1988.

78. Marcoux, S., Brisson, J., and Fabia, J., Calcium intake from dairy products and supplements and the risks of preeclampsia and gestational hypertension, *Am. J. Epidemiol.*, 133, 1266, 1991.

79. Richardson, B. E. and Baird, D. D., A study of milk and calcium supplement intake and subsequent preeclampsia in a cohort of pregnant women, *Am. J. Epidemiol.*, 141, 667, 1995.

80. Mikami, H., Ogihara, T., and Tabuchi, Y., Blood pressure response to dietary calcium intervention in humans, *Am. J. Hypertens.*, 3(Suppl.), 147s, 1990.

81. Allender, P. S., Cutler, J. A., Follmann, D., Cappuccio, F. P., Pryer, J., and Elliott, P., Dietary calcium and blood pressure: a meta-analysis of randomized clinical trials, *Ann. Intern. Med.*, 124, 825, 1996.

82. Bucher, H. C., Cook, R. J., Guyatt, G. H., Lang, J. D., Cook, D. J., Hatala, R., and Hunt, D. L., Effects of dietary calcium supplementation on blood pressure: a meta-analysis of randomized controlled trials, *JAMA*, 275, 1016, 1996.

83. Bucher, H. C., Guyatt, G. H., Cook, R. J., Hatala, R., Cook, D. J., Lang, J. D., and Hunt, D., Effect of calcium supplementation on pregnancy-induced hypertension and preeclampsia, *JAMA*, 275, 1113, 1996.

84. Bucher, H. C., Guyatt, G. H., and Cook, R. J., Dietary calcium and blood pressure, *Ann. Intern. Med.*, 126, 492, 1997.

85. Resnick, L. M., Nicholson, J. P., and Laragh, J. H., Calcium metabolism in essential hypertension: relationship to altered renin system activity, *Fed. Proc.*, 45, 2739, 1986.

86. Grobbee, D. E., and Hofman, A., Effect of calcium supplementation on diastolic blood pressure in young people with mild hypertension, *Lancet*, 2, 703, 1986.

87. Strazzullo, P., Siani, A., Guglielmi, S., DiCarlo, A., Galletti, F., Cirillo, M., and Mancini, M., Controlled trial of long-term oral calcium supplementation in essential hypertension, *Hypertension*, 8, 1084, 1986.

88. Resnick, L., DiFabio, B., Marion, R. M., James, G., and Laragh, J., Dietary calcium modifies the pressor effects of dietary salt intake in essential hypertension, *J. Hypertens.*, 4(Suppl. 6), 679s, 1986.

89. Zemel, M. B., Gualdoni, S. M., and Sowers, J. R., Reductions in total and extracellular water associated with calcium-induced natriuresis and the antihypertensive effect of calcium in blacks, *Am. J. Hypertens.*, 1, 70, 1988.

90. Vaughan, L. A., Manore, M. M., Russo, M. E., Swart, A., Carroll, S. S., and Felicetta, J. V., Blood pressure responses of mild hypertensive Caucasian males to a metabolic diet with moderate sodium and two levels of dietary calcium, *Nutr. Res.*, 17, 215, 1997.

91. Hojo, M. and August, P., Calcium metabolism in normal and hypertensive pregnancy, *Semin. Nephrol.*, 15, 504, 1995.

92. Repke, J. T. and Villar, J., Pregnancy-induced hypertension and low birth weight: the role of calcium, *Am. J. Clin. Nutr.*, 54(Suppl.), 237s, 1991.

93. Belizan, J. M., Villar, J., Gonzalez, L., Campodonico, L., and Bergel, E., Calcium supplementation to prevent hypertensive disorders of pregnancy, *N. Engl. J. Med.*, 325, 1399, 1991.

94. Knight, K. B. and Keith, R. E., Calcium supplementation on normotensive and hypertensive pregnant women, *Am. J. Clin. Nutr.*, 55, 891, 1992.

95. Villar, J. and Repke, J. T., Calcium supplementation during pregnancy may reduce preterm delivery in high-risk populations, *J. Obstet. Gynecol.*, 163, 1124, 1990.

96. McCarron, D. A. and Hatton, D., Dietary calcium and lower blood pressure: we can all benefit, *JAMA*, 275, 1126, 1996.

97. Levine, R. J., Hauthy, J. C., Curet, L. B., Sibai, V. M., Catalano, P. M., Morris, C. D., DerSimonian, R., Esterlitz, J. R., Raymond, E. G., Bild, D. E., Clemens, J. C., and Cutler, J. A., Trial of calcium for prevention of preeclampsia, *N. Engl. J. Med.*, 337, 69, 1997.

98. Roberts, J., Prevention or early treatment of preeclampsia, *N. Engl. J. Med.*, 337, 124, 1997.

99. Belizan, J. M., Villar, J., Bergel, E., del Pino, A., DiFulvio, S., Galliano, S. V., and Kattan, C., Long term effect of calcium supplementation during pregnancy on the blood pressure of offspring: follow up of a randomised controlled trial, *Br. Med. J.*, 315, 281, 1997.

100. McGarvey, S. T., Zinner, S. H., Willett, W. C., and Rosner, B., Maternal prenatal dietary potassium, calcium, magnesium, and infant blood pressure, *Hypertension*, 17, 218, 1991.

101. Bierenbaum, M. L., Wolf, E., Bisgeier, G., and Maginnis, W. P., Dietary calcium: a method of lowering blood pressure, *Am. J. Hypertens.*, 1(Suppl.), 149s, 1988.

102. Van Beresteijn, E. C. H., Van Schaik, M., and Schaafsma, G., Milk: does it affect blood pressure? a controlled intervention study, *J. Intern. Med.*, 228, 477, 1990.

103. Zemel, M. B., Bedford, B. A., Zemel, P. C., Marwah, O., and Sowers, J. R., Altered cation transport in non-insulin-dependent diabetic hypertension: effects of dietary calcium, *J. Hypertens.*, 6(Suppl. 4), 228s, 1988.

104. Van Beresteyn, E. C. H., Schaafsma, G., and de Waard, H., Oral calcium and blood pressure: a controlled intervention trial, *Am. J. Clin. Nutr.*, 44, 883, 1986.

105. Kynast-Gales, S. A. and Massey, L. K., Effects of dietary calcium from dairy products on ambulatory blood pressure in hypertensive men, *J. Am. Diet. Assoc.*, 92, 1497, 1992.

106. Zemel, M. B., Dietary pattern and hypertension: the DASH study, *Nutr. Rev.*, 55, 303, 1997.

107. Takagi, Y., Fukase, M., Takata, S., Fujimi, T., and Fujita, T., Calcium treatment of essential hypertension in elderly patients evaluated by 24H monitoring, *Am. J. Hypertens.*, 4, 836, 1991.

108. McCarron, D. A., A consensus approach to electrolytes and blood pressure. Could we all be right? *Hypertension*, 17(Suppl. I), 170s, 1991.

109. Orwoll, E. S. and Oviatt, S., Relationship of mineral metabolism and long-term calcium and cholecalciferol supplementation to blood pressure in normotensive men, *Am. J. Clin. Nutr.*, 52, 717, 1990.

110. The Trials of Hypertension Prevention Collaborative Research Group, The effects of nonpharmacologic interventions on blood pressure of persons with high normal levels: results of the Trials of Hypertension Prevention, Phase 1., *JAMA*, 267, 1213, 1992.

111. Gruchow, H. W., Sobocinski, K. A., and Barboriak, J. J., Calcium intake and the relationship of dietary sodium and potassium to blood pressure, *Am. J. Clin. Nutr.*, 48, 1463, 1988.

112. Weinberger, M. H., Wagner, U. L., and Fineberg, N. S., The blood pressure effects of calcium supplementation in humans of known sodium responsiveness, *Am. J. Hypertens.*, 6, 799, 1993.

113. Zemel, P., Gualdoni, S., and Sowers, J. R., Racial differences in mineral intake in ambulatory normotensives and hypertensives, *Am. J. Hypertens.*, 1, 1465, 1988.

114. Zemel, M. B., Gualdoni, S. M., Walsh, M. F., Komanicky, P., Standley, P., Johnson, D., Fitter, W., and Sowers, J. R., Effects of sodium and calcium on calcium metabolism and blood pressure regulation in hypertensive black adults, *J. Hypertens.*, 4(Suppl.), 364s, 1986.

115. Hamet, P., Mongeau, E., Lambert, J., Bellavance, F., Daignault-Gelinas, M., Ledoux, M., and Whissell-Cambiotti, L., Interactions among calcium, sodium, and alcohol intake as determinants of blood pressure, *Hypertension*, 17(Suppl. I), 150s, 1991.

116. Hamet, P., Daignault-Gelinas, M., Lambert, J., Ledoux, M., Whissell-Cambiotti, L., Bellavance, F., and Mongeau, F., Epidemiological evidence of an interaction between calcium and sodium intake impacting on blood pressure, a Montreal study, *Am. J. Hypertens.*, 5, 378, 1992.

117. Saito, K., Sano, H., Furuta, Y., and Fukuzaki, H., Effect of oral calcium on blood pressure response in salt-loaded borderline hypertensive patients, *Hypertension*, 13, 219, 1989.

118. Ely, D. L., Overview of dietary sodium effects on and interactions with cardiovascular and neuroendocrine functions, *Am. J. Clin. Nutr.*, 65(Suppl.), 594s, 1997.

119. Van Hooft, I. M. S., Grobbee, D. E., Frolich, M., Pols, H. A. P., and Hofman, A., Alterations in calcium metabolism in young people at risk for primary hypertension, The Dutch Hypertension and Offspring Study, *Hypertension*, 21, 267, 1993.

120. He, J., Tell, G. S., Tang, Y.-C., Mo, P.-S., and He, G.-Q., Relation of electrolytes to blood pressure in men, The Yi people study, *Hypertension*, 17, 378, 1991.

121. Criqui, M. H., Langer, R. D., and Reed, D. M., Dietary alcohol, calcium, and potassium: independent and combined effects on blood pressure, *Circulation*, 80, 609, 1989.

122. Resnick, L. M., Dietary calcium and hypertension, *J. Nutr.*, 117, 1806, 1987.

123. Linas, S. L., The role of potassium in the pathogenesis and treatment of hypertension, *Kidney Int.*, 39, 771, 1991.

124. Haddy, F. J., Roles of sodium, potassium, calcium, and natriuretic factors in hypertension, *Hypertension*, 18(Suppl. III), 179s, 1991.

125. Tobian, L., Dietary sodium chloride and potassium have effects on the pathophysiology of hypertension in humans and animals, *Am. J. Clin. Nutr.*, 65(s), 606s, 1997.

126. Sacks, F. M., Willett, W. C., Smith, A., Brown, L. E., Rosner, B., and Moore, T. J., Effect on blood pressure of potassium, calcium, and magnesium in women with low habitual intake, *Hypertension*, 31(part 1), 131, 1998.

127. Barden, A., Beilin, L. J., and Vandongen, R., Effect of potassium supplementation on blood pressure and vasodilator mechanisms in spontaneously hypertensive rats, *Clin. Sci.*, 75, 527, 1988.

128. Wu, X., Ackermann, U., and Sonnenberg, H., Potassium depletion and salt-sensitive hypertension in Dahl rats: effect on calcium, magnesium, and phosphate excretions, *Clin. Exper. Hypertens.* 17, 989, 1995.

129. Tobian, L., High potassium diets markedly protect against stroke deaths and kidney disease in hypertensive rats - a possible legacy from prehistoric times, *Can. J. Physiol. Pharmacol.*, 64, 840, 1986.

130. Intersalt Cooperative Research Group, Intersalt: an international study of electrolyte excretion and blood pressure: results for 24 hour urinary sodium and potassium excretion, *Br. Med. J.*, 297, 319, 1988.

131. Stamler, R., Implications of the INTERSALT Study, *Hypertension*, 17(Suppl. I), 16s, 1991.

132. Joffres, M. R., Reed, D. M., and Yano, K., Relationship of magnesium intake and other dietary factors to blood pressure: the Honolulu heart study, *Am. J. Clin. Nutr.*, 45, 469, 1987.

133. Geleijnse, J. M., Grobbee, D. E., and Hofman, A., Sodium and potassium intake and blood pressure change in childhood, *Br. Med. J.*, 300, 899, 1990.

134. Sinaiko, A. R., Gomez-Marin, O., and Prineas, R. J., Effect of low sodium diet or potassium supplementation on adolescent blood pressure, *Hypertension*, 21, 989, 1993.

135. Khaw, K. T. and Barrett-Connor, E., Dietary potassium and stroke-associated mortality: a 12-year prospective population study, *N. Engl. J. Med.*, 316, 235, 1987.

136. Xie, J. X., Saski, S., Joossens, J. V., and Kesteloot, H., The relationship between urinary cations obtained from the INTERSALT study and cerebrovascular mortality, *J. Hum. Hypertens.*, 6, 17, 1992.

137. Whelton, P. K., He, J., Cutler, J. A., Brancati, F. L., Appel, L. J., Follmann, D., and Klag, M. J., Effects of oral potassium on blood pressure: meta-analysis of randomized controlled clinical trials, *JAMA*, 277, 1624, 1997.

138. Brancati, F. L., Appel, L. J., Seidler, A. J., and Whelton, P. K., Effect of potassium supplementation on blood pressure in African Americans on a low-potassium diet, *Arch. Intern. Med.,* 156, 61, 1996.

139. Fotherby, M. D. and Potter, J. F., Long-term potassium supplementation lowers blood pressure in elderly hypertensive subjects, *Int. J. Clin. Practice,* 51, 219, 1997.

140. Siani, A., Strazzullo, P., Giacco, A., Pacioni, D., Celentano, E., and Mancini, M., Increasing the dietary potassium intake reduces the need for antihypertensive medication, *Ann. Intern. Med.*, 115, 753, 1991.

141. Langford, H. G., Cushman, W. C., and Hsu, H., Chronic affect of KCl on black-white differences in plasma renin activity, aldosterone, and urinary electrolytes, *Am. J. Hypertens.*, 4, 399, 1991.

142. Grimm, R. H., Jr., Neaton, J. D., Elmer, P. J., Svendsen, K. H., Levin, J., Segal, M., Holland, L., Witte, L. J., Clearman, D. R., Kofron, P., LaBounty, R. K., Crow, R., and Prineas, R. J., The influence of oral potassium chloride on blood pressure in hypertensive men on a low-sodium diet, *N. Engl. J. Med.*, 322, 569, 1990.

143. Kaplan, N. M. and Ram, C. V. S., Potassium supplements for hypertension, *N. Engl. J. Med.*, 322, 623, 1990.

144. Geleijnse, J. M., Witteman, J. C. M., den Breeijen, J. H., Hofman, A., de Jong, P. T. V. M., Pols, H. A. P., and Grobbee, D. E., Dietary electrolyte intake and blood pressure in older subjects: the Rotterdam Study, *J. Hypertens.*, 14, 737, 1996.

145. Paolisso, G. and Barbagallo, M., Hypertension, diabetes mellitus, and insulin resistance. The role of intracellular magnesium, *Am. J. Hypertens.* 10, 346, 1997.

146. Berthelot, A., Luthringer, C., Meyers, E., and Exinger, A., Disturbances of magnesium metabolism in the spontaneously hypertensive rat, *J. Am. Coll. Nutr.*, 6, 329, 1987.

147. Wallach, S. and Verch, R. L., Tissue magnesium in spontaneously hypertensive rats, *Magnesium*, 5, 33, 1986.

148. Matuura, T., Kohno, M., Kanayama, Y., Murakawa, K., Takeda, T., Ishimori, K., Morishima, I., and Yonesawa, T., Decreased intracellular free magnesium in erythrocytes of spontaneously hypertensive rats, *Biochem. Biophys. Res. Commun.*, 143, 1012, 1987.

149. Berthelot, A. and Esposito, J., Effects of dietary magnesium on the development of hypertension in the spontaneously hypertensive rat, *J. Am. Coll. Nutr.*, 4, 343, 1983.

150. Altura, B. M., Altura, B. T., Gebrewold, A., Ising, H., and Gunther, T., Magnesium deficiency and hypertension, correlation between magnesium deficient diets and microcirculatory changes in situ., *Science*, 223, 1315, 1984.

151. Wolf, P., Luthringer, C., Berthelot, A., and Berthelay, S., Blood pressure and plasma renin activity after magnesium supplementation in the spontaneously hypertensive rat: a study during developing and established hypertension, *Magnesium*, 6, 243, 1987.

152. Laurant, P., Kantelip, J.-P., and Berthelot, A., Dietary magnesium supplementation modifies blood pressure and cardiovascular function in mineralocorticoid-salt hypertensive rats but not in normotensive rats, *J. Nutr.*, 125, 830, 1995.

153. Whelton, P. K. and Klag, M. J., Magnesium and blood pressure: review of the epidemiologic and clinical trial experience, *Am. J. Cardiol.*, 63(Suppl. G), 26s, 1989.

154. Resnick, L. M., Laragh, J. H., Sealey, J. E., and Alderman, M. H., Divalent cations in essential hypertension, relations between serum ionized calcium, magnesium and plasma renin activity, *N. Engl. J. Med.*, 309, 888, 1983.

155. Ma, J., Folsom, A. R., Melnick, S. L., Eckfeldt, J. H., Sharrett, A. R., Nabulsi, A. A., Hutchinson, R. G., and Metcalf, P. A., Associations of serum and dietary magnesium with cardiovascular disease, hypertension, diabetes, insulin, and carotid arterial wall thickness: the ARIC study, *J. Clin. Epidemiol.*, 48, 927, 1995.

156. Zemel, P. C., Zemel, M. B., Urberg, M., Douglas, F. L., Geiser, R., and Sowers, J. R., Metabolic and hemodynamic effects of magnesium supplementation in patients with essential hypertension, *Am. J. Clin. Nutr.*, 51, 665, 1990.

157. Witteman, J. C. M., Grobbee, D. E., Derkx, F. H. M., Bouillon, R., de Bruijn, A. M., and Hofman, A., Reduction of blood pressure with oral magnesium supplementation in women with mild to moderate hypertension, *Am. J. Clin. Nutr.*, 60, 129, 1994.

158. Resnick, L. M., Magnesium in the pathophysiology and treatment of hypertension and diabetes mellitus: where are we in 1997? *Am. J. Hypertens.* 10, 368, 1997.

159. Devine, A., Prince, R. L., and Bell, R., Nutritional effect of calcium supplementation by skim milk powder or calcium tablets on total nutrient intake in postmenopausal women, *Am. J. Clin. Nutr.*, 64, 731, 1996.

160. Barger-Lux, M. J., Heaney, R. P., Packard, P. T., Lappe, J. M., and Recker, R. R., Nutritional correlates of low calcium intake, *Clinics in Applied Nutr.*, 2(4), 39, 1992.

161. Chan, G. M., Hoffman, K., and McMurray, M., Effects of dairy products on bone and body composition in pubertal girls, *J. Pediatr.*, 126, 551, 1995.

162. Cadogan, J., Eastell, R., Jones, N., and Barker, M. E., Milk intake and bone mineral acquisition in adolescent girls: randomized, controlled intervention trial, *Br. Med. J.*, 315, 1255, 1997.

163. Badenhop, N. E., Ilich, J. Z., Skugor, M., Landoll, J. D., and Matkovic, V., Changes in body composition and serum leptin in young females with high vs. low dairy intake, *J. Bone Miner. Res.*, 12(Suppl. I), 487s, 1997 (Abst.# S 537).

164. Swales, J. D., Salt substitutes and potassium intake, *Br. Med. J.*, 303, 1084, 1991.

CHAPTER 4

Dairy Foods and Colon Cancer

I. INTRODUCTION

Colorectal cancer is the third leading cause of cancer morbidity and mortality for both men and women in the U.S. In 1998, an estimated 131,600 Americans developed this disease (95,600 colon cancer; 36,000 rectum cancer) and 56,500 died from it (47,700 colon cancer; 8,800 rectum cancer).[1] An equal number of men and women are affected by colorectal cancer.

Both genetic and environmental factors contribute to cancer.[1-5] Among environmental factors, diet is estimated to be responsible for 30 to 60% of all cancers.[4] Colorectal cancer is thought to be caused by an interaction between environmental factors such as diet and genetic predisposition.[6] Since the cause(s) of cancers of the colon and rectum presumably is the same, these cancers will be treated as one in this chapter.

Although some dietary factors are suspected of contributing to specific cancers, others may be protective.[3,5] Recently it has begun to be appreciated that several components in dairy foods, specifically calcium and vitamin D, bacterial cultures (e.g., *Lactobacillus acidophilus*), a class of fatty acids known as conjugated dienoic derivatives of linoleic acid (CLA), sphingolipids, butyric acid, and milk proteins may protect against colon cancer.[7,8] Further, new clinical findings in humans indicate that increasing intake of lowfat dairy foods may reduce the risk of colon cancer.[9]

II. TOTAL FAT INTAKE, DAIRY FOODS, AND COLON CANCER

Dietary fat has been implicated as a promoter of colon carcinogenesis, although the extent of its exact role in this disease is uncertain.[4,6,10-21] Ecologic or descriptive epidemiological studies often associate diets high in total fat (and low in fiber) with increased risk of developing colon cancer.[4] A comparison of dietary data and the incidence of colon cancer in 37 countries indicated a positive association between fat intake and colon cancer.[11] Within the United States, Seventh Day

Adventists consume a lowfat diet and experience a low incidence of and mortality from colon cancer.[11]

Case-control and prospective (cohort or follow-up) epidemiological studies indicate a less consistent association between fat intake and colon cancer. In a review of case-control studies of fat intake and colon cancer, six studies supported a positive association between total and saturated fat and colon cancer, whereas five studies failed to find a positive association.[14] In a recent combined analysis of 13 case-control studies of colorectal cancer, Howe et al.[19] reported no increased risk of this disease with higher dietary fat intake after adjusting for total energy intake. In a case-control study involving French Canadians in Quebec, both total fat and saturated fatty acids were inversely associated with colon cancer, but the relationship was not statistically significant.[22] Other reviews point to inconsistent findings from case-control studies of fat intake and colon cancer.[4,17,20,21]

Prospective epidemiological studies also indicate an inconsistent association between dietary fat intake and colorectal cancer. In a 19-year prospective study of Chicago men, dietary fat accounted for 42% of total energy intake in patients with colon cancer and 43% in the control subjects.[23] In a 7-year prospective study involving 14,727 women enrolled in the New York University Women's Health Study, no association was found between intake of total or specific types of fat or total calories and colorectal cancer risk.[24] Likewise, in a prospective cohort study of over 35,000 women aged 55 to 69 living in Iowa, fat intake was not associated with colon cancer.[25] When dietary intake and the incidence of colon cancer were examined in a cohort of 47,949 U.S. male health professionals for six years, intakes of total fat, saturated fat, and animal fat were not related to colon cancer risk.[26]

In contrast to the above, Willett et al.[27] found a positive association between consumption of animal fat, at least from red meat but not from dairy products, and colon cancer in a large, well-controlled prospective study of nurses. This 6-year study identified 150 cases of colon cancer in a cohort of 89,494 women participating in the Nurses Health Study. A significant association was found between fat intake and colon cancer, but not vegetable fat after adjustment for energy intake. Red meat intake was positively associated with colon cancer but whole milk, cheese, and ice cream, foods which contributed to the total animal fat intake, were not significantly related to the risk of colon cancer.[27] Other epidemiological studies have associated a high intake of total fat and animal fat (from red meat or dairy products) or a "Western-style" diet high in red meat and low in fruits and vegetables with increased risk of colon cancer.[12,28-30] When dietary factors and risk of colorectal adenomas were examined in more than 7000 male health professionals, risk of colorectal adenomas was positively associated with intake of red meat (p = .03) and dairy fat (p = .04). The association between colon cancer risk and dairy food intake may be influenced by the specific dairy food consumed.[29] In a case-control study involving over 4600 subjects, more frequent intake of whole milk was associated with increased risk of colon cancer, whereas intake of 2% reduced fat and fluid milks appeared to be protective.[29]

The relationship between total fat and dairy fat in particular and colon cancer in epidemiological studies is unclear. In many epidemiological studies, it is difficult to clearly separate the effects of fat from those of calories.[6,20,30,31] Excess calories may be more important than total fat in the pathogenesis of colon cancer.[18,30] According to a recent case-control study involving over 4400 U.S. adults, consuming an extra 500 calories per day increased colon cancer risk by 15% in men and by 11% in women after controlling for physical activity and body weight.[32] Individual sources of energy (i.e., dietary fat, protein, carbohydrate) did not affect colon cancer risk beyond the risk associated with energy intake. Also, failure to demonstrate an association between fat intake and colon cancer in some epidemiological studies may be explained by a narrow range of fat intake and/or protective factors in the diet. Based on a review of 40 case-control and cohort studies, Giovannucci and Goldin [20] concluded that total fat intake or dairy foods are not associated with colon cancer risk.

In experimental animals, colon cancer develops more readily in animals fed a high fat diet than a lowfat diet, especially when carcinogens are administered concurrently.[11,16,33,34] As reviewed by Reddy,[16] carcinogen-induced colon tumor incidence was higher in rats fed high fat (23% by weight) semipurified diets containing corn oil, safflower oil, lard or beef tallow than in animals fed lowfat (5% by weight) diets containing these same fats. High fat diets containing coconut oil, olive oil, or trans fatty acids had no colon tumor enhancing effect. When fat intake is low (<4 to 5%), polyunsaturated fatty acids are more effective than saturated fats in enhancing tumorigenesis, apparently because of the requirement for the essential fatty acid, linoleic acid.[35] Once this requirement is satisfied, it is the total amount of dietary fat, not the type of fat, that appears to be more important in tumorigenesis. Dietary fat appears to promote, rather than initiate, carcinogenesis.[11,13,16] In a recent review of fat and colon cancer in experimental animals, Klurfeld and Bull[36] suggest that total dietary fat generally increases colon tumorigenesis; however, other confounding factors such as total energy intake and the interaction of fat with other nutrients influence this relationship. No one specific type of fat appears to promote colon cancer in experimental animals except linoleic acid when dietary fat intake is low.

Experimental animal studies suggest mechanisms by which fat may affect colon cancer risk.[11,16] Dietary fat intake increases free fatty acids and bile acid secretion which subsequently leads to a rise in the concentration of potentially toxic secondary bile acids (e.g., deoxycholic acid, lithocholic acid) in the colonic lumen.[37] Studies in experimental animals show that free fatty acids and secondary bile acids can induce mucosal cell damage, increase epithelial cell proliferation rates, and enhance carcinogenesis by acting as tumor promoters.[37-41] These findings support epidemiological studies that indicate that fecal bile acid concentrations are elevated in populations with a high incidence of colon cancer, especially those which consume a high fat, Western-style diet.[6]

Findings of an *in vitro* study indicate that dietary lipids and bile acids might act together to affect the production of diacylglycerol (DAG), a metabolite of phospholipid metabolism by bacteria in the intestinal lumen.[42] DAG in turn may enter the colonic epithelium and activate protein kinase C (an enzyme involved in cell signaling and growth), thus increasing cell proliferation. More research is needed to clarify the contribution of an interaction between dietary lipids, bile acids, and specific bacteria in colon cancer development.[42]

III. PROTECTIVE COMPONENTS IN DAIRY FOODS

A. Calcium, Vitamin D, and Colon Cancer

Numerous epidemiological, experimental animal, *in vitro*, and clinical studies in humans have investigated the protective effect of calcium vitamin D and dairy foods against colon cancer.[43-46]

1. Epidemiological Studies

Nearly two decades ago Garland and Garland[47] proposed that calcium and vitamin D could reduce the risk of colon cancer. Since that time, a number of epidemiological studies have examined this hypothesis.[21,48] Calcium intake has been demonstrated to be inversely associated with colon cancer incidence and mortality in human population studies conducted both within the United States and among different countries (Figure 4.1).[11,12,49,50] Similar types of studies demonstrate an inverse relationship between vitamin D (which increases calcium absorption) and colon cancer. Vitamin D is obtained through synthesis in the body from exposure to sunlight and by consuming vitamin D containing foods such as vitamin D fortified milk. In ecologic studies, geographic variations in colon cancer mortality rates are associated with differences in latitudes and exposure to sunlight.[17,23,47] At low latitudes where exposure to sunlight (and hence vitamin D) is high, colon cancer is uncommon.[17]

A number of case-control epidemiological studies suggest a protective effect for calcium and/or vitamin D against colon cancer.[17,22,32,49,51-54] In a case-control study in Utah in which male and female subjects were interviewed two years prior to the onset of cancer, Slattery et al.[49] found that a high intake of dietary calcium (i.e., >800 mg daily) was associated with reduced risk of colon cancer, particularly in males. In a more recent case-control study involving over 4000 adults in California, Utah, and Minnesota, risk of colon cancer was lower in subjects who consumed diets higher in calcium.[32] In this study, consuming diets high in calcium reduced the risk of colon cancer associated with a high intake of energy. Likewise, a case-control study in Sweden supports a protective effect of calcium against colon cancer.[52] Findings of a preliminary study in Australia involving 34 patients with colorectal cancer or at risk of this disease and 35 healthy controls indicated that fecal calcium levels were lower in the patients than in the control subjects.[55] This finding is consistent with the hypothesis that calcium protects against colon cancer. In a case-control study involving 1070 adults in Montreal, Quebec, dietary calcium intake was inversely associated with colon cancer.[22]

Calcium intake was associated with a significant decrease in colorectal cancer in a case-control study in Uruguay involving 282 patients with adenocarcinomas of the colon and rectum and 564 hospitalized controls.[54] Higher intakes of vitamin D were also associated with reduced risk of colorectal cancer. Martinez et al.[56] reported that a calcium intake of nearly 1400 mg/day was protective against adenomatous polyps. In another case-control study involving middle-aged men in Finland, the relative risk of colorectal cancer decreased with increasing blood levels of

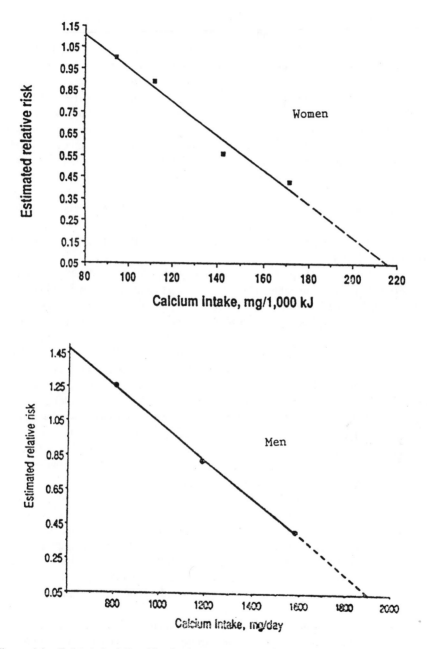

Figure 4.1   Estimated relative risk of colon cancer according to calcium intake per 1000 KJ
in adults aged 40-79 y, Utah, 1979-1982. (From Slattery, M.L., Sorenson, A.W.,
and Ford, M.H., *Am. J. Epidemiol.*, 128, 504, 1988. With permission.)

25-hydroxyvitamin D, an indicator of overall vitamin D status.[57] The results of a
recent case-control study of dietary intakes and other lifestyle factors for hyperplastic
polyps in over 500 adults indicate that high intakes of calcium (> 1000 mg per day)

may be protective.[58] Hyperplastic polyps may be markers for the subsequent development of adenomas or carcinomas.

Results of a large case-control study (746 matched pairs) in Los Angeles County, California demonstrated that increased calcium intake, and to a lesser extent vitamin D, are significantly associated with reduced risk of colon cancer after adjusting for total calories.[51] Moreover, when specific foods and cancer risk were examined, yogurt was found to protect against colon cancer, particularly in the distal colon, in men and women.[51] The protective effect of yogurt was independent of its calcium content and remained significant after adjustments for sources of calories and non-dietary risk factors. This finding suggests that yogurt reduces the incidence of colon cancer by a factor other than just its calcium content. When calcium was omitted from the statistical model, milk was protective against colon cancer in both males and females.[51] In contrast, a case-control study in the Netherlands failed to support a protective effect of dietary calcium or unfermented or fermented (e.g., yogurt, buttermilk) dairy foods against colon cancer after adjusting for potential confounding factors.[59]

Prospective (cohort) epidemiological studies also support a beneficial effect of calcium and vitamin D in colon cancer.[15,60,61] In a 19-year prospective study of 1954 men working at the Western Union Electric company in Chicago, the incidence of colorectal cancer was reduced by 75% in men who consumed 1200 mg or more of calcium a day and by 50% in those whose intake of vitamin D exceeded 3.75 μg (150 IU) a day.[15] Based on these findings, Newmark and Lipkin[44] suggested that calcium intakes of over 1800 mg and 1500 mg per day for men and women, respectively, are necessary to reduce the incidence of colon cancer. These amounts of calcium exceed current recommendations of 1000 to 1200 mg calcium/day for most adults.[62] In a four-year prospective study of over 35,000 Iowa women aged 55 to 69 years without a history of cancer, calcium and vitamin D intakes were associated with a modest reduction in colon cancer risk.[60] In an eight-year prospective study in Maryland, Garland et al.[63] reported an inverse association between serum 25-hydroxyvitamin D and the incidence of colon cancer.

The Antioxidant Polyp Prevention Study, a prospective study involving more than 700 adults found that increased intake of dietary calcium, but not calcium supplements, was associated with a reduced risk of recurrent colorectal adenomas.[61] Adults who consumed more than two servings of dairy foods a day had a slightly lower incidence of recurrent colon cancer than adults who consumed less than one-half serving of dairy foods a day.[61] Dietary calcium appeared to have a more beneficial effect on colon cancer risk in individuals with a high fat diet than those with a lowfat diet.[61]

Other more recent prospective studies are less supportive of a protective effect of calcium against colon cancer. Findings from the Nurses' Health Study, a six-year prospective study in the U.S. involving over 89,000 women, revealed no consistent, significant association between calcium intake and risk of colon or rectal cancers.[64] However, a possible protective effect of vitamin D was observed, especially for rectal cancer. In the Health Professionals Follow-up Study cohort, men who consumed higher intakes of calcium and vitamin D exhibited a slight, but statistically insignificant, reduction in risk of colon cancer compared to men who consumed lower intakes of these nutrients.[65] This study followed 47,935 male U.S. health professionals for six years, during which 203 men developed colon cancer. Intake of milk and fermented milk products was not significantly associated with colon cancer risk.[65]

A meta-analysis of 24 epidemiological studies (16 case-control and 8 prospective) of calcium and colon and/or rectal cancer or polyps failed to support the hypothesis that calcium protects against colorectal cancer.[48] The authors suggest that other dietary factors which affect calcium absorption and metabolism (e.g., vitamin D, phosphate, fiber) may influence the findings. Also, whether calcium has a protective effect only during a specific time of cancer development or at a specific subsite of the large bowel cannot be ruled out.[48]

Epidemiological studies have also investigated the possible protective effect of dairy foods, the major source of calcium and vitamin D, against colon cancer.[22,24,26,51,53,60,66-68] As mentioned above, yogurt may protect against colon cancer.[51] An earlier investigation in southern California, where milk is routinely fortified with vitamin D and where there is high exposure to sunlight, identified an inverse association between milk intake and risk of colon cancer.[68] This study of Seventh-Day Adventists who, on the average, have a low incidence of colorectal cancer, indicates a protective effect of vitamin D fortified milk.[68] Intake of dairy foods (and calcium) was inversely associated with colorectal cancer in a seven-year prospective study involving 14,727 women aged 34 to 65 years participating in the New York University Women's Health Study.[24] In a case-control study in Utah, Slattery et al.[49] observed an inverse association between risk of colon cancer in both men and women and intake of milk and other dairy foods. When the milk consumption habits of 3334 cancer patients and 1300 control subjects were compared, Mettlin et al.[29] found that 2% reduced fat and milks protected against colon cancer.

Similar observations have been reported outside the United States. For example, case-control studies in Russia support a protective effect of increased milk consumption against colorectal cancer.[53] Earlier studies found that Finnish men who consumed the highest amounts of dairy foods ranked lowest in terms of colorectal cancer risk, whereas Danish men who consumed lower amounts of dairy foods ranked high in colorectal cancer incidence.[66,67] Most of these studies have observed a slight, nonsignificant inverse association between dairy food intake and colon cancer risk. In other investigations there is no association between dairy food intake and colon cancer risk.[65,69,70]

Although many epidemiological studies support an inverse association between calcium, vitamin D, dairy food intake, and colon cancer, it is difficult to draw conclusions from these studies. The relative homogeneity of diets within populations, confounding dietary factors, and imprecise measurement of dietary intake in large population studies are among several variables that contribute to inconsistencies in the findings. However, despite these limitations, epidemiological studies appear to be weakly supportive of a protective effect of calcium, vitamin D, and colorectal cancer.

2. Animal Studies

A protective role for calcium and vitamin D in colon carcinogenesis is supported by many experimental animal studies.[17,33,43,71-77] In most of these studies, the effects of calcium and vitamin D on tumors induced in animals by chemicals (e.g., injections of 1,2-dimethylhydrazine [1,2 DMH]) are examined.[11]

Potential mechanisms underlying the protective effect of calcium against colon cancer are suggested from animal studies.[38,45,76] Dietary fat increases levels of bile acids and free fatty acids in the colonic lumen, resulting in damage to the colonic epithelium and increased epithelial proliferation. Increasing dietary calcium in rats fed high fat diets has been shown to reduce bile acid and free fatty acid excretion.[37,38,40,76-80] Intraluminal calcium chelates unconjugated bile acids and/or free ionized fatty acids, especially in a basic pH environment, forming relatively insoluble (nontoxic) calcium complexes of fatty acids/bile acids. Binding of calcium to fatty acids in the small bowel prevents the reabsorption of fatty acids/bile acids and increases free fatty acid excretion. Calcium complexes of fatty acids are less toxic to the colorectal mucosa than are free fatty acids.[38,76,78,79] Thus, increasing calcium may counteract any cancer-promoting effect of fat.

Direct evidence of this effect of calcium in experimental animals has been provided by Appleton et al.[78] These investigators showed that the fecal content of bile acids decreased 33% and total fecal concentrations of free fatty acids increased 117% in laboratory rats fed a calcium-enriched diet. And when the effects of three different concentrations of calcium on organ cultures of rat colonic explants were examined, crypt cell production fell by 43% when calcium was doubled, and by an additional 43% when calcium was increased three-fold (Figure 4.2).[78] Skrypec[80] found that bile acid excretion increased and lower tumor incidence occurred in laboratory animals fed increased dietary calcium. Likewise, Lupton et al.[76] observed that when rats were fed a high fat diet and a calcium intake equivalent to 1600 mg a day for humans, fecal excretion of bile acids and certain individual bile acids were reduced to a level found in the feces of rats fed a lowfat diet. However, the effect on indices of colonic proliferation was minimal (Figure 4.3).[76]

Hyperproliferation of colonic epithelial cells is a consistent and early marker of increased risk of colon cancer.[44, 81] Increased calcium intake inhibits hyperproliferation of colon epithelial cells induced by carcinogens or high levels of fatty acids or bile acids present in the colon.[37,72,82-86] In a study in which rats were fed a high fat (40% of energy) diet supplemented with calcium phosphate, total fatty acid and bile acid concentration in the feces increased and proliferation of colonic epithelium decreased compared to control animals which did not receive calcium phosphate.[75] Van der Meer [37] also found that in experimental animals the hyperproliferative effect of fat is inversely related to the amount of dietary calcium. On a low calcium diet, fat significantly increases colonic epithelial proliferation, whereas on a high calcium diet the hyperproliferative effect of fat is dramatically reduced (Figure 4.4).[37] The antiproliferative effect of dietary calcium phosphate has been demonstrated to be greater in the presence of saturated than polyunsaturated fat (Figure 4.5).[75]

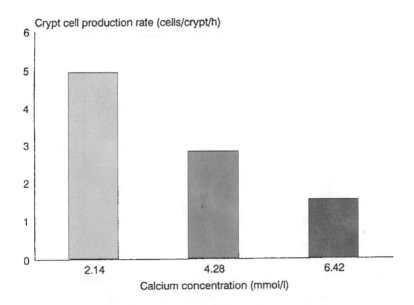

Figure 4.2 Doubling calcium concentrations reduced crypt cell production by 43%; tripling calcium concentrations caused an additional 43% fall in crypt cell production. (From Appleton, G.V.N., et al., *Gut*, 32, 1374, 1991. With permission.)

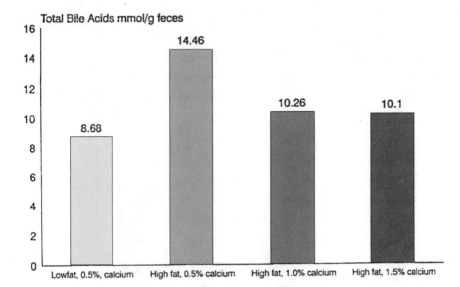

Figure 4.3 Effect of dietary calcium on fecal bile acid excretion in rats. Note that the high fat, low calcium diet resulted in the highest excretion of total fecal bile acids. As the amount of calcium increased in the high fat diet, total bile acid excretion fell to a level approaching that in rats fed the lowfat diet. (Based on Lupton, J.R., et al., *J. Nutr.*, 124, 188, 1994. With permission.)

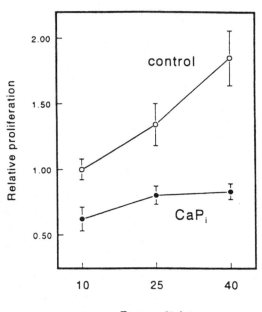

Figure 4.4   Effects of increasing amounts of fat and of calcium phosphate in purified diets of rats on colonic epithelial cell proliferation. The results are given relative to those for 10% of energy as fat on the low calcium control diet (mean ±SE; n = 6). (Reprinted from *Cancer Lett.*, 114, Van der Meer, et al., Mechanisms of the intestinal effects of dietary fats and milk products on colon carcinogenesis, Elsevier, 79, 1997. With permission.)

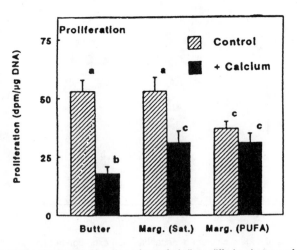

Figure 4.5   Colonic epithelial proliferation of rats fed diets differing in type of dietary fat and amount of CaHPO$_4$. Values are means of six rats ±SEs. Bars not sharing the same superscript are significantly different: P < 0.05. Control diets contain 25 μmol CaHPO$_4$/g diet, and diets with supplemental calcium contain 225 μmol CaHPO$_4$/g diet. (From Lapré, J.A., et al., *Cancer Res.*, 53, 784, 1993. With permission.)

Several investigators have shown that increasing dietary calcium and/or vitamin D reduces carcinogen-induced tumors in experimental animals.[72,80,86-92] Wargovich et al.[90] found that a calcium-enriched diet (equivalent to an intake of 2000 mg calcium by humans) suppressed azoxymethane-induced colon cancer at the promotional stage.

When laboratory rats injected with a single dose of 1,2 DMH were fed a diet high in fat (20% corn oil), calcium, and vitamin D, colon tumor incidence decreased by 45%.[87] In this study, neither calcium nor vitamin D independently reduced tumor incidence. Both calcium and vitamin D were required for the anticarcinogenic effect, suggesting that these nutrients may act synergistically to protect against colon cancer.[87] The anticarcinogenic effect of calcium and vitamin D was most pronounced in the distal colon, as opposed to the entire or proximal colon, of the animals.[87,92]

Sitrin et al.[91] examined the role of supplemental calcium alone or in combination with vitamin D on colonic tumorigenesis in rats receiving multiple injections of the carcinogen, 1,2 DMH. Dietary calcium decreased the number and size of tumors, but only when adequate vitamin D was present in the diet.[91] Vitamin D deficiency abolished the protective effects of calcium on colon cancer.

In contrast to the above, Pence and Buddingh[72] found that the combination of calcium and vitamin D was less effective in reducing tumorigenesis than either nutrient alone. These investigators used a $2 \times 2 \times 2$ factorial design in rats to examine the effects of dietary fat, calcium, and vitamin D on colon tumors induced by multiple injections of 1,2 DMH. Tumor incidence was reduced more in the animals fed a high fat, low vitamin D diet containing 1% calcium than in rats fed the same diet containing half as much calcium (0.5%). Calcium was not protective in rats fed lowfat or high vitamin D diets.[72] The reason for the conflicting findings regarding the relationship between calcium and vitamin D and carcinogenesis is unknown. However, Pence and Buddingh,[72] as well as other investigators,[33,90,92] generally agree that the anticarcinogenic effect of calcium and/or vitamin D is most pronounced when animals are fed a high fat, rather than a lowfat, diet. In a recent study investigating the effectiveness of two sources of calcium, elemental calcium (calcium carbonate) and dairy calcium (nonfat dried milk), in inhibiting chemically induced colon tumors in laboratory rats, the lowest incidence of cancer occurred when calcium was fed in conjunction with a high fat (20%) diet rather than a lowfat (5%) diet.[33] Both sources of calcium were equally effective in reducing fecal bile acid concentrations and colon tumors. The researchers concluded that the ability of dietary calcium to protect against cancer depends in part on the fat content of the diet.[33] Vitamin D's ability to inhibit chemically induced colon cancer appears to depend on a certain minimum amount of calcium.[87,93]

Other researchers have provided evidence that colonic epithelial cell hyperproliferation is decreased in laboratory animals fed increased calcium and vitamin D.[40,43,45,71-74,78,86,89,94] As mentioned above, dietary lipids can accelerate colonic epithelial proliferation. Calcium appears to reduce the tumor-promoting effects of dietary fat in the colon by binding with cytotoxic bile acids and/or free fatty acids.[45]

Appleton et al.[71,86] found that dietary calcium (calcium lactate) inhibited hyperproliferation of colonic epithelium in rats at high risk of colon cancer. Risk of colon cancer in these animals increased as a result of a surgical procedure (i.e., removal of a portion of the small bowel) to impair the uptake and reabsorption of bile acids, or exposure to the chemical carcinogen, azoxymethane.

Calcium has been demonstrated to restrict the tumor-promoting effects of dietary fat in the colon of rats or mice treated with ionized bile acids or free fatty acids such as deoxycholic acid or oleic acid, as well as different types and levels of fat.[39,85,90,95] When mice and rats were fed a Western-style "nutritional stress" diet high in fat (40%) and phosphate (i.e., equivalent to 700 mg in human diets) and low in calcium (i.e., equivalent to 440 to 600 mg in human diets) and vitamin D (i.e., equivalent to slightly higher than 200 IU for human adults), colonic hyperplasia and hyperproliferation were induced in the absence of a carcinogen.[73,74] However, when calcium intake was increased (i.e., to an amount equivalent to 3000 mg in a 2400 kcal diet for humans), hyperproliferation of epithelial cells in colonic crypts was reduced to almost control levels.[74] Of interest in this experimental animal study was the observation that calcium's effects on epithelial cell proliferation were greater in the sigmoid than in the ascending colon (i.e., the area of the colon where most human colon tumors occur) (Table 4.1).[74] Risio et al.[77] reported that when mice were fed a Western-style diet high in fat and phosphate and low in calcium and vitamin D for two years, advanced dysplastic morphological changes in the colon related to tumor development and progression occurred. Specifically, this diet triggered and sustained the early phases of tumorigenesis in the colonic mucosa, inducing significant changes in cell renewal, apoptosis (programmed cell death), and genetic instability of the epithelium. The gross colonic lesions and other changes in the colon induced by the Western-style diet were similar to those produced by a chemical carcinogen.[77]

Rafter et al.[79] showed that when the calcium content of a fluid containing bile acids was increased and perfused into rat colons, calcium inhibited the damaging effects of the bile acids. Calcium bound the bile acids, rendering them non-toxic to epithelial tissues. This protective effect of calcium on bile or fatty acid-induced hyperproliferation in animal models has been demonstrated by other investigators.[96]

Reshef et al.[89] showed that calcium reduced colonic epithelial hyperproliferation in rats during the initiation (induction) phase of colon cancer induced by the carcinogen, N-methyl-N-nitro-N-nitrosoguanidine, even when the animals received a lowfat diet. This beneficial effect of calcium on colon carcinogenesis in the presence of lowfat diets suggests that the effect of calcium on tumorigenesis may include other mechanisms. The source of calcium used (i.e., calcium lactate or calcium carbonate) did not influence the results.

Studies in experimental animals suggest that there are subclasses of tumors defined by particular genetic lesions which differ in their response to calcium and vitamin D.[97] Calcium, alone or in combination with vitamin D, may influence the frequency or type of K-ras and H-ras gene mutations in tumors. Calcium completely suppressed K-ras oncogene mutations in the colon of rats treated with the carcinogen, DMH, whereas, vitamin D appeared to abolish the protective effect of calcium.[97] A study in rats demonstrated that calcium precipitates cytotoxic surfactants (e.g., bile acids, fatty acids, phospholipids) in the colonic lumen, thereby resulting in decreased cytotoxicity of fecal water.[98] Calcium carbonate, calcium phosphate, and milk

Table 4.1 High Calcium Intake Reduces Colonic Hyperproliferation Induced in Animals by a Western-Style Diet High in Fat and Phosphate and Low in Calcium and Vitamin D

	Control diet	Stress diet 1	Stress diet 2	Control vs. diet 1	Control vs. diet 2	Diet 1 vs. diet 2
Calcium (mg/kcal)	1.4	0.22	1.3			
Phosphorus (mg/kcal)	1.1	0.8	0.8			
Vit D (IU/kcal)	0.3	0.1	0.1			
Corn oil						
% kcal	12	40	40			
kcal/g	3.6	4.5	4.5			
Sigmoid-colon results						
Rats						
Labeling index (%)	7.2 ± 0.7*†	9.9 ± 0.7	8.6 ± 0.4	P < 0.02	NS	NS
Cells/crypt	36.9 ± 0.9†	37.4 ± 0.9	36.2 ± 0.5	NS	NS	NS
Labeled cells/crypt	2.6 ± 0.2†	3.7 ± 0.3	3.1 ± 0.1	P < 0.02	NS	NS
Mice						
Labeling index (%)	4.1 ± 0.3	6.1 ± 0.4	4.3 ± 0.4	P < 0.001	NS	P < 0.01
Cells/crypt	18.6 ± 0.6	21.1 ± 0.5	19.5 ± 0.2	P < 0.01	NS	P < 0.01
Labeled cells/crypt	0.8 ± 0.06	1.3 ± 0.09	0.9 ± 0.09	P < 0.001	NS	P < 0.01
Ascending colon results						
Rats						
Labeling index (%)	8.0 ± 0.5†	7.5 ± 0.8	7.0 ± 0.8	NS	NS	NS
Cells/crypt	30.1 ± 2.0†	29.7 ± 4.2	32.7 ± 1.9	NS	NS	NS
Labeled cells/crypt	2.5 ± 0.2†	2.3 ± 0.6	2.3 ± 0.2	NS	NS	NS
Mice						
Labeling index (%)	6.5 ± 0.7	8.7 ± 0.8	6.5 ± 1.0	P = 0.05	NS	P < 0.05
Cells/crypt	15.9 ± 1.8	18.2 ± 1.9	16.6 ± 1.0	NS	NS	NS
Labeled cells/crypt	1.0 ± 0.1	1.6 ± 0.1	1.1 ± 0.1	P = 0.01	NS	P < 0.02

* 1 ± SEM; n = 6 for rats and mice, except where indicated.
† n = 5

From Newmark, H.L., Lipkin, M., and Maheshwari, N., *Am. J. Clin. Nutr.*, 54, 209S, 1991. With permission.

calcium elicited similar antiproliferative effects indicating that calcium in milk is responsible for this effect.

3. In Vitro Studies

Cell proliferation, differentiation, and apoptosis are critical in tissue homeostasis and carcinogenesis. Substances inducing cell proliferation are considered to be tumor promoters, whereas many antitumor agents induce cell differentiation and apoptosis.[84] The potential role of calcium in cell cycling and carcinogenesis has been investigated by *in vitro* studies. [84,99] *In vitro* studies of animal and human colonic mucosa cell cultures indicate that increasing dietary calcium intake decreases hyperproliferation of mucosal colonic epithelial cells and protects against the damaging effects of bile acids and fatty acids on colonic epithelial cells. However, when colonic epithelial cell proliferation is normal, calcium appears to have little, if any, effect on proliferation rates. *In vitro* studies also demonstrate that calcium phosphate precipitates hydrophobic bile acids and fatty acids in fecal water which decreases their concentrations and cytotoxicity, thus inhibiting epithelial cell damage and colonic proliferation. [98]

In vitro studies indicate that early calcium intervention may be particularly effective in preventing colon cancer in individuals at high risk of this disease.[78,83,100-102] According to findings of an *in vitro* study conducted by Buset et al.,[100] levels of extracellular calcium equivalent to those found in the blood of humans inhibited colonic epithelial cell proliferation, but not after the cells had progressed to adenomas (precursors of cancer) and carcinomas. The researchers hypothesized that sensitivity to calcium may be lost once colonic cells become malignant.

To determine if colonic cells lose their sensitivity to calcium once they progress to adenomas and carcinomas, Guo et al.[102] measured the direct effects of calcium on the growth of established colonic cancer cell lines *in vitro*. These researchers found that, in contrast to normal cells, colon cancer cell lines continued to grow in the presence of low concentrations of extracellular calcium, but that increasing the concentration of calcium specifically and directly inhibited growth of human and mouse colon cancer cells. Thus, increased intake of dietary calcium may reduce the risk of developing colon cancer by a direct inhibiting effect on the growth of colonic cancer cells. A potential role for calcium in apoptosis is under investigation. An increase in intracellular free calcium appears to trigger apoptosis induced by some agents.[99,103] Further, the role of calcium in regulation of apoptosis may be dependent on dietary vitamin D_3.[104]

4. Clinical Trials

Clinical intervention trials in humans generally support a protective effect of calcium and vitamin D against colon cancer.[44,84,101,105-108] Calcium intake has been shown to reduce colonic epithelial hyperproliferation in individuals at risk of colon cancer. When Lipkin and Newmark[82] examined epithelial cell proliferation in the colonic mucosa of 10 patients from families with non-polyposis colon cancer, those whose diets were supplemented with 1250 mg calcium (as carbonate) a day for two to three months experienced a significant reduction in colonic epithelial cell proliferation activity. Thus calcium reversed abnormal colonic epithelial cell proliferation known to be associated with increased risk of colon cancer.[82] These findings were later confirmed by the same investigators in a study employing a larger number of persons at high risk for colorectal cancer.[83] In this study, calcium (1300 to 1500 mg/day) given for several days decreased and normalized hyperproliferation of whole colonic crypts in individuals whose colonic proliferative activity was high, but not in those whose proliferative activity was close to normal.[83]

Wargovich et al.[105] add further support that calcium regulates the proliferative behavior of colonic epithelium in individuals at high risk for colon cancer. In a placebo-controlled, single-blinded cross-over study of the effect of calcium (2000 mg/day as carbonate) for 30 days on proliferation of rectal epithelium in subjects with sporadic adenomas, calcium markedly suppressed proliferation rates during the calcium phase of the study, but not during the placebo phase. These investigators also showed in two pilot clinical trials that 1500 mg supplemental calcium/day (in

addition to about 700 mg dietary calcium for a total of 2200 mg) for 90 days failed
to significantly reduce rectal epithelial cell proliferation in six subjects with sporadic
adenoma, whereas 2000 mg supplemental calcium/day (i.e., total of 2700 mg) in
another six patients was effective (Table 4.2).[105] Likewise, O'Sullivan et al.[106] found

Table 4.2   Effect of Calcium Supplements on Biomarker Response
             in Subjects at High Risk for Colon Cancer

Calcium Dose and Duration	Effect on Biomarker	
1500 mg/d for 90 d ($n = 6$)	20% reduction in LI*	P**
2000 mg/d for 30 d ($n = 6$)	29% reduction in LI	0.08
2000 mg/d vs. placebo crossover for 4-30 d ($n = 20$)	Lower LI on calcium but not on placebo	0.004

* Labeling Index from *in vitro* tritated thymidine uptake.
**Two-sided + test.

From Wargovich, M.J., et al. *Gastroenterol.*, 103, 92, 1992. With permission.

that while 1000 mg supplemental calcium (i.e., total of 2549 mg from diet and
supplement) reduced colonic crypt cell proliferation (indicated as the relative number
of labeled cells) in patients with adenomatous polyps of the large bowel, 2000 mg
of supplemental calcium was necessary to return proliferation rates to normal levels
(Figure 4.6). Thus, a critical amount of calcium may be necessary to reduce risk of

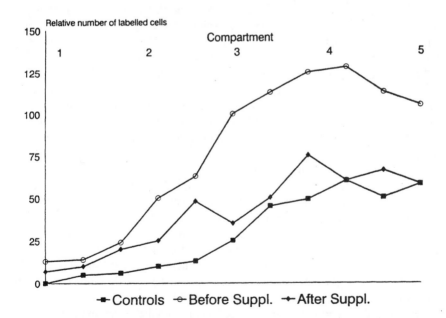

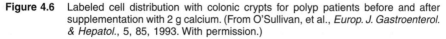

Figure 4.6   Labeled cell distribution with colonic crypts for polyp patients before and after
supplementation with 2 g calcium. (From O'Sullivan, et al., *Europ. J. Gastroenterol.
& Hepatol.*, 5, 85, 1993. With permission.)

colon cancer in some individuals. Studies failing to show a calcium-induced reduction in colonic proliferation, such as the one reported by Gregoire et al.[109] which used 1200 mg calcium/day, may be explained by the low amount of calcium fed and the fact that the study subjects had portions of their colons surgically removed. Gregoire et al.,[109] however, found that increased calcium intake by patients at risk of colon cancer resulted in a higher fecal pH and enhanced fecal bile acid concentration. Cats et al.[110] found that in individuals already consuming an adequate intake of dietary calcium, calcium supplementation has only a modest protective effect on cell proliferation. This was demonstrated in a randomized, double-blind placebo-controlled trial in individuals with a family history of colon cancer. Increasing calcium intake by 1500 mg/day in individuals who were already consuming 1250 mg calcium/day resulted in only a minor, insignificant reduction in epithelial cell proliferation. [110]

Although Kampman et al.[111] found no statistically significant effect of milk, fermented dairy foods, or calcium on colorectal adenomas, a slight anti-cancer effect was noted in men and women consuming a high saturated fat intake. This prospective study indicates that dairy products (including whole milk) do not increase and may slightly decrease the risk of colorectal adenoma.[111] The fact that other studies find a significant protective effect of dairy products and calcium on more mature forms of colon cancer suggests that dairy foods may be more protective at later stages than at earlier stages of colon cancer development.

Researchers in Arizona[112] found that increasing calcium intake by 1500 mg/day for nine months significantly reduced fecal bile acids by 35% and deoxycholic fecal bile acid by 36% in patients with resected colon adenomas. In another investigation which involved 22 patients with a history of resected adenocarcinomas of the colon but who were currently free of cancer, increasing calcium intake by 2000 to 3000 mg/day for 16 weeks produced a "healthier" bile acid profile with respect to cancer.[113] Compared with baseline levels, calcium supplementation significantly decreased the proportion of water in the stool, doubled fecal excretion of calcium, increased excretion of organic phosphate, and decreased the proportion of the primary bile acid chenodeoxycholic acid in the bile and the ratio of lithocholate to deoxycholate in feces.[113]

Buset et al.[100] found that a daily intake of 1500 mg calcium for 4 to 8 weeks reduced cellular hyperproliferation in six of nine patients with colon cancer or adenomas or with a family history of colon cancer. The three nonresponders may have had relatively quiescent epithelial cells similar to that in normal cells and which would not be further slowed by increased calcium.[100] Heterogeneity in response to calcium also may be explained by genetics.[114-116] Increased cellular calcium concentration may influence the expression of genetic mutations for predisposition for colon cancer.[115] Thus, early calcium intervention may delay the development of colon cancer in individuals who carry the gene for this disease.

Rozen et al.[117] reported a significant reduction in epithelial cell hyperproliferation (as indicated by the labeling index or LI) in the colonic mucosa when 1250 to 1500 mg calcium (as carbonate or a gluconate-lactate-carbonate preparation) was given for three months to 26 first degree relatives of colorectal cancer patients and nine patients with sporadic adenomas. Calcium had no significant effect on epithelial proliferation in individuals with normal proliferation rates. The different sources of calcium used in this study did not influence the findings. After calcium treatment was discontinued for six to eight weeks, colonic proliferation returned to high levels in individuals at risk of colon cancer (Figure 4.7).[117] Barsoum et al.[101] found that increased calcium intake (1250 mg/day) significantly reduced mucosal cell proliferation (measured by crypt cell production rate) in patients with adenomatous polyps (i.e., patients at risk of developing colorectal cancer) (Figure 4.8).

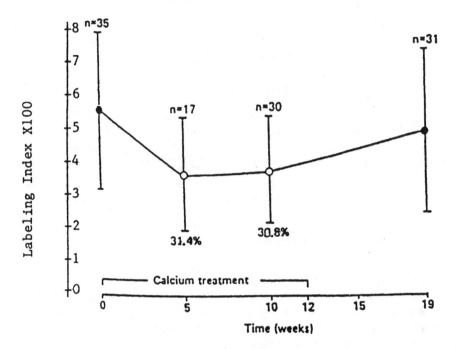

Figure 4.7   A significant (p <0.001) fall in LI (mean[sd]) at five and 10 weeks, of 31.4% and 30.8%, respectively (comparing each to their own basal values), during calcium treatment and its reversal after cessation of treatment. (From Rozen, P., Fireman, Z., Fine, N., Wax Y., and Ron, E., *Gut*, 30, 650, 1989. With permission.)

Further evidence of calcium's role in regulation of mucosal cell proliferation is provided by measurement of ornithine decarboxylase. This enzyme is elevated in colon cancer. Dietary calcium (2500 mg/day) has been shown to suppress mucosal ornithine decarboxylase activity in elderly patients with adenomatous polyps,[118] thus supporting findings in experimental animals.[44,88]

Using another biomarker of cell differentiation, Yang et al.[119] demonstrated that soybean agglutinin (SBA) lectin binding of carbohydrate residues was greater in human colon biopsies of normal colonic epithelial cells than in colonic carcinomas. Quantitation of SBA lectin binding before and after supplementation of calcium (1500 mg/day, as calcium carbonate) was studied. In subjects with initial low SBA lectin binding, calcium supplementation for less than three months led to a nonsignificant increase in binding rates. When calcium supplementation continued for more than three months, there was a significant increase in SBA lectin binding

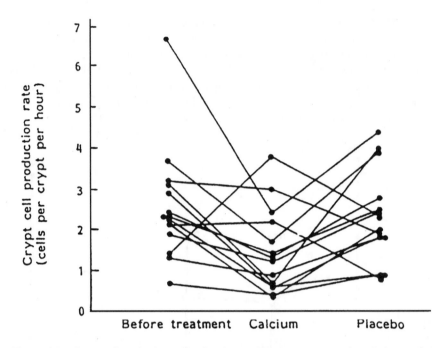

Figure 4.8   Crypt cell production rates of patients with adenomatous polyps, before and after treatment with calcium or placebo. (From Barsoum, G.H., et al., *Br. J. Surg.*, 79, 581, 1992. With permission.)

towards levels observed in normal colonic epithelial cells.[119] Calcium supplementation had no effect on SBA lectin binding in subjects who had normal binding levels prior to calcium supplementation. This study not only demonstrates that calcium is beneficial for individuals at risk for colon cancer, but it also identifies a marker for people at increased risk of this disease.

Further support for a protective effect of calcium on colon cancer comes from studies which have examined other risk markers for this disease.[107,108,120,121] Calcium has been demonstrated to normalize the distribution of proliferating cells within colorectal crypts.[107] In a randomized, double-blind, placebo-controlled trial, patients with sporadic colorectal adenomas received either a placebo or 1000 mg or 2000 mg calcium/day for six months. Increasing calcium intake normalized the distribution of proliferating cells within colorectal crypts without affecting the proliferation rate.[107] That is, calcium shifted the zone of proliferation from one that included the entire crypt to one that was confined to the lower 60%, or normal proliferative zone, of the crypt.

Calcium or dairy foods may also reduce the risk of colon cancer by decreasing the cytotoxicity of fecal water.[37,108,120,121] Substances such as bile acids and other surfactants in stool water have direct contact with the colonic mucosa where they can damage the epithelium and stimulate the proliferation of crypt cells. When 18 healthy adults received either a dairy product-rich or a dairy product-free diet for one week each in a cross-over study, the cytotoxicity of fecal water increased when dairy products were excluded from the diet.[121] The subjects consuming the dairy-free diet consumed less calcium (i.e., from about 1500 mg to 400 mg/day), phosphate, vitamin D, and total and saturated fat than those who consumed the dairy product-rich diet. The researchers[121] suggest that the significant decrease in calcium and/or phosphate intake in the dairy-free diet likely contributed to the increase in cytotoxicity of fecal water. This explanation is supported by a study in the Netherlands which demonstrated that calcium in milk products precipitates cytotoxic surfactants in the colonic lumen, thereby inhibiting colonic cytotoxicity.[37,108] In this double-blind, cross-over metabolic study, 13 healthy males consumed a typical Western-type diet containing either calcium-depleted milk products or calcium-rich milk products for one week each.[37,108] Subjects consumed 765 mg of calcium/day on the calcium-depleted diet and 1820 mg calcium/day on the diet with calcium-rich milk products. Milk calcium significantly increased fecal pH and the fecal excretion of phosphate, total fat, free fatty acids, and bile acids. These findings indicate that milk calcium precipitates luminal bile acids and free fatty acids inhibiting their absorption. Milk calcium also decreased fecal water concentration of long chain fatty acids, secondary bile acids, neutral sterols, and phospholipids by about half (Figure 4.9). The cytotoxicity of fecal water was reduced from 68% to 28% in subjects who consumed the diet high in dairy calcium.

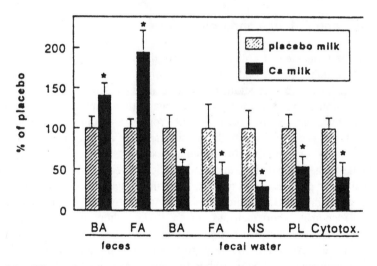

Figure 4.9   Effects of calcium milk versus placebo milk in healthy subjects on fecal and fecal water bile acids (BA), and fatty acids (FA), on neutral sterols (NS), and phospholipids (PL) in fecal water and on cytotoxicity of fecal water (mean ± SE; n = 13; *p<0.05 vs. placebo). (Reprinted from *Cancer Lett.*, 114, Van der Meer, et al., Mechanisms of the intestinal effects of dietary fats and milk products on colon carcinogenesis, Elsevier, 80, 1997.)

A recent randomized, double-blind study involving 930 patients who previously had a colorectal adenoma removed (a non-cancerous tumor which is a precursor of colon cancer) found that increasing calcium intake for four years reduced the risk of recurring colorectal adenomas.[122] The patients were randomized to receive either calcium carbonate (i.e., 1200 mg elemental calcium) or a placebo. In patients receiving the increased calcium, risk of return of single tumors was reduced by 17% and the number of adenomas decreased by 25%.[122]

Intake of lowfat dairy foods may reduce the risk of colon cancer, according to a recent randomized, single-blind controlled study.[9] Seventy adults at risk of colon cancer because of previous colonic adenomas were randomized into two groups. The control group consumed conventional diets, whereas the experimental group increased their intake of dairy foods to reach 1500 mg calcium a day. Participants were monitored for one year to evaluate changes in epithelial cells lining the colon and in other biomarkers of colon cancer. At both 6 and 12 months, significant positive changes were observed in the group receiving the increased intake of lowfat dairy foods. In this group, excess proliferative activity of colonic epithelial cells was reduced and normal differentiation-associated cell properties were restored.[9] The experimental group increased their calcium intake by a mean of 872 mg a day, bringing total calcium intake to nearly 1500 mg a day. Although increased calcium intake was the major nutrient change, the researchers acknowledge that the beneficial effect of lowfat dairy foods on colon cancer risk may also be explained by other components in dairy foods such as vitamin D, butyrate, sphingomyelin, and conjugated linoleic acid (CLA).[9]

B. Dairy Food Cultures and Colon Cancer

Intake of fermented or culture-containing dairy foods may reduce the risk of colon cancer, although the findings are not entirely consistent and may depend in part on such factors as the strain of bacteria used in dairy foods. As mentioned above, consuming yogurt as infrequently as one to three times a month was associated with protection against colon cancer.[51] Yogurt, a common component of the diet in Finland, may contribute to the low incidence of colon cancer in that country where per capita consumption of fat is high. In contrast, findings from a case-control study in the Netherlands do not support a beneficial effect of commercially available fermented dairy products (e.g., yogurt, buttermilk) against colon cancer.[59] A prospective study in the U.S. indicates a small protective effect of yogurt against colorectal adenomas in both men and women.[111] The authors suggest that the findings may have been significant if the study had included more participants and a wider range of intake of yogurt.[111] While yogurt intake could simply reflect a healthful lifestyle, components in yogurt (other than calcium) may protect against colon cancer. For example, the anticarcinogenic effect of cultured-containing dairy foods may be due to specific lactic acid bacteria.[123-129]

Consumption of *Lactobacillus* products containing viable lactic acid bacteria may lower risk of colon cancer directly by reducing procarcinogenic substances or indirectly by reducing the level of enzymes that convert procarcinogens to carcinogens in the intestine.[128] During the fermentation of milk by *S. thermophilus* and *L. bulgaricus*, metabolites possessing antimutagenic activity are produced.[130]

Lactic acid bacteria have been shown to decrease the proliferation of tumor cells in experimental animals implanted with tumor cells. When laboratory rats were fed *Lactobacillus acidophilus*, the most common bacteria added to milk to make yogurt, the induction time for experimental colon cancer was increased.[124] Friend and Shahani[127] reported that rats intraperitoneally injected with 1,2 DMH developed fewer chemically induced colon tumors when fed "sour" milk compared to when they received artificially acidified milk. Takano et al.[131] also found that feeding "sour" milk to carcinogen-induced (DMH) rats reduced the proliferation of colon tumors.

Another strain of *Lactobacillus*, specifically *Lactobacillus GG*, has been demonstrated to decrease colon tumor incidence or the number of tumors in DMH-treated laboratory rats.[132] Based on the time of feeding, it appears that this *Lactobacillus* species interferes with the initiation of early promotional stages of chemically induced carcinogenesis. Its effect also is more pronounced in animals fed a high fat (20% corn oil) diet than a lowfat (5% corn oil) diet. [132]

Bifidobacterium longum, a lactic acid-producing bacteria in the human colon, has also been demonstrated to inhibit colon tumor development in experimental animals.[133-135] Colon tumors were completely blocked in rats treated with a chemical carcinogen and fed a high fat diet supplemented with 5% *B. longum*.[133] In a more recent study, dietary intake of lypholized cultures of *B. longum* significantly suppressed colon tumor incidence and multiplicity and reduced tumor volume in carcinogen-treated rats.[134] *B. longum* also reduced carcinogen-induced cell proliferation, the activity of colonic mucosal and tumor ornithine decarboxylase, and the expression of ras-p21 oncoprotein.[134] Increased activity of ornithine decarboxylase, a rate limiting enzyme in the metabolism of polyamines, has been observed in colon adenomas and carcinomas, reflecting colonic mucosa hyperproliferation. Ras activation is an early and frequent genetic alteration associated with cancers, especially colon cancer.

In a recent investigation to determine whether *lactobacilli* and/or *bifidobacteria* reduce colon cancer risk in laboratory animals, as measured by the number of colonic aberrant crypts (precancerous lesions), the findings were inconsistent.[136] The authors attribute this inconsistency to differences in response to the chemical carcinogen based on the animals' age, as well as the species or strains of bacteria administered.[136] Other researchers have demonstrated that species of lactic acid bacteria can differ in their anticarcinogenic effect under *in vivo* conditions.[129]

In humans, *Lactobacillus acidophilus* supplements have been demonstrated to decrease activities of fecal bacterial B-glucuronidase and nitroreductase, enzymes that may convert procarcinogens to proximal carcinogens.[125,126] These enzymes returned to baseline levels 30 days after intake of the *Lactobacillus acidophilus* supplements ceased. Similar findings are reported by investigators in Finland.[137] When healthy female adults supplemented their normal omnivorous diet with yogurt containing viable *Lactobacillus GG* for four weeks, fecal beta-glucuronidase, nitroreductase, and glycocholic acid hydrolase activities decreased.[137] The activities of these enzymes returned to baseline levels after *Lactobacillus GG* treatment was discontinued.[137]

C. Other Protective Components in Dairy Foods

1. Conjugated Linoleic Acid (CLA)

CLA is a collective term to describe one or more positional and geometric isomers of the essential fatty acid, linoleic acid.[7,138] While linoleic acid stimulates carcinogenesis, *in vitro* and experimental animal studies indicate that CLA inhibits the development of a variety of tumors, particularly mammary tumors.[7,138-140] Animal products, specifically dairy products (milk, butter, yogurt, cheese), are the principal dietary source of CLA (Table 4.3).[141,142] Moreover, 90% of the CLA in dairy foods is in the cis-9, trans-11 isomeric form which is thought to be the biologically active CLA isomer.[141] As little as 0.5% CLA, an amount found in most dairy foods, reduces the formation of some cancers in experimental animals fed a chemical carcinogen.[143]

Table 4.3   Conjugated Dienoic Isomers Of Linoleic Acid (CLA) in Dairy Products

Number Foodstuff[a]	Total CLA[b] of Samples	c-9,t-11[c] (mg/g fat)	%
Homogenized milk	3	5.5 ± 0.30	92
Condensed milk	3	7.0 ± 0.29	82
Cultured buttermilk	3	5.4 ± 0.16	89
Butter	4	4.7 ± 0.36	88
Butter fat	4	6.1 ± 0.21	89
Sour cream	3	4.6 ± 0.46	90
Ice cream	3	3.6 ± 0.10	86
Nonfat frozen dairy dessert	2	0.6 ± 0.02	n.d.[d]
Lowfat yogurt	4	4.4 ± 0.21	86
Custard style yogurt	4	4.8 ± 0.16	83
Plain yogurt	2	4.8 ± 0.26	84
Nonfat yogurt	2	1.7 ± 0.10	83
Frozen yogurt	2	2.8 ± 0.20	85
Sharp Cheddar	3	3.6 ± 0.18	93
Cream cheese	3	3.8 ± 0.08	88
Colby	3	6.1 ± 0.14	92
Cottage cheese	3	4.5 ± 0.13	83
Cheez whiz™	4	5.0 ± 0.07	92
Velveeta™	2	5.2 ± 0.03	86

[a] Samples were from commercially available, uncooked edible portions.
[b] Values are means ± standard error for the number of samples indicated. [c] Values are means for the number of samples indicated. All standard error values are less than 3%. Data were expressed as % of total CLA isomers. [d]n.d. = not detectable.

From Chin, S.F., et al., *J. Food Composition & Analysis*, 5, 185, 1992. With permission.

In cell culture studies, physiologic concentrations of CLA have been demonstrated to inhibit the proliferation of human malignant colorectal cancer cells.[140] In experimental animals, feeding CLA markedly reduced the incidence of chemically induced aberrant crypt foci (a precancerous marker) in the colon.[144] The mechanism(s) by which CLA influences carcinogenesis is under investigation and may differ according to the site, age, duration of exposure, and stage of carcinogenesis.[7] CLA was once thought to protect against cancer by acting as an antioxidant.[139] More recently, research has indicated that CLA per se may not possess antioxidant properties,[145] but may protect against cancer by other means such as by modifying the fluidity of cell membranes, decreasing prostaglandin synthesis, and/or enhancing the immune response.[7,146]

CLA appears to reduce cancer risk by a mechanism different from that by which linoleic acid promotes cancer.[143] Although feeding Cheddar cheese (112 g/day) for four weeks has been demonstrated to increase plasma CLA levels in humans by 19 to 27%[147] and CLA exhibits cancer-inhibitory effects *in vitro* and in experimental animals, there is no direct evidence that CLA protects against cancer, including colon cancer, in humans. However, findings of more consistent protective effects of dairy foods on colon cancer than calcium alone provide indirect evidence that other components in dairy foods such as CLA may contribute to this food's potential cancer inhibitory effect.[9]

2. Sphingolipids

Sphingolipids, an important type of fat found in milk and other dairy foods, may protect against colon cancer.[148-150] Sphingolipids are combinations of different compounds that include ceramides, sphingomyelin, cerebrosides, sulfatides, and gangliosides.[148-150] These compounds have a long-chain (sphingoid) base as the backbone. In the body, sphingolipids modulate cell growth, differentiation, and transformation, and are important in cell-to-cell communication.[149-151] There has been no systematic study of the sphingolipid content of food. However, sphingomyelin, the most common sphingolipid, is found in cow's milk.[150] Sphingomyelin makes up about one-third of total milk phospholipids, although it can vary according to season and the cow's stage of lactation.[7] Milk, butter, and cheese contain approximately 1 umol sphingolipids per gram.[150] Because sphingolipids are found mainly in cell membranes, rather than in fat droplets, nonfat, lowfat, and full fat dairy products are all sources of sphingolipids.[7]

Studies indicate that sphingolipids influence cell regulation pertaining to carcinogenesis. According to *in vitro* investigations, sphingosine inhibits protein kinase C which is thought to promote tumors.[152] Sphingosine also appears to reduce the metastatic potential and growth of several human cancer cell lines.[149,153] Studies demonstrate that sphingomeylin is broken down into biologically active compounds (i.e., ceramid and sphingosine) throughout the gastrointestinal tract.[154]

Studies in laboratory mice indicate a protective effect of dietary sphingomyelin on colon cancer.[148,155,156] In a preliminary study in which mice were fed a carcinogen and sphingomyelin isolated from nonfat dried milk, the incidence of colon tumors (20%) was less than half that in the control animals fed the carcinogen only (47%).[148] These findings were confirmed in another study which demonstrated that milk sphingolipids (1% of the diet) reduced the number of aberrant colonic crypt foci by 70% and aberrant crypts per focus by 30% (i.e., early indicators of colon carcinogenesis) (Figure 4.10).[155] Athough the sphingomyelin-fed mice developed the same number of tumors as the mice which did not consume this compound, 31% of the tumors which formed in the

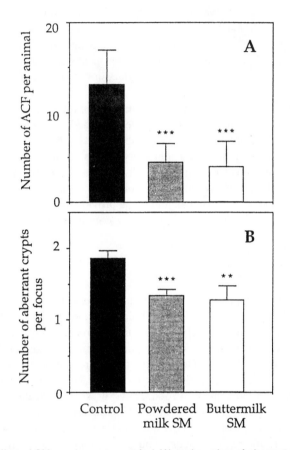

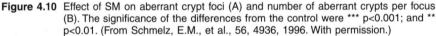

Figure 4.10 Effect of SM on aberrant crypt foci (A) and number of aberrant crypts per focus (B). The significance of the differences from the control were *** p<0.001; and ** p<0.01. (From Schmelz, E.M., et al., 56, 4936, 1996. With permission.)

sphingomyelin-fed mice were of the less dangerous form (i.e., adenomas), whereas all of the tumors which formed in the mice not fed sphingomyelin were the more dangerous type (i.e., adenocarcinomas).[155] The anticarcinogenic effect of sphingolipids is due to sphingomyelin and not to a contaminate.[156]

The mechanism(s) by which dietary sphingolipids protect against cancer is unknown. Researchers propose that sphingolipids inhibit the growth and metastasis of tumor cells and transform precancerous cells to more normal cells.[148] The chemo-protective properties of sphingolipids may also involve their effect on calcium[157] and vitamin D metabolism.[158] Sphingolipids can increase calcium release from intracel-lular stores.[157] This finding is important given calcium's protective effect against colon cancer. Research also indicates that sphingolipids mediate some of the cellular responses to vitamin D metabolites.[158]

3. Butyric Acid

Butyric acid, a four carbon short-chain fatty acid in milkfat, may protect against colon cancer, at least according to *in vitro* and experimental animal studies.[7,159] In a variety of cancer cell lines including colon, butyrate inhibits the proliferation and induces differentiation and programmed cell death (i.e., apoptosis).[7,160-164] At the molecular level, butyrate is associated with down-regulation or inactivation of the expression of cancer genes.[7,159] Butyrate also may inhibit tumor invasiveness and metastasis.[7,159]

In addition to its presence in milkfat, butyrate results from bacterial fermentation of unabsorbed carbohydrate (fiber) in the lower intestine.[7,159] Several studies indicate an anticarcinogenic effect of butyrate against colon cancer.[99,162-166] In *in vitro* studies, the addition to butyrate to colon cells from mice genetically at risk of colon cancer reduced cell proliferation by 28% and enhanced cell death by 350% compared to cell cultures not exposed to butyrate.[166] When human cancer cell lines were treated with sodium butyrate, the proliferation of cancer cells was inhibited and morphological changes consistent with cell death occurred.[162,163]

In laboratory animals fed a high fiber diet and a carcinogen, the presence of high levels of butyrate in the distal colon significantly reduced colon tumors.[167] The mechanism involved in the anticarcinogenic effect of butyric acid in milkfat is unknown. Milk short-chain fatty acids such as butyric acid are released in the upper gastrointestinal tract where they are immediately absorbed, processed, and released into circulation for transport to the liver where most of it is metabolized.[7,159] Because butyric acid from milkfat never reaches the lower intestine, it is unknown whether this source of butyric acid, unlike butyric acid derived from fiber, plays a protective role against cancer at this site.

4. Milk Proteins

Findings from experimental animal and cell culture studies indicate that milk proteins, such as casein and especially whey proteins, may protect against colon cancer.[8,168] Casein, which makes up nearly 80% of the protein in cow's milk, has been demonstrated to have anti-carcinogenic properties.[8,168-170] When different protein diets (20 g protein/100 g diet) were fed to Spraque-Dawley male rats administered a chemical carcinogen, casein produced fewer colon tumors than red meat (kangaroo skeletal muscle) or soybean protein.[168] Casein has been demonstrated to inhibit fecal beta-glucuronidase, an enzyme produced by intestinal bacteria, which deconjugates pro-carcinogenic glucuronides to carcinogens.[8] Casein may also protect against colon cancer by its affect on the immune system, specifically by its ability to stimulate phagocytic activities and increase lymphocytes.[8] *In vitro* studies indicate that casein-derived peptides isolated from the microbial fermentation of milk inhibit colon cancer by altering cell kinetics.[169] Other researchers suggest that the molecular structure of casein contributes to its anticarcinogenic properties.[170]

Whey proteins in particular appear to have a potentially beneficial role in protecting against colon cancer.[8] Both experimental animal and *in vitro* studies demonstrate a protective effect of whey proteins against colon cancer.[8,168] Whey proteins are rich in sulfur amino acids, cysteine and methionine, which are precursors of glutathionine, an important cancer protective agent. Glutathionine is a substrate for two classes of enzymes, specifically selenium-dependent glutathione peroxidase and glutathione transferase, which appear to have anti-cancer activity.[8] Glutathione peroxidase may reduce substances such as hydrogen peroxide and free radicals that damage DNA.[8] Glutathione transferase may help eliminate mutagens and carcinogens from the body. Whey proteins may also protect against colon cancer by enhancing humoral and cell-mediated immune responses.[8] Minor whey proteins such as lactoferrin, an iron-binding glycoprotein, also may have potential anti-cancer properties.[8]

Few studies have investigated the role of milk proteins on colon cancer in humans. However, a recent prospective study of colon cancer in women found that protein primarily from dairy foods, followed by red meat, poultry, fish, and shellfish, was inversely associated with colon cancer.[24] The researchers speculate that the amino acid methionine may protect against colon cancer.[24] As mentioned above, whey protein is a rich source of cysteine and methionine which are precursors of the anticarcinogenic tripeptide glutathionine.

IV. SUMMARY

Dietary recommendations to reduce cancer emphasize a reduction in total fat intake, especially from high fat foods.[21,171] This recommendation should be interpreted cautiously to ensure that recommended intakes of animal foods such as dairy foods are not jeopardized. Although a high fat or calorie intake is associated with increased risk of colon cancer, there is no scientific evidence that dairy foods contribute to this disease. On the contrary, components in dairy foods such as calcium, vitamin D, bacterial cultures (e.g., *Lactobacillus acidophilus*), CLA, sphingolipids, and others may protect against colon cancer.

Findings from epidemiological, experimental animal, *in vitro*, and clinical studies support the hypothesis that increased calcium and vitamin D intake reduce the hyperproliferation and cancer-promoting effects associated with a Western-style diet. In individuals at risk for colon cancer, hyperproliferation of colon epithelium is reduced towards normal by increased dietary calcium. Based on the evidence to date, meeting recommended intakes for calcium (1200 mg for adults over 50 years)[62] and vitamin D (10 to 15 μg/day for adults over 50 years)[62], especially from dairy foods which are major sources of these nutrients in our diets, appears to be a prudent measure to reduce the risk of colon cancer.[172] Unfortunately, calcium intake in the United States generally is lower than recommended. According to data from USDA's 1994 and 1995 Continuing Survey of Food Intakes by Individuals,[173] about 60% of U.S. adults over 50 years of age are not meeting 100% of the 1200 mg calcium/day currently recommended.[62]

New findings from a clinical trial indicate that increasing intake of lowfat dairy foods to reach 1500 mg calcium/day may reduce the risk of colon cancer.[9] There is also suggestive evidence that intake of culture-containing dairy foods such as yogurt may protect against colon cancer, although more research is needed to confirm this finding, as well as to delineate the potential anticarcinogenic role of CLA, sphingolipids, and other components in dairy foods. Dairy foods are an important source of calcium, vitamin D, CLA, sphingolipids, and, if cultured, bacterial cultures, as well as proteins each of which have been suggested to protect against colon cancer.[7,8] For this reason, all individuals, and particularly those at high risk of colon cancer, should consume the recommended number of servings from the milk and other food groups each day. Four servings a day of foods from the Milk Group can provide about 1200 mg calcium, the amount currently recommended for adults over 50 years of age.[62] Although most research on dairy foods and cancer prevention has focused on colon cancer, accumulating scientific evidence indicates that intake of dairy foods such as milk may also reduce the risk of breast cancer.[174-176] These findings provide an additional reason to consume dairy foods.

REFERENCES

1. American Cancer Society, *Cancer Facts & Figures–1998*, American Cancer Society, Atlanta, GA, 1998.
2. Committee on Comparative Toxicity of Naturally Occurring Carcinogens, *Carcinogens and Anticarcinogens in the Human Diet,* National Academy Press, Washington, D.C., 1996.
3. Ames, B. N., Gold, L. S., and Willett, W. C., The causes and prevention of cancer, *Natl. Acad. Sci. U.S.A.*, 92, 5258, 1995.
4. Doll, R., The lessons of life: keynote address to the nutrition and cancer conference, *Cancer Res.*, 52(Suppl.), 2024, 1992.
5. Doll, R., Nature and nuture: possibilities for cancer control, *Carcinogenesis*, 17, 177, 1996.
6. Potter, J. D., Nutrition and colorectal cancer, *Cancer Causes and Control*, 7, 127, 1996.
7. Parodi, P. W., Cows' milk fat components as potential anticarcinogenic agents. *J. Nutr.*, 127, 1055, 1997.
8. Parodi, P. W., A role for milk proteins in cancer prevention, *Austr. J. Dairy Technol.*, 53, 37, 1998.
9. Holt, P. R., Atillasoy, E. O., Gilman, J., Guss, J., Moss, S. F., Newmark, H., Fan, K., Yang, K., and Lipkin, M., Modulation of abnormal colonic epithelial cell proliferation and differentiation by lowfat dairy foods, *JAMA*, 280, 1074, 1998.
10. Bruce, W. R., Recent hypothesis for the origin of colon cancer, *Cancer Res.*, 47, 4237, 1987.
11. Burnstein, M. J., Dietary factors related to colorectal neoplasms, *Surg. Clin. N. Am.*, 73(1), 13, 1993.
12. Rose, D. P., Boyar, A. P., and Wynder, E. L., International comparisons of mortality rates for cancer of the breast, ovary, prostate, and colon, and per capita food consumption, *Cancer*, 58(11), 2363, 1986.

13. Birt, D. F., The influence of dietary fat on carcinogenesis: lessons from experimental models, *Nutr. Rev.*, 48, 1, 1990.

14. Willett, W., The search for the causes of breast and colon cancer, *Nature*, 338, 389, 1989.

15. Wynder, E. L., Reddy, B. S., and Weisburger, J. H., Environmental dietary factors in colorectal cancer: some unresolved issues, *Cancer*, 70, 1222, 1992.

16. Reddy, B. S., Dietary fat and colon cancer: animal model studies, *Lipids*, 27, 807, 1992.

17. Garland, C. F., Garland, F. C., and Goreham, E. D., Can colon cancer incidence and death rates be reduced with calcium and vitamin D?, *Am. J. Clin. Nutr.*, 54(Suppl.), 193, 1991.

18. Food and Nutrition Board, Committee on Diet and Health, Commission on Life Sciences, National Research Council, *Diet and Health. Implications for Reducing Chronic Disease Risk*, National Academy Press, Washington, D.C., 1989.

19. Howe, G. R., Aronson, K. J., Benito, E., et al., The relationship between dietary fat intake and risk of colorectal cancer: evidence from the combined analysis of 13 case-control studies, *Cancer Causes & Control*, 8, 215, 1997.

20. Giovannucci, E. and Goldin, B., The role of fat, fatty acids, and total energy intake in the etiology of human colon cancer, *Am. J. Clin. Nutr.*, 66(s), 1564, 1997.

21. American Institute for Cancer Research, *Food, Nutrition and the Prevention of Cancer: A Global Perspective*, American Institute for Cancer Research, Washington, D.C., 1997.

22. Ghadirian, P., Lacroix, A., Maisonneuve, P., Perret, C., Potvin, C., Gravel, D., Bernard, D., and Boyle, P., Nutritional factors and colon carcinoma: a case-control study involving French Canadians in Montreal, Quebec, Canada, *Cancer*, 80, 858, 1997.

23. Garland, C., Shekelle, R. B., Barrett-Connor, E., Criqui, M. H., Rossof, A. R., and Paul, O., Dietary vitamin D and calcium and risk of colorectal cancer: a 19-year prospective study in men, *Lancet*, 1, 307, 1985.

24. Kato, I., Akhmedkhanov, A., Koenig, K., Toniolo, P. G., Shore, R. E., and Riboli, E., Prospective study of diet and female colorectal cancer: The New York University Women's Health Study, *Nutr. & Cancer*, 28, 276, 1997.

25. Bostick, R. M., Potter, J. D., Kushi, L. H., Sellers, T. A., Steinmetz, K. A., McKenzie, D. R., Gapstur, S. M., and Folsom, A. R., Sugar, meat, and fat intake, and non-dietary risk factors for colon cancer incidence in Iowa women (United States), *Cancer Causes & Control*, 5, 38, 1994.

26. Giovannucci, E., Rimm, E. B., Stampfer, M. J., Colditz, G. A., Ascherio, A., and Willett, W. C., Intake of fat, meat, and fiber in relation to risk of colon cancer in men, *Cancer Res.*, 54, 2390, 1994.

27. Willett, W. W., Stampfer, M. J., Colditz, G. A., Rosner, B. A., and Speizer, F. E., Relation of meat, fat, and fiber intake to the risk of colon cancer in a prospective study among women, *N. Engl. J. Med.*, 323, 1664, 1990.

28. Giovannucci, E., Stampfer, M. J., Colditz, G., Rimm, E. B., and Willett, W. C., Relationship of diet to risk of colorectal adenoma in men, *J. Natl. Cancer Inst.*, 84, 91, 1992.

29. Mettlin, C. J., Schoenfeld, E. R., and Natarajan, N., Patterns of milk consumption and risk of cancer, *Nutr. Cancer*, 13, 89, 1990.

30. Slattery, M. L., Boucher, K. M., Caan, B. J., Potter, J. D., and Ma, K. N., Eating patterns and risk of colon cancer, *Am. J. Epidemiol.*, 148, 4, 1998.

31. Shike, M., Body weight and colon cancer, *Am. J. Clin. Nutr.*, 63(s), 442, 1996.

32. Slattery, M. L., Caan, B. J., Potter, J. D., Berry, T. D., Coates, A., Duncan, D., and Edwards, S.L., Dietary energy sources and colon cancer risk, *Am. J. Epidemiol.*, 145, 199, 1997.

33. Pence, B.C., Dunn, D.M., Zhao, C., Patel, V., Hunter, S., and Landers, M., Protective effects of calcium from nonfat dried milk against colon carcinogenesis in rats, *Nutr. Res.*, 25, 35, 1996.

34. Rijnkels, J. M., Hollanders, V. M., Woutersen, R. A., Koeman, J. H., and Alink, G. M., Interaction of dietary fat with a vegetables-fruit mixture on 1,2-dimethylhydrazine-induced colorectal cancer in rats, *Nutr. & Cancer*, 27, 261, 1997.

35. Erickson, K. L. and Hubbard, N. E., Dietary fat and tumor metastasis, *Nutr. Rev.*, 48, 6, 1990.

36. Klurfeld, D. M. and Bull, A. W., Fatty acids and colon cancer in experimental models, *Am. J. Clin. Nutr.*, 66(Suppl.), 1530, 1997.

37. Van der Meer, R., Lapre, J. A., Govers, M. J. A. P., and Kleibeuker, J. H., Mechanisms of the intestinal effects of dietary fats and milk products on colon carcinogenesis, *Cancer Lett.*, 114, 75, 1997.

38. Newmark, H. L., Wargovich, M. H., and Bruce, W. R., Colon cancer and dietary fat, phosphate, and calcium: a hypothesis, *J. Natl. Cancer Inst.*, 72, 1323, 1984.

39. Wargovich, M. J., Calcium and colon cancer, *J. Am. Coll. Nutr.*, 7, 295, 1988.

40. Wargovich, M. J., Eng, V. W. S., Newmark, H. L., and Bruce, W. R., Calcium ameliorates the toxic effects of deoxycholic acid on colonic epithelium, *Carcinogenesis*, 4, 1205, 1983.

41. Pariza, M. W., Ha, Y. L., Benjamin, H., Sword, J. T., Gruter, A., Chin, S. F., Storkson, J., Faith, N., and Albright, K., Formation and action of anticarcinogenic fatty acids. In *Nutritional and Toxicological Consequences of Food Processing*, Friedman, M., Ed., Plenum Press, NY, 1991, 269-272.

42. Morotomi, M., Guillem, J. G., LoGerfo, P., and Weinstein, I. B., Production of diacylglycerol, an activator of protein kinase C, by human intestinal microflora, *Cancer Res.*, 50, 3595, 1990.

43. Lipkin, M., Application of intermediate biomarkers to studies of cancer prevention in the gastrointestinal tract: introduction and perspective, *Am. J. Clin. Nutr.* 54(Suppl.), 188, 1991.

44. Newmark, H. L. and Lipkin, M., Calcium, vitamin D, and colon cancer, *Cancer Res.*, 52(Suppl.), 2067, 1992.

45. Wargovich, M. J., Lynch, P. M., and Liven, B., Modulating effects of calcium in animal models of colon carcinogenesis and short-term studies in subjects at increased risk for colon cancer, *Am. J. Clin. Nutr.*, 54(Suppl.), 202, 1991.

46. Van der Meer, R., Bovee-Oudenhoven, I. M. J., Sesink, A. L. A., and Kleibeuker, J. H., Milk products and intestinal health, *Int. Dairy J.*, 8, 163, 1998.

47. Garland, C. F. and Garland, F. C., Do sunlight and vitamin D reduce the risk of colon cancer?, *Int. J. Epidemiol.*, 9, 227, 1980.

48. Bergsma-Kadijk, J. A., Van't Veer, P., Kumpman, E., and Burema, J., Calcium does not protect against colorectal neoplasia, *Epidemiology*, 7, 590, 1996.

49. Slattery, M. L., Sorensen, A. W., and Ford, M. H., Dietary calcium intake as a mitigating factor in colon cancer, *Am. J. Epidemiol.*, 128, 504, 1988.

50. Sorensen, A. W., Slattery, M. L., and Ford, M. H., Calcium and colon cancer: a review, *Nutr. Cancer*, 11, 135, 1988.

51. Peters, R. K., Pike, M. C., Garabrant, D., and Mack, T. M., Diet and colon cancer in Los Angeles County, California, *Causes and Control*, 3, 457, 1992.

52. Arbman, G., Axelson, O., Ericsson-Begodzki, A.-B., Fredriksson, M., Nilsson, E., and Sjodahl, R., Cereal fiber, calcium, and colorectal cancer, *Cancer*, 69, 2042, 1992.

53. Zaridze, D., Filipchenko, V., Kustov, V., Serdyuk, V., and Duffy, S., Diet and colorectal cancer: results of two case-control studies in Russia, *Eur. J. Cancer*, 29A, 112, 1993.

54. De Stefani, E., Mendilaharsu, M., Deneo-Pellegrini, H., and Ronco, A., Influence of dietary levels of fat, cholesterol, and calcium on colorectal cancer, *Nutr. & Cancer*, 29, 83, 1997.

55. Frommer, D., Buchanan, M., Woodger, A., and Kalafatos, E., Can raised faecal calcium concentrations protect against colorectal neoplasms, *Gastrointestinal Oncology*, 104, (4, part 2), April 1993 (Abst).

56. Martinez, M. E., McPherson, R. S., Annegers, J. F., and Levin, B., Association of diet and colorectal adenomatous polyps: dietary fiber, calcium, and total fat, *Epidemiology*, 7, 264, 1996.

57. Tangrea, J., Helzlsouer, K., Pietinen, P., Taylor, P., Hollis, B., Virtamo, J., and Albanes, D., Serum levels of vitamin D metabolites and the subsequent risk of colon and rectal cancer in Finnish men, *Cancer Causes & Control*, 8, 615, 1997.

58. Martinez, M. E., McPherson, R. S., Levin, B., and Glober, G. A., A case-control study of dietary intake and other lifestyle risk factors for hyperplastic polyps, *Gastroenterology*, 113, 423, 1997.

59. Kampman, E., Van't Veer, P., Hiddink, G. J., Van Aken-Schneijder, P., Kok, F. J., and Hermus, R. J., Fermented dairy products, dietary calcium and colon cancer: a case-control study in the Netherlands, *Int. J. Cancer*, 59, 170, 1994.

60. Bostick, R. M., Potter, J. D., Sellers, T. A., McKenzie, D. R., Kushi, L. H., and Folsom, A. R., Relation of calcium, vitamin D, and dairy food intake to incidence of colon cancer among older women, *Am. J. Epidemiol*, 137, 1302, 1993.

61. Hyman, J., Baron, J. A., Dain, B. J., Sandler, R. S., Haile, R. W., Mandel, J. S., Mott, L. A., and Greenberg, E. R., Dietary and supplemental calcium and the recurrence of colorectal adenomas, *Cancer Epidemiol., Biomarkers and Prevention*, 7, 291, 1998.

62. IOM (Institute of Medicine), *Dietary Reference Intakes for Calcium, Phosphorus, Magnesium, Vitamin D, and Fluoride,* Standing Committee on the Scientific Evaluation of Dietary Reference Intakes, Food and Nutrition Board, National Academy Press, Washington, D.C., 1997.

63. Garland, C. F., Comstock, G. W., Garland, F. C., Hesling, K. J., Shaw, E. K., and Gorham, E. D., Serum 25-hydroxyvitamin D and colon cancer: eight-year prospective study, *Lancet*, 2, 1176, 1989.

64. Martinez, M. E., Giovannucci, E. L., Colditz, G. A., Stampfer, M. J., Hunter, D. J., Speizer, F. E., Wing, A., and Willett, W. C., Calcium, vitamin D, and occurrence of colorectal cancer among women, *J. Natl. Cancer Inst.*, 88, 1375, 1996.

65. Kearney, J., Giovannucci, E., Rimm, E. B., Ascherio, A., Stampfer, M. J., Colditz, G. A., Wing, A., Kampman, E., and Willett, W. C., Calcium, vitamin D, and dairy foods and the occurrence of colon cancer in men, *Am. J. Epidemiol.*, 143, 907, 1996.

66. Jensen, O. M., MacLennan, R., and Wahrendorf, J., Diet, bowel function, fecal characteristics, and large bowel cancer in Denmark and Finland, *Nutr. Cancer*, 4, 5, 1982.

67. Jensen, O. M. and MacLennan, R., Dietary factors and colorectal cancer in Scandinavia, *Israel J. Med. Sci.*, 15, 329, 1979.

68. Phillips, R. L., Role of life-style and dietary habits in risk of colon cancer among Seventh-Day Adventists, *Cancer Res.*, 35, 3513, 1975.

69. Negri, E., LaVecchia, C., D'Avanzo, B., and Franceschi, S., Calcium, dairy products and colorectal cancer, *Nutr. Cancer*, 13, 255, 1990.

70. Jain, M., Dairy foods, dairy fats, and cancer: a review of epidemiological evidence, *Nutr. Res.*, 18, 905, 1998.

71. Appleton, G. V. N., Bristol, J. B., and Williamson, R. C. N., Increased dietary calcium and small bowel resection have opposite effects on colonic cell turnover, *Br. J. Surg.*, 73, 1018, 1986.

72. Pence, B. C. and Buddingh, F., Inhibition of dietary fat-promoted colon carcinogenesis in rats by supplemental calcium or vitamin D_3, *Carcinogenesis*, 9, 187, 1988.

73. Newmark, H. L., Lipkin, M., and Maheshwari, N., Colonic hyperplasia and hyperproliferation induced by a nutritional stress diet with four components of Western-style diet, *J. Natl. Cancer Inst.*, 82, 491, 1990.

74. Newmark, H. L., Lipkin, M., and Maheshwari, N., Colonic hyperproliferation induced in rats and mice by nutritional-stress diets containing four components of a human Western-style diet (series 2), *Am. J. Clin. Nutr.*, 54(s), 209, 1991.

75. Lapré, J. A., DeVries, H. T., Koeman, J. H., and van der Meer, R., An antiproliferative effect of dietary calcium on colonic epithelium is mediated by luminal surfactants and dependent on the type of dietary fat, *Cancer Res.*, 53, 784, 1993.

76. Lupton, J. R., Chen, X-Q., Frolich, W., Schoeffler, G. L., and Peterson, M. L., Rats fed high fat diets with increased calcium levels have fecal bile acid concentrations similar to those of rats fed a lowfat diet, *J. Nutr.*, 124, 188, 1994.

77. Risio, M., Lipkin, M., Newmark, H., Yang, K., Rossini, F. P., Steele, V. E., Boone, C. W., and Kelloff, G. J., Apoptosis, cell replication, and Western-style diet-induced tumorigenesis in mouse colon, *Cancer Res.*, 56, 4910, 1996.

78. Appleton, G. N. V., Owen, R. W., Wheller, E. E., Challacombe, D. N., and Williamson, R. C. N., Effect of dietary calcium on the colonic luminal environment, *Gut*, 32, 1374, 1991.

79. Rafter, J. J., Eng, V. W. S., Furrer, R., Medline, A., and Bruce, W. R., Effects of calcium and pH on the mucosal damage produced by deoxycholic acid in the rat colon, *Gut*, 27, 1320, 1986.

80. Skrypec, D. J., Effect of dietary calcium on azoxymethane-induced intestinal carcinogenesis in male F344 rats fed high-fat diets, In *Calcium, Vitamin D, and Prevention of Colon Cancer*, Lipkin, M., Newmark, H. L., and Kelloff, G., Eds., CRC Press, Boca Raton, FL, 1991, 241-247.

81. Lipkin, M., Biomarkers of increased susceptibility to gastrointestinal cancer: new application to studies of cancer prevention in human subjects, Perspectives in Cancer Research, *Cancer Res.*, 48, 235, 1988.

82. Lipkin, M. D. and Newmark, H., Effect of added dietary calcium on colonic epithelial-cell proliferation in subjects at high risk for familial colonic cancer, *N. Engl. J. Med.*, 313, 1381, 1985.

83. Lipkin, M., Friedman, E., Winawer, S. J., and Newmark, H., Colonic epithelial cell proliferation in responders and nonresponders to supplemental dietary calcium, *Cancer Res.*, 49, 248, 1989.

84. Lipkin, M., Newmark, H. L., and Kelloff, G., Eds., *Calcium, Vitamin D, and Prevention of Colon Cancer*, CRC Press, Boca Raton, FL, 1991.

85. Wargovich, M. J., Eng, V. W. S., and Newmark, H. L., Calcium inhibits the damaging and compensatory proliferative effects of fatty acids on mouse colonic epithelium, *Cancer Lett.*, 23, 253, 1984.

86. Appleton, G. V. N., Davies, P. W., Bristol, J. B., and Williamson, R. C. N., Inhibition of intestinal carcinogenesis by dietary supplementation with calcium, *Br. J. Surg.*, 74, 523, 1987.
87. Beaty, M. M., Lee, E. Y., and Glauert, H. P., Influence of dietary calcium and vitamin D on colon epithelial cell proliferation and 1,2-dimethylhydrazine-induced colon carcinogenesis in rats fed high fat diets, *J. Nutr.*, 123, 144, 1993.
88. Behling, A. R., Kaup, S. M., Choquette, L. L., and Greger, J. L., Lipid absorption and intestinal tumour incidence in rats fed on varying levels of calcium and butterfat, *Br. J. Nutr.*, 64, 505, 1990.
89. Reshef, R., Rozen, P., Fireman, Z., Fine, N., Barzilai, M., Shasha, S. M., and Shkolnik, T., Effect of a calcium-enriched diet on the colonic epithelial hyperproliferation induced by N-methyl-N′-nitro-N-nitrosoquanidine in rats on a low calcium and fat diet, *Cancer Res.*, 50, 1764, 1990.
90. Wargovich, M. J., Allnutt, D., Palmer, C., Anaya, P., and Stephens, L. C., Inhibition of the promotional phase of azoxymethane-induced colon carcinogenesis in the F334 rat by calcium lactate: effect of simulating two human nutrient density levels, *Cancer Lett.*, 53, 17, 1990.
91. Sitrin, M. D., Halline, A. G., Abrahams, C., and Brasitus, T. A., Dietary calcium and vitamin D modulate 1,2-dimethylhydrazine-induced colonic carcinogenesis in the rat, *Cancer Res.*, 51, 5608, 1991.
92. Karkare, M. R., Clark, T. D., and Glauert, H. P., Effect of dietary calcium on colon carcinogenesis induced by a single injection of 1,2-dimethylhydrazine in rats, *J. Nutr.*, 121, 568, 1991.
93. Comer, P. F., Clark, T. D., and Glauert, H. P., Effect of dietary vitamin D_3 (cholecalciferol) on colon carcinogenesis induced by 1,2-dimethylhydrazine in male Fisher 344 rats, *Nutr. Cancer*, 19, 113, 1993.
94. Wargovich, M. J. and Lointier, P. H., Calcium and vitamin D modulate mouse colon epithelial proliferation and growth characteristics of a human colon tumor cell line, *Can. J. Physiol. Pharmacol.*, 65, 472, 1987.
95. Bird, R. P., Effect of dietary components on the pathobiology of colonic epithelium: possible relationship with colon tumorigenesis, *Lipids*, 21, 289, 1986.
96. Scalmati, A., Lipkin, M., and Newmark, H., Calcium, vitamin D, and colon cancer, *Clin. Appl. Nutr.*, 2, 67, 1992.
97. Llor, X., Teng, B., Jacoby, R., Davidson, N., Sitrin, M., and Brasitus, T. A., Dietary calcium and vitamin D modulate K-ras mutations in experimental colon cancer, *Gastroenterology*, 98, A 294, 1990.
98. Govers, M. J. A. P., Termont, D. S. M. L., and Van der Meer, R., Mechanism of the antiproliferative effect of milk mineral and other calcium supplements on colonic epithelium, *Cancer Res.*, 54, 95, 1994.
99. Marchetti, M. C., Migliorati, G., Moraca, R., Riccardi, C., Nicoletti, I., Fabiani, R., Mastrandrea, V., and Morozzi, G., Possible mechanisms involved in apoptosis of colon tumor cell lines induced by deoxycholic acid, short-chain fatty acids, and their mixtures, *Nutr. Cancer*, 28, 74, 1997.
100. Buset, M., Lipkin, M., Winawer, S., Swaroop, S., and Friedman, E., Inhibition of human colonic epithelial cell proliferation in vivo and in vitro by calcium, *Cancer Res.*, 46, 5426, 1986.
101. Barsoum, G. H., Hendrickse, C., Winslet, M. C., Youngs, D., Donovan, I. A., Neoptolemos, J. P., and Keighley, M. R. B., Reduction of mucosal crypt cell proliferation in patients with colorectal adenomatous polyps by dietary calcium supplementation, *Br. J. Surg.*, 79, 581, 1992.

102. Guo, Y.-S., Draviam, E., Townsend, Jr., C. M., and Singh, P., Differential effects of Ca2+ on proliferation of stomach, colonic, and pancreatic cancer lines in vitro, *Nutr. Cancer*, 14, 149, 1990.

103. Ichas, F. and Mazat, J. P., From calcium signaling to cell death: two conformations for the mitochondrial permeability transition pore. Switching from low-to high-conductance state, *Biochim. Biophys. Acta.*, 1366, 33, 1998.

104. Brenner, B. M., Russell, N., Albrecht, S., and Davies, R. J., The effect of dietary vitamin D_3 on the intracellular calcium gradient in mammalian colonic cypts, *Cancer Lett.*, 127, 43, 1998.

105. Wargovich, M. J., Isbell, G., Shabot, M., Winn, R., Lanza, F., Hochman, L. Larson, E., Lynch, P., Roubein, L. and Levin, B., Calcium supplementation decreases rectal epithelial cell proliferation in subjects with sporadic adenoma, *Gastroenterology*, 103, 92, 1992.

106. O'Sullivan, K. R., Mathias, P. M., Beattie, S., and O'Morain, C., Effect of oral calcium supplementation on colonic crypt cell proliferation in patients with adenomatous polyps of the large bowel, *Eur. J. Gastroenterol. Hepatol.*, 5, 85, 1993.

107. Bostick, R. M., Fosdick, L., Wood, J. R., Grambsch, P., Grandits, G. A., Lillemoe, T. J., Louis, T. A., and Potter, J. D., Calcium and colorectal epithelial cell proliferation in sporadic adema patients: a randomized, double-blinded, placebo-controlled clinical trial, *J. Natl. Cancer Inst.*, 87, 1307, 1995.

108. Govers, M. J. A. P., Tremont, D. S. M. L., Lapre, J. A., Kleibeuker, J. H., Vonk, R. J., and Van der Meer, R., Calcium in milk products precipitates intestinal fatty acids and secondary bile acids and thus inhibits colonic cytotoxicity in man, *Cancer Res.*, 56, 3270, 1996.

109. Gregoire, R. C., Stern, H. S., Yeung, K. S., Stadler, J., Langley, S., Furrer, R., and Bruce, W. R., Effect of calcium supplementation on mucosal proliferation in high risk patients for colon cancer, *Gut*, 30, 376, 1989.

110. Cats, A., Kleibeuker, J. H., Van der Meer, R., Kuipers, F., Sluiter, W. J., Hardonk, M. J., Oremus, E. Th. H. G. J., Mulder, N. H., and de Vries, E. G. E., Randomized, double-blinded, placebo-controlled intervention study with supplemental calcium in families with hereditary nonpolyposis colorectal cancer, *J. Natl. Cancer Inst.*, 87, 598, 1995.

111. Kampman, E., Giovannucci, E., van't Veer, P., Rimm, E., Stampfer, M. J., Colditz, G. A., Kok, F. J., and Willett, W.W., Calcium, vitamin D, dairy foods, and the occurrence of colorectal adenomas among men and women in two prospective studies, *Am. J. Epidemiol.*, 139, 16, 1994.

112. Alberts, D.-S., Ritenbaugh, C., Story, J. A., Aickin, M., Rees-McGee, S., Buller, M. K., Atwood, J., Phelps, J., Ramanujam, P. S., Bellapravalu, S., Patel, J., Bettinger, L., and Clark, L., Randomized, double-blinded, placebo-controlled study of effect of wheat bran fiber and calcium on fecal bile acids in patients with resected adenomatous colon polyps, *J. Natl. Cancer Inst.*, 88, 81, 1996.

113. Lupton, J. R., Steinbach, G., Chang, W. C., O'Brien, B. C., Wiese, S., Stoltzfus, C. L., Glober, G. A., Wargovich, M. J., McPherson, R. S., and Winn, R. J., Calcium supplementation modifies the relative amounts of bile acids in bile and affects key aspects of human colon physiology, *J. Nutr.*, 126, 1421, 1996.

114. Danes, B. S., Effect of increased calcium concentration on *in vitro* growth of human colonic mucosal lines, *Dis. Colon Rectum*, 34, 552, 1991.

115. Danes, B. S., de Angelis, P., Traganos, F., and Melamed, M. R., Heritable colon cancer: influence of increased calcium concentration on increased in vitro tetraploidy (IVT), *Med. Hypotheses*, 36, 69, 1991.

116. Llor, X., Jacoby, R. F., Teng, B.-B., Davidson, N. O., Sitrin, M. D., and Brasitus, T. A., K-ras mutations in 1,2-dimethylhydrazine-induced colonic tumors: effects of supplemental dietary calcium and vitamin D deficiency, *Cancer Res.*, 51, 4305, 1991.

117. Rozen, P., Fireman, Z., Fine, N., Wax, Y., and Ron, E., Oral calcium suppresses increased rectal epithelial proliferation of persons at risk of colorectal cancer, *Gut*, 30, 650, 1989.

118. Lans, J. I., Jaszewski, R., Arlow, F. L., Tureaud, J., Luk, G. D., and Majumdar, A. P. N., Supplemental calcium suppresses colonic mucosal ornithine decarboxylase activity in elderly patients with adenomatous polyps, *Cancer Res.*, 51, 3416, 1991.

119. Yang, K., Cohen, L., and Lipkin, M., Lectin soybean agglutinin: measurements in colonic epithelial cells of human subjects following supplemental dietary calcium, *Cancer Lett.*, 56, 65, 1991.

120. Lupton, J. R., Dairy products and colon cancer: mechanisms of the protective effect, *Am. J. Clin. Nutr.*, 66, 1065, 1997.

121. Glinghammar, B., Venturi, M., Rowland, I. R., and Rafter, J. J., Shift from a dairy product-rich to a dairy product-free diet: influence on cytotoxicity and genotoxicity of fecal water - potential risk factors for colon cancer, *Am. J. Clin. Nutr.*, 66, 1277, 1997.

122. Baron, J. A. and Beach, M., et al., for the Calcium Polyp Prevention Study Group, Calcium supplements for the prevention of colorectal adenomas, *N. Engl. J. Med.*, 340, 101, 1999.

123. Young, T. B. and Wolf, D. A., Case-control study of proximal and distal colon cancer and diet in Wisconsin, *Int. J. Cancer*, 42, 167, 1988.

124. Goldin, B. R. and Gorbach, S. L., Effect of *Lactobacillus acidophilus* dietary supplements on 1,2-dimethylhydrazine dihydrochloride-induced intestinal cancer in rats, *J. Natl. Cancer Inst.*, 64, 263, 1980.

125. Goldin, B. R., Swenson, L., Dwyer, J., Sexton, M., and Gorbach, S. L., Effect of diet and *Lactobacillus acidophilus* supplements on human fecal bacterial enzymes, *J. Natl. Cancer Inst.*, 64, 255, 1980.

126. Goldin, B. R. and Gorbach, S. L., The effect of milk and *lactobacillus* feeding on human intestinal bacterial enzyme activity, *Am. J. Clin. Nutr.*, 39, 756, 1984.

127. Friend, B. A. and Shahani, K. M., Antitumour properties of *lactobacilli* and dairy products fermented by *lactobacilli*, *J. Food Protect.*, 47, 717, 1984.

128. Fernandes, C. F., and Shahani, K. M., Anticarcinogenic and immunological properties of dietary *Lactobacilli*, *J. Food Protection*, 53(8), 704, 1990.

129. Pool-Zobel, B. L., Neudecker, C., Domizlaff, S., Schillinger, U., Rumney, C., Moretti, M., Vilarini, I., Scassellati-Sforzolini, R., and Rowland, I., *Lactobacillus*- and *bifidobacterium*-mediated antigenotoxicity in the colon of rats, *Nutr. Cancer*, 26, 365, 1996.

130. Bodana, A. R. and Rao, D. R., Antimutagenic activity of milk fermented by *Streptococcus thermophilus* and *Lactobacillus bulgaricus*, *J. Dairy Sci.*, 73, 3379, 1990.

131. Takano, T., Arai, K., Murota, I., Hayakawa, K., Mitzutani, T., and Mitsuoka, T., Effects of feeding sour milk on longevity and tumourigenesis in mice and rats, *Bifidobact. Microflora*, 4, 31, 1985.

132. Goldin, B. R., Gualtieri, L. J., and Moore, R. P., The effect of *Lactobacillus GG* on the initiation and promotion of DMH-induced intestinal tumors in the rat, *Nutr. Cancer*, 25, 197, 1996.

133. Reddy, B. S. and Rivenson, A., Inhibitory effect of *Bifidobacterium longum* on colon, mammary, and liver carcinogenesis induced by 2-amino-3-methylimidazo [4,5-f] quinoline, a food mutagen, *Cancer Res.*, 53, 3914, 1993.

134. Singh, J., Rivenson, A., Tomita, M., Shimamura, S., Ishibashi, N., and Reddy, B. S., *Bifidobacterium longum*, a lactic acid-producing intestinal bacterium inhibits colon cancer and modulates the intermediate biomarkers of colon carcinogenesis, *Carcinogenesis*, 18, 833, 1997.

135. Abdelali, H., Cassand, P., Soussotte, V., Daubeze, M., Bouley, C., and Narbonne, J. F., Effect of dairy products on initiation of precursor lesions of colon cancer in rats, *Nutr. Cancer*, 24, 121, 1995.

136. Gallaher, D. D., Stallings, W. H., Blessing, L. L., Busta, F. F., and Brady, L. J., Probiotics, cecal microflora, and aberrant crypts in the rat colon, *J. Nutr.*, 126, 1362, 1996.

137. Ling, W. H., Korpela, R., Mykkanen, H., Salminen, S., and Hanninen, O., *Lactobacillus* strain *GG* supplementation decreases colonic hydrolytic and reductive enzyme activities in healthy female adults, *J. Nutr.*, 124, 18, 1994.

138. Belury, M. A., Conjugated dienoic linoleate: a polyunsaturated fatty acid with unique chemoprotective properties, *Nutr. Rev.*, 53, 83, 1995.

139. Ha, Y. L., Storkson, J., and Pariza, M. W., Inhibition of benzo(a) pyrene-induced mouse forestomach neoplasia by conjugated dienoic derivatives of linoleic acid, *Cancer Res.*, 50, 1097, 1990.

140. Shultz, T. D., Chew, B. P., Seaman, W. R., and Luedecke, L. O., Inhibitory effect of conjugated dienoic derivatives of linoleic acid and B-carotene on the in vitro growth of human cancer cells, *Cancer Lett.*, 63, 125, 1992.

141. Chin, S. F., Liu, W., Storkson, J. M., Ha, Y. L., and Pariza, M. W., Dietary sources of conjugated dienoic isomers of linoleic acid, a newly recognized class of anticarcinogens, *J. Food Composition & Analysis*, 5, 185, 1992.

142. Lin, H., Boylston, T. D., Chang, M. J., Luedecke, L. O., and Schultz, T. D., Survey of the conjugated linoleic acid contents of dairy products, *J. Dairy Sci.*, 78, 2358, 1995.

143. Ip, C. and Scimeca, J. A., Conjugated linoleic acid and linoleic acid are distinctive modulators of mammary carcinogenesis, *Nutr. & Cancer*, 27, 131, 1997.

144. Liew, C., Schut, H. A. J., Chin, S. F., Pariza, M. W., and Dashwood, R. H., Protection of conjugated linoleic acid against 2-amino-3-methylimidazo[4,5-f]quinoline-induced colon carcinogenesis in the F344 rat: a study of inhibitory mechanisms, *Carcinogenesis*, 16, 3037, 1995.

145. Van den Berg, J. J. M., Cook, N. E., and Tribble, D. L., Reinvestigation of the antioxidant properties of conjugated linoleic acid, *Lipids*, 30, 599, 1995.

146. Havek, M. G., Meydani, S. N., Han, S. N., Wu, D., Dorsey, J. L., Meydani, M., and Smith, D. E., The effect of conjugated linoleic acid (CLA) on the immune response of young and old mice, *FASEB J.*, February 28, A580, 1997.

147. Huang, Y.-C., Luedecke, L. O., and Shultz, T. D., Effect of cheddar cheese consumption on plasma conjugated linoleic acid concentrations in men, *Nutr. Res.*, 14, 373, 1994.

148. Dillehay, D. L., Webb, S. K., Schmelz, E.-M., and Merrill, A. H., Jr., Dietary sphingomyelin inhibits 1,2-dimethylhydrazine-induced colon cancer in CF1 mice, *J. Nutr.*, 124, 615, 1994.

149. Merrill, A. H., Jr., Schmelz, E.-M., Wang, E., Schroeder, J. J., Dillehay, D. L., and Riley, R. T., Role of dietary sphingolipids and inhibitors of sphingolipid metabolism in cancer and other diseases, *J. Nutr.*, 125(Suppl.), 1677, 1995.

150. Merrill, A. H., Jr., Schmelz, E.-M., Wang, E., Dillehay, D. L., Rice, L. G., Meredith, F., and Riley, R. T., Importance of sphingolipids and inhibitors of sphingolipid metabolism as components of animal diets, *J. Nutr.*, 127(Suppl.), 830, 1997.

151. Merrill, A. H., Jr., Hannun, Y. A., and Bell, R. M., Sphingolipids and their metabolites in cell regulation, *Adv. Lipid Res.*, 25, 1, 1993.
152. Hannun, Y. A., Loomis, C. R., Merrill, A. H., Jr., and Bell, R. M., Sphingosine inhibition of protein kinase C activity and of phorbol bibutyrate binding in vitro and in human platelets, *J. Biol. Chem.*, 261, 12604, 1986.
153. Borek, C., Ong, A., Stevens, V. L., Wang, E., and Merrill, A. H., Jr., Long-chain (sphingoid) bases inhibit multistage carcinogenesis in mouse C3H/10T1/2 cells treated with radiation and phorbol 12-myristate-13-acetate, *Proc. Natl. Acad. Sci. U.S.A.*, 88, 1953, 1991.
154. Schmelz, E.-M., Crall, K. J., Larocque, R., Dillehay, D. L., and Merrill, A. H., Jr., Update and metabolism of sphingolipids in isolated intestinal loops of mice, *J. Nutr.*, 124, 702, 1994.
155. Schmelz, E. M., Dillehay, D. L., Webb, S. K., Reiter, A., Adams, J., and Merrill, A. H., Jr., Sphingomyelin consumption suppresses aberrant colonic crypt foci and increases the proportion of adenomas versus adenocarcinomas in CF1 mice treated with 1,2-dimethylhydrazine: implications for dietary sphingolipids and colon carcinogenesis, *Cancer Res.*, 56, 4936, 1996.
156. Schmelz, E. M., Bushnev, A. S., Dillehay, D. L., Liotta, D. C., and Merrill, A. H., Jr., Suppression of aberrant colonic crypt foci by synthetic sphingomyelins with saturated or unsaturated sphingoid base backbones, *Nutr. Cancer*, 28, 81, 1997.
157. Gosh, T. K., Bian, J., and Gill, D. L., Intracellular calcium release mediated by sphingosine derivatives generated in cells, *Science*, 248, 1653, 1990.
158. Okazaki, T., Bielawska, A., Bell, R. M., and Hannun, Y. A., Role of ceramide as a lipid mediator of 1-alpha, 25-dihydroxyvitamin D_3-induced HL-60 cell differentiation, *J. Biol. Chem.*, 265, 15823, 1990.
159. Smith, J. G. and German, J. B., Molecular and genetic effects of dietary derived butyric acid, *Food Technol.*, 49, 87, 1995.
160. Chen, Z. and Breitman, T., Tributyrin: a prodrug of butyric acid for potential clinical application in differentiation therapy, *Cancer Res.*, 54, 3494, 1994.
161. Pouillart, P., Cerutti, G., Ronco, G., Villa, P., and Chany C., Enhancement by stable butyrate derivatives of antitumor and antiviral actions of interferon, *Int. J. Cancer*, 51, 596, 1992.
162. Hague, A., Manning, A. M., Hanlon, K. A., Huschtscha, L. I., Hart, D., and Paraskeva, C., Sodium butyrate induces apoptosis in human colonic cell lines in a p53-independent pathway. Implications for the possible role of dietary fibre in the prevention of large bowel cancer, *Int. J. Cancer*, 55, 498, 1993.
163. Hague, A. and Paraskeva, C., This short-chain fatty acid butyrate induces apoptosis in colorectal tumor cell lines, *Eur. J. Cancer Prev.*, 4, 359, 1995.
164. Lupton, J. R., Butyrate and colonic cytokinetics: differences between *in vitro* and *in vivo* studies, *Eur. J. Cancer Prev.*, 4, 373, 1995.
165. Boffa, L. C., Lupton, J. R., Mariani, M. R., Ceppi, M., Newmark, H. L., Scalmati, A., and Lipkin, M., Modulation of colonic epithelial cell proliferation, histone acetylation, and luminal short chain fatty acids by variation of dietary fiber (wheat bran) in rats, *Cancer Res.*, 52, 5906, 1992.
166. Aukema, H. M., Davidson, L. A., Pence, B. C., Jiang, Y.-H., Lupton, J. R., and Chapkin, R. S., Butyrate alters activity of specific cAMP-receptor proteins in a transgenic mouse colonic cell line, *J. Nutr.*, 127, 18, 1997.
167. McIntyre, A., Gibson, P. R., and Young, G. P., Butyrate production from dietary fibre and protection against large bowel cancer in a rat model, *Gut*, 34, 386, 1993.

168. McIntosh, G. H., Regester, G. O., LeLeu, R. K., Royle, P. J., and Smithers, G. W., Dietary proteins protect against dimethylhydrazine-induced intestinal cancers in rats, *J. Nutr.*, 125, 809, 1995.

169. MacDonald, R. S., Thorton, W. H., Jr., and Marshall, R. T., A cell culture model to identify biologically active peptides generated by bacterial hydrolysis of casein, *J. Dairy Sci.*, 77, 1167, 1994.

170. Goeptar, A. R., Koeman, J. H., Van Boekel, M. A. J. S., and Alink, G. M., Impact of digestion on the antimutagenic activity of the milk protein casein, *Nutr. Res.*, 17, 1363, 1997.

171. The American Cancer Society 1996 Dietary Guidelines Advisory Committee, *Guidelines on Diet, Nutrition, and Cancer Prevention: Reducing the Risk of Cancer with Healthy Food Choices and Physical Activity*, American Cancer Society, Atlanta, GA, 1996.

172. National Institutes of Health, *Optimal Calcium Intake*, NIH Consensus Statement 12, 4, NIH, Bethesda, MD, 1994.

173. U.S. Department of Agriculture, Agricultural Research Service, *Data tables: Results from USDA's 1994–1996 Continuing Survey of Food Intakes by Individuals and 1996 Diet and Health Knowledge Survey*, ARS, Food Surveys Research Group. December, www.barc.usda.gov/bhnrc/foodsurvey/home.htm, 1997.

174. Knekt, P., Jarvinen, R., Seppanen, R., Pukkala, E., and Aromaa, A., Intake of dairy products and the risk of breast cancer, *Br. J. Cancer*, 73, 687, 1996.

175. Jarvinen, R., Knekt, P., Seppanen, R., and Teppo, L., Diet and breast cancer in a cohort of Finnish women, *Cancer Lett.*, 114, 251, 1997.

176. Xue, L., Newmark, H., Yang, K., and Lipkin, M., Model of mouse mammary gland hyperproliferation and hyperplasia induced by a Western-style diet, *Nutr. Cancer*, 26, 281, 1996.

CHAPTER 5

Dairy Foods and Osteoporosis

I. INTRODUCTION

Osteoporosis ("porous bones") is defined as "a metabolic bone disease characterized by low bone mass and microarchitectural deterioration of bone tissue leading
to enhanced bone fragility and a consequent increase in fracture risk."[1] Often called
a silent disease, osteoporosis develops gradually over many years before the occurrence of clinical symptoms such as loss of height, curvature of the spine, and
fractures, especially of the spine, hip, and wrist.[1] For many individuals, a skeletal
fracture is the first indication of osteoporosis.[1,2]

Osteoporosis is a major public health problem in the U.S., affecting 28 million
people, mostly women.[1,3] This disease is responsible for more than 1.5 million new
fractures a year, including more than 700,000 spine, 300,000 hip, 250,000 wrist
fractures, and 250,000 fractures at other sites.[1,4] Among older Caucasian women,
osteoporosis accounts for at least 90% of all hip and spine fractures.[5] Hip fracture,
the most devastating manifestation of osteoporosis, is associated with 12 to 20%
mortality.[1,2] Moreover, many older patients with osteoporotic hip fractures fail to
regain their former mobility. A woman's risk of developing a hip fracture is equal
to her combined risk of breast, uterine, and ovarian cancer.[4]

In addition to the considerable morbidity, mortality, loss of independence, and
decreased quality of life associated with osteoporosis, the economic burden of this
disease in the U.S. is staggering, amounting to an estimated $13.8 billion in 1995.[1,6]
Because osteoporosis increases with age and the proportion of the U.S. population
aged 65 years and older is escalating, this disease can be expected to impose an
even greater burden on health care expenditures and medical resources in coming
years.[1,7] By the year 2030, the cost of osteoporosis is expected to exceed $60 billion.[1]
Prevention is considered the only cost-effective approach to osteoporosis. Further,
prevention is critical considering the inability of current interventions to restore bone
once it is lost.[1]

The cause(s) of osteoporosis, similar to other chronic diseases, is multifactorial,
involving both genetic and environmental factors.[8-16] Lifestyle factors have received

considerable attention in recent years, especially since they can be manipulated. Because more than 99% of the total calcium content of the body is found in the skeleton, it is not surprising that considerable interest lies in the role of calcium and vitamin D (which enhances calcium absorption) in bone health.

Accumulating scientific evidence indicates that a sufficient intake of calcium throughout life protects against osteoporosis by achieving genetically programmed peak bone mass reached by 30 years of age or earlier and reducing postmenopausal and age-related bone loss.[17-19] The Food and Drug Administration (FDA), in response to provisions of the Nutrition Labeling and Education Act of 1990, has authorized the use of health claims relating to an association between calcium intake and osteoporosis on the labels of foods.[20] The FDA has concluded that a lifetime of "adequate calcium intake is important for maintenance of bone health and may help reduce the risk of osteoporosis particularly for individuals at greatest risk."[20] This food labeling health claim is supported by research compiled by the Life Sciences Research Office of FASEB.[21]

Dairy foods are the major source of calcium in the U.S. food supply, providing 73% of the calcium available in 1994 (Figure 5.1).[22] Vitamin D-fortified milk also is an important source of vitamin D for many people.[17,23] While optional, nearly all fluid milk marketed in the U.S. is fortified with vitamin D to obtain the standardized amount of 400 IU (10 μg) per quart of milk.[23] Incidences of over- or under-fortification of milk with vitamin D in the early 1990s [24] have led to more careful monitoring of the vitamin D content of milk, enforcement of the upper limit of vitamin D added to milk, and education efforts to better assure accurate fortification of milk.[25] The acceptable range allowed for vitamin D fortification of milk is not less than 100% and not more than 150% of label claims (i.e., 400 to 600 IU vitamin D).[25]

This chapter reviews recent studies confirming and extending previous research findings supporting the role of dairy foods or dairy food nutrients (i.e., calcium, vitamin D, etc.) in increasing peak bone mass and slowing age-related bone loss. It is important to appreciate that nutrition, particularly calcium and vitamin D, are among several factors influencing both optimal bone health and the development of osteoporosis.[17,21] Accumulating scientific evidence indicates that increasing calcium and/or vitamin D intake has a beneficial impact on bone health.[17-19] Recognizing the important role of these nutrients in bone health, the National Academy of Sciences (NAS)[17] recently raised the recommended calcium and vitamin D intakes for most age groups from the previous Recommended Dietary Allowances (RDAs).[26] It is difficult to obtain adequate intakes of these nutrients without consuming dairy products.[1,18,19,27] If calcium-rich foods such as dairy products are excluded, the usual American diet provides only about 200 to 300 mg calcium a day, an amount far less than the NAS recommendation of 1000 to 1200 mg per day (Table 5.1) for most adults. The NAS[17] presented its new calcium recommendations in terms of Adequate Intakes (AIs), not RDAs. The AI is provided instead of an RDA when sufficient scientific evidence is not available to determine an RDA. "If one were to estimate an RDA from the published AI figures, the RDA value would be about 20% higher than the AI," states Robert Heaney, M.D. (personal communication). Compared with

■ **Whole Milk**   ▒ **Lowfat Milk**   □ **Cheese**   ▨ **Other Dairy**   □ **Other**

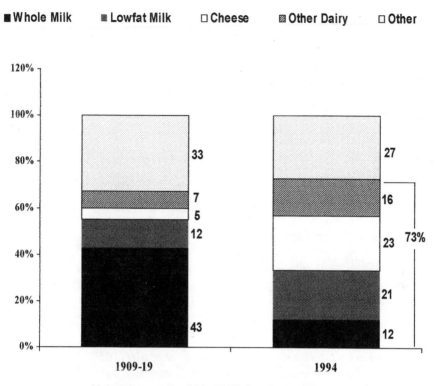

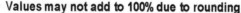

Values may not add to 100% due to rounding

Figure 5.1   Sources of calcium in the U.S. food supply. (Adapted from Gerrior, S. and Bente, L., USDA Center for Nutrition Policy Nutrient Content of the U.S. Food Supply 1909-94. Home Economics Research Project No. 53, 1997. With permission.)

this estimated RDA, a diet containing only 200 to 300 mg calcium/day would be even more limiting in this nutrient.

II. BONE BASICS

The skeleton is composed of two types of bone: cortical bone, or the dense compact outer layer of bone which is the predominant bone in the shafts of long bones, and trabecular (cancellous) bone which is the porous honeycomb-like structure in the interior of bones, especially in the vertebra and at the ends of all long bones.[1] About 80% of the adult skeleton is cortical (compact) bone, with the remaining 20% trabecular bone. However, the relative proportions of these two types of bone vary from one bone to another.

Throughout life, bone is constantly remodeled, a process important for self-repair of skeletal tissue.[1,28] Bone remodeling is a complex, highly ordered sequence of cellular events starting with activation of a quiescent bone surface, then a resorption phase whereby old bone is removed by osteoclasts, and finally bone formation and

Table 5.1   Recommended Calcium Intakes

Recommended Calcium Intakes (mg/day)			
NAS[1]		NIH[2]	
Ages			
Birth – 6 months	210	Birth – 6 months	400
6 months – 1 year	270	6 months – 1 year	600
1 – 3	500	1 – 10	800 – 1200
4 – 8	800	11 – 24	200 – 1500
9 – 13	1300	25 – 50	1000
14 – 18	1300	(women & men)	
19 – 30	1000	51 – 64	1000
31 – 50	1000	(women on ERT & men)	
51 - 70	1200	51 +	1400
70 or older	1200	(women not on ERT)	
		65 or older	1500
Pregnant or lactating	1000		
14 – 18	1300		
19 – 50	1000		

[1] National Academy of Sciences, 1997   [2] National Institutes of Health, 1994

From National Academy of Sciences, 1997; National Institutes of Health, 1994.

mineralization by osteoblasts.[2] At any one time, about 10 to 15% of bone surfaces are undergoing remodeling.[29] A number of interrelated hormonal, nutritional, mechanical, and genetic factors influence the bone remodeling rate and variance in bone mass.[1,28] For example, whenever dietary calcium is insufficient to meet adults' needs, the resorption component of bone remodeling exceeds the amount of new bone formed and increased amounts of calcium are drawn from bones to maintain a relatively constant concentration in the blood.[29]

Bone mass increases during infancy, childhood, and adolescence.[28] However, it does not stop when longitudinal growth or adult height is achieved. It generally is accepted that following completion of longitudinal growth, consolidation of bone density continues until peak bone mass is reached between 20 and 30 years of age,[1] or earlier.[30,31] Bone mass influences susceptibility to osteoporotic fractures.[28] Calcium increases in bone from about 25 g at birth to 900 to 1300 g at maturity paralleling the increase in bone mass (Table 5.2).[2] At menopause (i.e., between ages 45 and 55), bone loss accelerates (i.e., average of 3% a year) in women and remains elevated for about five years before slowing down to a rate similar to that of aging men. The sharp decline in estrogen production at menopause is responsible for the rapid loss of bone after menopause.[1,17] In men, bone loss generally occurs after age 50 but is not as rapid nor as great as women's.[1] Women's relatively lower peak bone mass and increased bone loss following menopause are a part of the reason why osteoporosis is more common in women than in men.[2] After age 65, women and men tend to lose bone at a similar rate. Decreases in hormones (e.g., testosterone, estrogen) likely contribute to reduced bone mass and increased fracture risk in men.[1,32]

Table 5.2   Skeletal Calcium Retention
             During Early Life

Age (Years)	Skeletal Calcium (g)	Retention (mg/day)
0	25	440
10	400	200
13	800 – 1100	400
17	800 – 1100	80
35	900 – 1300	15

From Christiansen, C., *J. Bone Min. Res.*, 8, Suppl. 2, S475, 1993. With permission.

Age-related bone loss in both sexes involves the gradual thinning of both cortex and trabeculae. The accelerated loss of bone postmenopausally is thought to be mediated mainly by osteoclasts. A gradual loss of cortical bone occurs with age and increases in women after menopause. The magnitude of peak bone mass and the rate and duration of postmenopausal and age-associated bone loss determine the likelihood of developing osteoporosis.[1] When bone mass is low, less trauma is necessary to cause a fracture. Although some age-related bone loss may be inevitable, osteoporosis is not a natural event. Throughout life, from early childhood through later adults years, measures can be taken to promote bone health.[1] For example, an adequate intake of calcium benefits bones at all ages.[1,33]

III. RISK FACTORS FOR OSTEOPOROSIS

A number of risk factors for osteoporosis have been identified (Table 5.3).[1,11,17] Both genetics and environmental, or lifestyle, factors influence the likelihood of developing this disease.[8-16] Genetics influence peak bone mass, skeletal structure, and metabolic activity.[34] Although multiple genes are likely involved, recent interest has focused on a vitamin D receptor (VDR) gene.[12-15] VDR gene polymorphisms may influence bone size; however, the VDR gene is responsible for only a small proportion of the population-level variation in bone mass.[12,15] Genetics and environmental factors interact in important ways on bone health. If heredity influences the efficiency of scarce nutrients such as calcium or vitamin D requirements, at marginal intakes of these nutrients there will be a "hereditary" difference in bone mass. However, when intakes of calcium and vitamin D are adequate, "hereditary" differences in bone mass will no longer be present.

Gender, ethnicity, age, hormonal status, and body frame/weight are other factors that influence bone mass and the development of osteoporosis.[1,17] Women, because of their generally smaller, lighter bones, rapid loss of bone at menopause, and lower calcium intake, are about four times more likely to develop osteoporosis than are men.[1] Caucasians, particularly those of northern European ancestry, and Asians of Japanese and Chinese descent are at significantly higher risk of developing osteoporosis than Hispanic women or African American women who generally have larger body frames. Although they are at lower risk, Hispanic and African American

Table 5.3   Risk Factors for Osteoporosis

Family History	If a family member has had osteoporosis, other members may be at risk
Gender	Osteoporosis is more common in women than in men
Ethnicity	Caucasian (white) and Asian women are most susceptible; Hispanic and African American women are also at significant risk
Age	Osteoporosis is found mostly in older adults
Hormonal Status	Estrogen deficiency at menopause or earlier (before age 45 years) in women, and hormonal reductions in men increase risk
Body Frame/Weight	A thin, small-boned frame increases risk of osteoporosis
Diet	A diet chronically low in calcium and vitamin D (if exposure to direct sunlight is limited) increases risk
Exercise	Lack of regular physical activity can reduce bone mass and in older adults also reduce muscle strength
Cigarette Smoking	Smoking is linked to increased risk
Alcohol	Excess alcohol intake increases risk
Medications	Certain medications such as glucocorticoids used to treat asthma or arthritis can increase risk

women are still at significant risk of developing osteoporosis.[1] According to data from NHANES III (1988–1994), the prevalence of osteoporosis of the total hip is higher among Caucasian women (21%) than among either Hispanic (16%) or African-American women (10%).[3] The risk of osteoporosis also increases with advancing age in both men and women, and with the loss of estrogen at menopause (either natural or surgical).[5,17] There is a linear decrease in calcium absorption efficiency from at least age 40, amounting to about 0.2% per year, with an additional 2.2% lost across menopause.[35] Between the ages of 40 and 60 years, the combination of increasing age and estrogen withdrawal reduces calcium absorption efficiency by 20 to 25%.[36] Age-related decreases in estrogen in women and testosterone and estrogen in men contribute to increased risk of osteoporosis in later years.[32,37] Young women with amenorrhea resulting from anorexia nervosa or excessive exercise are at high risk for osteoporosis.[1,38] Thin, small framed women or men are at greater risk of osteoporotic fractures than large-boned individuals. Also, following weight loss diets may increase the risk of osteoporotic fractures.[39] A recent investigation involving postmenopausal women found that increasing calcium intake by 1000 mg a day prevented the increase in bone turnover induced by a 10% loss in body weight.[39] In obese individuals, fracture risk is reduced.[1] Diseases, surgery, and some medications (e.g., corticosteroids, anticonvulsants, aluminum-containing antacids) also increase risk of osteoporosis.[1,2]

An individual's lifestyle may account for a substantial proportion of the variance in bone density and, in turn, fracture risk.[17,38,40] Lifestyle factors that increase risk of osteoporosis include cigarette smoking, excess alcohol intake, physical inactivity, and some dietary intakes, especially an inadequate intake of calcium. Although caffeine was once thought to adversely affect calcium status, new research indicates that it has a negligible effect on calcium metabolism, calcium status, or bone density.[41-43] Caffeine can induce an initial short-term increase in urinary calcium excretion, but there is no effect on integrated 24-hour calcium excretion.[42] A single cup of brewed coffee (i.e, 6 fluid ounces) causes a deterioration in calcium balance by about 4 mg/day, mainly by reducing calcium absorption.[42] However, this amount is readily offset by consuming one or two tablespoons of milk [42]

Cigarette smoking is associated with decreased bone density and increased risk of bone fractures.[44-46] Based on a cross-sectional study of 41 pairs of female twins with differing smoking habits, it was estimated that women who smoke one pack of cigarettes a day throughout their adult years will lose 5 to 10% of their bone density by the time they reach menopause.[44] A recent meta-analysis of 29 published cross-sectional studies linked smoking with a 50% greater risk of hip fractures.[46] In elderly Japanese-American men, risk of fractures of the distal radius increased 10 to 30% per decade of smoking.[45] Smoking may reduce calcium absorption or have a direct adverse effect on bone.[45,46] Bone loss associated with smoking can be reduced by cessation of smoking, even later in life.[47]

Excess alcohol intake is an important risk factor for osteoporosis.[38,48] Alcohol may damage bones directly and/or contribute to osteoporosis by its indirect effect on intake of calcium and other nutrients, liver damage, and/or by increasing predisposition to falls. With respect to physical activity, a sedentary lifestyle favors bone loss, whereas weight-bearing activities as well as regular moderate activities such as walking, increase bone mass.[17,49-52] Increased physical activity and adequate calcium intake have been demonstrated to increase bone density and decrease bone loss at various skeletal sites.[51,52] A review of 16 trials found that physical activity exerted beneficial effects on bone mineral density at the lumbar spine at high calcium intakes (i.e., >1000 mg/day), but not at calcium intakes less than 1000 mg/day.[51]

As reviewed below, low calcium intake increases the risk of osteoporosis. In addition, other nutrients or dietary components can influence risk of osteoporosis by their effect on the body's need for calcium. A high intake of sodium increases urinary calcium excretion.[17,38] In postmenopausal women, each 500 mg of sodium consumed increases urinary calcium excretion by about 10 mg.[17,38] According to a study by Matkovic et al.,[53] sodium intake was the main determinant of urinary calcium loss in adolescent girls aged 8 to 13 years, a finding leading the researchers to suggest a potential adverse effect on bone mass. In postmenopausal women, high urinary sodium excretion, which is a measure of sodium intake, was associated with increased bone loss from the hip and ankle.[54]

Similar to sodium, dietary protein (particularly purified proteins) increases urinary calcium excretion.[17,38,55-57] In metabolic studies, doubling protein intake increases urinary calcium excretion by 50%.[55] However, when protein is fed as foods such as dairy foods, there is little evidence that calcium balance is adversely affected.[58-60] An effect of protein on bone, if it exists, is likely to be small.

The presence of other components such as calcium, phosphorus, and potassium in protein-rich foods such as dairy foods appears to counterbalance or modify the calciuretic action of protein.[55,56,59,60] An adequate intake of calcium offsets calcium loss due to urinary excretion.[55] A recent investigation involving prepubescent girls found that increasing milk protein from 12 to 19 grams a day had no significant effect on urinary calcium excretion.[60] The body can adapt to protein-induced urinary calcium loss by absorbing more calcium. The actual amount of calcium absorbed depends on calcium intake. Therefore, it is useful to evaluate diets not on their protein intake per se, but on their calcium-to-protein ratios. A "good" calcium-to-protein ratio, or one that provides adequate protection for the skeleton, is 20:1 (mg:g) or higher.[58,59] Excess protein will not harm bone health if calcium intake is adequate. The calcium to protein ratio of cow's milk is approximately 36.

Dietary protein has many positive effects on bone.[59] Because of its content of essential amino acids, protein contributes to the building of new bone matrix. Also, food sources of protein provide other important bone-building nutrients such as calcium and zinc. For older adults, a group at high risk of osteoporosis, increasing protein intake can help prevent muscle atrophy which leads to falls, as well as reduce bone loss.[58,61] Increasing the protein intake (by 20 grams/day for six months) of older adults who experienced a recent osteoporotic hip fracture, reduced the loss of proximal femur bone and the patients' stay in a rehabilitation hospital, as well as raised their blood levels of insulin-like growth factor.[61] The higher calcium recommendations for the U.S. than for other less industrialized countries may be explained in part by Americans' typically higher protein and sodium intakes.[38,55]

Oxalate, found in spinach, inhibits the absorption of calcium from this food.[62] Only about 5% of the calcium in spinach is absorbed compared to about 30% of the calcium in milk.[62] In contrast, low oxalate vegetables (e.g., kale) have excellent calcium absorption. If consumed in large amounts, wheat bran can inhibit the absorption of coingested calcium.[63,64] However, at usual intakes of fiber (5 to 15 g/day), wheat bran's effect on calcium absorption is relatively small.[63] Phytate in wheat bran and together with oxalate in other foods such as beans (pinto, red, white) decreases the intestinal absorption of calcium from these foods. An individual would need to consume nearly 10 servings of red beans and 16 servings of spinach to obtain the same amount of absorbable calcium as in one cup of milk.[65]

IV. CALCIUM IMPORTANT AT EVERY AGE

A. Dietary Calcium Recommendations

The National Academy of Sciences (NAS), Institute of Medicine has issued new recommended intakes for calcium and related nutrients.[17] The NAS calcium recommendations, expressed as Adequate Intakes (AIs), reflect current scientific information.[17] The new recommendations are now more in line with calcium recommendations issued in 1994 by an advisory group on Optimal Calcium Intake for the National Institutes of Health (NIH)[18] (Table 5.1), and supported by the American Medical Association.[19]

For children and most adults, the NAS calcium recommendations are based on intakes consistent with desirable calcium retention, randomized clinical trials, and a factorial approach.[17] Desirable calcium retention is associated with increased bone mass and reduced risk of osteoporosis. Higher calcium intakes are recommended for many life-stage groups. For children (9 through 13) and adolescents (14 through 18), 1300 mg/day of calcium is recommended,[17] an amount higher than the 1989 RDA[26] of 800 mg/day for 7 through 10 years olds and 1200 mg/day for 11 through 18 year olds. These higher calcium recommendations coincide with peak calcium accretion rates in bone which occur at a mean age of 13 years for girls and 14.5 years for boys.[66]

For adults aged 19 through 50 years, 1000 mg/day of calcium is recommended, an amount higher than the previous recommendation of 800 mg/day for adults aged 25 to 50 years but lower for individuals 19 to 24 years.[17,26] For both men and women over age 50, 1200 mg calcium/day is recommended, or 400 mg/day more than previously recommended.[17,26] The age-related decline in calcium absorption, among other factors, supports the higher calcium recommendations for this age group.[17] Calcium recommendations are the same for pregnant/lactating females as for their nonpregnant/nonlactating counterparts because of adaptive changes in calcium homeostasis during pregnancy and lactation.[17]

B. Calcium Intake

Unfortunately, at a time when calcium recommendations are increased, many Americans fail to consume enough calcium to meet even the lower calcium recommendations (i.e., 1989 RDAs). A variety of surveys including Phase I of the Third National Health and Nutrition Examination Survey (NHANES III) (1988–91),[67] the Nationwide Food Consumption Survey,[68] the Continuing Survey of Food Intakes by Individuals (CSFII) 1994–96,[69] the Food and Drug Administration Total Diet Study,[70] and others[71-73] are fairly consistent in their calcium intake findings. In general, females (especially adolescents and older women) and older adults consume less calcium than recommended for this mineral. At all ages, males consume more calcium than females, partly because of males' higher energy intake (Figure 5.2). According to NHANES III, 1988–91,[67] the median daily calcium intake for all females in the U.S. is 652 mg/day, whereas for males it is 856 mg/day. This survey indicates that the following groups in particular consume low intakes of calcium: all adolescents except non-Hispanic white males, all females ages 12 and older, non-Hispanic black males 12 and older, and all males 60 years and older.[67] Non-Hispanic white males are more likely to meet their calcium recommendations than any other group. Among the ethnic groups, non-Hispanic blacks, both males and females, have lower calcium intakes than either non-Hispanic whites or Mexican Americans.[67] According to FDA's 1982–1991 Total Diet Study,[70] females 14 to 16 years, 25 to 30 years, and 60 to 65 years of age consumed, on average, only 61%, 72%, and 64%, respectively, of their recommended intake (1989 RDA) for calcium. A recent analysis on nutrient intakes concluded that even adequate *average* nutrient intakes can mask a significant prevalence of calcium deficiencies.[27] For example, although U.S. teenage males' average calcium intake in 1994 ranged from 95 to 114% of the 1989 RDA for calcium,[26] 31 to 46% of the males consumed less than 75% of the recommendation for calcium.[27]

Data from the 1994–96 CSFII (Figure 5.2) indicate that only 12% of females ages 12 to 19 and 32% of similar aged males are meeting 100% of the current recommendation (AI) of 1300 mg calcium per day.[69] This same survey indicates that only 16% of women ages 20 to 29 years, 14% of women ages 30 to 39 years, and 11.5% of women 40 to 49 years are meeting 100% of the AI of 1000 mg per day.[69] Although fewer than 15% of older adults are consuming 100% of the AI of 1000 mg per day, CSFII results indicate that more men are meeting the calcium recommendations. Approximately 15% of males ages 50 to 59, 13% of males ages 60 to

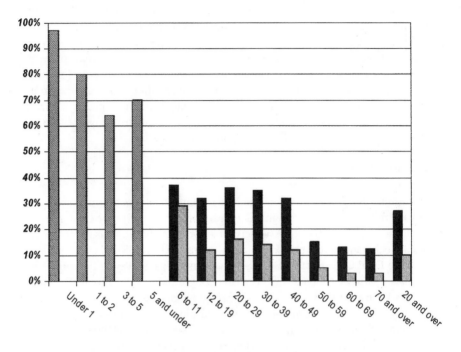

☒ Males and Females ■ Males ☐ Females

Figure 5.2 Calcium Intake % of AI (From USDA Continuing Survey of Food Intakes by Individuals, 1994–96. Personal Communication, 1998. With permission.)

69, and 13% of males over age 70 consume 100% of the calcium recommendations.[69] In contrast, only 5% of women ages 50 to 59, 4% of women ages 60 to 69, and 4% of women ages 70 and older consume 100% of the calcium recommendation.[69]

Low intake of dairy foods, which are the major source of calcium in the food supply,[22] contributes to low calcium intake.[27,72,74] While possible, it is improbable that adequate calcium intake will be obtained without including dairy foods in the diet.[27,74] According to an analysis of calcium consumption and food sources of calcium in the U.S., milk and milk products provided 83% of the calcium in the diets of young children, 77% of the calcium in adolescent females' diets, and between 65% and 72% of the calcium in the diets of adults.[75] In an investigation involving approximately 800 high school students, 79% of the students' calcium intake came from milk and other dairy foods (i.e., cheese, cottage cheese, yogurt, frozen yogurt, ice cream).[76] In this study, median calcium intake was 1016 mg/day for boys and 676 mg/day for girls. More girls (77.5%) than boys (61.0%) failed to meet 1200 mg/day of calcium recommended for adolescents (i.e., 1989 RDA).[76]

Several surveys indicate that female adolescents in particular consume low intakes of milk and/or other dairy foods.[69,72,77] In one study, women whose diets met their recommendations for calcium consumed more than three times as much lowfat milk as other women and more than six times as much fat-free milk.[74] Women who failed to meet their calcium recommendations consumed less milk and milk products and more sodas than women whose diets met their calcium recommendations.[74] A recent survey[78] conducted by the U.S. Department of Agriculture (USDA) found that the average American diet comes up short in servings from the Milk Group compared with USDA's *Food Guide Pyramid*.[79] Overall, Americans are consuming only an average of 1.5 servings per day from the Milk Group. According to USDA's *Healthy Eating Index 1994–96*,[80] fewer people consumed the recommended number of servings of dairy foods in 1996 than in 1989. In 1996, only 26% of people ate the recommended number of servings of milk products.[80]

The gap between intake and recommended servings of milk and other dairy foods may be even wider considering the increase in the number of servings of dairy foods being recommended.[81,82] Recognizing the higher calcium intakes recommended by the National Institutes of Health,[18] a recent American Academy of Pediatrics' publication[81] advises adolescents to consume five daily servings/day of milk and other dairy foods.[81] The American Heart Association recommends three to four servings of milk and other dairy foods a day.[82]

Numerous factors, physiological and sociodemographic, as well as lifestyle choices, knowledge, and attitudes influence intake of milk and milk products. Among these factors are:

- Taste. According to a study of social and demographic variables affecting adolescents' intake of milk and milk products, those who enjoyed the taste consumed these foods more often and consequently were more likely to have a higher intake of calcium.[76] A study of young and older women in New Zealand also identified taste as the most important factor influencing intake of milk and milk products.[83]
- Fat and Weight Concerns. The misperception that milk is fattening coupled with strong societal pressures to be thin prevents many adolescent and adult females from consuming calcium-rich milk and milk products.[83,84] However, recent research indicates that young females and adults can increase their calcium intake to recommended levels with milk and dairy foods without excessive fat or calorie intake, weight gain, or adversely affecting blood lipids.[85-90]
- Lactose Maldigestion. Low calcium intake may occur in some people who have lactose maldigestion or believe that they are lactose intolerant.[91] A recent study in Finland involving more than 11,000 women links self-reported lactose intolerance with both lower intakes of calcium from dairy foods (570 mg/day vs. 850 mg/day) and increased risk of fractures.[91] New research indicates that many individuals who are lactose maldigesters can consume the amount of lactose in one or two cups of milk, especially in divided doses with meals, without developing symptoms (see Chapter 8 on Lactose Intolerance).[92-94]
- Knowledge and Awareness. Many people do not know how much calcium they need and many mistakenly believe that they are consuming an adequate intake of calcium.[84] Data from the CSFII 1994-96 found that 51% of women ages 20 and older perceive their calcium intake to be "about right" even though many are failing to meet current recommendations for this nutrient.[69] Lack of awareness of the protective effect of calcium on bone health may also contribute to low calcium intakes.[95,96] In a recent study involving 472 women aged 50 years and over, those who knew that calcium protects bone health consumed more calcium than women who were unaware of this association.[95] Similar findings were observed in an investigation involving 1117 adolescents in Rhode Island.[96] In this study, adolescents who were knowledgeable

about their recommended intake of calcium, the beneficial effect of calcium on bone health, and the importance of adolescence as a time to build bone mass consumed more calcium than adolescents who were unaware of these facts.[96] Overall, only 10% of the adolescents knew the calcium content of various dairy foods and only 19% knew that they should consume four servings of dairy foods a day.[96]

- Other. Other factors such as image, family influence, and eating away from home can influence intake of dairy foods, and hence calcium intake. Adolescents in particular are more likely to consume milk if their friends and family drink this beverage.[76] If mothers drink milk, their daughters are also likely to consume milk throughout their lives.[97] Eating more meals in restaurants also may contribute to decreased milk intake because milk is consumed more often at home.[74,98] Also, a variety of milks, including lowfat, is usually not available on restaurant menus.

C. Prevention of Osteoporosis

There is general agreement that optimizing peak bone mass and reducing age-related bone loss later in life, especially after menopause, protects the skeleton and reduces fracture risk.[17-19,21,38] Variations in calcium status early in life may account for a 5 to 10% difference in peak bone mass which in turn contributes to more than a 50% difference in rates of hip fractures later in life.[28] Reviewed later are studies indicating that consuming an adequate intake of calcium throughout life, from periods of skeletal accumulation to maturity and beyond, protects against osteoporosis. The bulk of evidence supports the hypothesis that consuming an adequate intake of calcium is more protective of bone than a lower one. However, some studies fail to demonstrate a positive association between calcium intake and bone health. As reviewed by Heaney,[38] reasons for such inconsistencies include the following:

- The multifactorial nature of bone strength. As mentioned previously, many factors (e.g., hormonal status, physical activity, smoking, medications) in addition to calcium intake influence bone health. Manipulating a single variable such as calcium may be ineffective if calcium is not the limiting factor.[1,21,99] For example, a high calcium intake alone cannot protect against bone loss caused by estrogen deficiency or physical inactivity.[38]
- The multifactorial nature of calcium deficiency. In addition to calcium intake, calcium absorption and excretion also contribute to calcium status.[21,99] In general, fractional absorption of calcium is about 30%, although it varies with intake.[21,99] Some individuals may need to consume higher amounts of calcium because of their low absorption of this nutrient.[38] Dietary and nondietary factors influence calcium absorption and excretion and thus the need for this nutrient.[21,38,99,100] The decline in calcium absorption associated with aging may be explained in part by low body stores of vitamin D,[17,23,101] as well as the age-related decline in gut mass which generally is associated with decreased food intake. High intakes of sodium and protein can increase urinary calcium excretion.[21,23]
- The menopausal effect. In the early postmenopausal years, bone loss is specifically related to the cessation of estrogen production.[17,21,36,38,99,100,102-104] Calcium intake has a greater influence on bone mass after the first five years of the onset of menopause.

- The threshold effect of calcium. Several studies indicate threshold or saturation points above which the effect of additional calcium is reduced.[21,99,100,105] Individuals with an adequate calcium intake cannot be expected to derive further bone-preserving benefit from additional calcium intake. That is, the nutritional response in terms of calcium balance or bone mass will occur at intakes below the threshold, but not above. For example, the lack of an association between calcium intake and bone density reported in a study of healthy elderly women over 70 years may be explained by the women's average calcium intake of 921 mg a day from dairy foods.[106] The number of participants in this study with a calcium intake below the threshold likely was too small to detect an effect.[106] Further evidence for a calcium intake threshold is obtained from a recent investigation involving prepubertal girls.[107] In girls whose usual calcium intake was low (<700 mg/day), 1300 mg calcium/day was the least amount of calcium to achieve maximal calcium retention. In contrast, increasing calcium intake resulted in little additional benefit in the girls whose calcium intake was already adequate.[107]
- Heterogeneity of the calcium response. Skeletal sites differ in their degree of response to dietary calcium.[21,99]
- Duration of the study. Because of the nature of bone remodeling, a period of at least two years and preferably longer is necessary to establish a positive effect of calcium on bone density.[108-110]
- Difficulties in measuring bone mass and accurately determining calcium intake. The weakness of existing tools to accurately estimate calcium intake (e.g., food frequency questionnaires, 24-hour dietary recall) may contribute to a negative or inconsistent association between calcium intake and bone health. In many epidemiological studies, particularly observational studies, dietary calcium intake may be under- or overestimated.[111,112] Errors in food frequency questionnaires or dietary recalls, portion size estimations, and variability in the nutrient content of particular foods all contribute to inaccuracies in estimating actual calcium intake.[21,112] In addition, the bioavailability of calcium influences how much of a given nutrient is effectively used.[112] Calcium balance studies with or without isotopes are used to estimate calcium needs and to provide information on changes in calcium metabolism (e.g., urinary output, absorption). Direct measurements of bone mass indicate net retention of calcium over a long period. The advantage of the maximum calcium retention approach is that systematic errors of the balance method do not influence the ability to define the threshold value. A number of different noninvasive methods such as single and dual energy x-ray absorptiometry (DXA), peripheral dual energy absorptiometry, radiographic absorptiometry, quantitative computed tomography, and ultrasound are available to determine bone mass or density safely, conveniently, accurately, and at a relatively low cost.[1,17] Measurement of bone mineral density can detect osteoporosis before a fracture occurs, predict an individual's risk of fracture, and monitor the effectiveness of osteoporosis treatment.[1]

1. Childhood and Adolescence

Childhood and adolescence are critical times to begin building optimal bone mass. Bone mass is important to future risk of osteoporosis. For this reason, a logical attempt to reduce the prevalence of this disease later in life is to optimize bone accretion during childhood and adolescence.[17,31,113] Low dietary intake of calcium during childhood and adolescence may jeopardize attainment of genetically-determined optimal peak bone mass.[17-19,66] Although osteoporosis is typically a disease of older adults, its prevention begins in childhood by maximizing calcium retention and bone mass in the growing years.[114]

The NAS recently updated calcium recommendations for children and adolescents to 800 mg a day for 4 to 8 year olds and 1300 mg a day for 9 through 18 year olds.[17] Previous recommendations (i.e., 1989 RDAs) were 800 mg calcium a day for 7 to 10 year olds and 1200 mg a day for 11 to 19 year olds.[26]

Numerous studies indicate that increasing calcium intake during childhood and/or puberty benefits bone health.[87,107,115,116] In a study at Indiana University involving 22 pairs of twins averaging 7 years of age, bone mass accumulation was 3 to 5% higher among children who consumed 1600 mg calcium a day than those who had an intake of 900 mg a day (Figure 5.3).[115] In this three-year, double-blind, placebo-controlled study of the effect of increased calcium intake, one twin served as the control for the other. The findings of this study led the authors to suggest that increasing calcium intake of prepubertal children may reduce the risk of osteoporotic fractures later in life.[115] As expected for a nutrient present in insufficient quantities in the basal diet, this positive effect of calcium on bones appears to persist only as long as the high calcium intake is maintained.[110,117] Other investigations indicate that at least 1250 mg calcium per day is needed to improve bone health in 6 to 10 year old children.[107,118,119] According to a recent placebo-controlled, double-blind study involving 149, 8 year old Caucasian females, increasing calcium intake from approximately 900 to 1750 mg per day for one year increased bone mineral density in the

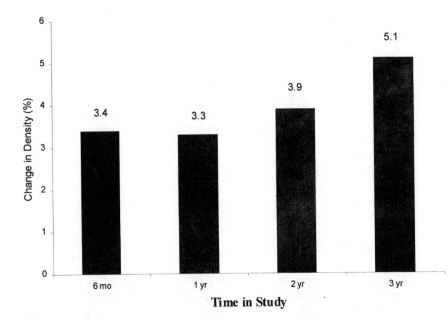

Figure 5.3   Mean differences within prepubertal twin pairs in the bone mineral density of the midshaft radius. (From Johnston, C. C., Jr., et al., *N. Engl. J. Med.*, 327, 82, 1992. With permission.)

arm and hip, and, to a lesser degree, the spine.[107] This increase in bone mass in response to increased calcium intake was markedly dependent upon habitual calcium intake. There was a 3.5-fold (2.1 vs. 0.6% per year) greater benefit for below average calcium consumers (<850 mg/day) than for above average calcium consumers.[107] This finding is explained by the fact that, at high calcium intakes, a larger fraction of the treated subjects will be replete, and therefore will not show any additional benefit from added calcium.

During adolescence, about 45% or more of the body's total skeletal mass is formed.[31,113,118] Although bone mass may accumulate through the third decade of life, peak adult bone density may be reached as early as late adolescence in certain bones (proximal femur and vertebrae).[17,31] Lu et al.[120] found that bone mineral density of the total body, lumbar spine, and femoral neck increased significantly until 17.5 years in males and 15.8 years in females. New research indicates that peak calcium accretion rate occurs at approximately age 13 for females and 14.5 years for males.[66]

In addition to this high rate of skeletal growth, calcium absorption during childhood and adolescence is much lower[36,121] than previously assumed.[26] One study demonstrated that calcium absorption was 32% in adolescents consuming 1332 mg calcium a day.[121] Calcium absorption appears to be more efficient in the early pubertal period than in prepubertal or late pubertal periods.[122,123] The dramatic increase in skeletal mass during adolescence and the inefficient absorption of calcium contribute to the recommendation of 1300 mg calcium a day for children and adolescents 9 through 18 years of age.[17]

Calcium intervention trials and calcium balance studies[87,118,119,123-129] support a calcium intake of at least 1300 mg per day for adolescents and perhaps closer to the upper optimal calcium intake of 1500 mg a day recommended by the NIH[18] and supported by the AMA.[19] According to an 18-month double-blind, placebo-controlled trial in Pennsylvania involving 94 healthy Caucasian 12 year old girls, increasing calcium intake from 935 mg a day to 1370 mg a day significantly increased total and spine bone mineral density (Figure 5.4).[126] Thus, increasing calcium intake by the amount of calcium (i.e., 300 mg) in one cup serving of milk or yogurt, or $1^{1}/_{2}$ ounces of hard cheese increased skeletal mass between 1 and 3%.[126] Jackman et al.[127] found that adolescent females aged 12 to 15 years needed to consume at least 1300 mg calcium per day to maximize body calcium retention. This study of 35 girls found that a calcium intake of 1200 mg per day resulted in only 57% of maximum calcium retention.[127]

Chan et al.[87] reported that, in a controlled study in Utah involving 48 pubertal girls (9 to 13 years), increasing calcium intake from 728 mg per day to 1437 mg per day with dairy foods for a year significantly increased total and spinal bone mineral density (Figure 5.5). The additional intake of dairy foods increased the girls' intake of calcium, phosphorus, vitamin D, and protein, but not their intake of total or saturated fat.[87] Body weight and fatness were similar between the dairy group and the controls.[87] Similar findings are reported by Cadogan and coworkers.[90] These investigators found that bone mineral content and bone mineral density were significantly increased in 80 girls aged 12 years who consumed additional calcium in the form of whole or lowfat milk (i.e., two extra cups) for 18 months. Mean calcium in the milk group was 1125 mg per day compared with the baseline calcium intake of

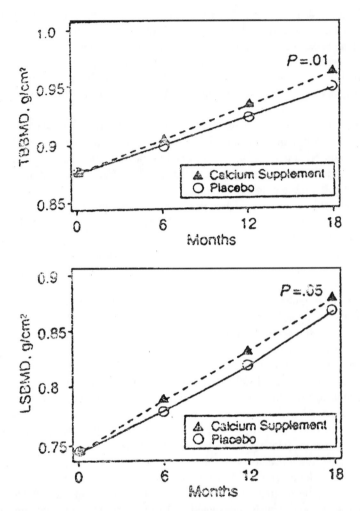

Figure 5.4 Total body bone mineral density (TBBMD) and lumbar spine bone mineral density (LSBMD) are shown for the 18-month study period. The *P* values shown are for the differences in linear terms. (From Lloyd, T., et al., *JAMA*, 270, 841, 1993. With permission.)

746 mg per day.[90] Compared to the control group, the girls who increased milk intake gained an additional 37 g of bone mineral. No significant differences in height gain, weight gain, lean body mass, or fat mass were evident between the groups.[90] The milk group significantly increased their protein, phosphorus, magnesium, zinc, riboflavin, and thiamin intakes.[90]

In a two-year longitudinal trial involving 31 healthy adolescent females initially aged 14 years, bone mass and bone density tended to be higher (2 to 5%) at almost all sites measured in those whose usual calcium intake of more than 850 mg/day was increased to 1640 mg with either milk or calcium carbonate supplements compared to the low calcium group (<850 mg/day).[125] In another controlled

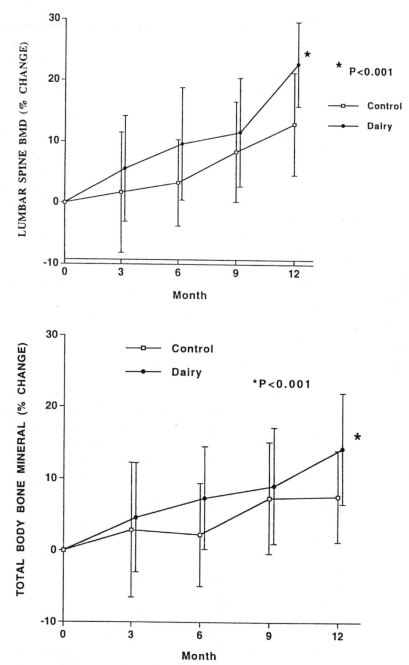

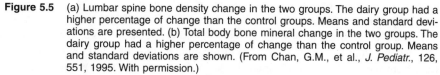

Figure 5.5 (a) Lumbar spine bone density change in the two groups. The dairy group had a higher percentage of change than the control groups. Means and standard deviations are presented. (b) Total body bone mineral change in the two groups. The dairy group had a higher percentage of change than the control group. Means and standard deviations are shown. (From Chan, G.M., et al., *J. Pediatr.*, 126, 551, 1995. With permission.)

intervention trial, a calcium intake of 1450 mg/day was estimated to optimize bone mass in adolescents.[119] Nieves et al.[128] report that a calcium intake of 1600 mg /day during adolescence was associated with increased hip bone density in women aged 30 to 39 years. These gains in bone mass, if maintained, could potentially offer some protection against future hip fractures. A recent Australian study involving 42 pairs of 17 year old twins found that increasing calcium intake from about 800 mg a day to more than 1600 mg a day for 18 months increased spinal and hip bone mineral densities.[129] In the twins who consumed the additional calcium (i.e., 1000 mg per day), bone density increased by 1.3% at the hip and 1.5% at the spine.[129]

In addition to the Chan et al.[87] and Cadogan et al.[90] investigations discussed above, other studies indicate that intake of milk and other dairy foods during childhood and adolescence is an important determinant of bone mass.[89,130-135] When children 7 to 9 years of age consumed an additional $3/4$ cup of milk every day for two years, bone density 14 years later was higher than in children who did not consume extra calcium.[133] A comparison of two rural communities in Yugoslavia which differed in their milk and dairy food consumption (and therefore calcium intake) identified a higher peak bone mass in residents of the community with a high milk intake than in those with a low milk intake.[130] Calcium intake of the one area (950 mg/day) was about twice that of the other area (450 mg/day). The greater bone mass and bone density reached by age 35 in residents of the high calcium district was maintained throughout life and was attributed to their larger bone mass formed in childhood (Figure 5.6). Of most importance, the incidence of hip fractures was lower among subjects in the high calcium district than in subjects in the low calcium district (Figure 5.7).[130]

Several retrospective studies link increased milk intake during the early years with greater bone density in adulthood.[131,134-138] Middle-aged women who reported drinking milk with every meal during childhood and adolescence had a higher bone mass in middle age than those who reported drinking milk infrequently (Figure 5.8).[131] Likewise, another retrospective study among middle-aged and elderly women found that bone mineral density in the hip and spine was significantly higher in women who reported drinking one or more servings of milk a day up to age 25.[134] Soroko et al.[135] reported that milk intake during adolescence was positively associated with increased bone mineral density at the spine and midradius in postmenopausal women. The findings of a beneficial effect of milk intake in early life on bone health in later years in these two studies were independent of other factors such as age, body mass, smoking, and physical activity.[134,135]

In another investigation, higher reported intakes of calcium from milk and milk products during childhood and adolescence were linked to both higher bone mineral density and a lower risk of osteoporosis in adulthood.[137] More recently, New et al.[138] reported higher bone densities in premenopausal women who consumed more than $2^{1}/_{2}$ cups of milk per day during their childhood and early teenage years than in those who reported low milk intakes (1 cup or less per day).

Compelling evidence indicates that adolescence is a critical time to optimize genetically-determined peak bone mass.[139-141] However, on average, U.S. children and teenagers fail to consume the current recommendation of 1300 mg per day.[69,73] Data from the 1994-96 CSFII[69] indicate that U.S. males ages 6 to 11 and 12 to 19

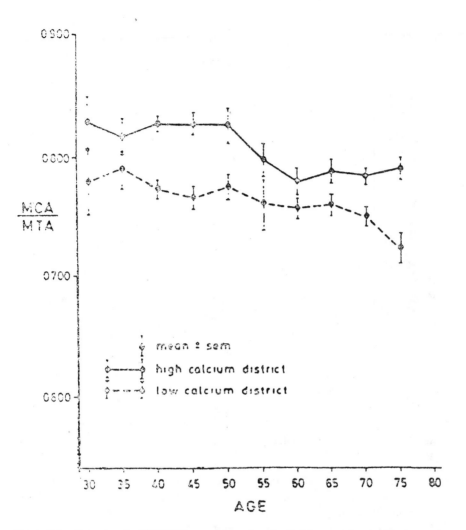

Figure 5.6   Bone density (MCA/MTA = metacarpal cortical/total area ratio of subjects accustomed to different calcium intakes over lifetime). (From Matkovic et al., *Am. J. Clin. Nutr.*, 32, 540, 1979. With permission.)

consume, on average, only 970 mg and 1145 mg of calcium per day, respectively. U.S. females ages 6 to 11 and 12 to 19 consume, on average, only 857 mg and 771 mg calcium per day, respectively.[69] USDA's Food Guide Pyramid[79] recommends two to three servings from the Milk Group. The American Heart Association's *Healthy Heart Food Pyramid* recommends two to four servings per day of skim milk and lowfat dairy products.[82] Recognizing adolescents' increased needs for calcium, an American Academy of Pediatrics' publication[81] includes a modified Food Guide Pyramid for adolescents that recommends five servings from the Milk Group. To meet their increased calcium needs, children and adolescents should be encouraged to increase their intake of milk and other dairy foods. Doing so will improve the overall nutritional quality of their diet,[75] without contributing to excess body weight

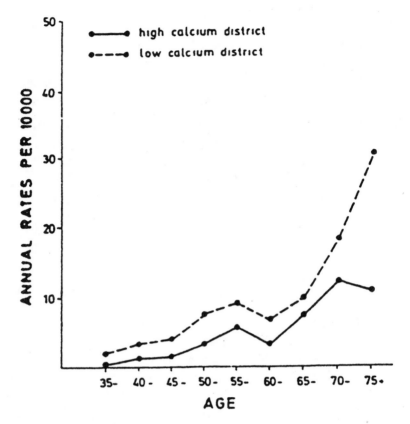

Figure 5.7   Annual hip fracture rates of subjects accustomed to different calcium intake over lifetime. (From Matkovic et al., *Am. J. Clin. Nutr.*, 32, 540, 1979. With permission.)

or body fat.[87,89,90] Recent findings indicating adolescents' lack of knowledge about how much calcium they need and the calcium content of various dietary sources of this mineral support the need for more education about calcium targeted to this group.[96]

2. Adulthood

a. Young Adulthood

In the early adult years (19 through 30), there is continued accumulation of bone mass. This retention of bone mass occurs for approximately 10 years after longitudinal growth has stopped, but generally at a lower rate than during adolescence.[17,142] However, calcium absorption efficiency during the early adult years is lower than during adolescence.[140] Although data are limited, 1000 mg calcium per day is recommended for men and women aged 19 through 30 years to maximize calcium retention.[17] Several studies indicate that a calcium intake of at least 1000 mg per day is optimal for young adults.[124,142-146] A review of both prospective and cross-sectional studies of the effects of calcium intake on bone mineral content in females

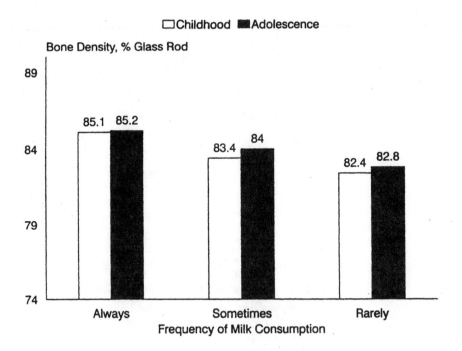

☐Childhood ■Adolescence

Bone Density, % Glass Rod

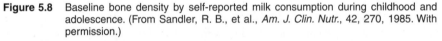

Figure 5.8 Baseline bone density by self-reported milk consumption during childhood and adolescence. (From Sandler, R. B., et al., *Am. J. Clin. Nutr.*, 42, 270, 1985. With permission.)

between the ages of 20 and 40 years indicates a positive effect of calcium intakes at or greater than 1000 mg per day on bone health.[146]

A high daily dietary calcium (i.e., 1000 mg) intake and physical activity (i.e., >90 minutes of moderate activity a week) increased radial bone mineral content and density in 24 to 28 year old Caucasian women participating in a cross-sectional study.[143] In a longitudinal prospective study (up to 5 years) involving 156 healthy women in their 20s (18 to 26 years), increasing dietary calcium intake to 1400 mg or higher and increasing physical activity both had a positive effect on bone density (Table 5.4).[142]

Intake of dairy foods is beneficial to bones in young adults.[144,145,147] When factors related to peak bone mass were examined in 421 women ages 25 to 34 living in Hawaii, milk intake was positively associated with forearm bone mass index.[147] In healthy Asian women aged 19 to 25 years, bone mineral density was positively associated with milk intake during childhood.[144] Among women with the lowest bone mineral density, 22% did not drink milk during childhood. Females who drank milk throughout life had a significantly higher bone mineral density (0.36 plus or minus 0.05 g/cm^2) than those who did not drink milk during childhood (0.32 plus or minus 0.06 g/cm^2) or adolescence (0.34 plus or minus 0.05 g/cm^2) (Figure 5.9).[144] The findings led the authors to suggest that "…high milk consumption, good supply of calcium for bone formation in childhood, increases the peak bone mass."[144]

Table 5.4   Estimated Effect of Activity or Diet Calcium on Percentage of Change in Spinal Bone Mineral Density in the Third Decade*

Activity, Counts/Hour	Calcium, mg/day	Change %
Calcium intake held constant, activity varies		
3	800	+0.26
4	800	+2.29
5	800	+4.32
6	800	+6.34
7	800	+8.37
Activity held constant, calcium intake varies		
5	220	−1.05
5	700	+3.39
5	1,000	+6.17
5	1,400	+9.87
5	2,106	+16.41

* Age = 25 years; protein intake = 65 g/day.
From Recker, R.R., et al., *JAMA*, 268, 2403, 1992. With permission.

Similarly, in a study of 705 healthy, Caucasian college women (18 to 22 years), radial bone mineral content and density were positively associated with intake of milk and cheese.[145] Distal radial bone mineral content and density were 1.8% and 2.7% higher, respectively, in women with high long-term calcium intakes (i.e., calcium intakes close to 1200 mg per day both during high school and college) than in women who consumed less than one serving of milk or cheese a day since age 14 (Figure 5.10).[145] Findings of this study also indicate a significant positive association between long-term physical activity patterns (>4 hours a week for 8 or more months of the year) and distal bone mineral content and bone mineral density. Moderate long-term calcium intake combined with moderate long-term physical activity was especially beneficial to bone mass. Conversely, a low calcium intake was most detrimental to bone mass when physical activity also was low (<1 hour a week). "Both regular physical activity and adequate calcium intake may be positive modulators of the distal radius from the perimenarcheal period through mid-adulthood," concluded Tylavsky et al.[145] Other more recent findings support the beneficial effect of increased calcium and physical activity on bone health.[51,52]

b. Between Peak Bone Mass and Menopause

Adequate calcium intake continues to be important to offset calcium losses and maintain bone health in the years after peak bone mass has been reached and before menopause.[38,132,148] For premenopausal women ages 31 through 50 years, 1000 mg calcium per day is recommended to maximize calcium retention.[17] According to a meta-analysis of 27 well-designed cross-sectional studies involving women between

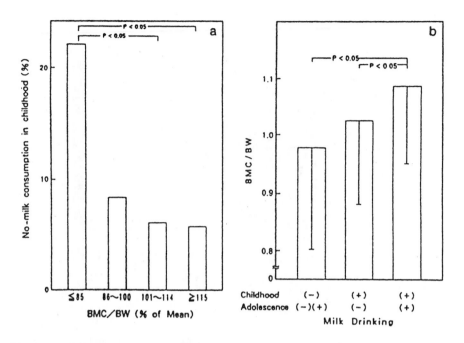

Figure 5.9 Milk consumption in childhood and bone mineral density. a: the percentage of subjects who did not drink milk in childhood, by BMD [bone mineral content (BMC)/bone width (BW)] group; b: BMDs for nonmilk drinkers in childhood, nonmilk drinkers in adolescence, and milk drinkers throughout life; $\bar{x} \pm$ SD. (From Hirota, T., et al., *Am. J. Clin. Nutr.*, 55, 1168, 1992. With permission.)

18 and 50 years of age, a calcium intake of approximately 1000 mg/day or higher is positively associated with bone mass.[149]

Increasing calcium intake from dairy products benefits bone health in premenopausal women.[138,150] In a three-year prospective trial involving premenopausal women 30 to 42 years of age, 20 women were randomly assigned to consume more dairy products (an increase of 610 mg calcium for a total of 1572 mg plus or minus 920 mg), while 17 women continued their usual diet (810 mg plus or minus 367 mg calcium).[150] Vertebral bone mineral density was significantly greater in the women consuming the higher than lower calcium diets.[150] Based on these findings, the authors suggested that the increase in the bone mass of women entering menopause might reduce their risk of osteoporosis as they age.[150] As mentioned earlier, premenopausal women ages 45 to 49 years who consumed more than two cups of milk a day during childhood and young adulthood had higher spinal and hip bone mineral densities than women who consumed one cup or less of milk a day.[138] A recent 12-year prospective study of 77,761 registered nurses ages 34 to 59 years found no evidence that higher intakes of milk or calcium from food sources reduced bone fractures.[151] However, this type of study (i.e., observational) cannot adequately control for confounding factors and therefore is unable to indicate a causal association.[112] Observational studies are useful for generating hypotheses for subsequent testing in stronger designs, but cannot produce definitive results. Further, this type

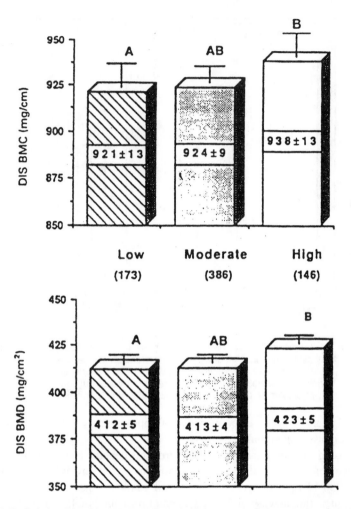

Figure 5.10 Relationship of long-term milk and cheese consumption to distal radial BMC and BMD values for white college-aged females (LS mean ± SEM), adjusted for age of menarche and BMI. Different superscripts over the bars indicate significantly different values using a Bonferroni adjustment ($p<0.017$). Numbers (n) of subjects are in parenthesis. Low <287 mg calcium during high school and < 209 mg calcium during college; moderate between high and low; high >842 mg calcium during high school and >660 mg calcium during college. (From Tylavsky, F. A., et al., *Osteop. Int.*, 2, 232, 1992. With permission.)

of study cannot negate the evidence produced from randomized controlled intervention trials.[112] This study[151] depended on a food frequency questionnaire to estimate calcium intake which is limited in its ability to accurately determine how much calcium or milk the subjects actually consumed or the relationship of calcium intake to bone mass and fractures.[112]

c. Early Postmenopausal Years

There is general agreement that calcium has a variable effect on bone health in women during early postmenopausal years, the period of most rapid bone loss.[17,105] Due to the loss of estrogen at menopause, women lose bone mineral at a rate of about 3% a year for about five years after menopause and then more slowly (1% a year) thereafter.[152] During the first five years of menopause, calcium is less effective in protecting the skeleton than in the premenopausal and late menopause years.[38,102,104,105] In an eight-year study of 154 healthy women with a mean age of 53 years, rate of cortical bone loss was unaffected by habitual calcium intake (75% derived from dairy products) ranging from less than 800 mg to more than 1350 mg in early postmenopausal years.[153] In contrast, dietary calcium influenced bone mass in women more than five years postmenopausal (Figure 5.11). Dawson-Hughes et al.[105] also showed that increasing calcium intake had little or no benefit on bone health in women during the first five years of menopause, but provided substantial protection thereafter. The profound and rapid loss of estrogen in the early postmenopausal years is responsible for the bone loss at this time. As a result of the initial rapid decline in estrogen at menopause, women lose about 15% of the bone they had before menopause.[38] Estrogen replacement therapy is effective in preventing postmenopausal bone loss from all skeletal sites and in reducing fracture risk.[103,104]

Although increased calcium intake has only a modest effect on the rapid bone loss that occurs immediately after menopause, studies indicate that even early postmenopausal women benefit from calcium intakes at or greater than recommended intakes.[104,105,154,155] Riis and colleagues[104] showed that an additional 2000 mg calcium a day had a modest effect on bone loss in the proximal radius, but had no effect in the spine or distal radius in early postmenopausal women whose normal dietary calcium intake was high. Calcium supplementation during menopause may be more important for cortical than trabecular bone.[154] In a controlled two-year trial of calcium supplementation (i.e., 1000 and 2000 mg elemental calcium/day) in 286 Dutch women 46 to 55 years old whose calcium intake was already high (average of 1150 mg/day), bone loss from the lumbar spine was reduced in the first year of supplementation but not in the second. The authors concluded that calcium supplementation reduces lumbar bone loss in the first year of calcium supplementation by reducing bone turnover.[154] At the end of two years of calcium supplementation, lumbar bone loss was reduced by 1.9% and 3.0% in the groups receiving 1000 mg calcium and 2000 mg calcium, respectively.[154]

Further support for a beneficial effect of increased calcium intake on bone health in the early postmenopausal years is provided by Aloia et al.[155] In this study, 118 healthy Caucasian women between three and six years past menopause were randomly assigned to one of three treatment groups for three years: 1) 1700 mg calcium a day from diet and calcium carbonate supplement; 2) estrogen-progesterone replacement therapy plus 1700 mg calcium a day; and 3) placebo. All subjects received 400 IU of vitamin D a day. The placebo group lost bone density in the arm, spine, and three areas of the hip.[155] However, increased calcium intake slowed age-related

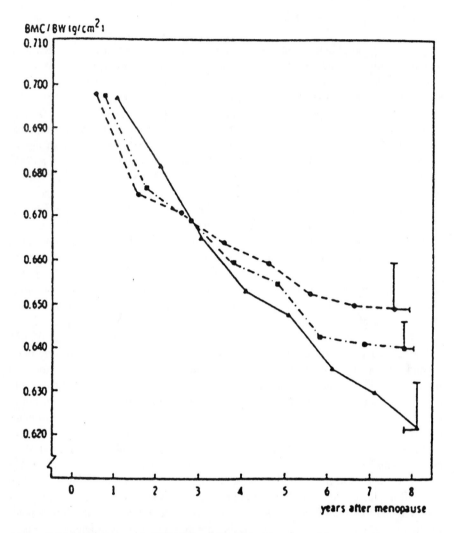

Figure 5.11 Mean changes in BMC/BW as a function of the mean of the years after menopause in 154 perimenopausal women subdivided according to habitual dietary calcium intake. Bars are 1 SEM. (BMC/BW first measured in 1980.) (●) Ca intake <800 mg/day (n = 28); (■) Ca intake 800-1350 mg/day (n = 95); (▲) Ca intake > 1350 mg/day (n = 31). (From van Beresteijn, E. C. H., et al., *Calcif. Tissue Int.*, 47, 338, 1990. With permission.)

bone loss in the skeletal sites measured. The estrogen-progesterone-calcium treatment was more effective in reducing bone loss and improving calcium balance than calcium alone. The findings nevertheless support a significant beneficial effect of calcium in reducing bone loss, especially in the neck of the femur, around the time of menopause (Figure 5.12).[155] Although calcium is less effective than estrogen in slowing the rapid bone loss that occurs immediately after menopause, consuming an adequate intake of calcium (1200 mg/day) during the early postmenopausal period is important to bone health. As discussed below under treatment, studies indicate

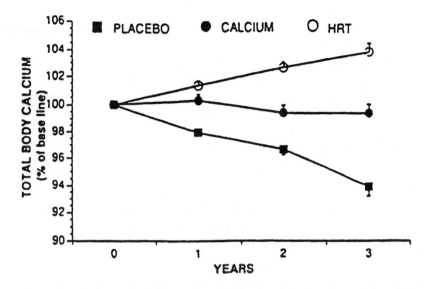

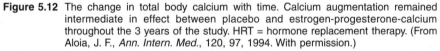

Figure 5.12 The change in total body calcium with time. Calcium augmentation remained intermediate in effect between placebo and estrogen-progesterone-calcium throughout the 3 years of the study. HRT = hormone replacement therapy. (From Aloia, J. F., *Ann. Intern. Med.*, 120, 97, 1994. With permission.)

that calcium plus estrogen reduces bone loss more than either calcium or estrogen alone.[156,157] For example, Nieves et al.[157] recently found that calcium improves the effectiveness of estrogen replacement therapy on bone.

d. Later Postmenopausal Years

Beginning about five years after the onset of menopause, calcium once again resumes relatively more importance in bone health than in the early postmenopausal years.[17,40,105,158] The difference in calcium's role in bone health between early and late menopause can best be explained by the effect of estrogen on the bone mass "set point." When estrogen declines at menopause, bone initially adjusts its mass downward releasing calcium. The result is that during the first few years after menopause, there is a modest dependence on external (dietary) calcium sources.[38] However, after a period of adjustment dependence on dietary calcium increases.[38]

For postmenopausal women ages 51 through 70 years, 1200 mg of calcium per day is recommended.[17] This calcium recommendation is 200 mg per day higher than for 31 through 50 year adults because of the decrease in calcium absorption with advancing age.[17] According to the NAS,[17] evidence is insufficient to support different calcium recommendations for women depending on their menopausal status or use of hormone replacement therapy.[17]

Findings from calcium balance studies and calcium intervention trials support a calcium recommendation of at least 1200 mg per day for postmenopausal women.[17,158-162] According to an investigation of 122 healthy postmenopausal New Zealand women, increasing calcium intake from 750 mg a day to 1750 mg a day (i.e., 1000 mg calcium from calcium lactate-gluconate and calcium carbonate) for two years reduced age-related bone loss by one-third to one-half in several bones as compared with the placebo group.[158] Increasing calcium intake reduced the rate of loss of total body mineral density by 43%.[158] At most skeleton sites, the placebo group lost bone at a rate of approximately 1% a year. When 86 postmenopausal women participated in a two-year extension to this study, a sustained beneficial effect on bones over the four years occurred with calcium supplementation.[159] However, the effect of increased calcium differed according to the specific bone site.[159] In the lumbar spine and femoral neck, bone loss was reduced in the calcium group in the first year with only a small positive effect of increased calcium over the remaining years. In contrast, the rate of bone loss of total body bone mineral density in the calcium group was maintained over the four years (Figure 5.13).[159]

Findings of a recent four-year follow-up study involving 84 women aged 54 to 74 years who were more than 10 years past menopause indicate that a calcium intake of almost 2 g/day may be necessary to slow or stop bone loss and reduce fracture risk.[160] Women consuming 1988 mg calcium/day for four years did not lose bone at the hip or ankle, whereas significantly more bone was lost from these sites in the control group which consumed 952 mg calcium/day (Figure 5.14).[160] In 49 women who were treated with increased calcium for two years, but then stopped, bone loss at the ankle site was significant.[160] Therefore, continuation of the increased calcium intake is important to maintain this positive effect on bone density. The researchers suggest that the findings are consistent with a growing body of evidence indicating that over 1500 mg of calcium/day is associated with bone health and reduced risk of fractures.[160] An earlier two-year, placebo-controlled study in women 10 years past menopause by these same investigators demonstrated that calcium supplementation (1800 mg/day) as milk powder or as tablets completely prevented bone loss at some areas of the hip.[161]

Michaelsson et al.[162] recently found that bone mineral density in postmenopausal women significantly improved in women who consumed more than 1400 mg calcium per day. This four-year prospective study divided 115 women into the following three groups based on their estimated mean dietary intakes of calcium: low (465 mg), medium (1006 mg), and high (1645 mg).[162] The group with the highest calcium intake had significantly greater hip, lumbar spine, and total body bone mineral densities than women in either the low or the intermediate calcium groups.[162]

Not only calcium alone, but also calcium combined with physical activity or estrogen-replacement therapy, benefits bone health in postmenopausal women.[49,51,102,103,128,161-164] Nelson et al.[49] found that a dietary calcium intake of approximately 1450 mg/day and moderate exercise (i.e., a one year program of walking briskly 15 to 40 minutes/day for three days/week) slowed bone loss at various skeletal sites in postmenopausal women. A two-year placebo-controlled study involving 168 postmenopausal women in Australia found that increasing calcium intake from 800 mg per day to 1800 mg per day by consuming either milk powder or calcium supplements reduced bone loss in the hip and leg.[161] Adding an extra four hours a week of weight-bearing exercise to increased calcium intake was more effective in reducing hip bone loss than calcium alone.[161] The findings led the authors to conclude that " ... a lifestyle regimen of increased dietary intake of

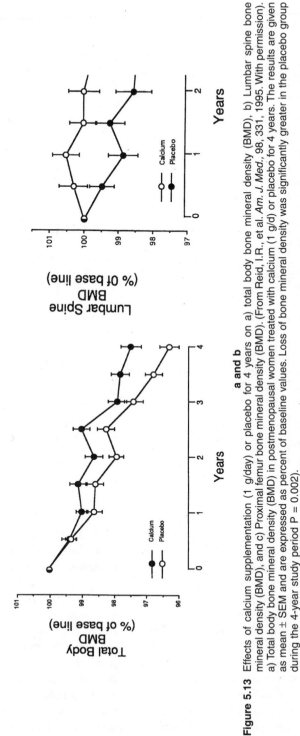

Figure 5.13 Effects of calcium supplementation (1 g/day) or placebo for 4 years on a) total body bone mineral density (BMD), b) Lumbar spine bone mineral density (BMD), and c) Proximal femur bone mineral density (BMD). (From Reid, I.R., et al. *Am. J. Med.*, 98, 331, 1995. With permission).

a) Total body bone mineral density (BMD) in postmenopausal women treated with calcium (1 g/d) or placebo for 4 years. The results are given as mean ± SEM and are expressed as percent of baseline values. Loss of bone mineral density was significantly greater in the placebo group during the 4-year study period P = 0.002).

b) Lumbar spine bone mineral density (BMD) in postmenopausal women treated with calcium supplementation or placebo for 4 years. Bone loss was reduced in the calcium group in year 1 (P = 0.004) and over the entire study period (P = 0.03).

c) (on next page) Proximal femur bone mineral density in postmenopausal women treated with calcium supplementation or placebo for 4 years. There was a significant difference between the groups in the femoral neck (P = 0.03) and trochanter (P = 0.01) over the 4-year study period.

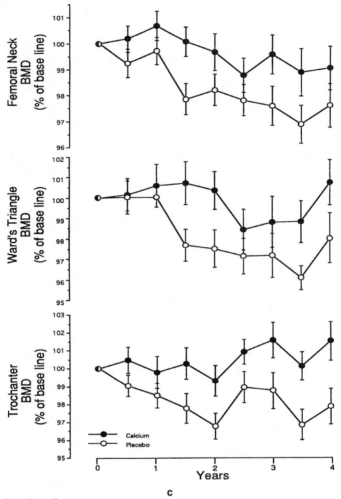

Figure 13 (continued)

calcium to ~1.8 g of calcium/day plus an exercise regimen of a 10% increase in the average exercise undertaken will significantly reduce bone loss at the clinically important hip site."[161] Researchers in England also demonstrated that both calcium intake and physical activity benefit bone health in women 5 to 12 years into menopause.[164] Specker[51] reported that the beneficial effects of physical activity on bone mineral density are dependent on a calcium intake of more than 1000 mg per day.

A high calcium intake may lower the dosage of estrogen necessary to prevent bone loss in postmenopausal women.[102,103] In an 18-month study of postmenopausal women aged 40 to 58 years, calcium intake (>1000 mg/day) was associated with a reduced loss of spinal trabecular bone density and a lowered amount of estrogen necessary to protect against bone loss.[103] A study in Hong Kong indicated a significant increase in hip bone mass in postmenopausal women receiving calcium and estrogen compared to estrogen alone.[163] A similar complementary effect of calcium

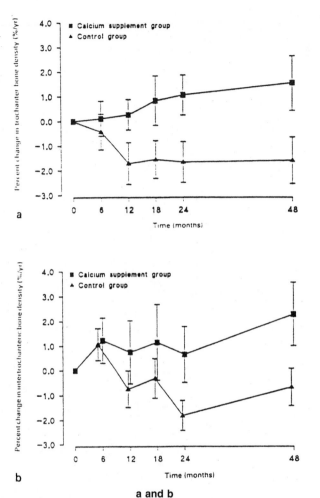

a and b

Figure 5.14 Percentage change in bone density at (a) trochanter, (b) intertrochanteric, (c) femoral neck, and (d) total hip sites. Results are the mean plus or minus SEM. The 4-year change in bone density determined from the slope of the least squares regression analysis was significantly different between the control group (▲; n = 21) and calcium supplemented group (■; n = 14). (From Devine, A., et. al., *Osteoporosis Int.,* 7, 23, 1997. European Foundation for Osteoporosis and the National Osteoporosis Foundation. Reprinted with permission from Sanger-Verlag London Ltd.) (c and d on next page).

and estrogen on the bone health of postmenopausal women is reported by Nieves et al.[128]

There is substantial evidence that increasing calcium intake protects against bone loss in postmenopausal women. Further, the data examining the association between dairy food intake and bone health in this population have been positive. In a study published by Recker and Heaney[165] more than a decade ago, increased milk intake (24 ounces/day) improved calcium balance in 13 healthy postmenopausal women compared to 9 control subjects who did not receive the milk supplement. Milk

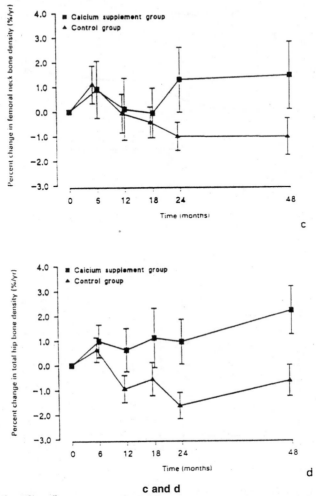

Figure 5.14 (continued)

consumption also was observed to result in less bone remodeling than that found with calcium supplements.[165]

Studies in Japan, Italy, and China indicate that intake of dairy foods is associated with increased bone mass in postmenopausal women.[166-169] In a cross-sectional study of 178 Japanese women living in Japan, current milk intake, but not calcium intake, was positively associated with midradial bone mineral content in postmenopausal women, ages 55 to 60 years.[166] In a more recent investigation involving 4573 adults in Japan, reported low milk intake was associated with increased risk of hip fractures.[162] In an investigation in Italy, current milk intake of postmenopausal women was positively associated with bone mineral content.[167] Postmenopausal Italian women who consumed at least one cup of milk a day exhibited higher bone density than those who consumed less than a cup of milk a day (Figure 5.15). The authors

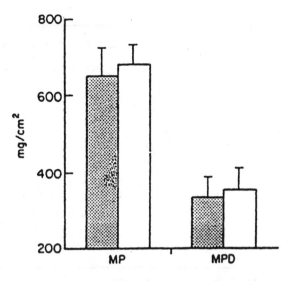

Figure 5.15 Bone mineral content as middle point (MP) and modified distal point (MDP) density in postmenopausal women consuming less than (■) and more than (□) 250 mg/day of milk. MP: P<0.02; MDP: P<0.07. (From Callegari, C., et al., *J. Hum. Nutr. & Dietetics.*, 3, 159, 1990. With permission.)

suggested that "... low milk intake represents a risk factor for the development of osteoporosis, probably through diminished calcium intake ...."[167]

Further support for a beneficial effect of dairy foods on bone health is provided by a recent study in China.[168] In this study, associations between dietary calcium from both dairy and nondairy sources and bone status were examined in 843 Chinese women aged 35 to 75 years and living in five different counties where dietary calcium varied widely. Peak bone mass at skeletal maturity was the same for the women before menopause (Figure 5.16). However, women in pastoral and semipastoral areas who consumed higher dairy calcium had a slower decline in bone mass after menopause than women residing in nonpastoral areas without dairy calcium.[168] Women in dairy calcium areas lost 8.6% bone per decade, whereas bone loss in women in non-dairy areas was 9.2%. As shown in Figure 5.16, women in pastoral counties had higher bone mass at the distal radius than did women residing in nonpastoral counties. Differences in dairy calcium were held responsible for the differences in the rate of bone loss. Dairy calcium was more significantly associated with bone mass than was nondairy calcium.[168] There was no association between nondairy calcium and bone variables after adjustment for age and/or body weight. In a separate analysis involving women living in pastoral areas, bone mineral content and density at the distal and midradius were positively associated with intake of milk, hard cheese, and other dairy foods. The above findings indicate that dietary calcium, especially from dairy sources, increases bone mass in postmenopausal women and helps to reduce risk of osteoporosis. Low milk intake (and low calcium intake) during either childhood, adulthood, and/or the recent past was associated with increased risk of hip fractures according to an epidemiological study.[9] This study of

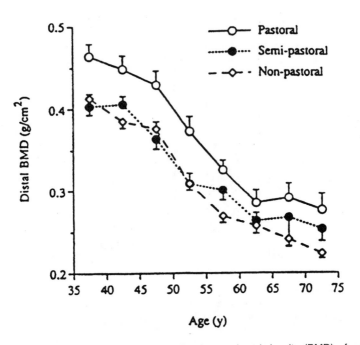

Figure 5.16 Age-related changes in distal radius bone mineral density (BMD) of women in pastoral, semipastoral, and nonpastoral areas ($\bar{x} \pm$ SEM). (From Hu, J.-F., et al., *Am. J. Clin. Nutr.*, 58, 219, 1993. With permission.)

risk factors for hip fractures involved more than 5600 women 50 years of age and older from six countries in Southern Europe.

V. PREVENTION AND TREATMENT OF OSTEOPOROSIS

A. Later Years

Osteoporosis and related fractures are a major cause of morbidity and mortality in the aging population.[17,170,171] The important role of calcium and vitamin D in decreasing bone loss and osteoporotic fractures in elderly men and women is widely recognized. Many older adults have low bone mass and continue to lose bone (i.e., 0.5 to 1.0%/year) with further aging.[38] Moreover, calcium deficiency and low vitamin D nutriture are frequently identified in this population.[17,67-69] Accumulating scientific evidence indicates that increasing intake of calcium and vitamin D in later years can slow the rate of bone loss and reduce risk of osteoporotic fractures.[105,172-178]

1. Men At Risk

Although more prevalent in women, osteoporosis also occurs in older men.[1,179-184] Women lose bone mass rapidly during the first few years of menopause (3%/year), however by age 65 or 70, women and men lose bone mass at the same slower rate of about 1%/year.[1,182] About 20% of all osteoporotic fractures occur in men.[1,19] However, the mortality rate in men after hip fractures is reported to be nearly twice that of women.[184] The lower risk of osteoporosis in men than in women is explained by men's larger bones and higher bone mineral content, their shorter lifespan (i.e., less time to lose bone), and hormonal changes.[1,179] Similar to women, men with low peak bone mass are vulnerable to osteoporosis.[1,183] Also, peak bone mass and subsequent bone loss in men, like in women, are influenced by genetics and certain lifestyle factors including physical activity, alcohol consumption, smoking, disease, and use of some medications.[183,184]

Studies examining the relationship between calcium (and vitamin D) intake and bone health in men are limited.[149] In one double-blind longitudinal placebo-controlled trial, 77 healthy men were given calcium, vitamin D_3, or a placebo for three years.[185] Although neither calcium nor vitamin D influenced bone loss at the radius or spine, the men already were consuming 1159 mg calcium. Thus, many men would not have been responsive and the benefit to the other men was likely overridden by the nonresponders. In contrast, a study in Australia associated a higher dietary intake of calcium in adult men with greater mineral density of bone in the lumbar spine and femoral neck (Figure 5.17).[180] Kroger and Laitinen[186] reported that hip bone mineral density, but not spinal bone density, was higher in Finnish men who consumed calcium intakes greater than 1200 mg/day than in those whose calcium intake was less than 800 mg/day. Because negative calcium balance can accompany aging in men as a result of low calcium intake, reduced efficiency of intestinal calcium absorption, and low synthesis of 1,25-dihydroxyvitamin vitamin D_3 (i.e., the metabolically active form of vitamin D), it is important that men consume recommended intakes of calcium and vitamin D.[178] As there are few data suggesting that the calcium and vitamin D needs of men are different from those of women, recommendations for these nutrients are the same for similar aged men and women.[17] The NAS recommends 1300 mg calcium/day for men 9 through 18 years, 1000 mg/day for 19 through 50 year olds, and 1200 mg/day for men 51 years and older. [17] Vitamin D recommendations are 200 IU/day for men 9 through 50 years, 400 IU/day for men 51 through 70 years, and 600 IU/day for those >70 years.[17]

Relatively little information is available regarding the effect of dairy food intake on bone health in men. An analysis of the Health Professionals Follow-up Study that followed more than 43,000 men aged 40 to 75 years for eight years linked higher reported intakes of calcium from dairy foods in general (but not from milk) with decreased risk of forearm and hip fractures.[187] Researchers at the University of Pittsburgh reported that bone mineral density was higher in men who drank milk from ages 18 to 50, and/or after age 50 than for men who drank milk less frequently.[188]

2. Calcium

Several recent studies[111,160,173-176,178,189] indicate that a calcium intake of at least recommended intakes of 1200 mg/day and 1500 mg/day[18,19] is necessary to protect older adults' bone health.

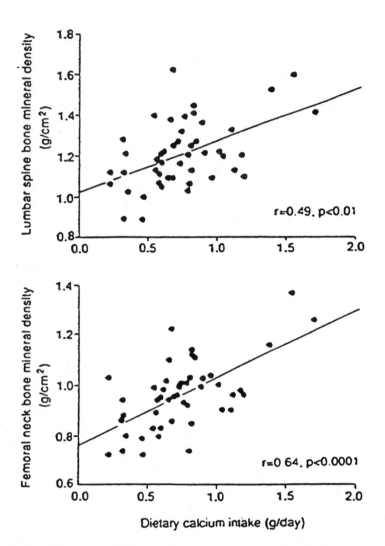

Figure 5.17 Relation between dietary calcium and bone mineral density at lumbar spine and femoral neck in normal men. (From Kelly, P. J., et al., *Br. Med. J.*, 300, 1361, 1990. With permission.)

According to a double-blind, placebo-controlled investigation in France involving 1765 ambulatory elderly women 69 to 106 years of age (mean age of 84), women who increased their calcium intake from 500 mg to 1700 mg/day and consumed an additional 800 IU of vitamin D_3 (cholecalciferol) for 18 months increased their hip bone density, and reduced the rate of hip fractures by 41% and other nonvertebral fractures by 30% (Figure 5.18).[174] Hip bone density continued to decrease at a rate of more than 3%/year in elderly women who did not consume additional calcium and vitamin D.[174] When this study was extended for an additional 18 months, risk of hip fractures was reduced by 29% and risk of all nonvertebral fractures was reduced by 24%.[189] These studies clearly indicate the peril that low calcium intake

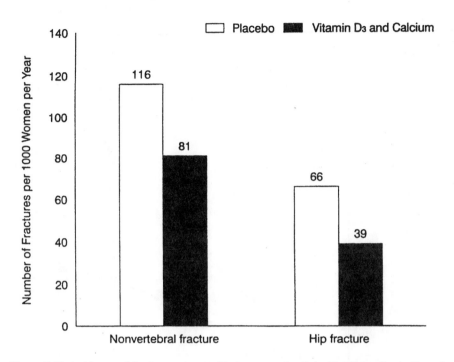

Figure 5.18 Incidence of fractures among elderly women treated with either vitamin D_3 and calcium or a placebo after 12-18 months of follow-up. (Adapted from Chapuy, M. C., et al., *N. Engl. J. Med.*, 327, 1637, 1992. With permission.)

presents for older adults and the importance of consuming adequate intakes of calcium and vitamin D to prevent bone loss and subsequent fractures even in the very old.

Recker et al.,[176] in a four year randomized controlled trial in vitamin D replete elderly women (mean age 73.5 years), found that increasing calcium intake by 1200 mg/day (total of about 1600 mg/day) reduced both femoral bone loss and the incidence of vertebral fractures. Women who experienced a previous fracture and were not treated with calcium were 2.8 times more likely to experience a fracture than other women.[176] Similar findings are reported by Chevalley et al.[175] In this study involving vitamin D replete elderly women, some of whom had suffered a hip fracture, increasing calcium intake by 800 mg/day (total of 1500 mg/day) for 18 months reduced femoral bone loss and the rate of vertebral fractures.

A more recent study by Dawson-Hughes et al.[178] found that increasing calcium intake by 500 mg/day (total of about 1400 mg/day) and vitamin D by about 700 IU/day for three years reduced bone loss in the hip, spine, and total body and nonvertebral fractures by 50% in adults 65 years and older (Figure 5.19). According to a recent meta-analysis of seven calcium intervention studies and 30 epidemiological trials in elderly women, increasing calcium intake by 1000 mg/day decreased hip fracture risk by 24%.[111] The researchers state that this translates into "… an 8% reduction in hip fracture risk for every glass of milk [consumed] per day."[111]

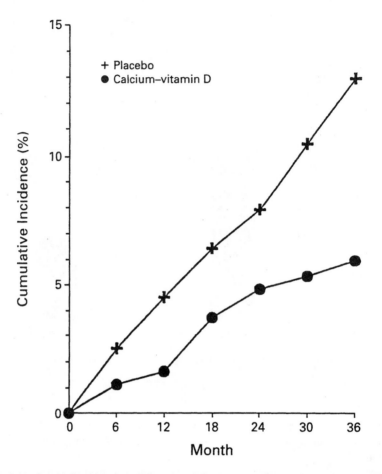

Figure 5.19 Cumulative percentage of all 389 subjects with a first nonvertebral fracture, according to study group. By 36 months, 26 of 202 subjects in the placebo group and 11 of 187 subjects in the calcium-vitamin D group had had a fracture (P = 0.02). (From Dawson-Hughes et al., *N. Engl. J. Med.,* 337, 670, 1997. With permission.)

The importance of adequate calcium intake in later years is supported by studies of age-related changes in the calcium economy.[189,190] Elevated blood levels of parathyroid hormone, which increases bone resorption, are thought to be typical of advancing age. However, in elderly women who had abnormally high blood levels of parathyroid hormone, increasing calcium intake by 1200 mg/day normalized blood parathyroid hormone levels.[189] Likewise, in another study, increasing elderly women's calcium intake to more than 2400 mg/day normalized parathyroid hormone levels and decreased bone resorption.[190]

Studies have examined the effect of dairy food intake on bone health of older adults. Bauer et al.,[173] in a comprehensive, cross-sectional study of over 9700 women over 65 years of age, found a positive association between current calcium intake from food, but not from supplements, and bone mass.[173] Women who reported drinking milk at every meal between the ages of 18 and 50 had a 3.1% higher bone mass after age 65 than women who reported rarely or never drinking milk.[173] Several other retrospective studies indicate that a higher bone density in later life is associated with a higher intake of milk in the early years.[9,134,135,191] Hu et al.[168] found that increasing dietary calcium, especially from dairy sources, increased bone mass in elderly women.

3. Vitamin D

It is recognized that vitamin D enhances calcium absorption and that a deficiency of this nutrient increases the risk for osteoporosis.[17,21,23,38,100] Numerous studies indicate that many older adults, especially those who do not get enough sun exposure because they are housebound, residents of nursing homes, or live in northern climates, are at risk of vitamin D deficiency.[17,23,172,192-197] The NAS[17] has issued new intake recommendations for vitamin D (Table 5.5). These recommendations are twice as high for adults 51 through 70 years (i.e., 10 µg or 400 IU/day) and three times higher for adults over 70 years (i.e., 15 µg or 600 IU/day) than in earlier adulthood and childhood years[17] or as previously recommended.[26] These higher dietary vitamin D recommendations, which assume limited availability from sun exposure, are intended to help reduce older adults' risk of bone-related disorders and fractures.[17]

Table 5.5   Vitamin D
Recommendations

Life-Stage Group	Adequate Intake (µg/day)
0 – 6 months	5
6 – 12 months	5
1 – 3 years	5
4 – 8 years	5
9 – 13 years	5
14 – 18 years	5
19 – 30 years	5
11 – 50 years	5
51 – 70 years	10
>70 years	15
Pregnancy	
<18 years	5
19 – 50 years	
Lactation	
<18 years	5
19 – 50 years	

From National Academy of Sciences, 1997.

Vitamin D is obtained from the diet as well as from cutaneous synthesis upon exposure to sunlight.[23,198] Important food sources of vitamin D include vitamin D enriched milk, eggs, fish oils, and liver.[23] Currently, 98% of the U.S. milk supply is voluntarily fortified with vitamin D at the level of 10 μg (400 IU) per quart. Fortified cow's milk is an important source of vitamin D for older adults because of its high acceptance and use by this population.[23] The importance of milk as a source of vitamin D was recently demonstrated in a multicenter osteoporosis trial involving 376 women aged 65 to 77 years.[199] In this trial, higher intakes of calcium from milk, but not from non-milk foods, were associated with increased levels of vitamin D and lower blood levels of parathyroid hormone.[199] The researchers attributed the findings to the fact that milk is a good source of vitamin D, accounting for 51% of dietary vitamin D intake in this study.[199] Vitamin D_3 (cholecalciferol) is synthesized from 7-dehydrocholesterol in the epidermis when the skin is exposed to ultraviolet light. Cholecalciferol then is successively hydroxylated in the liver and kidney to 1,25-dihydroxyvitamin D_3, the metabolically active form of vitamin D which stimulates intestinal absorption of calcium.[23,198] Skin biosynthesis of vitamin D is influenced by a number of factors including latitude, sun (UV) exposure, age, dress, season of the year, and skin melanin pigment.[17,23,195,198,200]

The aging population, especially institutionalized or in nursing homes, may be at risk for vitamin D deficiency because of inadequate dietary intake and/or limited exposure to sunlight without a compensatory increase in dietary vitamin D.[193-200] Also, several age-related physiological changes in vitamin D metabolism potentially compromise vitamin D status and/or increase the requirement for this vitamin. Low intake of vitamin D due to decreased consumption of vitamin D enriched dairy products can contribute to suboptimal vitamin D status in some older adults. Recent research indicates that vitamin D deficiency may be more widespread than previously suspected. Thomas et al.[201] reported that more than half of 290 hospitalized patients were deficient in vitamin D, even including some patients with high intakes of vitamin D. These findings indicate that even higher vitamin D intakes (i.e., 800 to 1000 IU/day) than currently recommended[17] may be beneficial for some individuals.[202]

Several studies indicate that increasing vitamin D intake of older adults enhances calcium absorption and reduces age-related bone loss or osteoporotic-related bone fractures.[101,172,174,192,203,204] In healthy postmenopausal women living in Boston, increasing vitamin D by 400 and 700 IU/day raised blood calcidiol levels (an index of vitamin D status) and reduced net bone loss from the spine[192] and hip during the winter months.[101] In another investigation, increasing vitamin D intake by 400 to 800 IU/day reduced vitamin D-induced secondary hyperparathyroidism and improved bone density in older adults.[204] A protective effect of vitamin D was demonstrated in two large controlled investigations of older adults in Europe, one of calcium and vitamin D[174] and the other of vitamin D alone.[203] As discussed above, nonvertebral and hip fractures were reduced by 30% and 41%, respectively, within two years in healthy ambulatory elderly women (mean age 84 years) in nursing homes in France who were supplemented with 800 IU (20 μg) vitamin D and 1200 mg calcium (Figure 5.18).[174] In a study in Finland where vitamin D deficiency among the aging population is common during the winter months, intramuscular vitamin D injections of single yearly doses equivalent to 400 to 800 IU/day maintained blood levels of 25-hydroxyvitamin D and significantly reduced the incidence of fractures.[203]

Based on available evidence, assuring an adequate intake of both calcium and vitamin D throughout life is estimated to reduce the fracture burden due to osteoporosis by 50% or more.[38] Vitamin D fortified milk is a major dietary source of both of these nutrients.

4. Treatment

An adequate intake of calcium and vitamin D is considered to be the mainstay of osteoporosis treatment.[100,205] All patients with this disease are encouraged to consume intakes of calcium and vitamin D meeting at least the amounts recommended by the NAS[17] or the NIH consensus levels.[18] Moreover, calcium is an important adjunct to treatment with medications such as alendronate (trade name Fosamax), calcitonin, and estrogen.[100,155-157,204,206] According to a recent meta-analysis of 31 estrogen studies and 7 calcitonin (an antiresorptive drug) trials, an adequate calcium intake potentiates the beneficial effect of estrogen and possibly calcitonin on bone mass.[157] In postmenopausal women who took estrogen combined with calcium (1183 mg/day) to treat osteoporosis, bone mass increased by 3.3% per year in the lumbar spine, by 2.4% per year in the femoral neck, and by 2.1% per year in the forearm (Figure 5.20).[157] Thus, bone mass increased two to five times more when the women taking estrogen also consumed nearly 1200 mg calcium/day. The findings indicate that the effectiveness of osteoporosis treatments such as estrogen is not fully realized unless adequate calcium is consumed. The results also underscore the conclusion that women taking estrogen after menopause need just as much calcium

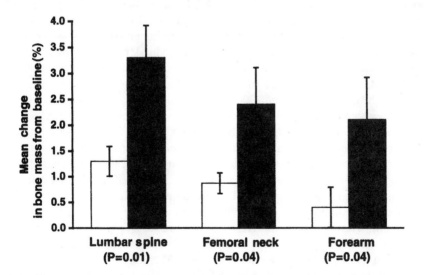

Figure 5.20 Mean (±SEM) annual percentage change in bone mass at the lumbar spine, femoral neck, and forearm in postmenopausal women treated with estrogen alone (□: total average calcium intake: 563 mg/d) compared with women treated with estrogen and calcium (■: total average calcium intake: 1183 mg/d). (From Nieves, J.W., et al., *Am. J. Clin. Nutr.*, 67, 18, 1998. With permission.)

as women not taking estrogen.[207] This is contrary to the 1994 consensus guidelines from the NIH[18] that recommended less calcium for postmenopausal women receiving hormone replacement therapy. The NAS[17] recently concluded that calcium recommendations for postmenopausal women are the same (i.e., 1200 mg/day) regardless of whether or not they are taking estrogen.

VI. SUMMARY

Because many available, approved treatments for osteoporosis do not significantly restore previous lost bone and/or have side effects, emphasis is placed on prevention of osteoporosis.[1] Research indicates that it is never too early or too late to reduce the risk of osteoporosis.[1,174] Prevention of this disease involves increasing peak bone mass at skeletal maturity which is reached by age 30 or earlier and reducing the rate of bone loss after menopause in women and in later years in both sexes. A variety of factors including diet, especially calcium and vitamin D, influence both peak bone mass and age-related bone loss. Meeting needs for these two nutrients, which are readily found in vitamin D fortified dairy products, is critical considering their important role in bone health and the economic advantages of reducing the risk of osteoporosis. In 1995, osteoporosis-related expenses amounted to $13.8 billion in the U.S. and are expected to exceed $60 billion by the year 2030 if preventive measures are not taken.[1]

Although the "optimal" calcium intake for skeletal health and prevention of osteoporosis is unknown, the Institute of Medicine, National Academy of Sciences (NAS) has released new calcium recommendations.[17] These calcium recommendations are based on intakes consistent with desirable calcium retention, which in turn, is associated with increased bone mass and reduced risk of osteoporosis. The NAS calcium recommendations are as follows: 800 mg/day for children 4 through 8 years, 1300 mg/day for children and adolescents 9 through 18 years, 1000 mg/day for adults 19 through 50 years, and 1200 mg/day for adults 51 years and over. Although the NAS calcium recommendations differ slightly from the 1994 NIH [18] "optimal" calcium intakes which are supported by the AMA[19] (Table 5.1), both sets of calcium recommendations support higher calcium intakes than the 1989 Recommended Dietary Allowances (RDAs).[26] Unfortunately, many Americans, particularly females of all ages, and older adults, do not consume recommended intakes of calcium.[67-73]

Major changes have been made in the recommendations for vitamin D in recognition of the importance of this vitamin in enhancing calcium absorption and maintaining a healthy skeleton.[17] The NAS recommends 5 µg (200 IU)/day of vitamin D for all adults 51 years of age and younger.[17] The vitamin D recommendation increases to 10 µg (400 IU)/day for adults ages 51 through 70 years, a level twice as high as in earlier adulthood and childhood years, or the 1989 RDAs. For adults over 70 years, 15 µg (600 IU)/day of vitamin D is recommended, or three times more than for individuals through age 50 or previously recommended (Table 5.5).[17,26] These higher vitamin D recommendations are intended to help reduce the risk of bone related disorders and osteoporotic fractures. However, many older adults are vitamin D deficient. Failure to consume sufficient servings of foods such as vitamin

D fortified milk contributes to deficiencies of vitamin D and calcium and increased risk of developing osteoporosis.

Foods are recognized as the best source of nutrients for bone and overall health.[18,19,88,176,205,208-210] A nutritionally balanced diet containing a variety of foods is recommended to meet the needs for calcium and other nutrients that may protect against osteoporosis. The NIH consensus statement on Optimal Calcium Intakes[18] states that " ... the preferred approach to attaining optimal calcium intake is through dietary sources." The AMA[19] concurs, stating that "... the preferred source of calcium is through calcium-rich foods such as dairy products." The 1995 *Dietary Guidelines for Americans*[208] states that "Many women and adolescent girls need to eat more calcium-rich foods to get the calcium needed for healthy bones throughout life. By selecting lowfat or fat-free milk products and other lowfat calcium sources, they can obtain adequate calcium and keep fat intake from being too high." The NAS,[17] in its new dietary recommendations for calcium and related nutrients, recognizes the importance of "unfortified foodstuffs" as the major source of calcium. The NAS explains that meeting calcium needs from foods offers the advantage of providing intakes of other beneficial nutrients and unidentified food components and possibly enhancing the body's use of nutrients through nutrient interactions.[17] For some individuals at high risk of osteoporosis who have difficulty meeting their calcium needs from foods either naturally containing this nutrient or fortified, use of calcium supplements may be desirable.[17]

Milk and other dairy foods are the major food source of calcium in the U.S. diet (Figure 5.1).[22] Dairy products such as fluid milk, cheese, and yogurt provided 73% of the calcium in the food supply in 1994.[22] Not only are milk and other dairy foods calcium-dense foods providing about 300 mg calcium per serving, but these foods also contain other nutrients important to bone health such as vitamin D (if fortified), protein, phosphorus, magnesium, vitamin A, vitamin B_6, and trace elements such as zinc.[88,209,211] Few foods other than milk and dairy products provide such a concentrated source of calcium that is readily available for absorption. The calcium from vegetables such as broccoli, bok choy, and kale is absorbed as well as or better than calcium from milk and milk products, but these foods have a significantly lower amount of calcium per serving.[65] Further, some plant sources of calcium may contain substances such as phytate (in wheat bran) and oxalate (in spinach) which reduce the availability of calcium.[17-19,38,62,65] In addition to calcium, vitamin D fortified dairy foods are a major source of vitamin D.[23,198] Also, because milk and milk products are a good source of other nutrients such as protein, phosphorus, magnesium, vitamin A, vitamin B_{12}, and trace elements such as zinc, their intake improves the overall quality of the diet.[74,75,86,88,212,213] Guthrie[74] reports that women whose diets meet their calcium recommendation consume significantly more servings of milk and milk products and more of several essential nutrients than women whose diets do not meet their calcium needs.

Diets low in calcium are commonly low in other essential nutrients as well and reflect overall poor dietary quality.[85-87,212,213] According to a study in Omaha, Nebraska in which 272 healthy Caucasian women kept food diaries for seven consecutive days, women consuming low calcium diets had lower intakes of many of the essential nutrients often delivered by dairy foods, vitamins A, C, B_6, B_{12}, thiamin, riboflavin, iron, magnesium, protein, and phosphorus.[212] An investigation in Portland, Oregon revealed that adults who included more dairy foods in their diet for at least 12 weeks increased not only their intake of calcium, but also magnesium, phosphorus, potassium, thiamin, riboflavin, and vitamins C and D.[87] In young females 13 to 18 years, milk drinkers had higher intakes of calcium, vitamin A, folate, riboflavin, B_6, B_{12}, magnesium, and potassium than non-milk drinkers.[75] More recently, postmenopausal women in Australia who increased their calcium intake to about 1600 mg/day with skim milk powder, also increased their intakes of protein, potassium, magnesium, phosphorus, riboflavin, thiamin, and zinc.[88] Dairy foods are good sources of many of these nutrients and, for this reason, their intake improves the overall nutritional adequacy of the diet.

Moreover, increasing calcium intake through dairy foods can easily be done without necessarily increasing calorie or fat intake, body weight, or percent body fat.[86-90] For example, Devine et al.[88] recently found that postmenopausal women could increase their calcium intake to 1600 mg/day by consuming skim milk powder without increasing their total fat or saturated fat intake. Similarly, studies in children and adolescents demonstrate that a high dairy food intake does not increase body weight or dietary fat intake.[87,89,90] When 9 to 12 year old girls increased their calcium intake to 1437 mg/day by consuming additional servings of dairy foods, including some higher-fat versions, they did not gain more weight or body fat, or increase the total fat content of their diets compared to those who ate their usual lower calcium diets (728 mg/day).[87]

Increasing dietary intake of calcium and vitamin D by consuming more servings of dairy foods is beneficial to bone health and is safe. The NAS has recently established Tolerable Upper Intake Levels (ULs) or the maximum intake of a nutrient or food component that is unlikely to pose risks of adverse health effects in almost all individuals in a specific group.[17] The ULs for calcium and vitamin D are 2500 mg/day and 50 µg/day, respectively.[17] Although calcium intakes up to 2500 mg/day are considered safe for almost all healthy individuals, Whiting and Wood[214] suggest that a high intake of calcium as obtained from calcium supplements or calcium-fortified foods may reduce the bioavailability of some minerals. However, other investigators have demonstrated that high calcium intakes do not interfere with the absorption of nutrients such as iron, zinc, and magnesium, especially over the long-term and when individuals are replete in these minerals.[17,215]

A high dietary intake of calcium has been suspected of increasing the risk of kidney stones. However, several studies indicate just the opposite, namely that a low calcium intake increases the risk of developing calcium oxalate kidney stones.[216-221] In a four-year prospective study involving over 45,000 men 40 to 75 years of age with no history of kidney stones, the incidence of kidney stones was 44% lower in men consuming the highest calcium intake (i.e., 1336 mg/day) than in those with the lowest calcium intakes (i.e., 516 mg/day).[216] Similarly, in a study of nearly 92,000 nurses with no history of kidney stones who participated in the Nurses' Health Study, those who consumed the most calcium from dairy foods (>1098 mg calcium/day) over 12 years were 35% less likely to develop stones than women who consumed less than 500 mg/day from their diets.[218] In this study, a greater intake of dairy products, the major source of dietary calcium, was associated with decreased risk of kidney stones.[218] Urinary oxalate is more important than urinary calcium for kidney stone formation.[217,219,221] When 21 adults with a history of kidney stones and normal urine calcium levels substituted $1^1/_2$ cups of skim milk for apple juice, urinary oxalate levels decreased by 18%.[219] Consuming milk and oxalate-rich foods (e.g., vegetables, beans, whole grains) at the same meal allows the calcium in milk to bind with oxalate rendering it unavailable for absorption.[219] The result is that urinary oxalate excretion and risk of kidney stones are reduced.[219] Findings of the above studies support the message that kidney stone patients should not restrict calcium intake, but should consume at least the recommended two to three servings of dairy foods, as indicated in USDA's *Food Guide Pyramid*.[79]

This chapter emphasizes the critical role of calcium and vitamin D, of which dairy foods are a major source, in protecting against osteoporosis. However, many other nutrients play a role in bone health. For example, trace elements may contribute to bone health,[211,222] certain fatty acids including those in milkfat may enhance bone growth,[223,224] and whey protein may increase bone health.[225] Dietary recommendations for bone health should therefore focus on the total diet rather than on single nutrients. An emphasis on a single nutrient rather than foods within the context of the total diet may perpetuate or create other nutritional problems.[33] To optimize bone health, a total healthful diet including recommended servings from a variety of foods from all the major food groups[79] and maintenance of a healthful lifestyle are advised.[33]

REFERENCES

1. National Osteoporosis Foundation, *Boning Up On Osteoporosis*, National Osteoporosis Foundation, Washington, D.C., 1997.
2. Christiansen, C., Skeletal osteoporosis, *J. Bone Miner. Res.*, 8(Suppl. 2), 475, 1993.
3. Looker, A. C., Orwoll, E. S., Johnston, C. C., Jr., Lindsay, R. L., Wahner, H. W., Dunn, W. L., Calvo, M. S., Harris, J. B., and Heyse, S. P., Prevalence of low femoral bone density in older U.S. adults from NHANES III, *J. Bone Miner. Res.*, 12, 1761, 1997.
4. Riggs, B. L. and Melton, L. J., III, The worldwide problem of osteoporosis: insights afforded by epidemiology. *Bone*, 17, 505s, 1995.
5. Melton, L. J., III, Thamer, M., Ray, N. F., Chan, J. K., Chesnut, C. H., III, Einhorn, T. A., Johnston, C. C., Jr., Raisz, L. G., Silverman, S. L., and Siris, E. S., Fractures attributable to osteoporosis: report from the National Osteoporosis Foundation, *J. Bone Miner. Res.*, 12, 16, 1997.
6. Ray, N. F., Chan, J. K., Thamer, M., and Melton, L. J., III, Medical expenditures for the treatment of osteoporotic fractures in the United States in 1995: Report from the National Osteoporosis Foundation, *J. Bone Miner. Res.*, 12, 24, 1997.
7. Gullberg, B., Johnell, O., and Kanis, J. A., World-wide projections for hip fracture, *Osteoporosis Int.*, 7, 407, 1997.
8. Krall, E. A. and Dawson-Hughes, B., Heritable and life-style determinants of bone mineral density, *J. Bone Miner. Res.*, 8, 1, 1993.
9. Johnell, O., Gullberg, B., Kanis, J. A., Allander, E., Elffors, L., Dequeker, J., Dilsen, G., Gennari, C., Vaz, A. L., Lyritis, G., Mazzuoli, G., Miravet, L., Passeri, M., Cano, R. P., Rapado, A., and Ribot, C., Risk factors for hip fracture in European women: The MEDOS study, *J. Bone Miner. Res.*, 10, 1802, 1995.

10. Salamone, L. M., Glynn, N. W., Black, D. M., Ferrell, R. E., Palermo, L., Epstein, R. S., Kuller, L. H., and Cauley, J. A., Determinants of premenopausal bone mineral density: the interplay of genetic and lifestyle factors, *J. Bone Miner. Res.*, 11, 1557, 1996.

11. Hopper, J. L., Green, R. M., Nowson, C. A., Young, D., Sherwin, A. J., Kaymakci, B., Larkins, R. G., and Wark, J. D., Genetic, common environment, and individual specific components of variance for bone mineral density in 10- to 26-year-old females: a twin study, *Am. J. Epidemiol.*, 147, 17, 1998.

12. Eisman, J. A., Vitamin D polymorphisms and calcium homeostasis: a new concept of normal gene variants and physiologic variation, *Nutr. Rev.*, 56, 22s, 1998.

13. Riggs, B., Vitamin D-receptor genotypes and bone density, *N. Engl. J. Med.*, 337, 125, 1997.

14. Sainz, J., Van Tornout, J. M., Loro, M. L., Sayre, J., Roe, T. F., and Gilsanz, V., Vitamin D-receptor gene polymorphisms and bone density in prepubertal American girls of Mexican descent, *N. Engl. J. Med.*, 337, 77, 1997.

15. Wishart, J. M., Horowitz, M., Need, A. G., Scopacasa, F., Morris, H. A., Clifton, P. M., and Nordin, B. E. C., Relations between calcium intake, calcitriol, polymorphisms of the vitamin D-receptor gene, and calcium absorption in premenopausal women, *Am. J. Clin. Nutr.*, 65, 798, 1997.

16. O'Brien, K. O., Abrams, S. A., Liang, L. K., Ellis, K. J., and Gagel, R. F., Bone turnover response to changes in calcium intake is altered in girls and adult women in families with histories of osteoporosis, *J. Bone Miner. Res.*, 13, 491, 1998.

17. IOM (Institute of Medicine), *Dietary Reference Intakes for Calcium, Phosphorus, Magnesium, Vitamin D, and Fluoride*, Standing Committee on the Scientific Evaluation of Dietary Reference Intakes, Food and Nutrition Board, National Academy Press, Washington, D.C., 1997.

18. U.S. Department of Health and Human Services, Public Health Service, National Institutes of Health, *Consensus Development Conference Statement, Optimal Calcium Intake*, June 6-8, 12(4), 1, 1994.

19. American Medical Association, Council on Scientific Affairs, Intake of dietary calcium to reduce the incidence of osteoporosis, *Arch. Fam. Med.*, 6, 495, 1997.

20. U.S. Department of Health and Human Services, Food and Drug Administration, Food labeling: health claims; calcium and osteoporosis, *Fed. Register*, 58(3) (Jan 6), 2665, 1993.

21. Heaney, R. P., Evaluation of publicly available scientific evidence regarding certain nutrient-disease relationships: 3. calcium and osteoporosis, Life Sciences Research Office, Federation of American Societies for Experimental Biology, Bethesda, MD, December 1991.

22. Gerrior, S. and Bente, L., *Nutrient Content of the U.S. Food Supply, 1909-94.* Home Economics Research Report No. 53, Washington, D.C., U.S. Department of Agriculture, Center for Nutrition Policy and Promotion, 1997.

23. Anderson, J. J. B. and Toverud, S. U., Diet and vitamin D: a review with an emphasis on human function, *J. Nutr. Biochem.*, 5, 58, 1994.

24. Chen, T. C., Heath, H., III, and Holick, M. F., An update on the vitamin D content of fortified milk from the United States and Canada, *N. Engl. J. Med.*, 329, 1507, 1993.

25. U.S. Department of Health and Human Services, Public Health Service, Food and Drug Administration, *Grade "A" Pasteurized Milk Ordinance, 1995 Revision*, Publ. No. 229, Washington, D.C., USDHHS, PHS, FDA, 1995.

26. Food and Nutrition Board, *Subcommittee on the Tenth Edition of the RDAs, National Research Council, Recommended Dietary Allowances*, 10th Edition, National Academy Press, Washington, D.C., 1989.
27. Kennedy, E. and Powell, R., Changing eating patterns of American children: a view from 1996, *J. Am. Coll. Nutr.*, 16, 524, 1997.
28. Matkovic, V., Nutrition, genetics and skeletal development, *J. Am. Coll. Nutr.*, 15, 556, 1996.
29. Heaney, R. P., Calcium in the prevention and treatment of osteoporosis, *J. Intern. Med.*, 231, 169, 1992.
30. Haapasalo, H., Kannus, P., Sievanen, H., Pasanen, M., Uusi-Rasi, K., Heinonen, A., Oja, P., and Vuori, I., Development of mass, density, and estimated mechanical characteristics of bones in Caucasian females, *J. Bone Miner. Res.*, 11, 1751, 1996.
31. Matkovic, V., Tomislav, J., Wardlaw, G. M., Ilich, J. Z., Goel, P. K., Wright, J. K., Andon, M. B., Smith, K. T., and Heaney, R. P., Timing of peak bone mass in Caucasian females and its implication for the prevention of osteoporosis, *J. Clin. Invest.*, 93, 799, 1994.
32. Bilezikian, J. P., Estrogens and postmenopausal osteoporosis: was Albright right after all? *J. Bone Miner. Res.*, 13, 774, 1998.
33. Miller, G. D., Groziak, S. M., and DiRienzo, D., Age considerations in nutrient needs for bone health, *J. Am. Coll. Nutr.*, 15, 553, 1996.
34. Raisz, L. G., The osteoporosis revolution, *Ann. Intern. Med.*, 126, 458, 1997.
35. Heaney, R. P., Recker, P. R., Stegman, M. R., and Moy, A. J., Calcium absorption in women: relationships to calcium intake, estrogen status, and age, *J. Bone Miner. Res.*, 4, 469, 1989.
36. Weaver, C. M., Age-related calcium requirements due to changes in absorption and utilization, *J. Nutr.*, 124, 1418s, 1994.
37. Greendale, G. A., Edelstein, S., and Barrett-Connor, E., Endogenous sex steroids and bone mineral density in older women and men: The Rancho Bernardo Study, *J. Bone Miner. Res.*, 12, 1833, 1997.
38. Heaney, R. P., Bone mass, nutrition, and other lifestyle factors, *Nutr. Rev.*, 54(4), 3, 1996.
39. Ricci, T. A., Chowdhury, H. A., Heymsfield, S. B., Stahl, T., Pierson, R. N., Jr., and Shapses, S. A., Calcium supplementation suppresses bone turnover during weight reduction in postmenopausal women, *J. Bone Miner. Res.*, 13, 1045, 1998.
40. Dawson-Hughes, B., Krall, E. A., and Harris, S., Risk factors for bone loss in healthy postmenopausal women, *Osteoporosis Int.*, Suppl. 1, 27s, 1993.
41. Barrett-Connor, E., Chang, J. C., and Edelstein, S. L., Coffee-associated osteoporosis offset by daily milk consumption, *JAMA*, 271, 280, 1994.
42. Barger-Lux, M. J. and Heaney, R. P., Caffeine and the calcium economy revisited, *Osteoporosis Int.*, 5, 97, 1995.
43. Lloyd, T., Rollings, N., Eggli, D. E., Kieselhorst, K., and Chinchilli, V. M., Dietary caffeine intake and bone status of postmenopausal women, *Am. J. Clin. Nutr.*, 65, 1826, 1997.
44. Hopper, J. L. and Seeman, E., The bone density of female twins discordant for tobacco use, *N. Engl. J. Med.*, 330, 387, 1994.
45. Vogel, J. M., Davis, J. W., Nomura, A., Wasnich, R. D., and Ross, P. D., The effects of smoking on bone mass and the rates of bone loss among elderly Japanese-American men, *J. Bone Miner. Res.*, 12, 1495, 1997.

46. Law, M. R. and Hackshaw, A. K., A meta-analysis of cigarette-smoking, bone mineral density and risk of hip fracture: recognition of a major effect, *Br. Med. J.*, 315, 841, 1997.

47. Hollenbach, K. A., Barrett-Connor, E., Edelstein, S. L., and Holbrook, T., Cigarette smoking and bone mineral density in older men and women, *Am. J. Publ. Health*, 83, 1265, 1993.

48. Hirsch, P. E. and Peng, T. C., Effects of alcohol on calcium homeostasis and bone, In *Calcium and Phosphorus in Health and Disease*, Anderson, J.J.B. and Garner, S.C. Eds., CRC Press, Boca Raton, FL, 1996, 289-300.

49. Nelson, M. E., Fisher, E. C., Dilmanian, F. A., Dallal, G. E., and Evans, W. J., A 1-y walking program and increased dietary calcium in postmenopausal women: effects on bone, *Am. J. Clin. Nutr.*, 53, 1304, 1991.

50. Prince, R. L., Smith, M., Dick, I. M., Price, R. I., Webb, P. G., Henderson, N. K., and Harris, M. M., A comparative study of exercise, calcium supplementation, and hormone-replacement therapy, *N. Engl. J. Med.*, 325, 1189, 1991.

51. Specker, B. L., Evidence for an interaction between calcium intake and physical activity on changes in bone mineral density, *J. Bone Miner. Res.*, 11(10), 1539, 1996.

52. Uusi-Rasi, K., Sievanen, H., Vuori, I., Pasanen, M., Heinonen, A., and Oja, P., Associations of physical activity and calcium intake with bone mass and size in healthy women at different ages, *J. Bone Miner. Res.*, 13(1), 133, 1998.

53. Matkovic, V., Ilich, J. Z., Andon, M. D., Hsieh, L. C., Tzagournis, M. A., Lagger, B. J., and Goel, P. K., Urinary calcium, sodium and bone mass of young females, *Am. J. Clin. Nutr.*, 62, 417, 1995.

54. Devine, A., Criddle, R. A., Dick, I. M., Kerr, D. A., and Prince, R. L., A longitudinal study of the effect of sodium and calcium intakes on regional bone density in post-menopausal women, *Am. J. Clin. Nutr.*, 62, 740, 1995.

55. Heaney, R. P., Protein intake and the calcium economy, *J. Am. Diet. Assoc.*, 93, 1259, 1993.

56. Whiting, S. J., Anderson, D. J., and Weeks, S. J., Calciuric effects of protein and potassium bicarbonate but not of sodium chloride or phosphate can be detected acutely in adult women and men, *Am. J. Clin. Nutr.*, 65, 1465, 1997.

57. Itoh, R., Nishiyama, N., and Suyama, Y., Dietary protein intake and urinary excretion of calcium: a cross-sectional study in a healthy Japanese population, *Am. J. Clin. Nutr.*, 67, 438, 1998.

58. Massey, L. K., Does excess dietary protein adversely affect bone? Symposium overview, *J. Nutr.*, 128, 1048, 1998.

59. Heaney, R. P., Dietary protein may not adversely affect bone, *J. Nutr.*, 128, 1054, 1998.

60. Duff, T. L. and Whiting, S. J., Calciuric effects of short-term dietary loading of protein, sodium chloride and potassium citrate in prepubertal girls, *J. Am. Coll. Nutr.*, 17, 148, 1998.

61. Schurch, M.-A., Rizzoli, R., Slosman, D., Vadas, L., Vergnaud, P., and Bonjour, J.-P., Protein supplements increase serum insulin-like growth factor-1 levels and attenuate proximal femur bone loss in patients with recent hip fracture, *Ann. Intern. Med.*, 128, 801, 1998.

62. Heaney, R. P., Weaver, C. M., and Recker, R. R., Calcium absorbability from spinach, *Am. J. Clin. Nutr.*, 47, 707, 1988.

63. Weaver, C. M., Heaney, R. P., Martin, B. R., and Fitzsimmons, M. L., Human calcium absorption from whole-wheat products, *J. Nutr.*, 121, 1769, 1991.

64. Weaver, C. M., Heaney, R. P., Teegarden, D., and Hinders, S. M., Wheat bran abolishes the inverse relationship between calcium load size and absorption fraction in women, *J. Nutr.*, 126, 303, 1996.

65. Weaver, C. M. and Plawecki, K. L., Dietary calcium: adequacy of a vegetarian diet, *Am. J. Clin. Nutr.*, 59s, 1238, 1994.

66. Martin, A. D., Bailey, D. A., McKay, H. A., and Whiting, S., Bone mineral and calcium accretion during puberty, *Am. J. Clin. Nutr.*, 66, 611, 1997.

67. Alaimo, K., McDowell, M. A., Briefel, R. R., Bischof, A. M., Caughman, C. R., Loria, C. M., and Johnson, C. L., Dietary intake of vitamins, minerals, and fiber of persons ages 2 months and over in the United States: Third National Health and Nutrition Examination Survey, Phase I, 1988-91. Advance Data from Vital and Health Statistics, No. 258, National Center for Health Statistics, Hyattsville, MD, 1994.

68. Enns, C. W., Goldman, J. D., and Cook, A., Trends in food and nutrient intakes by adults: NFCS 1977-78, CSFII 1989-91, and CSFII 1994-95, *Family Econ. Nut. Rev.*, 10, 2, 1997.

69. U.S. Department of Agriculture, Agricultural Research Service, Data tables: Results from USDA's 1994-96 Continuing Survey of Food Intakes by Individuals and 1994-96 Diet and Health Knowledge Survey, 1997, ARS Food Surveys Research Group, www.barc.usda.gov/bhnrc/foodsurvey/home.htm, December 1997.

70. Pennington, J. A. T., Intakes of minerals from diets and foods: is there a need for concern? *J. Nutr.*, 2304s, 1996.

71. Federation of American Societies for Experimental Biology, Life Sciences Research Office, Prepared for the Interagency Board for Nutrition Monitoring and Related Research, *Third Report on Nutrition Monitoring in the United States: Executive Summary.* U.S. Government Printing Office, Washington, D.C., 1995.

72. Lin, B.-H., Guthrie, J., and Blaylock, J. R., The diets of America's children, *Agricultural Economic Report No. 746*, December 1996.

73. Albertson, A. M., Tobelmann, R. C., and Marquart, L., Estimated dietary calcium intake and food sources for adolescent females: 1980–92, *J. Adol. Health*, 20, 20, 1997.

74. Guthrie, J. E., Dietary patterns and personal characteristics of women consuming recommended amounts of calcium, *Family Econ. and Nutr. Rev.*, 9, 33, 1996.

75. Fleming, K. H. and Heimbach, J. T., Consumption of calcium in the U.S.: food sources and intake levels, *J. Nutr.*, 124(8)s, 1426s, 1994.

76. Barr, S. I., Associations of social and demographic variables with calcium intakes of high school students, *J. Am. Diet. Assoc.*, 94, 260, 269, 1994.

77. Schwenk, N. E., Children's diets, *Family Econ. and Nutr. Rev.*, 10, 34, 1997.

78. U.S. Department of Agriculture, Agricultural Research Service, Pyramid Servings Data, Results from USDA's 1995 and 1996 Continuing Survey of Food Intakes by Individuals, Riverdale, MD: U.S. Department of Agriculture, www.barc.usda.gov/bhnrc/foodsurvey/home.htm, 1997.

79. U.S. Department of Agriculture, Human Nutrition Information Service, *The Food Guide Pyramid.* Home and Garden Bulletin No. 52, Government Printing Office, Washington, D.C., 1992.

80. Bowman, S. A., Lino, M., Gerrior, S. A., and Basiotis, P. P., *The Healthy Eating Index: 1994–96,* U.S. Department of Agriculture, Center for Nutrition Policy and Promotion, CNPP-5, July 1998.

81. Skiba, A., Loghmani, E., and Orr, D. P., Nutritional screening and guidance for adolescents, *Adol. Health Update*, 9, 1, 1997.

82. American Heart Association, *AHA Healthy Heart Food Pyramid*, American Heart Association, 1997.

83. Horwath, C. C., Govan, C. H., Campbell, A. J., Busby, W., and Scott, V., Factors influencing milk and milk product consumption in young and elderly women with low calcium intakes, *Nutr. Res.*, 15(2), 1735, 1995.

84. Chapman, K. M., Chan, M. W., and Clark, C. D., Factors influencing dairy calcium intake in women, *J. Am. Coll. Nutr.*, 14, 336, 1995.

85. Miller, G. D., Steinbach, T. T., and Jarvis, J. K., The challenge: motivating women to increase calcium intake from dairy foods, *J. Am. Coll. Nutr.*, 14, 309, 1995.

86. Karanja, N., Morris, C. D., Rufolo, P., Snyder, G., Illingworth, D. R., and McCarron, D. A., Impact of increasing calcium in the diet on nutrient consumption, plasma lipids, and lipoproteins in humans, *Am. J. Clin. Nutr.*, 59, 900, 1994.

87. Chan, G. M., Hoffman, K., and McMurray, M., Effects of dairy products on bone and body composition in pubertal girls, *J. Pediatr.*, 126, 551, 1995.

88. Devine, A., Prince, R. L., and Bell, R., Nutritional effect of calcium supplementation by skim milk powder or calcium tablets on total nutrient intake in postmenopausal women, *Am. J. Clin. Nutr.*, 64, 731, 1996.

89. Badenhop, N. E., Ilich, J. Z., Skugor, M., Landoll, J. D., and Matkovic, V., Changes in body composition and serum leptin in young females with high vs. low dairy intake, *J. Bone Miner. Res.*, 12, 487s, 1997 (Abst. # S537).

90. Cadogan, J., Eastell, R., Jones, N., and Barker, M. E., Milk intake and bone mineral acquisition in adolescent girls: randomized, controlled intervention trial, *Br. Med. J.*, 315, 1255, 1997.

91. Honkanen, R., Kroger, H., Alhava, E., Turpeinen, P., Tuppurainen, M., and Saarikoski, S., Lactose intolerance associated with fractures of weight-bearing bones in Finnish women aged 38-57 years, *Bone*, 21, 473, 1997.

92. Suarez, F. L., Savaiano, D. A., and Levitt, M. D., A comparison of symptoms after the consumption of milk or lactose-hydrolyzed milk by people with self-reported severe lactose intolerance, *N. Engl. J. Med.*, 333, 1, 1995.

93. Suarez, F. L., Savaiano, D., Arbisi, P., and Levitt, M. D., Tolerance to the daily ingestion of two cups of milk by individuals claiming lactose intolerance, *Am. J. Clin. Nutr.*, 65, 1502, 1997.

94. McBean, L. D. and Miller, G. D., Allaying fears and fallacies about lactose intolerance, *J. Am. Diet. Assoc.*, 98, 671, 1998.

95. Tepper, B. J. and Nayga, R. M., Jr., Awareness of the link between bone disease and calcium intake is associated with higher dietary calcium intake in women aged 50 years and older: results of the 1991 CSFII-DHKS, *J. Am. Diet. Assoc.*, 98, 196, 1998.

96. Harel, Z., Riggs, S., Vaz, R., White, L., and Menzies, G., Adolescents and calcium: what they do and do not know and how much they consume, *J. Adol. Health*, 22, 225, 1998.

97. Ulrich, C. M., Georgiou, C. G., Snow-Harter, C. M., and Gillis, D. E., Bone mineral density in mother-daughter pairs: relations to lifetime exercise, lifetime milk consumption, and calcium supplements, *Am. J. Clin. Nutr.*, 63, 72, 1996.

98. Haines, P. S., Hungerford, D. W., Popkin B. M., and Guilkey, D. K., Eating patterns and energy and nutrient intakes of U.S. women, *J. Am. Diet. Assoc.*, 92, 698, 1992.

99. Heaney, R. P., Nutritional factors in bone health in elderly subjects: methodological and contextual problems, *Am. J. Clin. Nutr.*, 50, 1182, 1989.

100. Heaney, R. P., Nutritional factors in osteoporosis, *Annu. Rev. Nutr.*, 13, 287, 1993.

101. Dawson-Hughes, B., Harris, S. S., Krall, E. A., Dallal, G. E., Falconer, G., and Green, C. L., Rates of bone loss in postmenopausal women randomly assigned to one or two dosages of vitamin D, *Am. J. Clin. Nutr.*, 61, 1140, 1995.

102. Ettinger, B., Genant, H. K., and Cann, C. E., Postmenopausal bone loss is prevented by treatment with low-dosage estrogen with calcium, *Ann. Intern. Med.*, 106, 40, 1987.

103. Ettinger, B., Genant, H. K., Steiger, P., and Madvig, P., Low-dosage micronized 17B-estradiol prevents bone loss in postmenopausal women, *Am. J. Obstet. Gynecol.*, 166, 479, 1992.

104. Riis, B., Thomsen, K., and Christiansen, C., Does calcium supplementation prevent postmenopausal bone loss? *N. Engl. J. Med.*, 316, 173, 1987.

105. Dawson-Hughes, B., Dallal, G. E., Krall, E. A., Sadowski, L., Sahyoun, N., and Tannenbaum, S., A controlled trial of the effect of calcium supplementation on bone density in postmenopausal women, *N. Engl. J. Med.*, 323, 878, 1990.

106. Ooms, M. E., Lips, P., van Lingen, A., and Valkenburg, H. A., Determinants of bone mineral density and risk factors for osteoporosis in healthy elderly women, *J. Bone Miner. Res.*, 8, 669, 1993.

107. Bonjour, J.-P., Carrie, A.-L., Ferrari, S., Clavien, H., Slosman, D., Theintz, G., and Rizzoli, R., Calcium-enriched foods and bone mass growth in prepubertal girls: a randomized, double-blind, placebo-controlled trial, *J. Clin. Invest.*, 99, 1287, 1997.

108. Heaney, R. P., The bone remodeling transient: implications for the interpretation of clinical studies of bone mass change, *J. Bone Miner. Res.*, 9, 1515, 1994.

109. Lee, W. T. K., Leung, S. S. F., Leung, D. M. Y., and Cheng, J. C. Y., A follow-up study on the effects of calcium-supplement withdrawal and puberty on bone acquisition of children, *Am. J. Clin. Nutr.*, 64, 71, 1996.

110. Lee, W. T. K., Leung, S. S. F., Leung, D. M. Y., Wang, S.-H., Xu, Y.-C., Zeng, W.-P., and Cheng, J. C. Y., Bone mineral acquisition in low calcium intake children following the withdrawal of calcium supplement, *Acta Paediatr.*, 86, 570, 1997.

111. Cumming, R. G. and Nevitt, M. C., Calcium for prevention of osteoporotic fractures in postmenopausal women, *J. Bone Miner. Res.*, 12, 1321, 1997.

112. Heaney, R. P., Nutrient effects: discrepancy between data from controlled trials and observational studies, *Bone*, 21, 469, 1997.

113. Matkovic, V., Calcium and peak bone mass, *J. Intern. Med.*, 231, 151, 1992.

114. Fassler, A.-L. and Bonjour, J.-P., Osteoporosis as a pediatric problem, *Pediatr. Clin. N. Am.*, 42, 811, 1995.

115. Johnston, C. C., Jr., Miller, J. Z., Slemenda, C. W., Reister, T. K., Hui, S., Christian, J. C., and Peacock, M., Calcium supplementation and increases in bone mineral density in children, *N. Engl. J. Med.*, 327, 82, 1992.

116. Lee, W. T. K., Leung, S. S. F., Wang, S. H., Xu, Y. C., Zeng, W. P., Lau, J., Oppenheimer, S. J., and Cheng, J., Double-blind controlled calcium supplementation and bone mineral accretion in children accustomed to low calcium diet, *Am. J. Clin. Nutr.*, 60, 744, 1994.

117. Slemenda, C. W., Peacock, M., Hui, S., Zhou, L., and Johnston, C. C., Jr., Reduced rates of skeletal remodeling are associated with increased bone density during the development of peak skeletal mass, *J. Bone Miner. Res.*, 12, 676, 1997.

118. Matkovic, V. and Heaney, R. P., Calcium balance during human growth: evidence for threshold behavior, *Am. J. Clin. Nutr.*, 55, 992, 1992.

119. Andon, M. B., Lloyd, T., and Matkovic, V., Supplementation trials with calcium citrate malate: evidence in favor of increasing the calcium RDA during childhood and adolescence, *J. Nutr.*, 124, 1412s, 1994.

120. Lu, P. W., Briody, J. N., Ogle, G. D., Morley, K., Humphries, I. R., Allen, J., Howman-Giles, R., Sillence, D., and Cowell, C. T., Bone mineral density of total body, spine, and femoral neck in children and young adults: a cross-sectional and longitudinal study, *J. Bone Miner. Res.*, 9, 1451, 1994.

121. Weaver, C. M., Martin, B. R., Plawecki, K. L., Peacock, M., Wood, O. B., Smith, D. L., and Wastney, M. E., Differences in calcium metabolism between adolescent and adult females, *Am. J. Clin. Nutr.*, 61, 577, 1995.

122. Abrams, S. A. and Stuff, J. E., Calcium metabolism in girls: current dietary intakes lead to low rates of calcium absorption and retention during puberty, *Am. J. Clin. Nutr.*, 60, 739, 1994.

123. Abrams, S. A., Grusak, M. A., Stuff, J., and O'Brien, K. O., Calcium and magnesium balance in 9-14-y-old children, *Am. J. Clin. Nutr.*, 66, 1172, 1997.

124. Matkovic, V., Calcium metabolism and calcium requirements during skeletal modeling and consolidation of bone mass, *Am. J. Clin. Nutr.*, 54(Suppl.), 245, 1991.

125. Matkovic, V., Fontana, D., Tominac, C., Goel, P., and Chesnut, C. H., III, Factors that influence peak bone mass formation: a study of calcium balance and the inheritance of bone mass in adolescent females, *Am. J. Clin. Nutr.*, 52, 878, 1990.

126. Lloyd, T., Andon, M. B., Rollings, N., Martel, K., Landis, R., Demers, L. M., Eggli, D. F., Kieselhorst, K., and Kulin, H. E., Calcium supplementation and bone mineral density in adolescent girls, *JAMA*, 270, 841, 1993.

127. Jackman, L. A., Millane, S. S., Martin, B. R., Wood, O. B., McCabe, G. P., Peacock, M., and Weaver, C. M., Calcium retention in relation to calcium intake and postmenarcheal age in adolescent females, *Am. J. Clin. Nutr.*, 66, 327, 1997.

128. Nieves, J. W., Golden, A. L., Siris, E., Kelsey, J. L., and Lindsay, R., Teenage and current calcium intakes are related to bone mineral density of the hip and forearm in women aged 30-39, *Am. J. Epidemiol.*, 141, 342, 1995.

129. Nowson, C. A., Green, R. M., Hopper, J. L., Sherwin, A. J., Young, D., Kaymakci, B., Guest, C. S., Smid, M., Larkins, R. G., and Wark, J. D., A co-twin study of the effect of calcium supplementation on bone density during adolescence, *Osteoporosis Int.*, 7, 219, 1997.

130. Matkovic, V., Kostial, K., Simonovic, I., Buzina, R., Brodarec, A., and Nordin, B. E. C., Bone status and fracture rates in two regions of Yugoslavia, *Am. J. Clin. Nutr.*, 32, 540, 1979.

131. Sandler, R. B., Slemenda, C. W., LaPorte, R. E., Cauley, J. A., Schramm, M. M., Barresi, M. L., and Kriska, A. M., Postmenopausal bone density and milk consumption in childhood and adolescence, *Am. J. Clin. Nutr.*, 42, 270, 1985.

132. Halioua, L. and Anderson, J. J. B., Lifetime calcium intake and physical activity habits: independent and combined effects on the radial bone of healthy premenopausal Caucasian women, *Am. J. Clin. Nutr.*, 49, 534, 1989.

133. Fehily, A. M., Coles, R. J., Evans, W. D., and Elwood, P. C., Factors affecting bone density in young adults, *Am. J. Clin. Nutr.*, 56, 579, 1992.

134. Murphy, S., Kay-Tee, K., May, H., and Compston, J. E., Milk consumption and bone mineral density in middle aged and elderly women, *Br. Med. J.*, 308, 939, 1994.

135. Soroko, S., Holbrook, T. L., Edelstein, S., and Barrett-Connor, E., Lifetime milk consumption and bone mineral density in older women, *Am. J. Public Health*, 84, 1319, 1994.

136. Kerstetter, J. E. and Insogna, K., Do dairy products improve bone density in adolescent girls? *Nutr. Rev.*, 53, 328, 1995.

137. Stracke, H., Renner, E., Knie, G., Leidig, G., Minne, H., and Federlin, K., Osteoporosis and bone metabolic parameters in dependence upon calcium intake through milk and milk products, *Europ. J. Clin. Nutr.*, 47, 617, 1993.

138. New, S. A., Bolton-Smith, C., Grubb, D. A., and Reid, D. M., Nutritional influences on bone mineral density: a cross-sectional study in premenopausal women, *Am. J. Clin. Nutr.*, 65, 1831, 1997.

139. Matkovic, V. and Ilich, J. Z., Calcium requirements for growth: are current recommendations adequate? *Nutr. Rev.*, 51: 171, 1993.

140. Weaver, C. M., Martin, B. R., Plawecki, K. L., Peacock, M., Wood, O. B., Smith, D. L., and Wastney, M. E., Differences in calcium metabolism between adolescent and adult females, *Am. J. Clin. Nutr.*, 61, 577, 1995.

141. Miller, G. D. and Weaver, C. M., Required versus optimal intakes: a look at calcium, *J. Nutr.*, 124, 1404s, 1994.

142. Recker, R. R., Davies, K. M., Hinders, S. M., Heaney, R. P., Stegman, M. R., and Kimmel, D. B., Bone gain in young adult women, *JAMA*, 268, 2403, 1992.

143. Metz, J. A., Anderson, J. J. B., and Gallagher, P. N., Jr., Intakes of calcium, phosphorus, and protein, and physical activity level are related to radial bone mass in young adult women, *Am. J. Clin. Nutr.*, 58, 537, 1993.

144. Hirota, T., Nara, M., Ohguri, M., Manago, E., and Hirota, K., Effect of diet and lifestyle on bone mass in Asian young women, *Am. J. Clin. Nutr.*, 55, 1168, 1992.

145. Tylavsky, F. A., Anderson, J. J. B., Talmage, R. V., and Taft, T. N., Are calcium intakes and physical activity patterns during adolescence related to radial bone mass of white college-age females? *Osteoporosis Int.*, 2, 232, 1992.

146. Anderson, J. J. B. and Rondano, P. A., Peak bone mass development of females: can young adult women improve their peak bone mass? *J. Am. Coll. Nutr.*, 15, 570, 1996.

147. Davis, J. W., Novotny, R., Ross, P. D., and Wasnich, R. D., Anthropometric, lifestyle and menstrual factors influencing size-adjusted bone mineral content in a multiethnic population of premenopausal women, *J. Nutr.*, 126, 2968, 1996.

148. Anderson, J. J. B., Calcium, phosphorus, and human bone development, *J. Nutr.*, 126, 1153, 1996.

149. Welten, D. C., Kemper, H. C. G., Post, G., and Van Staveren, W. A., A meta-analysis of the effect of calcium intake on bone mass in young and middle aged females and males, *J. Nutr.*, 125, 2802, 1995.

150. Baran, D., Sorensen, A., Grimes, J., Lew, R., Karellas, A., Johnson, B., and Roche, J., Dietary modification with dairy products for preventing vertebral bone loss in premenopausal women: a three-year prospective study, *J. Clin. Endocrinol. Metab.*, 70, 264, 1990.

151. Feskanich, D., Willett, W. C., Stampfer, M. J., and Colditz, G. A., Milk, dietary calcium, and bone fractures in women: a 12-year prospective study, *Am. J. Public Health*, 87, 992, 1997.

152. Dawson-Hughes, B., Calcium and vitamin D nutritional needs of elderly women, *J. Nutr.*, 126, 1165s, 1996.

153. van Beresteijn, E. C. H., van't Hof, M. A., Schaafsma, G., de Waard, H., and Duursma, S. A., Habitual dietary calcium intake and cortical bone loss in perimenopausal women: a longitudinal study, *Calcif. Tissue Int.*, 47, 338, 1990.

154. Elders, P. J. M., Netelenbos, J. C., Lips, P., van Ginkel, F. C., Khoe, E., Leeuwenkamp, O. R., Hackeng, W. H. L., and van der Stelt, P. F., Calcium supplementation reduces vertebral bone loss in perimenopausal women: a controlled trial in 248 women between 46 and 55 years of age, *J. Clin. Endocrinol. Metab.*, 73, 533, 1991.

155. Aloia, J. F., Vaswani, A., Yeh, J. K., Ross, P. L., Flaster, E., and Dilmanian, F. A., Calcium supplementation with and without hormone replacement therapy to prevent postmenopausal bone loss, *Ann. Intern. Med.*, 120, 97, 1994.

156. Davis, J. W., Ross, P. D., Johnson, N. E., and Wasnich, R. D., Estrogen and calcium use among Japanese-American women: effects upon bone loss when used singly and in combination, *Bone*, 17(4), 369, 1995.

157. Nieves, J. W., Komar, L., Cosman, F., and Lindsay, R., Calcium potentiates the effect of estrogen and calcitonin on bone mass: review and analysis, *Am. J. Clin. Nutr.*, 67, 18, 1998.

158. Reid, I. R., Ames, R. W., Evans, M. C., Gamble, G. D., and Sharpe, S. J., Effect of calcium supplementation on bone loss in postmenopausal women, *N. Engl. J. Med.*, 328, 460, 1993.

159. Reid, I. R., Ames, R. W., Evans, M. C., Gamble, G. D., and Sharpe, S. J., Long-term effects of calcium supplementation on bone loss and fractures in postmenopausal women: a randomized controlled trial, *Am. J. Med.*, 98, 331, 1995.

160. Devine, A., Dick, I. M., Heal, S. J., Criddle, R. A., and Prince, R. L., A 4-year follow-up study of the effects of calcium supplementation on bone density in elderly post-menopausal women, *Osteoporosis Int.*, 7, 23, 1997.

161. Prince, R., Devine, A., Dick, I. M., Criddle, A., Kerr, D., Kent, N., Price, R., and Randell, A., The effects of calcium supplementation (milk powder or tablets) and exercise on bone density in postmenopausal women, *J. Bone Miner. Res.*, 10, 1068, 1995.

162. Michaelsson, K., Bergstrom, R., Holmberg, L., Mallmin, H., Wolk, A., and Ljunghall, S., A high dietary calcium intake is needed for a positive effect on bone density in Swedish postmenopausal women, *Osteoporosis Int.*, 7, 155, 1997.

163. Haines, C. J., Chung, T. K. H., Leung, P. C., Hsu, S. Y. C., and Leung, D. H. Y., Calcium supplementation and bone mineral density in postmenopausal women using estrogen replacement therapy, *Bone*, 16, 529, 1995.

164. Suleiman, S., Nelson, M., Li, F., Buxton-Thomas, M., and Moniz, C., Effect of calcium intake and physical activity level on bone mass and turnover in healthy, white, postmenopausal women, *Am. J. Clin. Nutr.*, 66, 937, 1997.

165. Recker, R. R. and Heaney, R. P., The effect of milk supplements on calcium metabolism, bone metabolism and calcium balance, *Am. J. Clin. Nutr.*, 41, 254, 1985.

166. Lacey, J. M., Anderson, J. J. B., Fujita, T., Yoshimoto, Y., Fukase, M., Tsuchie, S., and Koch, G. G., Correlates of cortical bone mass among premenopausal and post-menopausal Japanese women, *J. Bone Miner. Res.*, 6, 651, 1991.

167. Callegari, C., Lami, F., Levantesi, F., Andreacchio, A. M., Tatali, M., Miglioli, M., Gnudi, S., and Barbara, L., Post-menopausal bone density, lactase deficiency and milk consumption, *J. Human Nutr. & Dietetics*, 3, 159, 1990.

168. Hu, J.-F, Zhao, X.-H., Jia, J.-B., Parpia, B., and Campbell, T. C., Dietary calcium and bone density among middle-aged and elderly women in China, *Am. J. Clin. Nutr.*, 58, 219, 1993.

169. Fujiwara, S., Kasagi, F., Yamada, M., and Kodama, K., Risk factors for hip fracture in a Japanese cohort, *J. Bone Miner. Res.*, 12, 998, 1997.

170. Prince, R. L., Diet and prevention of osteoporotic fractures, *N. Engl. J. Med.*, 337, 701, 1997.

171. Heaney, R. P., Age considerations in nutrient needs for bone health: older adults, *J. Am. Coll. Nutr.*, 15, 575, 1996.

172. Tilyard, M. W., Spears, G. F. S., Thomson, J., and Dovey, S., Treatment of postmenopausal osteoporosis with calcitriol or calcium, *N. Engl. J. Med.*, 326, 357, 1992.

173. Bauer, D. C., Browner, W. S., Cauley, J. A., Orwoll, E. S., Scott, J. C., Black, D. M., Tao, J. L., and Cummings, S. R., Factors associated with appendicular bone mass in older women, *Ann. Intern. Med.*, 118, 657, 1993.

174. Chapuy, M. C., Arlot, M. E., DuBoeuf, F., Brun, J., Crouzet, B., Arnaud, S., Delmas, P. D., and Meunier, P., Vitamin D-3 and calcium to prevent hip fractures in elderly women, *N. Engl. J. Med.*, 327, 1637, 1992.

175. Chevalley, T., Rizzoli, R., Nydegger, V., Slosman, D., Rapin, C.-H., Michael, J.-P., Vasey, H., and Bonjour, J.-P., Effects of calcium supplements on femoral bone mineral density and vertebral fracture rate in vitamin D-replete elderly patients, *Osteoporosis Int.*, 4, 245, 1994.

176. Recker, R. R., Hinders, S., Davies, K. M., Heaney, R. P., Stegman, M. R., Lappe, J. M., and Kimmel, D. B., Correcting calcium nutritional deficiency prevents spine fractures in elderly women, *J. Bone Miner. Res.*, 11, 1961, 1996.

177. Baeksgaard, L., Andersen, K. P., and Hyldstrup, L., Calcium and vitamin D supplementation increases spinal BMD in healthy postmenopausal women, *Osteoporosis Int.*, 8, 255, 1998.

178. Dawson-Hughes, B., Harris, S. S., Krall, E. A., and Dallal, G. E., Effect of calcium and vitamin D supplementation on bone density in men and women 65 years of age or older, *N. Engl. J. Med.*, 337, 670, 1997.

179. Anderson, D. C., Osteoporosis in men, *Br. Med. J.*, 305, 489, 1992.

180. Kelly, P. J., Pocock, N. A., Sambrook, P. N., and Eisman, J. A., Dietary calcium, sex hormones, and bone mineral density in men, *Br. Med. J.*, 300, 1361, 1990.

181. Jackson, J. A. and Kleerekoper, M., Osteoporosis in men: diagnosis, pathology, and prevention, *Medicine*, 69, 137, 1990.

182. Hannan, M. T., Felson, D. T., and Anderson, J. J., Bone mineral density in elderly men and women: results from the Framingham Osteoporosis Study, *J. Bone & Miner. Res.*, 7, 547, 1992.

183. Niewoehner, C. B., Osteoporosis in men. Is it more common than we think? *Postgrad. Med.*, 93, 59, 1993.

184. Grisso, J. A., Kelsey, J. L., O'Brien, L. A., Miles, C. G., Sidney, S., Maislin, G., LaPann, K., Moritz, D., Peters, B., and the Hip Fracture Study Group, Risk factors for hip fracture in men, *Am. J. Epidemiol.*, 145, 786, 1997.

185. Orwoll, E. S., Oviatt, S. K., McClung, M. R., Deftos, L. J., and Sexton, G., The rate of bone mineral loss in normal men and the effects of calcium and cholecalciferol supplementation, *Ann. Intern. Med.*, 112, 29, 1990.

186. Kroger, H. and Laitinen, K., Bone mineral density measured by dual-energy x-ray absorptiometry in normal men, *Europ. J. Clin. Invest.*, 22, 454, 1992.

187. Owusu, W., Willett, W. C., Feskanich, D., Ascherio, A., Speigelman, D., and Colditz, G. A., Calcium intake and the incidence of forearm and hip fractures among men, *J. Nutr.*, 127, 1782, 1997.

188. Glynn, N. W., Meilahn, E. N., Charron, M., Anderson, S. J., Kuller, L. H., and Cauley, J. A., Determinants of bone mineral density in older men, *J. Bone Miner. Res.*, 10, 1769, 1995.

189. Chapuy, M. C., Arlot, M. E., Delmas, P. D., and Meunier, P. J., Effect of calcium and cholecalciferol treatment for three years on hip fractures in elderly women, *Br. Med. J.*, 308, 1081, 1994.

190. McKane, W. R., Khosla, S., Egan, K. S., Robins, S. P., Burritt, M. F., and Riggs, B. L., Role of calcium intake in modulating age-related increases in parathyroid function and bone resorption, *J. Clin. Endocrinol. Metab.*, 81, 1699, 1996.

191. Orwoll, E. S., Bauer, D. C., Vogt, T. M., and Fox, K. M., Axial bone mass in older women, *Ann. Intern. Med.,* 124, 187, 1996.

192. Dawson-Hughes, B., Dallal, G. E., Krall, E. A., Harris, S., Sokoll, L. J., and Falconer, G., Effect of vitamin D supplementation on wintertime and overall bone loss in healthy postmenopausal women, *Ann. Intern. Med.,* 115, 505, 1991.

193. Gloth, F. M., Gundberg, C. M., Hollis, B. W., Haddad, J. G., Jr., and Tobin, J. D., Vitamin D deficiency in homebound elderly persons, *JAMA,* 274, 1683, 1995.

194. Chapuy, M. C., Schott, A. M., Garnero, P., Hans, D., Delmas, P. D., and Meunier, P. J., Healthy elderly French women living at home have secondary hyperparathyroidism and high bone turnover in winter, *J. Clin. Endocrinol. Metab.,* 81, 1129, 1996.

195. Dawson-Hughes, B., Harris, S. S., and Dallal, G. E., Plasma calcidiol, season, and serum parathyroid hormone concentrations in healthy elderly men and women, *Am. J. Clin. Nutr.,* 65, 67, 1997.

196. Chapuy, M.-C., Preziosi, P., Maamer, M., Arnaud, S., Galan, P., Hercberg, S., and Meunier, P. J., Prevalence of vitamin D insufficiency in an adult normal population, *Osteoporosis Int.,* 7, 439, 1997.

197. Jacques, P. F., Felson, D. T., Tucker, K. L., Mahnken, B., Wilson, P. W. F., Rosenberg, I. H., and Rush, D., Plasma 25-hydroxyvitamin D and its determinants in an elderly population sample, *Am. J. Clin. Nutr.,* 66, 929, 1997.

198. Holick, M. F., Vitamin D and bone health, *J. Nutr.,* 126, 1159, 1996.

199. Kinyamu, H. K., Gallagher, J. C., Rafferty, K. A., and Balhorn, K. E., Dietary calcium and vitamin D intake in elderly women: effect on serum parathyroid hormone and vitamin D metabolites, *Am. J. Clin. Nutr.,* 67, 342, 1998.

200. Kinyamu, H. K., Gallagher, J. C., Balhorn, K. E., Petranick, K. M., and Rafferty, K. A., Serum vitamin D metabolites and calcium absorption in normal young and elderly free-living women and in women living in nursing homes, *Am. J. Clin. Nutr.,* 65, 790, 1997.

201. Thomas, M. K., Lloyd-Jones, D. M., Thadhani, R. I., Shaw, A. C., Deraska, D. J., Kitch, B. T., Vamvakas, E. C., Dick, I. M., Prince, R. L., and Finkelstein, J. S., Hypervitaminosis D in medical inpatients, *JAMA,* 338, 777, 1998.

202. Utiger, R. D., The need for more vitamin D, *N. Engl. J. Med.,* 338, 828, 1998.

203. Heikinheimo, R. J., Inkovaara, J. A., Harju, E. J., Haavisto, M. V., Kaarela, R. H., Kataja, J. M., Kokko, A. M., Kolho, L. A., and Rajala, S. A., Annual injection of vitamin D and fractures of aged bones, *Calcif. Tissue Int.,* 51(2), 105, 1992.

204. Ooms, M. E., Roos, J. C., Bezemer, P. D., Van der Vijch, W. J. F., Bouter, L. M., and Lips, P., Prevention of bone loss by vitamin D supplementation in elderly women: a randomized double blind trial, *J. Clin. Endocrinol. Metab.,* 80, 1052, 1995.

205. Packard, P. T. and Heaney, R. P., Medical nutrition therapy for patients with osteoporosis, *J. Am. Diet. Assoc.,* 97, 414, 1997.

206. McClung, M., Clemmesen, B., Daifotis, A., et al., for the Alendronate Osteoporosis Prevention Study Group, Alendronate prevents postmenopausal bone loss in women without osteoporosis, *Ann. Intern. Med.,* 128, 253, 1998.

207. Dawson-Hughes, B., Osteoporosis treatment and the calcium requirement, *Am. J. Clin. Nutr.,* 67, 5, 1998.

208. U.S. Department of Agriculture and U.S. Department of Health and Human Services, *Nutrition and Your Health: Dietary Guidelines for Americans.* 4th edition. Home and Garden Bulletin No. 232, Washington, D.C., USDA/DHHS, December 1995.

209. Heaney, R. P., Food: what a surprise! *Am. J. Clin. Nutr.,* 64, 791, 1996.

210. U.S. Department of Health and Human Services, Public Health Service, Healthy People 2000. National Health Promotion and Disease Prevention Objectives, DHHS Publ. No. (PHS) 91-50212, Superintendent of Documents, U.S. Government Printing Office, Washington, D.C., September 1991.

211. Saltman, P. D. and Strause, L. G., The role of trace minerals in osteoporosis, *J. Am. Coll. Nutr.*, 12(4), 384, 1993.

212. Barger-Lux, M. J., Heaney, R. P., Packard, P. T., Lappe, J. M., and Recker, R. R., Nutritional correlates of low calcium intake, *Clinics in Applied Nutr.*, 2(4), 39, 1992.

213. Holbrook, T. L. and Barrett-Conner, E., Calcium intake: covariates and confounders, *Am. J. Clin. Nutr.*, 53, 741, 1991.

214. Whiting, S. J. and Wood, R. J., Adverse effects of high-calcium diets in humans, *Nutr. Rev.*, 55, 1, 1997.

215. Minihane, A. M. and Fairweather-Tait, S. J., Effect of calcium supplementation on dairy nonheme-iron absorption and long-term iron status, *Am. J. Clin. Nutr.*, 68, 96, 1998.

216. Curhan, G. C., Willett, W. C., Rumm, E. B., and Stampfer, M. J., A prospective study of dietary calcium and other nutrients and the risk of symptomatic kidney stones, *N. Engl. J. Med.*, 328, 833, 1993.

217. Massey, L. K. and Sutton, R. A. L., Modification of dietary oxalate and calcium reduces urinary oxalate in hyperoxaluric patients with kidney stones, *J. Am. Diet. Assoc.*, 93, 1305, 1993.

218. Curhan, G. C., Willett, W. C., Speizer, F. E., Spiegelman, D., and Stampfer, M. J., Comparison of dietary calcium with supplemental calcium and other nutrients as factors affecting the risk for kidney stones in women, *Ann. Intern. Med.*, 126, 497, 1997.

219. Massey, L. K. and Kynast-Gales, S. A., Substituting milk for apple juice does not increase kidney stone risk in most normocalciuric adults who form calcium oxalate stones, *J. Am. Diet. Assoc.*, 98, 303, 1998.

220. Coe, F. L., Diet and calcium: the end of an era? *Ann. Intern. Med.*, 126, 553, 1997.

221. Liebman, M. and Chai, W., Effect of dietary calcium on urinary oxalate excretion after oxalate loads, *Am. J. Clin. Nutr.*, 65, 1453, 1997.

222. Strause, L., Saltman, P., Smith, K., Bracker, M., and Andon, M. B., Spinal bone loss in postmenopausal women supplemented with calcium and trace minerals, *J. Nutr.*, 124, 1060, 1994.

223. Seifert, M. F. and Watkins, B. A., Role of dietary lipid and antioxidants in bone metabolism, *Nutr. Res.*, 17, 1209, 1997.

224. Watkins, B. A., Shen, C.-L., McMurty, J. P., Xu, H., Bain, S. D., Allen, K. G. D., and Seifert, M. F., Dietary lipids modulate bone prostaglandin E_2 production, insulin-like growth factor-1 concentration and formation rate in chicks, *J. Nutr.*, 127, 1084, 1997.

225. Takada, Y., Matsuyama, H., Kato, K., Kobayashi, N., Yamamura, J.-I., Yahiro, M., and Aoe, S., Milk whey protein enhances the bone breaking force in ovariectomized rats, *Nutr. Res.*, 17, 1709, 1997.

CHAPTER 6

Bone Health and the Vegetarian

I. INTRODUCTION

Keeping bones healthy begins with establishing good nutrition and lifestyle habits that continue throughout life. When an individual adopts a healthy diet and lifestyle, the risk of developing the debilitating bone disease, osteoporosis, as well as other chronic health problems, is greatly reduced.

Proper diet and healthy lifestyle habits practiced throughout life can maximize bone growth and mass during childhood and adolescence, maximize the attainment of peak bone mass in young adulthood, and minimize bone loss later in life. To meet these goals an individual should (1) consume a diet adequate in calcium, phosphorus, vitamin D, and moderate in protein and sodium; (2) engage in weight-bearing exercise regularly; (3) and refrain from smoking and excessive alcohol intake. In addition, estrogen replacement therapy may be appropriate for some women. Many vegetarians currently practice diet and lifestyle habits that are conducive to bone health. For more detailed information about bone health, refer to the Bone Basics section in Chapter 5, "Dairy Foods and Osteoporosis."

In this chapter we will review the health effects of a vegetarian diet, focusing primarily on its impact on osteoporosis risk. When attempting to evaluate whether the vegetarian diet influences osteoporosis risk or the risk of other diseases, it is important to keep in mind the specific type of vegetarian diet being followed (e.g., lacto-ovo, vegan). Disease risk may be modulated not only by diet, but by other healthy lifestyle habits (i.e., exercising regularly, not smoking, using alcohol in moderation) often practiced by vegetarians. In studies evaluating mortality and disease prevention, it is often difficult to separate the effect of diet from the role of other lifestyle factors. We will also examine the impact of the amount and source of dietary protein, as well as other dietary factors including calcium, vitamin D, phosphorus, sodium, and fiber on bone health.

II. VEGETARIANISM

A. Types

A vegetarian generally is defined as one who abstains from meat, fish, and poultry. However, vegetarians exhibit a wide variety of eating habits. When reading the literature on the health effects of the vegetarian diet, keep in mind the specific type of diets that are being compared.

- A *semi-vegetarian* eats dairy products, eggs, chicken, and fish, but no other animal flesh.
- A *pesco-vegetarian* eats dairy products, eggs, and fish, but no other animal flesh.
- A *lacto-ovo-vegetarian* eats dairy products and eggs, but no animal flesh.
- A *lacto-vegetarian* eats dairy products, but no animal flesh or eggs.
- An *ovo-vegetarian* eats eggs, but no dairy products or animal flesh.
- A *pollo-vegetarian* eats dairy products, eggs, and poultry, but no other animal flesh.
- A *vegan* eats no animal products of any kind. Veganism is the most restrictive form of vegetarianism.

Most who follow a vegetarian diet do so for its potential health benefits, while others are motivated by religious beliefs, or by ecological or animal rights concerns.[1]

B. How Many Vegetarians are There?

Although the number of vegetarians (who eat no meat, poultry, or fish) has remained stable over the past several years, the interest in part-time vegetarianism, those who eat meatless dinners several times a week and look for vegetarian entrées in restaurants, appears to be growing. Depending on how "vegetarian" is defined, anywhere from 1 to 38 million Americans currently follow a vegetarian diet.

When strictly defined as those who *never* eat meat, fish, or fowl, a 1997 Roper Poll estimated the number of vegetarians to be about 1% of the population or 2 million people.[2] About one third to one half (0.3 to 0.5% of the population) of these vegetarians are vegans and eat no animal products of any kind. Even among those who don't consider themselves vegetarians, there is a trend for consumers to be more "vegetarian aware." A report in *Food Technology* cites survey results from 1983 and 1985 indicating that nearly three quarters of American households were firmly entrenched in a daily routine of meat and potatoes. By 1992, however, only 29% of shoppers believed it was necessary to eat meat every day.[3] Based on the results of several recent polls, the Vegetarian Resource Group estimates that currently between 20 and 30% of the population purchases natural and vegetarian foods regularly.[2]

Vegetarianism is gaining popularity among teens, apparently due to increased sensitivity about animals. A 1995 Roper poll of 8 to 17 year olds found that more teens than adults are following this dietary pattern.[4] Almost 2% of teens are vegetarian (never eat meat, fish, or fowl). Higher percentages of 8 to 12 year olds and 13 to 17 year olds when compared to adults "do not ever eat" meat (8%, 8%, and

6%, respectively), poultry (8%, 6%, and 3%, respectively), fish (19%, 17%, and 4%, respectively), eggs (9%, 8%, and 4%, respectively). These data, particularly when coupled with the finding that 4% of 8 to 12 year olds and 3% of 13 to 17 year olds avoid all dairy products, have sparked concern among health professionals.[5] Teens with an inadequate consumption of calcium and dairy foods are at risk for low peak bone density and osteoporosis later in life. It must be remembered, however, that while an estimated 2% of adults (from the 1997 poll)[2] and 3% of teenagers (from the 1995 poll)[4] avoid dairy products, all do not do so because they are vegetarian. Approximately $1/2$ of 1% of American adults avoid dairy products because they are following a vegan diet.

C. Health Effects of a Vegetarian Diet and Lifestyle

Vegetarian diets are often lower in saturated fat and cholesterol and higher in dietary fiber, folate, anti-oxidant vitamins (such as E and C), carotenoids, and phytochemicals, than most omnivorous diets.[6] The potential benefits of a vegetarian diet and lifestyle may include a lower risk of obesity, cardiovascular disease, hypertension, diabetes mellitus, and some forms of cancer, though differences in disease rates are often related to factors other than diet.[6]

Often those who choose a vegetarian diet embrace other healthy lifestyle habits, such as not smoking, engaging in regular exercise, and maintaining a healthy weight, which are associated with lower chronic disease risk.[7] Researchers in Britain recently investigated the role of dietary habits in mortality among 11,000 vegetarians and health conscious people.[8] Overall, the cohort had a mortality about half that of the general population. Daily consumption of fruit, not vegetarian status per se, was associated with reduced mortality from ischemic heart disease, cerebrovascular disease, and all causes combined. When comparing disease risk among vegetarians and omnivores, it is important to carefully evaluate the types of diets being compared (i.e., vegan, lacto-ovo, semi-vegetarian) and the composition of those diets, as well as how well lifestyle factors other than diet are controlled.

Often it is not the presence or absence of meat in the diet that attenuates disease risk and mortality rate. In some omnivorous populations that follow a "prudent" diet, the fat, saturated fat, and cholesterol content of the diet may be similar to that of vegetarians.[9] Investigators from Australia reviewed the evidence linking vegetarian diets to lower blood pressure.[10] Evidence that diet effectively lowers blood pressure, they conclude, has been seen most clearly in those who follow a strict lacto-ovo-vegetarian diet. Compared to a typical Western diet, the lacto-ovo-vegetarian diet is lower in saturated fat, higher in dietary fiber, fruits and vegetables, and dairy products. The review states that blood pressure is not influenced by the absence of meat protein per se. This conclusion has been supported by the results of the DASH (Dietary Approaches to Stop Hypertension) trial.[11] This study demonstrated that a low fat diet rich in fruits and vegetables and lowfat dairy foods was effective in reducing blood pressure. In fact, it was as effective as medication for those with mild hypertension.

Whether vegetarians live longer than nonvegetarians is difficult to determine, since few studies of all-cause mortality have been conducted that compare these groups. Two major studies of this kind had differing results.[12,13] A more recent study evaluated various lifestyle characteristics of 1904 German vegetarians to determine which might be associated with decreased mortality after 11 years of follow-up.[14] The majority of participants were lacto- or lacto-ovo-vegetarians; only 6% were vegan. In men, activity level and body mass index were the most important determinants of total mortality. For women, mortality was significantly reduced among moderate (ate fish or meat occasionally) vs. strict vegetarians (avoided fish and meat completely), and among those with a higher activity level. Body mass index did not affect mortality in females. Since moderate vegetarians, especially women, had a lower risk of death than strict vegetarians, the authors suggest that "the choice of a wide variety of foods and sound nutritional planning may be more important than an absolute avoidance of meat." In addition, a greater proportion of moderate vegetarians claimed to have chosen the vegetarian lifestyle to improve their overall health, so may have paid more attention to the nutritional adequacy of their diet.

There appears to be no overwhelming evidence that vegetarians live longer than nonvegetarians. Mortality rates may be affected by overall diet, socioeconomic differences, selective factors relating to who chooses to become and remain a vegetarian, and overall health consciousness.[15]

III. FACTORS INFLUENCING BONE HEALTH

Both heredity and environmental factors (including diet and exercise) influence bone density. While one cannot change the genetic determinants of bone structure or other uncontrollable factors that influence bone mass, such as gender, ethnicity, age, hormonal status, and body frame size/weight,[16] there are many things one can do to improve bone health.

A. Heredity

Investigators estimate the role of heredity in determining bone density to be 50 to 80%. Krall and Dawson-Hughes compared bone density among family members (men and women) of 40 families, and examined the association between bone density and environmental factors. They estimated that heredity and environmental factors exerted an equal effect on bone density.[17] Studies in twins indicate that about 75% or 80% of the variability in bone density, size, and bone turnover is explained by genetic factors.[18,19]

Experimental data support the hypothesis that peak bone size, bone mass, and bone density in young women are strongly influenced by genetic factors from fathers as well as from mothers. By the age of 16 years, daughters had attained 90% to 97% of the bone size, mass, and density of their premenopausal mothers.[20] Inheritance may influence both the level of peak bone mass and the rate at which bone is lost after menopause.[21] Since bone mass is partly hereditary, young women whose mothers have been diagnosed with osteoporosis may be at increased risk themselves, and should be especially careful to control the environmental factors affecting bone. Johnston and Slemenda, in a review of the determinants of peak bone mass, say,

"Genetic factors are important in determining peak bone mass, but environmental factors such as calcium nutrition and exercise are important in maximizing the genetic potential."[22]

B. Environment

1. Diet

Building and maintaining healthy bones requires adequate amounts of many nutrients, including calcium, vitamin D, phosphorus, zinc, and magnesium. Manganese and copper are needed in smaller amounts as well.[23] Calcium is the major building block of bone; adequate amounts are needed throughout life to maintain a healthy skeleton. Vitamin D, manufactured in the body from sunlight or obtained in the diet, facilitates calcium absorption and the incorporation of calcium into bone. The primary dietary source of vitamin D is vitamin D fortified milk. Excessive sodium, protein, and fiber intake can decrease the amount of calcium that is available to build and remodel bone, either by decreasing calcium absorption or increasing calcium excretion.[23] Though these excesses are not particularly harmful in themselves when calcium intake is adequate, they will aggravate calcium deficiency if calcium intake and/or absorption is low. Increasing calcium in the diet will neutralize the negative effects of any of these excesses. Sodium, protein, and fiber will be discussed in more detail later in this chapter.

2. Lifestyle

Exercise and physical work increase bone density and strength. Both weight-bearing and resistance exercises are important for building and maintaining bone mass and density.[16] Weight-bearing exercises include walking, jogging, impact aerobics, stair climbing, dancing, and hiking. Swimming and bicycling are not weight-bearing. The usual prescription for maintaining bone health is brisk walking; however, many women over the age of 75 who have led a sedentary lifestyle, do not have the aerobic capacity to engage in a walking program.[24] This loss of strength can be reversed by a carefully planned progressive exercise program.

It is estimated that increasing physical activity will have an overall benefit of 4 to 8% on bone mass, depending on the type of exercise and the skeletal site measured.[22] Exercise has many advantages as a therapy, since it is inexpensive, readily available, and enjoyable. A small percentage increase in bone mass can have a large effect on fracture reduction. For example, for every percentage point of bone lost, the risk of fracture increases by 8 to 10%. Increasing an individual's muscular strength and balance to prevent falls is probably the most important contribution of exercise overall.

There is evidence that exercise should be encouraged in childhood, adolescence, and young adulthood, to improve the attainment of peak bone mass and help reduce the risk of osteoporosis later in life. Sports activities had a positive effect on the bone density of the spine and hip among pubertal girls[25] and boys ages 4 to 20.[26] The results of recent cross-sectional studies in college age and young adult women, showed that at least moderate exercise along with adequate calcium intake had a positive effect on bone mineral density.[27,28] French researchers, studying the determinants of bone mineral density in children and adolescents, found that weekly sports activity significantly influenced both vertebral and femoral bone density, especially in girls during puberty.[25] Calcium intake was also a significant, independent determinant of bone density for both sexes. A majority of the participants found to have low bone mass, had calcium intakes below 1,000 mg/d (the Recommended Dietary Allowance in France for 10 to 12 year olds). A review of the effects of physical activity on bone mineral density in postmenopausal women concludes that a calcium intake of at least 1000 mg/d is needed in order for physical activity to have a positive effect on bone.[29]

Studies have shown that moderate intensity, low or high impact exercise three days per week[30] or walking for 50 min. 4 days per week[31] for one year improved bone density in postmenopausal women. A review of both cross-sectional and prospective studies of bone density and exercise concludes that an exercise regimen should include both vigorous strength and aerobic training.[32] The National Osteoporosis Foundation recommends weight-bearing exercise four times a week and resistance training two to three times a week.[16]

Cigarette smoking increases by about 50% a person's risk of osteoporosis leading to fracture. Compared to nonsmokers, women smokers have lower levels of estrogen, possibly producing lower bone density. Estrogen replacement therapy is less effective in smokers, so shouldn't be relied upon to counteract the damage to bone caused by cigarette smoking.[33] In order to evaluate the effect of cigarette smoking on bone density, a group of Australian researchers compared the bone density in the spine, leg, and hip of 41 pairs of female twins who had differing smoking habits.[34] In the 20 twin pairs whose smoking habits differed the most, the heaviest smoking twin had bone density 9.3% lower in the spine, 6.5% lower in the leg, and 5.8% lower in the hip. The authors conclude that women who smoke one pack of cigarettes per day throughout adulthood can expect to lose an average of 5 to 10% in bone density by the time of menopause.[34]

Consuming alcohol to excess is also damaging to bone, perhaps more so than cigarette smoking. Excess alcohol intake may harm the bones by reducing calcium absorption, decreasing calcium intake (and that of other nutrients), and causing liver damage, which alters calcium metabolism.[35]

A low calcium intake will further aggravate the negative effects of inactivity, smoking, or excessive alcohol intake. However, taking extra calcium will not neutralize the effects of any of these excesses.

3. Lifestage or Disease State

Age and certain diseases can increase a person's need for calcium. Dietary adjustments should be made to meet the increased need for calcium. Elderly persons may need more calcium than younger adults because they have decreased vitamin D production and reduced calcium absorption.[36] A number of diseases common in older adulthood, such as gastrointestinal disorders and renal insufficiency, can decrease calcium absorption and/or increase calcium excretion, thereby increasing calcium need. Chronic laxative use, as well as other medications, can increase calcium need.

IV. THE VEGETARIAN DIET AND OSTEOPOROSIS RISK

Differences in the prevalence of osteoporosis between vegetarians and nonvegetarians are not well documented. Some cross-cultural studies have shown that people living in countries with low calcium intake and primarily vegetarian diets do not have the high incidence of fracture seen in Western cultures where calcium intake is higher.[37] However, actual calcium intake is difficult to obtain from these societies, and no doubt genetic, lifestyle, and other confounding factors unique to that population play an important role in determining osteoporosis risk. Therefore, only comparisons between groups *within* the same population will yield plausible and valid conclusions.[38]

Osteoporosis and other disease rates do not vary markedly between vegetarians and nonvegetarians in the U.S. when differences in lifestyle factors such as exercise, smoking, and alcohol habits are taken into account. Any claimed reductions in osteoporosis risk as a result of consuming a vegetarian diet are based on studies that contain no dietary data or assessment of lifestyle habits that affect bone.[39,40] The randomized, controlled trial is the "gold standard" for evaluating either therapeutic or nutritional interventions and for establishing causation.[41] However, the hypothesis that the avoidance of animal protein reduces osteoporosis risk is not supported by experimental data from well-controlled studies. Studies conducted in the U.S. in which dietary and other lifestyle factors were carefully assessed and controlled, and where calcium intake was at or above recommended levels, showed no difference in bone mineral density between lacto-ovo-vegetarian and omnivorous premenopausal or postmenopausal women.[42,43,44,45,46] Hunt et al. found that while bone density decreased steadily with age, it did not differ significantly between the lacto-ovo-vegetarian and omnivorous women studied (Figure 6.1).[43] Similarly Reed et al. (Table 6.1) found that neither distal nor mid-radial bone mineral content or density differed between 49 lacto-ovo-vegetarian and 140 omnivorous elderly women (average age 81 years).[45] Tylvasky and Anderson found no difference in bone mass between 88 lacto-ovo-vegetarian and 278 omnivorous postmenopausal women when adjusted for age.[46] Marsh et al. found no difference in bone mineral density between vegetarian and omnivorous men.[47] Barr et al., however, found that in a small group of Canadian women ages 20 to 40, vegetarians (lacto-ovo and vegan) had significantly lower bone mineral density of the spine than nonvegetarians.[48] The differences in bone mineral density between groups were explained by the vegetarian's lower bone mass and lower body weight/body fat and lower intake of some nutrients. The vegetarians had lower intakes of zinc, vitamin B_{12}, and calcium (vegans only) than did the nonvegetarians.

Lacto-vegetarians who have calcium intakes above recommended levels do not seem to be at risk for osteoporosis.[49] The vegan's low calcium intake, use of foods high in phytates, oxalates, and fiber, and tendency to be underweight are characteristics that likely increase this risk of osteoporosis. However, to our knowledge,

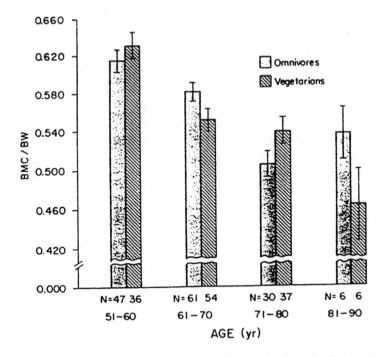

Figure 6.1 Bone mineral content/bone width (BMC/BW) of the cortical radius by decade of age (x ± SEM). No significant differences were found between omnivores and vegetarians within decades. The difference between decades was significant (*p* <0.0001, analysis of variance). Values are not shown for the small numbers of postmenopausal women aged ≤ 50 y (two omnivores and six vegetarians) and > 90 y (one omnivore and four vegetarians). (From Hunt, I. F., Murphy, N. J., Henderson, C., Clark, V. A., Jacobs, R. M., Johnston, P. K., and Coulson, A. H., *Am. J. Clin. Nutr.*, 50(3), 517, 1989. With permission.)

Table 6.1 Bone Variables of Study Groups: Unadjusted and Adjusted for Age and Lean Body Mass (LBM), 1988*

Variable	Unadjusted Means				Means Adjusted for Age and LBM			
	DBMC	DBMD	MBMC	MBMD	DBMC	MBMD	MBMC	MBMD
Lacto-ovo-vegetarian diet (n = 49)	709.3	323.1	673.9	530.2	802.9	351.2	728.0	543.0
Omnivorous diet (n = 140)	658.3	303.3	654.2	528.6	823.8	358.7	727.5	529.7

* DBMC, distal-bone mineral content; DBMD, distal-bone mineral density; MBMC, midradial-bone mineral content; MBMD, midradial-bone mineral density.

(From Reed, J. A., Anderson, J. J. B., Tylavsky, F. A., and Gallagher, Jr., P. N., *Am. J. Clin. Nutr.*, 59 (Suppl.), 1197s, 1994. With permission.)

sufficiently large controlled studies comparing bone density of vegans and nonvegetarians in the U.S. have not been conducted, possibly because there are few vegans from which to build a study population. A small number of strict vegetarians have been studied as part of a larger group. Marsh et al. found that vegans (n = 11) had lower bone densities than lacto-ovo or semi-vegetarians who included some fish, chicken, or meat in their diets; however, there were too few subjects in each group for statistical analysis.[50] Barr et al. found that vegan women (n = 8) did not have lower bone mineral density than lacto-ovo-vegetarian women, though their calcium intake was 300 mg/d lower.[48] However, no conclusions can be drawn from such a small sample. Vegetarians as a group, though, had lower bone density than nonvegetarians. The authors recommend that vegetarian women maintain a generous intake of calcium and other bone-related nutrients.

Reports on the bone density of the elderly Chinese provides good insight on the skeletal status of vegans, and the relative importance of calcium and protein in the diet.[51-54] Studies conducted by Zhao et al. and Hu et al. compare bone mass between individuals living in different areas of China whose diets vary widely, providing a unique opportunity to evaluate the impact of different dietary patterns on bone mass. If low calcium intake contributes to osteoporotic fracture, one would expect to find the evidence in populations that have a range of low to high calcium intakes, rather than in countries like the United States where intakes are predominantly higher (though well below requirements).[23] China provides ideal conditions for such a study. China is a vast country in which dietary patterns can vary widely, and people are not highly mobile. Therefore one may evaluate the impact of lifetime adherence to a particular diet.

A study conducted among 2169 subjects aged 45 to 75 years investigated the influence of diet on health problems occurring in the elderly in six areas of China, including rural farming, fishing, herding, and urban areas.[51] Bone status of males and females was evaluated as part of the larger survey. Chinese living in rural areas typically have low calcium intakes and obtain calcium and protein primarily from plant sources. The data revealed that bone density of the distal radius was higher among women living in pastoral areas of China where dairy foods comprise a large portion of the diet, when compared to those living in rural, nondairy consuming areas. Bone density of both the distal- and mid-radius was positively related to total calcium and dairy calcium intake. In 376 healthy elderly subjects, bone density was positively related to calcium intake. Those who had low calcium intakes (<700 mg/day) had the lowest bone density.

Associations between dietary calcium and bone status were investigated in 843 middle-aged and elderly (35 to 75 years) women who lived in five rural counties where eating patterns and calcium intakes varied.[52] Figure 6.2 shows the types of foods eaten in each county. County YA (Xianghuangqi) and WA (Tuoli) are located in two pastoral areas of China, but county WA is termed semi-pastoral, because the women only drank milk tea and consumed no cheese or other dairy products. The rest of the counties, CD (Jiexiu), SB (Cangxi), and LC (Changle) were selected from rural farming areas where no milk or dairy foods were available. A 3-day dietary survey was conducted in each household to determine usual food intakes for each subject. The average daily intake of selected nutrients of women in the five survey

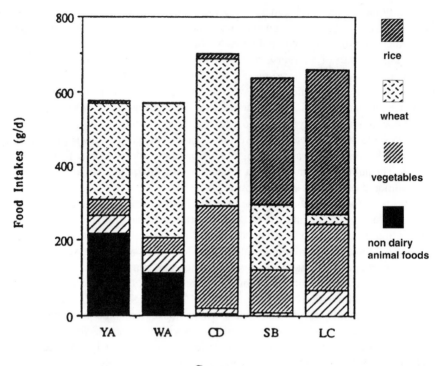

Figure 6.2   Dietary patterns of middle-aged and elderly women in the five survey counties:
YA, Xianghuangqi; WA, Tuoli; CD, Jiexiu; SB, Cangxi; LC, Changle. Intakes of milk
and dairy foods were expressed as grams dry weight per day. (From Hu, J.-F.,
Zhao, X.-H., Parpia, B., and Campbell, T. C., *Am. J. Clin. Nutr.*, 58, 398, 1993.
With permission.)

counties is presented in Table 6.2. Bone mass was measured at both the distal- and
mid-radius of the nondominant arm by a single-photon absorptiometer. Only in
county YA, where dairy products were consumed regularly, did the calcium intake
approach the Chinese recommended allowance of 800 mg/d.

The five survey counties were grouped into pastoral, semi-pastoral, and non-
pastoral based the frequency of dairy food consumption. Bone mass declined with
age in all areas, beginning as early as age 35; decline in bone mass accelerated after
age 50 (Figure 6.3). Women in the dairy-consuming county (pastoral) had a higher
peak bone mass at age 35. This suggests that the greater bone mass at each age was
primarily the result of differences in the attainment of peak bone mass, rather than
differences in bone mass later in life. This conclusion is supported by Matkovic et
al.[55] who demonstrated that calcium is an important determinant of peak bone mass.
In county YA (pastoral with a high consumption of dairy foods) dietary calcium
remained positively associated with all bone variables even after adjustment for age
and/or body weight. These women had a 20% greater bone mass at the distal radius,
than women in non-pastoral areas with lower calcium intakes.

Table 6.2   Average Daily Nutrient Intakes of Women in the Five Survey Counties*

	Xianghuangqi (n = 142)	Tuoli (n = 147)	Jiexiu (n = 156)	Cangxi (n = 151)	Changle (n = 168)
Energy (kJ)	6303 ± 1704[c]	6237 ± 1724[c]	7461 ± 1898[b]	10268 ± 3227[a]	7319 ± 1767[b]
Carbohydrate (g)	216 ± 59[c]	228 ± 64[c]	336 ± 93[b]	498 ± 164[a]	328 ± 84[b]
Fat					
(g)	38 ± 18[a]	42 ± 27[a]	24 ± 12[b]	26 ± 16[b]	27 ± 15[b]
(% of energy)	22.3 ± 6.7[b]	24.5 ± 10.3[a]	12.6 ± 5.6[c]	9.9 ± 5.2[d]	13.6 ± 5.1[c]
Protein					
(g)	75 ± 27[a]	51 ± 17[c]	57 ± 15[b]	57 ± 18[b]	49 ± 13[c]
(g/kg body wt)	1.5 ± 0.5[a]	1.0 ± 0.4[c]	1.1 ± 0.3[c]	1.3 ± 0.4[b]	1.0 ± 0.3[c]
Calcium (mg)	724 ± 333[a]	369 ± 153[b]	359 ± 159[b]	328 ± 133[b]	230 ± 104[c]
Dairy foods (g)[†]	217 ± 110[a]	113 ± 71[b]	5 ± 2[c]	0[c]	0[c]
Dairy calcium					
(mg)	516 ± 296[a]	152 ± 99[b]	6 ± 4[c]	0[c]	0[c]
(% of total calcium)	67.3 ± 14.2[a]	34.6 ± 11.9[b]	0.7 ± 0.3[c]	0[c]	0[c]
Phosphorus (mg)	1130 ± 360[a]	909 ± 235[c]	996 ± 261[b]	1003 ± 306[b]	689 ± 168
Calcium: phosphorus	0.6 ± 0.2[a]	0.4 ± 0.2[b]	0.4 ± 0.1[b]	0.3 ± 0.1[b]	0.3 ± 0.1[b]

*$x \pm SD$; n = 764. Means not sharing the same letter superscript are significantly different for the five counties. P < 0.05 (Duncan's multiple-range test).
[†]Dry weight.
From Hu, J., et al., *Am. J. Clin. Nutr.*, 58, 219, 1993. With permission.

The results of the study by Hu et al. provide important information about whether calcium from non dairy sources is as effective as calcium from dairy foods in maintaining bone mass. The women living in the semi-pastoral county of YA had an average calcium intake of 369 mg/d of which 34.6% came from dairy foods; the women living in the three non-pastoral counties had similar calcium intakes (Table 6.2), but none was provided by dairy foods. Dairy calcium was more significantly correlated with bone mass than was nondairy calcium. In fact, nondairy calcium showed no association with bone variables after adjustment for age and/or body weight. In a separate analysis, the consumption of milk, hard cheese, and other dairy foods by women in counties YA and WA, were positively associated with bone mineral content and bone mineral density at the distal- and mid-radius. The authors suggest that the nondairy calcium consumed by the Chinese women in this study may be less bioavailable due to binding with phytates and other components of vegetable foods. Further studies may help clarify this issue.

A recent study conducted among 258 postmenopausal Taiwanese vegetarian women, linked long-term adherence to a vegan diet with significantly lower bone mineral density of the hip (after controlling for other variables), when compared to those with a shorter or less strict adherence to a vegan diet.[53] Low BMI and protein intake contributed to bone loss in this population. In addition, the calcium intake of these women was extremely low (approximately 350 mg/d), less than

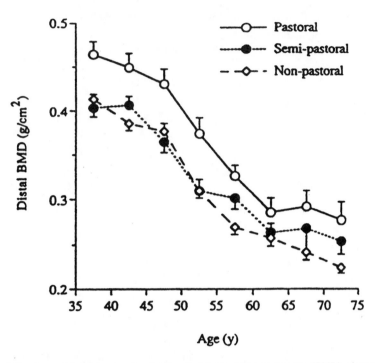

Figure 6.3 Age-related changes in distal radius bone mineral density (BMD) of women in pastoral, semipastoral, and nonpastoral areas ($x \pm$ SEM). (From Hu, J.-F., Zhao, X.-H., Jia, J.-B., Parpia, B., and Campbell, T. C., *Am. J. Clin. Nutr.*, 58, 219, 1993. With permission.)

50% of the level recommended in China. The authors conclude that to prevent osteoporosis in this population, nutritional supplementation of calcium and protein should be considered.

Lau et al. compared the bone density of elderly Chinese lacto-vegetarians, vegans, omnivores, and Caucasian vegetarians.[54] When compared to the omnivores, the bone mineral density of the hip of the vegetarians was significantly and consistently lower. Dietary energy, protein, and calcium intake were positively associated with bone mineral density at all sites. Urinary sodium/creatinine ratios were negatively correlated with bone mineral density of two sites within the hip. The average calcium intake of vegetarians in this study was quite low, 328 mg/d, and was likely below this population's threshold for maintaining bone mass. The bone mineral density of the lacto-vegetarians was not significantly different from that of the vegans. (The definition of a lacto-vegetarian is that they consumed milk at least once a month.) The authors suggested that although the calcium intake of the lacto-vegetarians was higher than that of the vegans, its beneficial effect may have been offset by the lower protein and energy intake (both below recommended levels). Adequate calories and protein are important for building bone mass. It is important to note that the diet of Chinese vegetarians differs considerably from that of Caucasian vegetarians. In this study, the dietary intake of calories, protein, fat, and calcium were much lower among Chinese vegetarians than among Caucasian vegetarians. The diet of the Chinese omnivores was similar to that of the Caucasian vegetarians in all respects except calcium. Chinese omnivores had an average calcium intake of only 334 mg/d, while the Caucasian vegetarians consumed an average of 819 mg of calcium daily.

Since the diets of the two cultures are so different, conclusions about the bone health status of Chinese vegetarians do not necessarily apply to vegetarians living in the United States. Although vegans living in China appear to be at high risk for low bone density and osteoporosis, studies among a large sample of U.S. vegans are needed to determine if they are at similar risk. Hip fracture rates in Hong Kong and other parts of Asia are rising, though they are still substantially lower than in the United States.[56] In addition to diet, other factors, such as bone mass, body weight, physical labor, latitude, reproductive history, femur anatomy, and differences in data collection, contribute to reported hip fracture risk.[57] Obviously, many factors contribute to fracture risk, but the data from China provide clear evidence that consuming adequate amounts of protein and calcium (particularly from dairy foods), is important to maintaining the bone health of vegetarians.

V. FACTORS OF VEGETARIAN DIETS THAT AFFECT BONE HEALTH

A. Calcium

1. Intake Recommendations and Consumption Patterns

There is widespread recognition that an adequate calcium intake throughout life helps to optimize peak bone mass and prevent age-related bone loss, and thus protects the skeleton from osteoporosis and fracture.[58,59] Adequate calcium intake may have the added benefits of decreased risk of developing hypertension and colorectal cancer.[60,61,62] (See Chapters 3 and 4.)

In 1997 the National Academy of Sciences (NAS) updated the recommendations for calcium intake, as well as the other bone related nutrients (vitamin D, phosphorus, magnesium, and fluoride).[59] (Table 6.3) The calcium recommendations were increased for several age groups. Children (9 through 13) and teens (14 through 18) are encouraged to consume 1300 mg of calcium/d to optimize peak bone mass. Calcium recommendations for adults were increased to 1000 mg/d (from 800 mg/d) for 19 through 50 year olds, and to 1200 mg/d (from 800 mg) for adults over age 50. Lacto-vegetarians can meet these recommendations by the consumption of 3 or 4 servings of milk and milk products daily. Vegans will use a combination of calcium-containing plant foods, calcium-fortified foods (Table 6.4), and supplements to meet calcium intake recommendations. The NAS recommendations for calcium intake, now expressed as Adequate Intakes (AI) rather than Recommended Dietary Allowances (RDA), are consistent with the amount of calcium needed for maximal calcium retention, increased bone mass, and reduced risk of osteoporosis. (Adequate Intakes are set when there is not enough data to establish an Estimated Average Intake upon which the RDA is set. They are used similarly as the RDAs, to establish intake goals for individuals.) The new NAS recommendations for calcium are more in line with those of The National Institutes of Health (NIH) Expert Panel on Optimal Calcium

Table 6.3   Dietary Reference Intakes for Bone-related Nutrients

Life-Stage Group	Calcium Adequate Intake mg/d	Phosphorus Recommended Dietary Allowance mg/d	Magnesium Recommended Dietary Allowance mg/dl		Vitamin D Adequate Intake μg/d
			Males	Females	
0–6 months	210	100*	30*	30*	5
6–12 months	270	275*	75*	75*	5
1–3 years	500	460	80	80	5
4–8 years	800	500	130	130	5
9–13 years	1,300	1,250	240	240	5
14–18 years	1,300	1,250	410	360	5
19–30 years	1,000	700	400	310	5
31–50 years	1,000	700	420	320	5
51–70 years	1,200	700	420	320	10
> 70 years	1,200	700	420	320	15
Pregnancy					
≤ 18 years	1,300	1,250		400	5
19–50 years	1,000	700			
19–30 years				350	
31–50 years				360	
Lactation					
≤ 18 years	1,300	1,250		360	5
19–50 years	1,000	700			
19–30 years				310	
31–50 years				320	

* Adequate Intake

Source: IOM, Dietary Reference Intakes for Calcium, Phosphorus, Magnesium, Vitamin D, and Fluoride, Food and Nutrition Board, National Academy Press, 1997. With permission.

Intake released in 1994[63] and supported by the American Medical Association.[64] The NIH Expert Panel recommends 800 mg calcium/day for children 1 to 10 years, 1200 to 1500 mg calcium/day for older children and young adults 11 to 24 years, 1000 mg calcium/day for adult men and women 25 to 50 years, 1000 to 1500 mg calcium/day for postmenopausal women, and 1500 mg calcium/day for all men and women over age 65.[63] The consensus statement issued by the panel indicated that calcium-rich foods such as dairy foods are the preferred source of calcium.

Vegetarians who consume a diet relatively low in protein and sodium and engage in regular weight-bearing exercise, may have a lower calcium requirement than those who consume the typical Western diet, upon which current calcium recommendations are based. However, calcium requirements for vegans have not been established. Therefore vegans are encouraged to meet the calcium requirements established for their age group by the National Academy of Sciences, Institute of Medicine.[6]

Table 6.4   Food Sources of Calcium and Vitamin D

Calcium	Milligrams per Serving
Dairy Foods	
Cow's milk, 1 cup	300
Yogurt, 1 cup	275–400
Cheddar cheese, $1^1/_2$ oz.	306
Legumes (1 c cooked)	
Chickpeas	78
Great northern beans	121
Navy beans	128
Pinto beans	82
Black beans	103
Vegetarian baked beans	128
Soyfoods	
Soybeans, 1 c cooked	175
Tofu, $1/_2$ c	120–350
Tempeh, $1/_2$ c	77
Textured vegetable protein	85
Soymilk, 1 c	84
Soymilk, fortified, 1 c	250–300
Soynuts, $1/_2$ c	252
Nuts and Seeds (2 Tbsp)	
Almonds	50
Almond butter	86
Vegetables (1/2 c cooked)	
Bok choy	79
Broccoli	89
Collard greens	178
Kale	90
Mustard greens	75
Turnip greens	125
Fruits	
Dried figs, 5	258
Calcium-fortified orange juice, 1 c	300
Other Foods	
Blackstrap molasses, 1 Tbsp	187

Table 6.4   Food Sources of Calcium and Vitamin D (continued)

Calcium	Milligrams per Serving
Vitamin D	**Micrograms per Servings**
Fortified cow's milk	2.5
Fortified ready-to-eat cereals, $^3/_4$ c	1.0–2.5
Fortified soymilk or other nondairy milk, 1 c	1.0–2.5

Sources: Package information and data from: Pennington J. Bowe's and Church's Food Values of Portions Commonly Used, 16 ed., Lippincott-Raven, 1994; Hytowitz, D. B., Matthews, R. H., *Composition of Foods: Legumes and Legume Products*, Washington, D.C., U.S. Department of Agriculture, 1986, Agriculture Handbook No. 8-16.
Adapted from: Position of The American Dietetic Association: Vegetarian Diets, *J. Am. Dietetic Assoc.*, 97(11), 1317, 1997. With permission.

Approximately 75% of Americans are not meeting current calcium recommendations.[65] Intakes of milk and milk group foods are similarly low, particularly among females and older adults. Americans are consuming an average of only 1.5 servings per day of Milk Group foods, which is slightly more than half the two to three servings recommended in USDA's *Food Guide Pyramid*.[66] Lacto-ovo-vegetarians have calcium intakes comparable to those of nonvegetarians[6], and their calcium utilization tends to be adequate.[67] There is some evidence that the calcium intakes of vegans is generally lower than that of the population in general.[59] For example, a study conducted among vegetarian and nonvegetarian women found that the mean calcium intake of vegans participating in the study (578 mg/d) was significantly lower than that of either the nonvegetarians (950 mg/d) or the lacto-vegetarians (875 mg/d).[68] The authors suggest that vegans consider supplementation with calcium.

2. Food Sources of Calcium and Absorption

How well dietary calcium is absorbed from the intestine is a major factor in determining how much calcium is available for the body to use. It has long been recognized that calcium absorption increases as intake decreases. For example, when healthy women reduced their calcium intake from 2000 mg/d to 300 mg/d (50 to 7.5 mmol/d), their fractional whole body retention of ingested calcium (an index of calcium absorption) increased from 27 to 37%.[69] Calcium absorption increases during times of increased need, such as pregnancy, and decreases with aging. Vitamin D, either synthesized from sunlight or provided by vitamin D-fortified milk products, facilitates calcium absorption.

Vegans are at greater risk for inadequate calcium nutrition because of low calcium intakes, coupled with the presence in many plant foods of several inhibitors of calcium absorption such as phytic and oxalic acids. Phytates and oxalates form insoluble salts with calcium, thereby reducing its absorbability. Calcium bioavailability from food depends on the combined effects of the total calcium content of the meal and the presence of elements that either enhance or inhibit its absorption.

In general, calcium absorption is inversely proportional to the oxalic acid content of the food. Therefore, calcium bioavailability is very low for both American and Chinese varieties of spinach and rhubarb, intermediate for sweet potatoes, and highest from low oxalate vegetables such as kale, broccoli, and bok choy.[70]

Weaver and colleagues in two separate articles, provide useful data on the bioavailability of calcium from a number of dairy and plant foods.[49,70] Using calcium absorption data, and the amount of calcium contained in a typical food serving, they translated this data into the number of servings an individual would need to consume to equal the amount of calcium absorbed from 240 ml of milk (Table 6.5).[49]

Milk and other dairy products are the richest food source of calcium. Dairy foods provide 73% of the calcium in the U.S. food supply.[71] Soybeans and green leafy vegetables such as kale, broccoli, and bok choy contain less calcium per serving than milk, but the calcium in these vegetables is absorbed as well or slightly better than calcium from milk. Almost no calcium is absorbed from spinach, and calcium from navy, pinto, or red beans (only fair sources of calcium) is absorbed only half as well as from milk. Based on this information, one must consume approximately $2 \frac{1}{2}$ cups of broccoli, 6 cups of pinto beans, or 30 cups of unfortified soy milk to deliver the same amount of calcium absorbed from one 8 ounce glass (240 ml) of milk. The authors state, "The low calcium content of common plant sources including most vegetables, fruits and cereal grains, makes it difficult for most Americans to meet their requirements exclusively through these foods, even when the bioavailability of calcium from these sources is high and the larger servings sizes of many vegetarians are taken into account."[70]

Results of a recent study indicate that, despite differences in diet composition between lacto-ovo-vegetarians and nonvegetarians (i.e., protein, sodium, fiber), young women with an adequate calcium intake were able to compensate for these differences to maintain mineral balance. Researchers at the USDA Agricultural Research Service studied zinc absorption, mineral balance, and blood lipid concentrations in 21 women (average age 33 years) consuming controlled lacto-ovo-vegetarian and nonvegetarian diets.[72] The calcium intake of both groups approached 1000 mg/d, the amount currently recommended for this age group. Apparent calcium absorption in the lacto-ovo-vegetarian women was decreased when compared to the nonvegetarians (22% vs. 30%), most likely due to the presence of inhibitors of calcium absorption (i.e., phytates, wheat bran). This was partially compensated for by a decrease in urinary calcium excretion. The net result was a slightly, but not significantly, lower calcium balance in the lacto-ovo-vegetarians. Similar homeostatic adjustments compensated for differences in intake of other minerals as well. Although the lacto-ovo-vegetarian's diet contained more copper, magnesium, and manganese than the nonvegetarians, mineral balance did not differ between groups. It remains to be determined whether homeostatic mechanisms can maintain calcium balance at the lower calcium intakes typical of the vegan diet.

B. Vitamin D

Vitamin D is essential for maintaining a healthy mineralized skeleton primarily by maintaining blood concentrations of calcium to a level necessary for deposition

Table 6.5   Food Sources of Bioavailable Calcium

Food[d]	Serving size (g)	Calcium[b] content (mg)	Fractional[c] absorption (%)	Estimated[a] absorbable Ca/serving (mg)	Servings needed to = 240 ml milk (n)
Milk	240	300	32.1	96.3	1.0
Almonds, dry roasted	28	80	21.2	17.0	5.7
Beans, pinto	86	44.7	17.0	7.6	12.7
Beans, red	172	40.5	17.0	6.9	14.0
Beans, white	110	113	17.0	19.2	5.0
Broccoli	71	35	52.6	18.4	5.2
Brussel sprouts	78	19	63.8	12.1	8.0
Cabbage, Chinese	85	79	53.8	42.5	2.3
Cabbage, green	75	25	64.9	16.2	5.9
Cauliflower	62	17	68.6	11.7	8.2
Citrus punch with CCM	240	300	50.0	150	0.64
Fruit punch with CCM	240	300	52.0	156	0.62
Kale	65	47	58.8	27.6	3.5
Kohlrabi	82	20	67.0	13.4	7.2
Mustard greens	72	64	57.8	37.0	2.6
Radish	50	14	74.4	10.4	9.2
Rutabaga	85	36	61.4	22.1	4.4
Sesame seeds, no hulls	28	37	20.8	7.7	12.2
Soy milk	120	5	31.0	1.6	60.4
Spinach	90	122	5.1	6.2	15.5
Tofu, calcium set	126	258	31.0	80.0	1.2
Turnip greens	72	99	51.6	51.1	1.9
Watercress	17	20	67.0	13.4	7.2

[a] Calcium content (mg) x Fx abs.

[b] An average was used for beans, broccoli, and mustard greens processed different ways.

[c] Adjusted for load; for milk, this is fractional absorption (Fx abs) = 0.889-0.0964 ln load; for low-oxalate vegetables, after adjusting by the ratio of fractional absorption determined for kale relative to milk at the same load, the equation becomes Fx abs = 0.959-0.0964 ln load. For tofu and soy milk, fractional absorption was assumed to be equal to high phytate soybeans. For sesame seeds and almonds, the ratio of fractional absorption of sesame and almonds compared with nonfat dry milk in rats was applied to calcium absorption from milk in humans. Calcium absorption from beans was calculated similarly from rat data. The ratio of fractional absorption from citrus punch (Sunny Delight Plus Calcium; Procter and Gamble, Cincinnati, OH) and fruit punch (Hawaiian Punch Plus Calcium; Procter and Gamble, Cincinnati, OH) was compared with fluid milk in rats and applied to calcium absorption from milk in humans.

[d] Based on 1/2-cup serving size except for milk, citrus punch, and fruit punch (1 cup) and almonds and sesame seeds (1 oz).

From Weaver, C. M. and Plawecki, K. L., *Am. J. Clin. Nutr.*, 59 (Suppl.), 1238s, 1994. With permission.

into bone. Vitamin D, in its active form $(1,25 [OH]_2 D)$, increases the efficiency of calcium absorption, especially when calcium intakes are low. Vitamin D insufficiency in adults decreases calcium absorption by up to 50%.[73] The major source of vitamin D is the exposure of the skin to sunlight. Vitamin D can also be obtained through foods, though very few foods naturally contain vitamin D (i.e., egg yolks, liver). The major dietary source of vitamin D is fortified milk. 98% of milk produced in the U.S. is voluntarily fortified to the level of 400 IU/quart. Vitamin D synthesis from sun exposure may not be adequate for persons in northern parts of the country in the winter, for those using sunscreen, or for elderly shut-ins.[73] Therefore, dietary sources of vitamin D such as vitamin D-fortified milk, cereals, and margarine, are important.

The results of a study conducted in Finland, where there is no ultraviolet B light from October to March to synthesize vitamin D, demonstrated that those following a strict vegan diet were at increased risk of vitamin D deficiency. Low serum 25(OH)D concentrations led to secondary hyperparathyroidism.[74] In this study, intakes of calcium and vitamin D, as well as serum concentrations of 25(OH)D and parathyroid hormone, were compared between middle-aged white vegetarians grouped according to dietary practices (1) strict vegetarians; (2) lacto-vegetarians; (3) lacto-ovo-vegetarians consuming some fish; (4) vegetarians taking vitamin D supplements or exposed to sunshine; and (5) omnivores. Strict vegetarians failed to meet the 1989 RDA for calcium (800 mg) and had a calcium intake significantly lower than the control group of omnivores (Figure 6.4). All vegetarians had a dietary vitamin D intake that was lower than the recommended dietary allowance of 5 µg (200 IU); it was significantly lower in all vegetarian groups than in the control group (Figure 6.5). Serum 25(OH)D concentration reflects nutritional vitamin D status. Figure 6.6 shows that the strict vegetarians have a significantly lower concentration

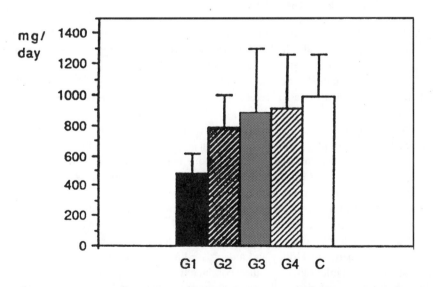

Figure 6.4   Dietary calcium intake ($x \pm$ SD) in the groups studied. G1 (group 1), strict vegetarians; G2 (group 2), lacto-vegetarians; G3 (group 3), lacto-ovo-vegetarians consuming some fish; G4 (group 4), vegetarians taking vitamin D supplements or exposed to sunshine; C, control group. Group 1 differs from the control group at $P < 0.000$. (From Lamberg-Allardt, C., Kärkkäinen, M., Seppänen, R., and Biström, H., *Am. J. Clin. Nutr.*, 58, 684, 1993. With permission.)

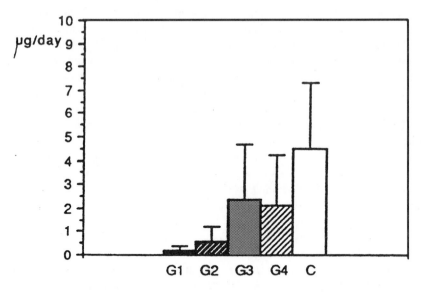

Figure 6.5   Dietary vitamin D intake ($x \pm$ SD) in the groups studied. G1 (group 1), strict vegetarians; G2 (group 2), lacto-vegetarians; G3 (group 3), lacto-ovo-vegetarians consuming some fish; G4 (group 4), vegetarians taking vitamin D supplements or
exposed to sunshine; C, control group. Group 1 differs from the control group at P
< 0.000, group 2 at P < 0.001, group 3 at P < 0.011, and group 4 at P < 0.006.
(From Lamberg-Allardt, C., Kärkkäinen, M., Seppänen, R., and Biström, H., *Am. J.
Clin. Nutr.*, 58, 684, 1993. With permission.)

of 25(OH)D than the control group; values for most subjects were below the lower
reference limit. Vegans also had higher serum concentrations of parathyroid hormone
(PTH) than in the control group, indicating secondary hyperparathyroidism (Figure
6.7). PTH was negatively correlated with serum concentrations of 25(OH)D. Serum
alkaline phosphatase was also elevated in vegans, indicating increased bone turnover
in these subjects.

Vitamin D fortification of dairy products is largely responsible for the elimination
of rickets in this country. However, rickets has reemerged as a public health problem
in vegan infants who are breast-fed for more than six months without access to
supplementary feedings or supplements that contain vitamin D, as well as in young
children of other vegetarians who use few or no vitamin D-fortified milk products.
Reliance on sunshine alone, especially in northern climates, is unlikely to provide
enough vitamin D to protect infants and young children against rickets.[15]

The elderly have the additional risk of both decreased rate of vitamin D (calcitriol) synthesis by the kidney and a decreased ability to form provitamin D_3 upon
exposure to ultraviolet light.[75] A study conducted in postmenopausal women showed
that daily supplementation of their diet with 400 International Units (IU) of vitamin
D reduced winter bone loss and improved spinal bone density.[76] Another study
showed that a single oral dose of 2.5 mg (100,000 IU) of vitamin D_3 was effective
in maintaining satisfactory vitamin D status of the elderly in the winter months.[77]
In addition, homebound elderly persons are likely to suffer from vitamin D deficiency.[78] In response to the growing body of evidence indicating that the elderly

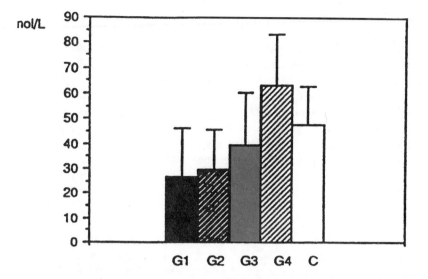

Figure 6.6 Serum 25-hydroxyvitamin D concentration ($x \pm$ SD) in the groups studied. G1 (group 1), strict vegetarians; G2 (group 2), lacto-vegetarians; G3 (group 3), lacto-ovo-vegetarians consuming some fish; G4 (group 4), vegetarians taking vitamin D supplements or exposed to sunshine; C, control group. Group 1 differs from the control group at $P < 0.01$. (From Lamberg-Allardt, C., Kärkkäinen, M., Seppänen, R., and Biström, H., *Am. J. Clin. Nutr.*, 58, 684, 1993. With permission.)

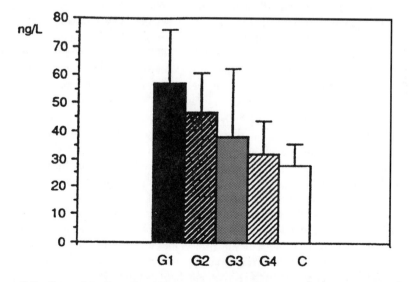

Figure 6.7 Serum intact parathyroid hormone concentration ($x \pm$ SD) in the groups studied. G1 (group 1, $n = 10$), strict vegetarians; G2 (group 2, $n = 6$), lacto-vegetarians; G3 (group 3, $n = 13$), lacto-ovo-vegetarians consuming some fish; G4 (group 4, $n = 14$), vegetarians taking vitamin D supplements or exposed to sunshine; C, control group ($n = 11$). Group 1 differs from the control group at $P < 0.000$. (From Lamberg-Allardt, C., Kärkkäinen, M., Seppänen, R., and Biström, H., *Am. J. Clin. Nutr.*, 58, 684, 1993. With permission.)

need higher levels of vitamin D to help maintain bone mass, in 1997 the National Academy of Sciences raised the recommendations for older Americans.[59] NAS recommends 400 IU/d for adults ages 51 to 70 and 600 IU/d for adults aged 71 or older; 200 IU/d is recommended for all other age groups (Table 6.3). These recommendations assume that vitamin D production from sunlight is limited.

Vegan diets may lack vitamin D, since vitamin D-fortified cow's milk is the major dietary source. Sunlight exposure is the most important factor in maintaining vitamin D status. If sunlight exposure is inadequate (less than 5 to 15 minutes/d on face, hands, and arms, two to three times a week), consumption of vitamin D-fortified foods or vitamin D supplements is recommended.[6]

C. Phosphorus

Phosphorus makes up about half the weight of bone mineral and is as important as calcium for bone health. Phosphorus must be provided in the diet in adequate quantity for both mineralization and maintenance of the skeleton.[23]

A homeostatic system maintains blood levels of calcium and phosphorus within narrow tolerance limits. This system consists of a feedback loop involving three major target organs, the intestine, the kidney, and bone, responding to hormonal signaling from parathyroid hormone (PTH), $1,25 \ (OH)_2 \ D_3$, and possibly calcitonin.[79]

Although the metabolism of calcium and phosphorus are closely linked, the NAS, upon evaluating the available data for bone-related nutrients, concluded that it is not necessary to maintain calcium and phosphorus intakes within a strict 1:1 ratio.[59] The report also states that it is doubtful whether phosphorus intakes within the range currently consumed in the U.S. adversely affect bone health.[59]

Phosphorus recommendations are no longer tied to calcium. The recommendations are based on the amount of dietary phosphorus needed to maintain serum inorganic phosphate levels necessary for cellular functions and bone formation.[59] The NAS recommends higher intakes of phosphorus for adolescents than for adults (1250 mg/d vs. 700 mg/d) (Table 6.3).

Phosphorus intake has increased about 10 to 15% over the past 20 years, likely due to higher consumption of soft drinks and an increased use of phosphates as additives in processed foods.[59] According to the 1994–96 Continuing Survey of Food Intakes by Individuals, the average phosphorus consumption in adults over age 20 is 1459 mg for males (twice the recommended level) and 1017 mg for females (about 1.5 times the recommended amount). Adolescent males 12 to 19 years have the highest phosphorus consumption, 1635 mg/d. Phosphorus intakes may be underestimated, however, since nutrient databases may not reflect the current increased use of phosphate salts in processed foods.[59] The NAS set an upper limit for phosphorus intake of 4 g/d for children and adolescents (9 to 18 years) and adults (19 to 70 years), and an upper limit of 3 g for toddlers and children (age 1 to 8 years) and adults over age 70.[59] It has been estimated that people who prefer processed or convenience foods, could have a phosphorus intake of 2.5 times the recommended amount.[80]

Milk and most dairy foods, except some processed cheeses, have nearly a 1:1 calcium to phosphorus ratio and provide about one third of the phosphorus in the food supply.[71] Most other foods have a much lower ratio. Meat, fish, and poultry have the greatest amount of phosphorus relative to calcium and provide about 25% of the phosphorus in the food supply.[71] Phosphorus is found in virtually every food. Even though vegetarians avoid meat, phosphorus is provided in the diet by vegetables, grains, dairy products (if used), and any processed foods or soft drinks they might consume. Studies that compare bone density between vegetarians and omnivores show little or no difference in calcium to phosphorus ratios between these groups.[55,56,57]

D. Protein

Dietary protein is necessary for the synthesis of new bone matrix. The amount of protein in the diet as well as the source of protein has an effect on the amount of calcium that will be retained by the body to build and remodel bones. Too little protein causes decreased absorption of calcium;[81] too much protein in the diet causes greater urinary calcium loss. An increase in dietary protein induces an increase in urinary calcium excretion, so that each additional gram of protein consumed results in a calcium loss of about 1 mg.[82] When the calcium intake is adequate, the amount of calcium absorbed is great enough to compensate for the increased obligatory losses in the urine caused by a higher protein intake, thereby preventing adverse affects on the skeleton.[38]

The amino acid profile of proteins, specifically the proportion of sulfur containing amino acids, determines to a large extent the protein's calciuric effect. The sulfur amino acids, methionine and cystine, produce an acidic urine causing calcium loss but this explains less than half of the increased calcium loss.[83] The increased filtering rate of the kidneys, as well as increases in certain hormone levels when dietary protein is increased, also contribute to urinary calcium loss. Vegetarian diets (including lacto-ovo) generally produce a more neutral or alkaline urine than do omnivorous diets and less calcium may be required to achieve calcium balance.[84]

Ball and Maughan compared the blood and urine acid-base status between 33 omnivorous and vegetarian premenopausal women.[85] Blood pH was higher and urine pH was lower, though not significantly so, in the omnivorous women when compared to the vegetarians. Calcium intakes between groups were similar and adequate (approximately 1000 mg/d). Omnivores had higher daily intakes of protein (69.9 gm vs. 55 gm), sodium (2691 mg vs. 2139 mg), and slightly higher excretion of calcium (154 mg vs. 128.8 mg) than the vegetarians. These differences were not statistically significant. Since both protein and sodium intakes were higher in the omnivores compared to the vegetarians, the authors state that "the interaction between these two factors could explain the increased excretion of calcium despite a similar dietary intake."[85] Nevertheless, the difference in calcium excretion was small (25.2 mg/d). The impact on bone was not measured. However, as pointed out previously, when the calcium intake is adequate (as in these study subjects), the body is better able to adapt to higher protein intakes without adversely affecting the skeleton.[38]

Gram for gram, milk, soybean, and vegetable protein have a lower amount of the sulfur containing (acid-producing) amino acids than do cereal grains, chicken, beef, or fish. For example, chicken, whole wheat flour, flank steak, milk, tofu, and broccoli contain 46, 40, 38, 34, 27, and 6 milligrams of methionine and cystine per gram of protein, respectively.[86] Following a vegetarian diet does not necessarily mean that intake of sulfur containing amino acids (or total protein) will be low. Wheat and cereal grains which are a dietary staple in many less developed countries are quite high in sulfur amino acids. In a study of dietary intakes and urinary calcium excretion in women in China, rice and millet were found to be positively correlated with urinary calcium probably due to their relatively high content of sulfur containing amino acids.[52] A vegetarian in this country who eats 1/2 cup of dry roasted soybean nuts (34 gm protein) will be getting more methionine and cystine (1008 mg) than in 3 ounces of flank steak (800 mg), and almost four times as much as in an 8 ounce glass of milk (275 mg). In free-living populations, urinary calcium excretion is most likely determined by the acid-base status of the total diet.[52] As Weaver, Proulx, and Heaney state in their discussion of this subject, "Following a vegetarian diet does not guarantee that significant differences in urinary calcium will exist between vegetarians and omnivores."[70]

1. Protein in Perspective

There is little evidence that high protein intakes reduce bone mass or increase fracture risk in free-living human beings.[38] The four well-controlled studies mentioned earlier involving premenopausal or postmenopausal women showed no difference in bone mineral density between lacto-ovo-vegetarians and nonvegetarians.[42-46] The diets of these subjects did not differ significantly in calcium or phosphorus content. No significant differences were seen in bone mineral density between the groups, even though the diets of the nonvegetarians were significantly higher in protein (averaging 63 to 77 g/day), and of course contained animal protein. Though bone density in both the vegetarians and omnivores decreased with age, bone mineral density did not differ between groups even for women 80 to 90 years of age.[43,45] More recently, Feskanich et al. found no association between protein intake and hip fractures in the U.S. Nurse's Health Study.[87]

The body of evidence from studies where diet and lifestyle factors were evaluated suggests that the source of protein in the diet is not a significant factor influencing bone density. If meat eating per se were a cause of significant calcium loss, one would find a difference in urinary calcium loss between vegetarians and nonvegetarians. However, urinary calcium concentrations were similar between vegetarian and omnivorous pre- and postmenopausal women.[42,44]

There is evidence that a low protein intake, especially by the very elderly, may contribute to the problem of osteoporosis.[23] A study by Reed et al. among elderly women reported that in fact protein exerted a slightly positive effect on bone density.[45] Bonjour et al. found that protein supplementation reduced further bone loss in elderly patients with hip fracture.[88]

2. A Matter of Balance

If bone health is to be maximized, amounts of protein, calcium, sodium, and phosphorus in the diet should be close to recommended levels.

Since the body needs more calcium when the diet is high in protein, some find it useful to speak in terms of a calcium to protein ratio for achieving the proper dietary balance of these nutrients. In a study which examined the rate of bone gain in college aged women, the calcium to protein ratio was the single most important determinant of bone gain.[89] The calcium to protein ratio predicted bone mineral density of the spine and hip in a group of Chinese women (ages 31 to 40) living in Hong Kong.[90] Based on this information, Heaney has recommended that the calcium to protein ratio be used to evaluate the adequacy of calcium intake.[82,38] Using the calcium to protein ratio adjusts for the counterbalancing effects of calcium and protein on the calcium economy. Though the ideal ratio has yet to be determined, a good reference point is probably the recommended level for both of these nutrients.[82] For an adult woman, the daily recommended level for calcium is 1000 mg and the RDA for protein is 50 g, yielding a ratio of 20:1 (mg/g). However, the average woman has a calcium to protein ratio of only 10:1 (635 mg of calcium/62.5 g of protein).[65]

There is evidence that current protein intakes should not be of concern for bone health if calcium consumption is adequate. For example, Baran et al. supplemented the diets of premenopausal women with an additional 500 to 600 mg of calcium with dairy foods (1500 mg/d total). Participants experienced no deterioration of calcium balance, even though their protein intake at the end of the 3-year study was 107 g/d (calcium to protein ratio of 14:1).[91] Hunt found that in postmenopausal women who consumed approximately 800 mg of calcium per day, a high meat intake (10 ounces/d) did not increase urinary calcium excretion or impair calcium balance or indexes of bone metabolism.[92] Duff and Whiting tested the acute effects of several dietary factors on calcium excretion in children.[93] Increasing milk protein from approximately 12 g to approximately 29 g did not increase urinary calcium excretion.

Calcium consumption is well below recommended levels for a large percentage of women, teenage girls, and older adults in the U.S. In a review of strategies for vegetarians to achieve an adequate calcium intake, Weaver et al. propose that those following a plant-based diet could either (1) consume a diet low in protein and/or low sulfur amino acid content, or (2) increase calcium consumption to offset the effect of a higher protein diet. According to the authors, the latter strategy is less restrictive and will be easier to continue long-term.[70]

Because milk and hard cheeses have a calcium to protein ratio in the range of 36:1, these foods are an excellent way to improve the calcium to protein ratio of the diet. Fruits and vegetables also provide a major source of alkali to the diet, and serve to buffer an acid load.[94] The recently published DASH study (that demonstrated that a diet rich in lowfat dairy foods, fruits, and vegetables can substantially lower blood pressure) found that adding additional servings of fruits and vegetables to a typical American diet decreased excretion of urinary calcium between 157 and 110 mg/d.[11] In an article that discusses how vegetarians can meet their calcium needs, Weaver states, "the lacto-ovo-vegetarian diet when evaluated on the basis of calcium to protein ratio appears to be the safest approach to minimizing protein-induced calcium losses and maximizing calcium balance."[70] In her evaluation of the effect of dietary protein on bone, Massey states, "Even if the major source of dietary protein is meat, adverse effects may be counterbalanced by generous amounts of calcium from other foods such as milk and increased consumption of fruits and vegetables, especially those rich in calcium."[94]

E. Sodium

A dietary excess of sodium increases urinary calcium loss and will therefore interfere with the body's ability to conserve calcium in response to a low calcium intake.[23] In fact, sodium may be the most important nutritional factor influencing urinary calcium loss (more important than protein or caffeine).[70] Sodium and calcium compete for reabsorption in the renal tubules. Among individuals whose plasma calcium and glomerular filtration rate are within the normal range, the main determinant of obligatory calcium excretion is the filtered load of sodium. Urinary calcium rises 0.5 to 1.5 mmol (11.5 to 34.5 mg) for every 100 mmol (2300 mg) increase in dietary sodium. The effect of dietary sodium on urinary calcium excretion is much more apparent when calcium intake is below 25 mmol/d (1000 mg).[95]

In order for optimal peak bone mass to be attained by young adulthood, children and young adults must maintain a positive balance between calcium intake and obligatory losses in feces, urine, and sweat. In normal children, the most important determinants of calcium retention in the body is dietary calcium intake and urinary excretion of calcium.[96] Matkovic et al. found that in early pubertal girls, dietary calcium had a positive and urinary calcium excretion a negative association with bone mineral density.[96] Sodium intake was the primary determinant of urinary calcium excretion. The authors conclude that sodium intake may influence the calcium requirement for adolescents. A short-term load test in prepubertal children, however, showed no association of sodium and urinary calcium excretion.[93]

Although discrepancies have been observed in the results between studies in free-living subjects and loading studies, the totality of evidence from both types of studies supports the conclusion of Nordin that for every 100 mmol (2300 mg) of sodium excreted by normal, healthy persons, there is approximately 1 mmol (23 mg) loss of urinary calcium.[97] This relationship was also recently observed in Japanese adults age 20 to 49 and 50 to 79.[98] In addition, excretion of hydroxyproline (marker for bone resorption) was positively and significantly correlated to urinary sodium excretion, a measurement of sodium intake.

Studies of sodium supplementation in men and women have shown a positive association between 24-hour urinary sodium excretion and urinary excretion of calcium.[99,100] Devine et al. found that a high sodium intake measured as urinary sodium excretion was associated with increased bone loss of the hip in postmenopausal women.[101] A calcium intake of about 1700 mg/d was required to achieve calcium balance in this population, who had a mean sodium intake of about 3 g. The authors state that calcium balance could also have been achieved at a sodium intake of 2300 mg/d (the RDI) and at the currently recommended calcium intake for this age group of 1200 mg/d.

Estrogen-deprived women excrete more calcium relative to sodium in the fasting state than do premenopausal or estrogen-replete women. It is thought that estrogen, as well as parathyroid hormone, promotes tubular reabsorption of calcium. The rise of urinary calcium at menopause may represent a "calcium leak" due to estrogen deficiency. A study evaluating the relationship between urinary sodium and urinary calcium in women found that when women increased their daily sodium intake from 50 mmol (1153 mg) to 150 mmol (3450 mg), obligatory loss of calcium increased by

1 mmol/d (40 mg).[102] Since obligatory calcium loss determines bone resorption, a high salt intake by postmenopausal women can be considered a risk factor for osteoporosis.[95]

To minimize the negative effects of a high sodium diet on bone, an individual has the following options (1) increase calcium intake to increase calcium absorption; this will allow the body to offset any extra urinary calcium loss; (2) decrease sodium intake to decrease urinary calcium loss; or (3) both increase calcium and decrease sodium a modest degree. The latter may be the easiest to achieve.[70] Although available evidence suggests that excessive salt consumption may contribute to bone loss, additional research is needed in order to make recommendations for the prevention or treatment of osteoporosis.[97]

F. Fiber

Vegetarians typically have higher fiber diets than nonvegetarians. High intakes of dietary fiber may interfere with calcium absorption as well as with the absorption of other minerals, probably because of associated inhibitors of mineral absorption. There seems to be agreement among most researchers that phytate, a compound found principally in the outer hull of cereal grains, interferes with mineral absorption.[23,103] Heaney estimates that if an adult doubled his intake of wheat bran fiber from 10 g to 20 g per day, he might expect a 6 to 10% decrease in calcium availability.[23] Wheat bran co-ingested with milk, reduces the absorbability of calcium in milk.[104] Weaver et al. found that consuming wheat bran cereal (16 g wheat bran) with calcium carbonate reduced the usual increase in calcium absorption that follows an increased calcium intake.[105] The authors conclude that the phytic acid and/or fiber in wheat bran cereal has a high capacity to bind calcium at "all reasonable calcium intake levels." Half of any amount of calcium added (five different calcium loads ranging from 0.5 to 15.5 mmol or 20 to 620 mg) was bound. A decrease in calcium absorption due to wheat bran is most significant for individuals with low calcium intake or for those most vulnerable to nutritional inadequacies, such as the very young, pregnant or lactating women, and the elderly. Increasing dietary calcium can easily compensate for this decrease in calcium availability.

A recent study in healthy young men demonstrated that supplementation with soluble (inulin) and partly soluble (sugar beet) fiber can enhance calcium balance as well as that of other minerals.[106] Inulin is a fructo-oligosaccharide currently used in various agro-food industries, including the dairy and cheese industry. Supplementation with inulin, when compared to the control diet, significantly increased the absorption of calcium. Presumably the fermentation process in the colon enhances the solubility of calcium and other minerals. Because of its high calcium (and magnesium) content, the quantity of calcium absorbed on the sugar beet fiber diet was significantly greater than that of the control diet, although the fractional absorption of the minerals studied was not altered. Sugar beet fiber increased the participant's calcium intake by about 30%. Increased ingestion of both fiber foods improved calcium balance in these subjects. The digestibility of calcium in calcium-rich foods, such as dairy products, can be improved by the addition of inulin.[106]

Elderly individuals following a high fiber vegetarian diet are at increased risk of calcium deficiency, since calcium absorption is already decreased at this age. For example, intestinal absorption of calcium was decreased by 13.5% in elderly volunteers who added 30 g of wheat bran to their usual diet.[107] More recently, elderly subjects fed a high fiber (10.5 g) meal experienced a 20% decrease in calcium absorption when compared with those fed a low fiber (0.5 g) meal. The authors concluded that calcium requirements may be increased in elderly individuals consuming a high fiber diet.[108]

Interpretation of studies examining calcium bioavailability under conditions of high and low fiber intake can be difficult. Results may be confounded when calcium in the test diet is contributed by a fiber source with low bioavailability such as wheat bran. Thirty grams of fiber is the amount recommended as the daily reference value (DRV) for a 2500 calorie diet. The results of these studies suggest that at this level of fiber intake, individuals should consume calcium at or above the recommended level.

VIII. SPECIAL CHALLENGES OF VEGETARIAN DIETS

A. Pregnancy and Lactation

Pregnancy and lactation place additional nutritional demands on the mother to provide for fetal growth and milk production.[109] While the nutrient and energy needs of pregnant women can be met with either a lacto-ovo-vegetarian or vegan diet,[6] pregnant vegans have increased nutritional challenges. Calcium and vitamin D (in addition to iron, zinc, vitamin B_{12}, and riboflavin) are nutrients of particular concern for vegan women during pregnancy and lactation.[67,109] A low calcium intake has been demonstrated to increase the risk of pregnancy-induced hypertension.[110] The American Dietetic Association recommends that vegan women who are pregnant eat adequate amounts of calcium-rich foods and supplement their diet with and 10 µg of vitamin D (if sun exposure is limited), and with vitamin B_{12} during pregnancy (2.0 µg) and lactation (2.6 µg).[6]

A review of studies conducted in lactating women consuming macrobiotic diets, found that vegetarian women had lower calcium intakes (486 mg/d vs. 1038mg/d), lower serum concentrations of 25(OH)D, and higher concentrations of 1,25(OH)$_2$D than did nonvegetarian women.[109] The differences in vitamin D status between vegetarian and nonvegetarian mothers were most apparent in the winter and spring months, when exposure to sunlight is minimal. Because parathyroid hormone levels were not elevated, it is unclear whether the elevated 1,25(OH)$_2$D concentrations indicate an adverse affect on bone, or whether adequate adaptation occurred (increased calcium absorption) to maintain calcium homeostasis.

Vegetarian mothers usually breastfeed their infants. Human milk from vegetarians, especially if the vegan diet is followed, is lower in vitamin D, as well as vitamin B_{12} and other water-soluble vitamins than that of nonvegetarian mothers. Therefore, vegan infants should be supplemented with those nutrients. Vegan mothers should use calcium-rich foods and/or calcium supplements during lactation to meet the current calcium recommendation of 1000 mg/d.[67]

B. Adolescence

Teens who adopt a vegetarian diet will need guidance in meal planning to assure nutritional adequacy during rapid growth.[6] Although adopting a vegetarian diet does not in itself lead to eating disorders, vegetarian diets are somewhat more common among adolescents with eating disorders than among adolescents in general.[111,68]

Researchers in Canada compared the dietary intakes of female adolescents (ages 14 to 19) who consumed vegetarian, semi-vegetarian, and omnivorous diets.[112] Lacto-ovo-vegetarians and semi-vegetarians were more at risk for nutrient inadequacies of protein, calcium, iron, zinc, and riboflavin than were omnivores, though omnivores were also at risk for inadequate intakes of iron and zinc. The researchers expressed concern that calcium intakes were below recommendations and may not be adequate to optimize bone mass. They emphasized that diets of vegetarian teens be well planned to ensure adequate nutrient density for growth.

Adequate calcium and optimal vitamin D status is necessary to optimize bone mass during stages of rapid growth. Researchers in the Netherlands investigated the influence of consuming a macrobiotic diet for at least 6 years on the development of peak bone mass in adolescents aged 9 to 15 years.[113] They found that children of both sexes who followed a macrobiotic diet had significantly lower bone mineral content at almost all sites measured, the total body, spine, femoral neck, radius, and the trochanter in girls, when compared to controls. The authors conclude that a low calcium intake and limited vitamin D status, along with other aspects of the macrobiotic diet contributed to low bone mass. Macrobiotic children also consumed less energy, protein, fat, riboflavin, and vitamin B_{12}, and more fiber, thiamin, and non-heme iron than controls. Although it was not possible to identify exactly which nutrients were responsible for the differences in bone mass, the authors recommend that children following a macrobiotic or vegan diet add dairy products (as a source of calcium) and fatty fish (as a source of vitamin D and vitamin B_{12}) to their diets.

IX. CALCIUM SUPPLEMENTS

If for whatever reason an individual does not wish to include dairy products in the diet, a calcium and vitamin D supplement may be needed. According to a *Vegetarian Times* survey, approximately 45% of all vegetarians take vitamin and/or mineral supplements.[114] The elderly, young children, and pregnant or lactating women are at greatest risk of deficiency. Therefore, these groups may have the greatest need for supplements of calcium or vitamin D. Calcium absorption from supplements (calcium carbonate and calcium lactate) is about the same as its absorption from dairy foods.[115,116,117] Calcium supplements vary greatly in solubility, as one supplement may be several thousand times more soluble than another. But when intestinal calcium absorption was tested in human subjects, very little difference was found between calcium carbonate, calcium phosphate, and calcium citrate.[118] Some supplements contain a higher percentage of calcium than others (calcium carbonate), requiring fewer tablets to meet the targeted intake.

The American Dietetic Association (ADA) as well as most health professional groups recommend that "the best strategy for promoting optimal health and reducing the risk of chronic disease is to obtain adequate nutrients from a wide variety of foods."[119] ADA acknowledges that nutrient supplementation can be useful in situations when dietary selection is limited, as in the vegan diet. They recommend supplementation for vegans with vitamin B_{12} and with vitamin D when exposure to sunlight is limited. They also recommend that practitioners assess the calcium intake for all individuals. Those with low calcium intakes should first be encouraged to increase their consumption of foods naturally rich in calcium, such as dairy foods. Calcium-fortified foods and/or calcium supplements may be recommended for those unwilling or unable to consume milk and milk products.

Supplement use increases the risk of nutrient imbalances and toxicity, which are less likely to occur when nutrients are obtained from foods.[119] Individuals choosing to use supplements should not take them at levels higher than recommended for their age/gender group, and their use should ideally be monitored by a physician or registered dietitian. For example, supplementing the diet with large amounts of calcium can reduce the amount of phosphorus absorbed and could lead to phosphate deficiency in those with a low phosphate intake (i.e., some elderly persons).[23]

X. BENEFITS OF CALCIUM-RICH FOODS

Foods contain a wide range of nutrients and other constituents that are not provided by a single supplement. Dietary patterns, rather than individual nutrients, are the most important determinants of nutritional adequacy. Calcium researchers from Creighton University found that adult women with a low calcium intake (less than two thirds of the 1989 RDA of 800 mg) also had significantly lower intakes of protein and 9 other vitamins and minerals. Over half (53%) of the women with a low calcium intake were judged to have "poor diets" (low intakes for five or more of the nine nutrients studied).[120] Fleming and Heimbach found similar nutrient deficits among teenage girls who did not drink milk.[121] They compared the diets of teenage girls (13 to 18 years) who drank milk with those who didn't. They found that girls who didn't drink milk had lower intakes of vitamins A, B_6, B_{12}, folate, riboflavin, calcium, magnesium, and potassium. Increasing the calcium intake through supplementation still leaves other nutrient deficiencies. A four-year longitudinal study among 64 postmenopausal women in Australia demonstrated that skim milk powder was superior to calcium supplements at improving diet quality.[122] When compared to the women who took a calcium supplement (1000 mg/d in addition to calcium provided by their diet), those who increased their calcium intake to 1600 mg/d with skim milk also significantly increased their intakes of protein, potassium, magnesium, phosphorus, riboflavin, thiamin, and zinc. They did so without increasing their total fat or saturated fat intake. According to Dr. Robert Heaney, a noted calcium researcher, "Food is always the best source of nutrition for our bodies because it helps meet total nutrient needs. When you drink milk, you're getting an entire nutrient package."[123]

A study conducted among pubertal girls (ages 9 to 13) in Utah demonstrated that increasing their consumption of dairy foods (choice of products) to meet calcium recommendations increased bone mineralization in the spine and total body without increasing fat intake, weight gain, or body fatness.[124] Compared to controls, those who ate extra dairy foods had higher intakes of calcium, phosphorus, vitamin D, and protein.

Researchers in Oregon demonstrated that it is feasible to increase food calcium to 1500 mg/d in free-living adults by increasing the consumption of calcium-rich foods, and that doing so improves the quality of the total diet.[125] Nutrient intake was compared between those who consumed 1500 mg of calcium per day primarily from dairy foods and those taking a 1000 mg calcium supplement or a placebo. Intake of calcium, magnesium, phosphorus, potassium, thiamine, riboflavin, and vitamins C and D increased in the diets of those consuming dairy foods, but not in those taking a calcium carbonate supplement (1000 mg/d) or the placebo. The authors state that "a diet that consistently excludes or limits dairy foods will not only provide less calcium, but may also limit those nutrients that track with calcium from foods." Increasing the amount of dairy foods in the diet for 12 weeks did not increase blood lipid levels or lead to weight gain.

The results of these studies clearly demonstrate that when adults or teens meet current calcium intake recommendations with food, particularly dairy foods, the nutritional quality of the diet is improved without increasing overall fat intake or causing weight gain. It is particularly important for health professionals to communicate this information to young women who exclude dairy foods from their diet due to concerns about weight gain.

XI. THE VALUE OF MILK AND MILK PRODUCTS IN VEGETARIAN DIETS

Dairy products are recommended as an important part of a vegetarian diet by researchers in bone mineral metabolism.[49,50] Evidence indicates that vegetarian women who have included milk and other dairy foods in their diet over a lifetime have the best chance of maintaining adequate bone density as they age. Soy beverage, even if fortified with calcium, is not nutritionally equivalent to cow's milk. An 8 ounce serving of soybean beverage contains no vitamin B_{12}, only about half the phosphorus, 40% of the riboflavin, and 10% of the vitamin A in a serving of cow's milk.[86]

Milk can be an important source of high quality protein in a vegetarian diet. A high percentage of milk protein is retained by the body for maintenance and growth; it contains all of the essential amino acids needed by the body and is easily digested. The amino acid distribution of milk is ideal for calcium utilization. Milk has a higher proportion of lysine, which enhances calcium utilization (increases intestinal absorption and renal conservation),[126] and a lower proportion of the sulfur containing amino acids, methionine and cystine, which decrease calcium utilization. The relative surplus of lysine in milk also makes it the perfect companion to vegetable proteins, particularly cereals, which are low in lysine.[127]

Lacto-vegetarians also reap the following benefits:

- Milk and milk products provide significant amounts of calcium, phosphorus, magnesium, and zinc in proportions important for bone health. Milk and milk products are the major source of calcium in the American diet.
- Milk, yogurt, and hard cheeses have a surplus of calcium relative to protein (approximately 36:1), making them ideal foods for maximizing bone health.
- Lacto-vegetarians are less likely to have deficiencies in calcium or vitamin D. Studies have shown that lacto-vegetarians have adequate bone density.
- Vitamin D-fortified dairy products can afford protection from calcium and vitamin D depletion during times of growth or increased need, such as with adolescents, elderly persons, or during pregnancy and lactation.
- Milk (as well as eggs) provides an easily digestible form of protein, and one that is of high biologic value. Milk and other dairy foods can supply a significant amount of the protein requirement of the vegetarian diet and are recommended in the diets of vegetarian athletes.[128]
- Including milk in the diet improves its overall nutritional quality because of the many nutrients it delivers (see Chapter 1).[120,121,122,125]

XII. CONCLUSION

Some prefer the vegetarian lifestyle for sociological, animal rights, or religious reasons. However, there is no bone health justification for insisting that nonvegetarians avoid animal foods such as meat and dairy products, just as there is no bone health justification for urging vegetarians to give up the vegetarian diet and lifestyle.[15]

Both vegetarians and nonvegetarians can achieve optimal bone health if they follow a few simple guidelines:

- Consume a diet adequate in calcium, phosphorus, vitamin D, and moderate in protein and sodium.
- Engage in regular exercise.
- Refrain from lifestyle habits like smoking and excessive alcohol consumption, both of which decrease bone density.

It is never too late to adopt good habits of diet and health. Although one cannot completely reverse years of neglect, benefits can be gained at any stage of life.

REFERENCES

1. National Restaurant Association, survey, *Interest in eating vegetarian foods in restaurants*, June 1991.
2. More notes from the Scientific Department – How many vegetarians are there?, *Vegetarian J.*, September/October 21, 1997.
3. Sloan, E., Minding the move to meatless, *Food Technol.*, February 1994.

4. Notes from the Scientific Department – Special Report: Vegetarian Resource Group conducts Roper poll on eating habits of youths, *Vegetarian J.*, November/December 6, 1995.

5. Ribadeneira, T., "More teenagers foresaking meat: diet's shortcomings draw concern, advice on healthy nutrition," *Boston Globe*, December 7, 23, 1997.

6. Messina, V. K. and Burke, K. I., Position of The American Dietetic Association: vegetarian diets, *J. Am. Diet. Assoc.*, 97(11), 1317, 1997.

7. Ball, M., Vegetarian, vegan or meat eater: the pros and the cons, *Australian Family Physician*, 26(11), 1269, 1997.

8. Key, T. J. A., Thorogood, M., Appleby, P. N., and Burr, M. L., Dietary habits and mortality in 11,000 vegetarians and health conscious people: results of a 17 year follow up, *Br. Med. J.*, 313, 775, 1996.

9. Melby, C. L., Goldflies, D. G., and Toohey, M. L., Blood pressure differences in older black and white long-term vegetarians and nonvegetarians, *J. Am. Coll. Nutr.*, 12(3), 262, 1993.

10. Beilin, L. J. and Burke, V., Vegetarian diet components, protein and blood pressure: Which nutrients are important?, *Clin. Exp. Pharmacol. Physiol.*, 22, 195, 1995.

11. Appel, L. J., Moore, T. J., Obarzanek, E., Vollmer, W. M., Svetkey, L. P., Sacks, F. M., Bray, G. A., Vogt, T. M., Cutler, J. A., Windhauser, M. M., Lin, P-H., and Karanja, N., A clinical trial of the effects of dietary patterns on blood pressure, *N. Engl. J. Med.*, 336, 1117, 1997.

12. Burr, M. L. and Sweetnam, P. M., Vegetarianism, dietary fiber, and mortality, *Am. J. Clin. Nutr.*, 36, 873, 1982.

13. Kahn, H. A., Phillips, R. L., Snowdon, D. A., and Choi, W., Association between reported diet and all cause mortality: twenty-one year follow up on 27,530 adult Seventh-Day Adventists, *Am. J. Epidemiol.*, 119, 775, 1984.

14. Chang-Claude, J. and Frentzel-Beyme, R., Dietary and lifestyle determinants of mortality among German vegetarians, *Inter. J. Epidemiol.*, 22(2), 228, 1993.

15. Dwyer, J. R., Health Aspects of Vegetarian Diets, *Am. J. Clin. Nutr.*, 48, 712, 1988.

16. National Osteoporosis Foundation, *Boning Up on Osteoporosis*, Washington, D.C., 1997.

17. Krall, E. A. and Dawson-Hughes, B., Heritable and life style determinants of bone density, *J. Bone Miner. Res.*, 8(1), 1, 1993.

18. Hopper, J. L., Green, R. M., Nowson, C. A., Young, D., Sherwin, A. J., Kaymakci, B., Larkins, R. G., and Wark, J. D., Genetic, common environment, and individual specific components of variance for bone mineral density in 10- to 26-year-old females: a twin study, *Am. J. Epidemiol.*, 147, 17, 1998.

19. Slemenda, C. W., Christian, J. C., Williams, C. J., Norton, J. A., and Johnston, C. C., Jr., Genetic determinants of bone mass in adult women: a re-evaluation of the twin model and the potential importance of gene interaction on heritability estimates, *J. Bone Miner. Res.*, 6, 561, 1991.

20. Matkovic, V., Fontana, D., Tominac, C., Goel, P., and Chesnut III, C. H., Factors that influence peak bone mass formation: a study of calcium balance and the inheritance of bone mass in adolescent females, *Am. J. Clin. Nutr.*, 52, 878, 1990.

21. Lutz, J. and Tesar, R., Mother-daughter pairs: spinal and femoral bone densities and dietary intakes, *Am. J. Clin. Nutr.*, 52, 872, 1990.

22. Johnston, C. C., Jr. and Slemenda, C. W., Determinants of peak bone mass, *Osteoporosis Int.*, Suppl. 1, S54, 1993.

23. Heaney, R. P., Nutritional Factors in Osteoporosis, *Ann. Rev. Nutr.*, 13, 287, 1993.

24. Drinkwater, B. L., Exercise in the prevention of osteoporosis, *Osteoporosis Int.*, Suppl. 1, S169, 1993.

25. Ruiz, J. C., Mandel, C., and Garabedian, M., Influence of spontaneous calcium intake and physical exercise on the vertebral and femoral bone mineral density of children and adolescents, *J. Bone Miner. Res.*, 10, 675, 1995.

26. Boot, A. M., Ridder, M. A. J., Pols, H. A. P., Krenning, E. P., Mink, A, and Keizer-Schrama, S. M. P. F., Bone mineral density in children and adolescents: Relation to puberty, calcium intake, and physical activity, *J. Clin. Endocrinol. Metab.*, 82, 57, 1997.

27. Tylavsky, F. A., Anderson, J. J. B., Talmage, R. V., and Taft, T. N., Are calcium intakes and physical activity patterns during adolescence related to radial bone mass of white college-age females?, *Osteoporosis Int.*, 2, 232, 1992.

28. Metz, J. A., Anderson, J. J. B., and Gallagher, P. N., Intakes of calcium, phosphorus, and protein, and physical activity level are related to radial bone mass in young adult women, *Am. J. Clin. Nutr.*, 58, 537, 1993.

29. Specker, B. L., Evidence for an interaction between calcium intake and physical activity on changes in bone mineral density, *J. Bone Miner. Res.*, 11(10), 1539, 1996.

30. Grove, K. A. and Londeree, B. R., Bone density in postmenopausal women: high impact vs. low impact exercise, *Med. Sci. Sports and Exer.*, 24(11), 1190, 1992.

31. Nelson, M. E., Fisher, E. C., Dilmanian, F. A., Dallal, G. E., and Evans, W., A 1-y walking program and increased dietary calcium in postmenopausal women: effects on bone, *Am. J. Clin. Nutr.*, 53, 1, 1991.

32. Gutin, B. and Kasper, M. J., Can vigorous exercise play a role in osteoporosis prevention?, *Osteoporosis Int.*, 2, 55, 1992.

33. Slemenda, C. W., Cigarettes and the skeleton, *N. Engl. J. Med.*, 330(6), 430, 1994.

34. Hopper, J. L. and Seeman, E., The bone density of female twins discordant for tobacco use, *N. Engl. J. Med.*, 330(6), 387, 1994.

35. Hirsch, P. E. and Peng, T. C., Effects of alcohol on calcium homeostasis and bone, In, *Calcium and Phosphorus in Health and Disease*, J.J.B. Anderson and S.C. Garner Eds., Boca Raton, FL, CRC Press, 1996.

36. Mitchell, M. K., Aging and older adults, In, *Nutrition Across the Lifespan*, W.B. Saunders Co., Philadelphia, 1997.

37. Hegsted, D. M., Calcium and osteoporosis, *J. Nutr.*, 116(11), 2316, 1986.

38. Heaney, R. P., Excess dietary protein may not adversely affect bone, *J. Nutri.*, 128, 1054, 1998.

39. Ellis, F. R., Pathol, F. R. C., Holesh, S., and Ellis, J. W., Incidence of osteoporosis in vegetarians and omnivores, *Am. J. Clin. Nutr.*, 25, 555, 1972.

40. U.S. Department of Health and Human Services/National Institutes of Health, Sanchez, T. V., Mickelsen, O., Marsh, A. G., Garn, S. M., and Mayor, G. H., Bone mineral in elderly vegetarian and omnivorous females, Proceedings: International Conference on Bone Measurement, University of Toronto, Ontario, Canada, June 1-3, NIH publication no. 80-1938, 1978.

41. Heaney, R. P., Nutrient effects: discrepancy between data from controlled trials and observational studies, *Bone*, 21(6), 469, 1997.

42. Tesar, R., Notelovitz, M., Shim, E., Kauwell, G., and Brown, J., Axial and peripheral bone density and nutrient intakes of postmenopausal vegetarian and omnivorous women, *Am. J. Clin. Nutr.*, 56, 699, 1992.

43. Hunt, I. F., Murphy, N. J., Henderson, C., Clark, V. A., Jacobs, R. M., Johnston, P. K., and Coulson, A. H., Bone mineral content in postmenopausal women: comparison of omnivores and vegetarians, *Am. J. Clin. Nutr.*, 50(3), 517, 1989.

44. Lloyd, T., Schaeffer, J. M., Walker, M. A., and Demers, L. M., Urinary hormonal concentrations and spinal bone densities of premenopausal vegetarian and nonvegetarian women, *Am. J. Clin. Nutr.*, 54, 1005, 1991.
45. Reed, J. A., Anderson, J. J. B., Tylavsky, F. A., and Gallagher, P. N., Comparative changes in radial-bone density of elderly female lacto-ovo-vegetarians and omnivores, *Am. J. Clin. Nutr.*, 59(Suppl.), 1197S, 1994.
46. Tylavsky, F. A. and Anderson, J. J. B., Dietary factors in bone health of elderly lacto-ovo-vegetarian and omnivorous women, *Am. J. Clin. Nutr.*, 48, 842, 1988.
47. Marsh, A. G., Sanchez, T. V., Chaffee, F. L., Mayor, G. H., and Mickelsen, O., Bone mineral mass in adult lacto-ovo-vegetarian and omnivorous males, *Am. J. Clin. Nutr.*, 37, 453, 1983.
48. Barr, S. I., Prior, J. C., Janelle, K. C., and Lentle, B.C., Spinal bone mineral density in premenopausal vegetarian and nonvegetarian women: cross-sectional and prospective comparisons, *J. Am. Diet. Assoc.*, 98(7), 760, 1998.
49. Weaver, C. M. and Plawecki, K. L., Dietary calcium: adequacy of a vegetarian diet, *Am. J. Clin. Nutr.*, 59(Suppl.), 1238S, 1994.
50. Marsh, A. G., Sanchez, T. V., Michelsen, O., Chaffee, F. L., and Fagal, S. M., Vegetarians' lifestyle and bone mineral density, *Am. J. Clin. Nutr.*, 48(3 Suppl.), 837, 1988.
51. Zhao, X. and Chen, X., Diet and bone density among elderly Chinese, *Nutr. Rev.*, 50(12), 395, 1992.
52 Hu, J., Zhao, X., Jia, J., Parpia, B., and Campbell, T. C., Dietary calcium and bone density among middle-aged and elderly women in China, *Am. J. Clin. Nutr.*, 58, 219, 1993.
53. Chiu, J.-F., Lan, S.-J., Yang, C.-Y., Wang, P.-W., Yao, W.-J., and Hsieh, C.-C., Long-term vegetarian diet and bone mineral density in postmenopausal Taiwanese women, *Calcified Tissue Int.*, 60, 245, 1997.
54. Lau, E. M. C., Kwok, T., Woo, J., and Ho, S. C., Bone mineral density in Chinese elderly female vegetarians, vegans, lacto-vegetarians and omnivores, *Eur. J. Clin. Nutr.*, 52(1), 60, 1998.
55. Matkovic, V., Kostial, K., Simonovic, I., Buzina, R., Brodarec, A., and Nordin, B. E. C., Bone status and fracture rates in two regions of Yugoslavia, *Am. J. Clin. Nutr.*, 32, 540, 1979.
56. Gullberg, B., Johnell, O., and Kanis, J. A., World-wide projections for hip fracture, *Osteoporosis Int.*, 7, 407, 1997.
57. Bason, W. E., Maggi, S., Looker, A., Harris, T., Nair, C. R., Giaconi, J., Honkanen, R., Ho, S. C., Peffers, K. A., Torring, O., Gass, R., and Gonzalez, N., International comparison of hip fracture rates in 1988-89, *Osteoporosis Int.*, 6, 69, 1996.
58. Heaney, R. P., *Evaluation of publicly available scientific evidence regarding certain nutrient-disease relationships: 3. Calcium and osteoporosis*, Life Sciences Research Office, Federation of American Societies for Experimental Biology, Bethesda, MD, December 1991.
59. IOM (Institute of Medicine), *Dietary Reference Intakes for Calcium, Phosphorus, Magnesium, Vitamin D, and Fluoride*, Standing Committee on the Scientific Evaluation of Dietary Reference Intakes, Food and Nutrition Board, National Academy Press, Washington, D.C., 1997.
60. Heaney, R. P. and Barger-Lux, M. J., ADSA Foundation Lecture, Low calcium intake: the culprit in many chronic diseases, *J. Dairy Sci.*, 77, 1155, 1994.

61. National Institutes of Health, *The Sixth Report of the Joint National Committee on Detection, Evaluation, and Treatment of High Blood Pressure*, National High Blood Pressure Education Program, National Heart, Lung, and Blood Institute, NIH, November 1997.

62. Martinez, M.E., McPherson, R.S., Annegers, J.F., and Levin, B., Association of diet and colorectal adenomatous polyps: dietary fiber, calcium, and total fat, *Epidemiology*, 7(3), 264, 1996.

63. U.S. Department of Health and Human Services, Public Health Service, National Institutes of Health, *Consensus Development Conference Statement, Optimal Calcium Intake*, June 6–8, 12(4), 1, 1994.

64. American Medical Association, Council on Scientific Affairs, Intake of dietary calcium to reduce the incidence of osteoporosis, *Arch. Fam. Med.*, 6, 495, 1997.

65. U.S. Department of Agriculture/Agricultural Research Service, *Continuing Survey of Food Intakes by Individuals*, Food Surveys Research Group, Beltsville Human Nutrition Research Center, 1994–96.

66. Cleveland, L. E., Cook, A. J., Wilson, J. W., Friday, J. E., Ho, J. W., and Chahil, P. S., Pyramid Serving Data, *Results from USDA's 1994 Continuing Survey of Food Intakes by Individuals, Food Surveys Group*, Beltsville Human Nutrition Research Center, Agricultural Research Service, U. S. Department of Agriculture, Riverdale, MD, March 1997.

67. Dwyer, J. R., Nutritional consequences of vegetarianism, in *Ann. Rev. Nutr.*, 11, Olson, R. E., Bier, D. M., and McCormick, D. B., Eds., Annual Reviews, Inc., Palo Alto, 1991.

68. Janelle, K. C. and Barr, S. I., Nutrient intakes and eating behavior scores of vegetarians and nonvegetarian women, *J. Am. Diet. Assoc.*, 95(2), 180, 1995.

69. Dawson-Hughes, B., Harris, S., Kramich, C., Dallal, G., Rasmussen, H. M., Calcium retention and hormone levels in black and white women on high- and low-calcium diets, *J. Bone Miner. Res.*, 8, 779, 1993.

70. Weaver, C. M., Proulx, W. R., and Heaney, R., Choices for achieving adequate dietary calcium within a vegetarian diet, *Am. J. Clin. Nutr.*, 74, 00, 1999.

71. Gerrior, S. and Bente, L., U.S. Department of Agriculture, Center for Nutrition Policy and Promotion, *Nutrient Content of the U.S. Food Supply, 1909–94*, Home Economics Research Report No. 53.

72. Hunt, J. R., Matthys, L. A., and Johnston, L. K., Zinc absorption, mineral balance, and blood lipids in women consuming controlled lacto-ovo-vegetarian and omnivorous diets for 8 weeks, *Am. J. Clin. Nutr.*, 67, 421, 1998.

73. Holick, M. F., Vitamin D and bone health, *J. Nutr.*, 126, 1159S, 1996.

74. Lamberg-Allardt, C., Kärkkäinen, M., Seppänen, R., and Biström, H., Low serum 25-hydroxyvitamin D concentrations and secondary hyperparathyroidism in middle-aged white strict vegetarians, *Am. J. Clin. Nutr.*, 58, 684, 1993.

75. Russell, R. M., Micronutrient requirements of the elderly, *Nutr. Rev.*, 50(12), 463, 1992.

76. Dawson-Hughes, B., Dallal, G. E., Krall, E. A., Harris, S., Sokoll, L. J., and Falconer, G., Effect of vitamin D supplementation on wintertime and overall bone loss in healthy postmenopausal women, *Ann. Inter. Med.*, 115, 505, 1991.

77. Khaw, K-T, Scragg, R., and Murphy, S., Single-dose cholecalciferol suppresses the winter increase in parathyroid hormone concentrations in healthy older men and women: a randomized trial, *Am. J. Clin. Nutr.*, 59, 1040, 1994.

78. Gloth, F. M., Gundberg, C. M., Hollis, B. W., Haddad, J. G., and Tobin, J. D., Vitamin D deficiency in homebound elderly persons, *J. Am. Med. Assoc.*, 274(21), 1683, 1995.

79. Lobaugh, B., Blood calcium and phosphorus regulation, in *Calcium and Phosphorus in Health and Disease*, Anderson, J.J.B., and Garner, S.C., Eds., CRC Press, Boca Raton, FL, 1996.

80. Anderson, J. J. B. and Barett, J. H., Dietary phosphorus: the benefits and the problems, *Nutr. Today*, March/April 29, 1994.

81. Kerstetter, J.E., O'Brien, K. O., and Insogna, K.L., Dietary protein affects intestinal calcium absorption, *Am. J. Clin. Nutr.*, 68, 859, 1998.

82. Heaney, R. P., Protein intake and the calcium economy, *J. Am. Diet. Assoc.*, 93(11), 1259, 1993.

83. Zemel, M. B., Schuette, S. A., Hegsted, M., and Linkswiler, H. M., Role of the sulfur-containing amino acids in protein-induced hypercalciuria in men, *J. Nutr.*, 111, 545, 1981.

84. Mickelsen, O. and Marsh, A. G., Calcium requirement and diet, *Nutr. Today*, 24(1), 28, 1989.

85. Ball, D. and Maughan, R. J., Blood and urine acid-base status of premenopausal omnivorous and vegetarian women, *Br. J. Nutr.*, 78, 683, 1997.

86. Agricultural Research Service, U.S. Department of Agriculture, *Composition of Foods*, Handbook 8–1, U.S. Government Printing Office, Washington, D.C., 1976.

87. Feslanich, D., Willett, W. C., Stampfer, J. J., and Colditz, G. A., Protein consumption and bone fractures in women, *Am. J. Epidemiol.*, 143, 472, 1996.

88. Bonjour, J.P., Schurch, M.-A., and Rizzoli, R, Nutritional aspects of hip fractures, *Bone*, 18, 139S, 1996.

89. Recker, R. R., Davies, K. M., Hinders, S. M., Heaney, R. P., Stegman, M. R., and Kimmel, D. B., Bone gain in young adult women, *J. Am. Med. Assoc.*, 268(17), 2403, 1992.

90. Ho, S. C., Leung, P. C., Swaminathan, R., Chan, C., Ghan, S. S. G., Fan, Y. K., and Lindsay, R., Determinants of bone mass in Chinese women aged 21-40 years, II. Pattern of dietary calcium intake and association with bone mineral density, *Osteoporosis Int.*, 4, 167, 1994.

91. Baran, D., Sorensen, A., Grimes, J., Lew, R., Karellas, A., Johnson, B., and Roche, J., Dietary modification with dairy products for preventing vertebral bone loss in premenopausal women: a three-year prospective study, *J. Clin. Endocrine Metab.*, 70(1), 264, 1990.

92. Hunt, J. R., Gallagher, S. K., Johnson, L. K., and Lykken, G. I., High-versus low-meat diets: effects on zinc absorption, iron status, and calcium, copper, iron, magnesium, manganese, nitrogen, phosphorus, and zinc balance in postmenopausal women, *Am. J. Clin. Nutr.*, 62, 621, 1995.

93. Duff, T. L. and Whiting, S. J., Calciuric effects of short-term dietary loading of protein, sodium chloride and potassium citrate in prepubescent girls, *J. Am. Coll. Nutr.*, 17(2) 148, 1998.

94. Massey, L. K., Does excess dietary protein adversely affect bone?, *J. Nutr.*, 128, 1048, 1998.

95. Nordin, B. E. C., Morris, H. A., and Horowitz, M., Sodium, calcium and osteoporosis, in *Nutritional Factors in Osteoporosis*, Burckhardt, P., and Heaney, R. P., Eds., Raven Press, New York, 1991.

96. Matkovic, V. Illich, J. Z., Andon, M. B., Hsieh, L. C., Tzagournis, M. A., Lagger, B. J., and Goel, P. K., Urinary calcium, sodium, and bone mass of young females, *Am. J. Clin. Nutr.*, 62, 417, 1995.

97. Massey, L. K. and Whiting, S. J., Dietary salt, urinary calcium, and bone loss, a review, *J. Bone Miner. Res.*, 11(6), 731, 1996.

98. Itoh, R. and Suyama, Y., Sodium excretion in relation to calcium and hydoxyproline excretion in a healthy Japanese population, *Am. J. Clin. Nutr.*, 63, 735, 1996.

99. Shortt, C., Madden, A., Flynn, A., and Morrissey, P. A., Influence of dietary sodium intake on urinary calcium excretion in selected Irish individuals, *Eur. J. Clin. Nutr.*, 42, 595, 1988.

100. Castenmiller, J. J. M., Mensink R. P., vander Heijden, L, Louwenhoven, T., Hautrast, J. G. A. J., de Leeuw, P. W., and Schasfsma, G., The effect of dietary sodium on urinary calcium and potassium excretion in normotensive men with different calcium intakes, *Am. J. Clin. Nutr.*, 41, 52, 1985.

101. Devine, A., Criddle, R. A., Dick, I. M., Kerr, D. A., and Ricnce, R. L., A longitudinal study of the effect of sodium and calcium intakes on regional bone density in post-menopausal women, *Am. J. Clin. Nutr.*, 62, 740, 1995.

102. Nordin, B. E., Need, A. G., Morris, H. A., and Horowitz, M., The nature and significance of the relationship between urinary sodium and urinary calcium in women, *J. Nutr.*, 123, 1615, 1993.

103. Gordon, D. T., Dietary fiber and mineral nutrition, presented at the Vahouny Fiber Symposium, Washington, D.C., April 13-16, 1992.

104. Weaver, C. M., Heaney, R. P., Martin, B. R., and Fitsimmons, M. L., Human calcium absorption from whole wheat products, *J. Nutr.*, 121, 1769, 1991.

105. Weaver, C. M., Heaney, R. P., Teegarden, D., and Hinders, S. M., Wheat bran abolishes the inverse relationship between calcium load size and absorption fraction in women, *J. Nutr.*, 126, 303, 1996.

106. Coudray, C., Bellanger, J., Castiglia-Delavaud, C., Remesy, C., Vermorel, M., and Rayssignuier,Y., Effect of soluble or partly soluble dietary fibres supplementation on absorption and balance of calcium, magnesium, iron and zinc in healthy young men, *Eur. J. Clin. Nutr.*, 51, 375, 1997.

107. Balasubramanian, R., Johnson, E. J., and Marlett, J. A., Effect of wheat bran on bowel function and fecal calcium in older adults, *J. Am. Coll. Nutr.*, 6(3), 199, 1987.

108. Knox, T. A., Kassarjian, Z., Dawson-Hughes, B., Golner, B. B., Dallal, G. E., Arora, S., and Russell, R. M., Calcium absorption in elderly subjects on high- and low-fiber diets: effect of gastric acidity, *Am. J. Clin. Nutr.*, 53, 1480, 1991.

109. Specker, B. L., Nutritional concerns of lactating women consuming vegetarian diets, *J. Am. Diet. Assoc.*, 59(Suppl.), 1182S, 1994.

110. Bucher, H. C., Guyatt, G. H., Cook, R. J., Hatala, R., Cook, D. J., Lang, D., and Hunt, D., Effect of calcium supplementation on pregnancy-induced hypertension and preeclampsia, *JAMA*, 275, 1113, 1996.

111. O'Connor, M. A., Touyz, S. W., Dunn, S. M., and Beaumont, P. J. V., Vegetarianism in anorexia nervosa? A review of 116 consecutive cases, *Med. J. Aust.*, 147, 540, 1987.

112. Donovan, U. M. and Gibson, R. S., Dietary intakes of adolescent females consuming vegetarian, semi-vegetarian, and omnivorous diets, *J. Adolescent Health*, 18, 292, 1996.

113. Parsons, T. J., Van Dussledorp, M. V., Van Der Vliet, M., Van de Werken, K., Schaafsma, G., and Van Staveren, A., Reduced bone mass in Dutch adolescents fed a macrobiotic diet in early life, *J. Bone Miner. Res.*, 12, 1486, 1997.

114. Krizmanic, J., Here's who we are: a new survey reveals some surprises about America's 12 million plus (and counting) vegetarians, *Vegetarian Times*, October, 1992.

115. Recker, R. R., Bammi, A., Barger-Lux, M. J., and Heaney, R. P., Calcium absorbability from milk products, an imitation milk, and calcium carbonate, *Am. J. Clin. Nutr.*, 47, 93, 1988.

116. Lewis, N. M., Marcus, M. S. K., Behling, A., and Greger, J. L., Calcium supplements and milk: effects on acid-base balance and on retention of calcium, magnesium, and phosphorus, *Am. J. Clin. Nutr.*, 49, 527, 1989.

117. Sheikh, M., Santa Ana, C. A., Nikar, M. J., Schiller, L. R., and Fordtran, J. S., Gastrointestinal absorption of calcium from milk and calcium salts, *New England J. Med.*, 317, 532, 1987.

118. Garcia-Lopez, S. and Miller, G. D., Bioavailability of calcium from four different sources, *Nutr. Res.*, 11, 1187, 1991.

119. Position of The American Dietetic Association: Vitamin and mineral supplementation, *J. Am. Diet. Assoc.*, 96(1), 73, 1996.

120. Barger-Lux, M. J., Heaney, R. P., Packard, P. T., Lappe, J. M., and Recker, R. R., Nutritional correlates of low calcium intake, *Clin. Appl. Nutr.*, 2(4), 39, 1992.

121. Fleming, K. and Heimbach, J. R., Availability and consumption of calcium in the U.S.: levels and sources, *J. Nutr.*, 124, 1426S, 1994.

122. Devine, A., Prince, R. L., and Roma, B., Nutritional effect of calcium supplementation by skim milk powder or calcium tablets on total nutrient intake in postmenopausal women, *J. Am. Diet. Assoc.*, 95(2), 180, 1995.

123. Heaney, R. P., Food: What a surprise!, *Am. J. Clin. Nutr.*, 64, 791, 1996.

124. Chan, G. M., Hoffman, K., and McMurry, M., Effects of dairy products on bone and body composition in pubertal girls, *J. Pediatr.*, 126, 551, 1995.

125. Karanja, N., Morris, C. D., Rufolo, P., Illingworth, D. R., and McCarron, D. A., The impact of increasing calcium through the diet on nutrient consumption, plasma lipids and lipoproteins in humans, *Am. J. Clin. Nutr.*, 59, 900, 1994.

126. Civitelli R., Villareal, D. T., Agnusdei, D., Dietary L-lysine and calcium metabolism in humans, *Nutrition*, 8, 400, 1992.

127. Mahan, K. L. and Arlin, M., Eds., *Krause's Food Nutrition and Diet Therapy, 8th edition*, W. B. Saunders Co., Philadelphia, 1992.

128. Houtkooper, L., Food selection for endurance sports, *Med. Sci. Sports Exer.*, 24(9), S349, 1992.

CHAPTER 7

Dairy Foods and Oral Health

I. INTRODUCTION

Dental caries (tooth decay) and periodontal (gum) diseases are the two most prevalent, but preventable, oral health diseases in industrialized nations.[1-3] Although the prevalence of dental caries in children and periodontal diseases in adults has been declining,[1] these diseases nevertheless remain major public health concerns and pose a substantial economic burden on Americans.[3,4] As shown in Figure 7.1, dental caries among children still exceeds the goals for the year 2000.[3] Forty-five percent of school-aged children have dental caries in their permanent teeth and 94% of adults display evidence of past or current tooth decay.[3] Some evidence of periodontal disease occurs in over 90% of people 13 years of age and older.[3] Cost of dental care amounted to $47.6 billion in 1996.[4]

Dental caries increases with age, at least until middle age. The elderly are at high risk of developing root caries and periodontal diseases.[2,5] Thirty percent of the elderly (>65 years) have lost all of their teeth.[3]

The cause of these chronic, infectious oral health disorders is multifactorial, involving genetic and environmental (e.g., diet) factors. For centuries, food intake has been recognized as a contributing factor to dental caries.

Nutrition or nutritional status systemically influences the pre-eruptive development of teeth and oral tissues (e.g., the composition, size, and morphology of teeth, and the quantity and composition of saliva).[2,6,7] Nutritional deficiencies during the pre-eruptive development of teeth could directly and indirectly influence caries susceptibility by affecting the formation of enamel, composition and function of saliva, and immunological responses.[8] Epidemiological studies have demonstrated that a single episode of mild to moderate malnutrition during the first year of life is associated with increased caries in both deciduous and permanent teeth.[7] It is therefore important that children consume sufficient amounts of tooth-forming nutrients such as calcium, phosphorus, magnesium, fluoride, trace minerals, and other nutrients such a vitamin D. This is especially true between birth and three years of age when mineralization of tooth enamel primarily occurs.[9] Once teeth have erupted,

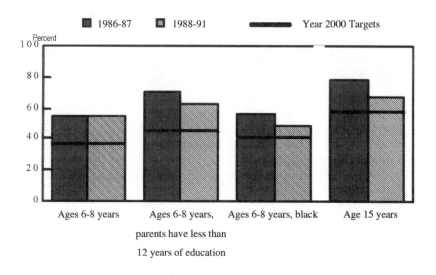

	1986-87	1988-91	Year 2000 Targets
Ages 6-8 years	54	54	35
Ages 6-8 years, parents have less than 12 years of education	70	62	45
Ages 6-8 years, black	56	48	40
Age 15 years	78	67	60

Figure 7.1 Prevalence of dental caries among children: United States, 1986-7, 1988-91, and year 2000 targets, (From National Center for Health Statistics. *Healthy People 2000 Review, 1995–96*. Hyattsville, Maryland: Public Health Service, 1996.)

it is the topical effect of food in the oral cavity that is critical to the development of oral diseases such as caries.

This chapter reviews scientific findings regarding the role of dairy foods in oral diseases. Research suggests that several varieties of cheese (e.g., aged Cheddar, Monterey Jack, Swiss) have caries protective properties and that milk is safe for teeth.

II. DENTAL CARIES

Foods per se do not cause dental caries. Dental caries is the result of complex interactions involving the host (e.g., nutrition, genetics, behavior, race, age), plaque bacteria, saliva flow and composition, and environment (Figure 7.2).[6] Diet is only one environmental factor in this process, albeit an important one.

The caries process is considered to be a dynamic equilibrium involving alternating periods of demineralization (i.e., release of calcium and phosphate from teeth) and remineralization (i.e., replacement of calcium and phosphate) (Figure 7.3). Following intake of food containing fermentable carbohydrates (e.g., sugars and cooked starches), bacteria in dental plaque on either smooth surfaces, or within pits

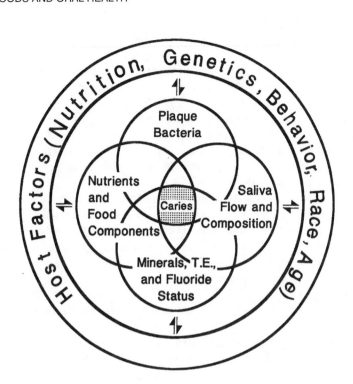

Figure 7.2 Multifactorial interactions in the etiology of dental caries. (From Navia, J.M., *Am. J. Clin. Nutr.*, 61(Suppl.), 407, 1995. With permission.)

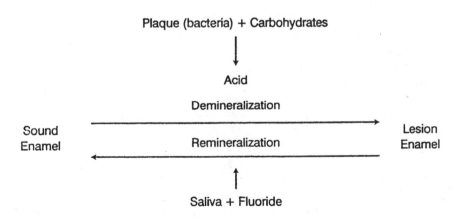

Figure 7.3 The caries process: an equilibrium of demineralization and remineralization.

and fissures, metabolize the carbohydrate producing organic acids. When organic acids cause plaque pH to fall from its usual level of around neutrality (i.e., pH 7.0) to a so-called "critical pH" of about 5.7, demineralization of tooth enamel occurs.

Over time (i.e., six months to two years), carious lesions result. Fortunately, caries is not a continuous process of mineral loss from the tooth. The protective effects of saliva, fluoride, and remineralization help to offset the many episodes of acid attack.

A number of factors influences both demineralization and remineralization. Dental caries results when the following conditions are present simultaneously: a susceptible tooth, cariogenic microorganisms in plaque, and a fermentable carbohydrate substrate especially if consumed frequently throughout the day. Prevention of caries involves increasing tooth resistance (e.g., by fluoride), reducing or interfering with oral microorganisms (e.g., by fluoride, oral hygiene), and changing the oral environment (e.g., dietary intervention).[2,10]

Food intake can affect the development of dental caries.[2] The cariogenic potential of simple sugars is well known.[2,8] However, it is not only the amount of fermentable carbohydrate in a food that influences its cariogenicity, but also the food's consistency, how often it is consumed, how long it remains in the mouth, and other foods with which it is consumed.[2,8] Sucrose in a retentive form (e.g., dried fruits) and eaten between meals is potentially more cariogenic than carbohydrates that are rapidly cleared from the mouth (e.g., in liquids such as chocolate milk).[2] The longer fermentable carbohydrates remain in the mouth or on tooth surfaces, the greater the risk of dental caries.

Some foods or food components have the potential to inhibit caries formation. As reviewed below, findings from laboratory animal and human (e.g., plaque pH, enamel demineralization/remineralization, epidemiological, clinical) studies indicate that dairy foods such as milk and cheese do not promote dental caries. Moreover, dairy foods, particularly certain cheeses, may even protect against this chronic oral health disease.[11,12]

A. Animal Studies

While findings from experimental animals cannot be casually extrapolated to humans, foods that are cariogenic for animals are generally thought to be cariogenic for humans.[13] Animal experiments also provide some evidence of the relative cariogenicity of different foods.[13]

Studies in laboratory animals indicate that several varieties of cheese inhibit the formation of caries even when the animals consume diets high in sugars or cooked starches. Few smooth surface carious lesions developed in laboratory rats when selected exposures to a high sucrose diet were followed by cheese intake.[14] Smooth surface caries has been demonstrated to be reduced in rats fed Cheddar cheese, a cheese spread, mozzarella cheese, and cream cheese.[14,15] Cheese intake also has been demonstrated to reduce the incidence of root caries, a common form of dental caries in older adults. When experimental desalivated animals (i.e., animals at high risk of caries because of their lack of saliva) were fed Cheddar- or Swiss-type cheeses, along with a cariogenic diet, the animals developed fewer and less severe caries on crowns and root surfaces than when fed cariogenic snacks alone or with no additional snacks.[16] These findings may be of relevance for elderly humans for whom root-surface caries is becoming of increasing concern.

Experimental animal studies not only indicate that cheese prevents dental caries, but also that milk is relatively noncariogenic (i.e., not caries promoting).[13,17-24] In 1961 Dreizen et al.[17] reported that non-fat dry cow's milk fed to laboratory rats was noncariogenic. In 1966, Stephan[18] identified whole milk as a noncariogenic food. Similar findings were obtained in 1981 by Reynolds and Johnson[20] who suggested that supplementation of a cariogenic diet with milk (4 to 5%) reduced the incidence of caries in rats. When three casein-free milk mineral concentrates with various levels of whey protein, calcium, and phosphate were included in a caries-producing diet containing 20% sucrose, significant reductions in caries occurred on the smooth surfaces of rat molars.[21]

When desalivated rats were given 2% milk (4% lactose) or lactose-reduced milk, the animals remained essentially caries free.[22] In contrast, animals who drank sucrose (10%) or lactose (4%) solutions developed some caries. This study demonstrates that milk with lactose, in contrast to sucrose, is either noncariogenic or minimally caries-promoting. The authors of the study suggest that because milk has many of the physical properties of saliva and is negligibly cariogenic, this food may be a good saliva substitute for older people who have decreased salivary flow (i.e., hyposalivation) and, as such, experience difficulty in chewing, tasting, and swallowing food. Hyposalivation can result from either use of medications or degenerative physiological changes.[10] Milk may serve as a saliva substitute by providing moisture and lubrication for dehydrated oral mucosa.[25] It also may buffer oral acidity, reduce enamel solubility, and contribute to enamel remineralization.[25] Individuals with hyposalivation may be able to sip milk to alleviate their discomfort without risk of developing caries.

Several studies demonstrate that milk exerts some protection against the cariogenic challenge of sucrose.[23,24] When the cariostatic properties of milk were examined in laboratory rats, the relative noncariogenicity of milk was maintained despite the addition of sucrose in concentrations of 2, 5, and 10%.[23] Animals given milk containing as much as 10% sucrose developed 70% less smooth surface caries than animals given a 10% aqueous solution of sucrose (Figure 7.4).[23] However, milk containing sucrose was more cariogenic than milk alone.[23] When desalivated rats received a sucrose solution (5%) or one of several commonly used infant formulas, or 2% milk, cow's milk was found to be the least cariogenic of all the products tested.[24] In contrast, sucrose was by far the most cariogenic.[24] In fact, sucrose was 2.5 times more cariogenic than the most cariogenic infant formulas and at least 20 times more cariogenic than milk.[24] Experimental animal studies have identified yogurt as a food with low cariogenic potential,[26] thus supporting earlier findings.[27]

B. Human Studies

1. Plaque pH

Plaque acidity studies, which indicate pH changes following food intake, are another important measure of relative food cariogenicity.[28] Human dental plaque pH studies have shown that a number of cheeses such as aged Cheddar, Swiss, blue,

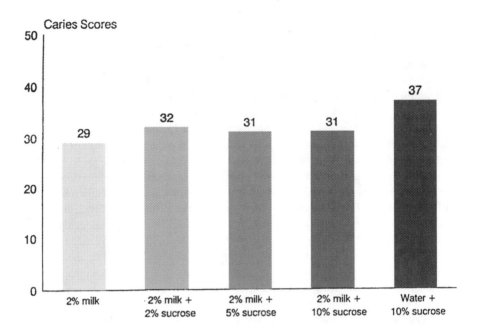

Figure 7.4   Sucrose-milk solutions are significantly less cariogenic in rats than a sucrose-water solution. Note that milk protects against the cariogenic challenge of sucrose. (Adapted from Bowen, W. H. and Pearson, S. K., *Caries Res.*, 27, 461, 1993. With permission.)

Table 7.1   Foods Which Do Not Cause the Interproximal Plaque pH to Fall to 5.5 Within 30 Minutes after Ingestion

Eggs	Chewing Gums
Cheeses	Mannitol
Blue	Sorbitol
Brie	Xylitol
Cheddar, aged	Meats
Gouda	Ham
Monterey Jack	Nuts
Mozzarella	Peanuts
Swiss	Walnuts
	Swiss Products*

* Approximately 90 sweet confectionary products formulated to be nonacidogenic in humans.

From Schachtele, C. F. and Harlander, S. K., *J. Can. Dent. Assn.*, 3, 213, 1984. With permission.

Monterey Jack, mozzarella, Brie, and Gouda produce little or no plaque acid (Table 7.1).[29-32] When a variety of foods were fed to humans and the production of inter-proximal plaque pH was measured by telemetry, all foods except aged Cheddar cheese and skim milk caused plaque pH to fall close to 4.0 (i.e., a pH conducive to caries).[30] Some cheeses, including aged Cheddar, Monterey Jack, and Swiss have been demonstrated to eliminate sucrose-induced decreases in plaque pH when consumed just prior to[30] or after[32] sucrose intake. A study of plaque pH changes demonstrated a beneficial effect of American processed cheese.[33] When processed cheese was eaten alone or before sucrose (10%), plaque pH stayed above 5.7, the "safe for teeth" level (Figure 7.5).[33]

Early studies evaluating changes in plaque pH in humans following intake of specific foods suggested that fat free milk is relatively noncariogenic.[31] When Dodds and Edgar[34] ranked seven foods (apple drink, caramel, chocolate, cookie, skimmed milk powder, snack cracker, and wheat flake) according to their plaque pH response in 12 volunteers, skimmed milk powder was ranked as the food with the lowest potential cariogenicity.

2. Demineralization/Remineralization Studies

Several studies suggest that dairy foods such as cheese and milk prevent de-mineralization of enamel and favor remineralization. Silva et al.,[35] using intraoral caries models (i.e., models that use sections of human or bovine enamel placed at interproximal sites in fixed appliances), found that consumption of 5 grams (g) of aged Cheddar cheese immediately following sucrose intake (i.e., a 10% sucrose challenge) reduced, by an average of 71%, sucrose-induced demineralization of experimental enamel slabs. Similarly, cheese[36] and a dairy product (derived from the whey of cow's milk) containing 26% calcium and 39% phosphorus[37] were identified as foods of low cariogenic potential in in vivo intraoral tests carried out in New Zealand. The enamel-softening effect of toasted breadcrumbs was substantially reduced when cheese was added.[36] Similarly, the addition of whey mineral to fruit juice reduced the enamel softening effect of fruit juice.[37] Processed cheese also has been shown to prevent demineralization and enhance remineralization of enamel and root lesions in a human in situ caries model.[33] In this model, processed cheese reduced carious lesions on root surfaces by 52%.

A study in Israel involving 10 subjects demonstrated that chewing hard cheese significantly increased in situ remineralization of previously softened (by a cola-type drink) tooth enamel surfaces.[38] The researchers speculated that the calcium and phosphate in cheese may be partly responsible for the remineralization. Likewise, using an in situ caries model developed by Featherstone and Zero,[39] enamel de-mineralization occurred in the absence of Cheddar cheese. In contrast, in the presence of cheese, a significant trend toward remineralization of enamel was evident.[39]

Early in vitro studies demonstrated that the presence of milk solids reduced the ability of a fermentable food to demineralize enamel.[27] Moreover, whole milk solids offered more protection against demineralization than skim milk solids,[27] possibly because of the inclusion of fat which has been demonstrated to have protective effects. Other investigations indicate that phosphoproteins in milk are adsorbed into

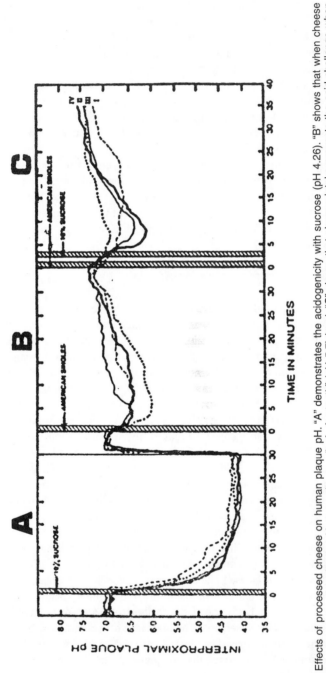

Figure 7.5 Effects of processed cheese on human plaque pH. "A" demonstrates the acidogenicity with sucrose (pH 4.26). "B" shows that when cheese is eaten alone, the plaque pH stays above a "safe for teeth" (pH 5.7) level. "C" shows that cheese intake prevents the acid challenge when followed by sucrose. (From Jensen, M. E. and Wefel, J. S., *Am. J. Dent.*, 3(5), 217, 1990. With permission.)

enamel *in vitro* and inhibit acid dissolution of enamel.[40,41] Milk also has been shown to remineralize enamel *in vitro*.[42] Gedalia and coworkers[43] reported that milk (and saliva) enhanced remineralization of previously softened tooth enamel surfaces.

When the relative potential of different foods to contribute to caries was assessed by a combination of tests (i.e., two plaque pH models, an experimental animal study, and an *in vitro* enamel demineralization model), skimmed milk was found to be the least cariogenic and apple juice the most cariogenic of the seven foods tested (i.e., apple juice, chocolate, caramel, wheat flake, cookie, cracker, skimmed milk).[28] Other researchers have identified dairy foods such as cheese and milk as foods with relatively low cariogenic potential.[44]

3. Epidemiological and Clinical Studies

Epidemiological studies associate intake of cheese and milk with a reduced incidence of caries.[45-48] An epidemiological study published in 1984 found that the only significant difference in the diets of 23 caries-prone and 19 caries-free English school children over a two year period was average intake of cheese.[45] The caries-free group consumed twice as much cheese (8 g daily) as did the caries-prone group (4 g daily).[45]

Milk intake has been associated with a low incidence of caries in 14-year-old Danish school children.[46] In a survey of preschool children of different ethnic origins in Fort Worth, Texas, average decayed, extracted, or filled teeth (DEF) decreased with increased daily milk intake (as determined by a 24-hour dietary recall), especially for black and Hispanic children.[47]

When the effect of milk intake on dental caries was studied in 6- to 11- year old Italian school children, it was found that milk protected against caries in children who did not use fluoride, whose oral hygiene was poor, and who frequently had a high daily sucrose intake.[48]

Epidemiological investigations support a protective effect of cheese against root caries.[44,49] Root caries affects about two thirds of the U.S. elderly.[44] Given that the size of this population is increasing, combined with the use of prescription drugs, many of which suppress saliva gland function, root caries can be expected to become an even greater problem. When food intake was assessed in 275 adults aged 44 to 64 years who were grouped according to their root caries status, those without root caries consumed more cheese, dairy foods, fruits and fruit juices, and less sugars and starches than did subjects with root caries.[49] In another investigation[44] of the relationship between diet and root caries in 141 adults aged 47 to 83 years, individuals in the lowest quartile for root caries consumed approximately twice as much cheese as those in the highest quartile (Table 7.2). The researchers reported that individuals who were free from root caries consumed 50% more cheese and 25% more of other dairy products than did subjects who experienced the most caries.[44] Additionally, caries-free subjects had higher intakes of fiber, protein, calcium, phosphorus, and magnesium and lower sugar intakes than subjects with caries (Table 7.3).[44]

A protective effect of cheese has also been demonstrated in a clinical trial involving 179 Israeli children aged 7 to 9 years.[50] In this two-year clinical trial, dental caries was significantly reduced (by 26%) in children who consumed 5 g of

Table 7.2 Frequency of Consumption of Specific Food Items (Based on the Food Diaries), With Groups Separated by Caries Experience[1]

Food item[2]	Lower quartile root DFS/100 teeth	Upper quartile root DFS/100 teeth
Liquid sugars	4.23 ± 5.74	8.50 ± 7.26
Sticky sugars	2.81 ± 1.81	8.41 ± 1.81[3]
Cheese	4.77 ± 3.00	2.20 ± 2.00[4]

[1] x± SD; n = 13, lower quartile; n = 16, upper quartile. DFS, decayed and filled surfaces.
[2] There were no differences in the total number of food items eaten by the two groups.
[3,4] Significantly different from lower quartile: [3] $P < 0.02$ [4] $P < 0.03$.

From Papas, A.S. et al., *Relationship of diet to root caries*, Am. J. Clin. Nutr., 61(Suppl:423s), 1995. With permission.

Table 7.3 Comparison of Intakes in Subjects With Root Caries Compared With Those Who Were Root-Caries Free[1]

	Subjects With Caries	Subjects Without Caries
Crude fiber (g)	4	5
Protein (g)	76	87
Calcium (mg)	727	828
Phosphorus (mg)	1136	1131[2]
Magnesium (mg)	241	297
Sucrose (g)	11	7[2]
Refined sugar (g)	22	15

[1] N = 66, with caries; n = 42, without caries
[2] Significantly different from caries-laden subjects, P = 0.02

From Papas, A.S. et al., *Relationship of diet to root caries*, Am. J. Clin. Nutr., 61(Suppl:423s), 1995. (With permission.)

Edam cheese a day following breakfast compared to children who did not consume this extra cheese (Table 7.4).

C. How Dairy Foods Inhibit Caries Formation

The mechanism(s) or protective factor(s) responsible for the cariostatic action of cheese and milk is unknown, although several possibilities have been proposed.[11,14,21,22,51,52] Cheese, for example, may stimulate the flow of alkaline saliva and reduce the number of plaque bacteria.[11,14] Enamel demineralization can be prevented by stimulation of the production of saliva, which increases plaque pH (i.e., increases its alkalinity) and the clearance of fermentable carbohydrate from the oral cavity (Figure 7.6).[29,35] However, the finding that cheese may inhibit dental caries in the absence of saliva indicates that there may be other mechanisms involved in addition to its effect on saliva.[16]

Components in cheese or milk such as protein (casein and whey), lipids, calcium, and phosphorus may be partly responsible for the beneficial effects of these foods

Table 7.4 **Mean and Number of DMF Surfaces For Groups 1 and 2 at the Start of the Study and After 2 Years**

Group	No. of Children	Baseline DMFS (SE)	At 2 Years DMFS (SE)	Caries Increment	% Reduction
Control	136	0.55[a] (0.16)	2.90 (0.31)	2.35[b] (0.35)	
Cheese	84	0.62[a] (0.25)	1.24 (0.15)	0.62[b] (0.19)	26.4

(SE) ± not standard error
[a] Not significant
[b] Significant, P < 0.001

From Gedalia, I. et al., *Dental caries protection with hard cheese consumption*, Am. J. Dent., 7, 6, December 1994. With permission.

on oral health.[11,21,22,51-55] Casein and whey proteins in dairy foods may be involved in the reduction of enamel demineralization.[11] Using an intraoral caries model, Reynolds[41] found that casein prevented enamel demineralization and that this effect was related to casein's incorporation into plaque. However, in a study of the effect of cheese fractions on enamel demineralization in humans, water-soluble protein in cheese did not exert a major role in protecting the enamel from demineralization.[51] Casein phosphopeptides in cheese and milk may be responsible for the anticariogenicity of these foods by concentrating calcium and phosphate in plaque.[11] The plaque pH effect of cheese has been attributed in part to the proteolysis of cheese proteins,

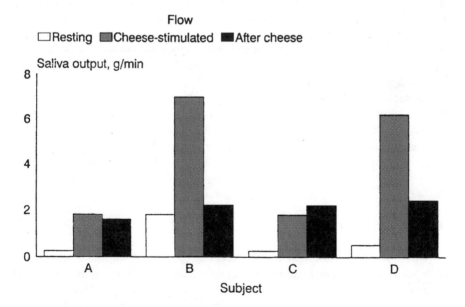

Figure 7.6 Salivary flow rate (g/min) for 4 subjects during pre-experimental resting period (3 min), during cheese stimulation (1 min), and during post-cheese period (2 min). (From Silva, M. F., de A., Jenkins, G. N., Burgess, R. C., and Sandham, H. J., *Caries Res.*, 20, 263, 1986. With permission.)

notably casein.[32] Reynolds and colleagues[54] have suggested that casein phosphopeptides released by the proteolysis of cheese on consumption stabilize calcium phosphate through the formation of casein phosphopeptide-calcium phosphate complexes (CPP-CP) and facilitate the uptake of calcium and phosphate by plaque. Studies in rats investigated the effect of CPP-CP on caries. Animals were fed a cariogenic diet free of dairy products and solutions of CPP-CP (0.1, 0.2, 0.5, and 1.0% w/v) were applied to molar teeth twice daily. Control groups received solutions of 500 ppm fluoride or non-phosphorylated peptides of a casein digest (0.5% w/v). The investigators reported that CPP-CP reduced caries in a dose response manner and that fluoride and CPP-CP worked synergistically to reduce caries.[54]

Milk proteins may protect against caries by inhibiting the ability of cavity-causing bacteria to adhere to tooth surfaces. Milk proteins, particularly kappa casein, have been demonstrated to reduce the adherence of *Streptoccocus mutans* to the saliva-coated hydroxyapatite surfaces of teeth.[55-57] Milk and the milk protein, kappa-casein, also may protect against caries by decreasing the activity of the plaque-promoting enzyme, glucosyltransferase produced by *S. mutans*, and the ability of this enzyme to adhere to tooth surfaces or saliva-coated hydroxyapatite.[57]

Lipids in cheese, by forming a protective coating on enamel surfaces, may retard the dissolution of enamel surfaces. An antibacterial effect of fatty acids in cheese also may explain cheese's protective effect against dental caries.[11,16]

The high calcium and phosphorus content of cheese and milk may contribute to the anticariogenic effect of these foods.[11,21,43,51,52] Cheese may be protective by increasing calcium and phosphorus concentrations in dental plaque thus favoring remineralization.[11,38,51,52] A significant increase in plaque calcium, but not plaque phosphate, was reported in subjects who ate 5 g of several different varieties of cheese (mild Cheddar, Cheshire, Danish blue, Double Glouster, Edam, Gouda, Stilton, Wensleydale) (Figure 7.7).[52] The findings led the authors to suggest that eating cheese at the end of a meal might be an effective way to reduce dental caries.[52]

In studies reported by Gedalia et al.,[38,43] the remineralizing effects of hard cheese and cow's milk on enamel surfaces previously softened by an acidic beverage were attributed to the uptake of calcium and phosphate salts by the surface enamel. These findings support earlier observations from *in vitro* and *in vivo* experiments that cheese's calcium and phosphorus content contributes to this food's ability to inhibit demineralization and favor remineralization, thus, reducing the cariogenicity of sucrose.[51]

D. Chocolate Milk

There is some evidence that foods containing cocoa, milk fat, and other components such as calcium and phosphorus found in chocolate milk may be less likely to contribute to dental caries than either sucrose alone or snack foods such as potato chips, cookies, and raisins.[58] Cocoa powder has been shown to be noncariogenic.[59,60] Water-soluble components of cocoa have been found to inhibit plaque accumulation and caries by reducing the biosynthesis of extracellular polysaccharide by selected human plaque-forming microorganisms (e.g., *Streptococcus mutans*).[60]

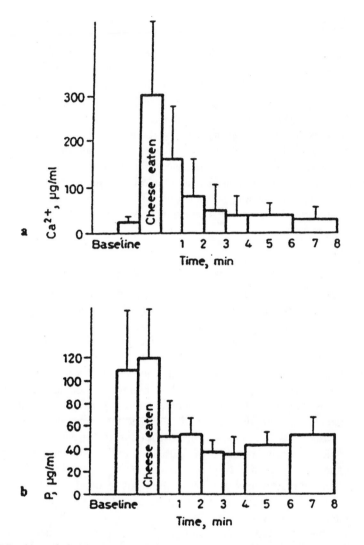

Figure 7.7   Mean Ca^{2+} (a) and soluble phosphate (b) concentrations in saliva before, during, and after eating 5 g of Edam cheese. (From Jenkins, G. N. and Hargreaves, J. A., *Caries Res.*, 23, 159, 1989. With permission.)

The moderate amount of sucrose in chocolate milk is no more likely to cause dental caries than other sugars such as lactose in milk or fructose in fruits.[47,61] As discussed above, the inclusion of sugar in milk is very much less likely to contribute to dental caries than sugar in water.[23,24] The cariogenicity of chocolate milk has yet to be established in humans. However, liquids such as chocolate milk tend to clear the mouth faster than carbohydrate-containing solids, and therefore may be less likely to cause tooth decay.

E. Nursing Bottle Caries

The belief that cow's milk causes nursing bottle caries is a myth that needs to be dispelled.[62] Nursing bottle caries is a rampant form of caries before three years of age which results from allowing infants and young children to use a nursing bottle containing a fermentable carbohydrate (e.g., juice) as a pacifier (e.g., while sleeping).[2,62,63] There is no epidemiological evidence to support the suggestion that milk intake contributes to this condition.[62] Repeated studies in laboratory animals, including desalivated animals, demonstrate that intake of cow's milk has a negligible, if any, effect on dental caries.[22-24,62] Other factors in addition to the contents of the nursing bottle such as the presence of the nipple in the mouth and intake of solid food may contribute to nursing bottle caries.[62] The nursing bottle can effectively block the tooth surfaces from saliva, thereby increasing the cariogenicity of any food remaining in the mouth.[62]

F. Milk as a Vehicle for Fluoridation

There is firm evidence that fluoride helps to prevent dental caries in individuals of all ages.[2,64] For this reason, community water supplies in many areas of the country are fluoridated. Of interest is whether or not the anticariogenic effect of sodium fluoride is more pronounced when administered in water or in milk. Milk has attracted attention as a vehicle for fluoridation because it is a universal food for growing children, it contains essential nutrients needed for growth and development, and it is consumed by many people, especially children.[9,65] As reviewed by Marino,[65] clinical trials over the past 30 years support a protective effect of fluoridated milk against dental caries. Recently, Pakhomov described the caries reducing effect of a community-based milk fluoridation project involving Bulgarian school children.[66] Also, the caries protective potential of fluoridated milk has been demonstrated in laboratory animals [67,68] as well as in *in vitro* studies of human dental enamel.[69] In a study in which laboratory rats were given frequent feedings of fluoridated milk, plain milk, fluoridated water, and plain distilled water via an automatic feeding machine, the lowest caries scores occurred in the animals given the fluoridated milk, followed by the plain milk.[67] The findings led the authors to conclude that the anticariogenic effect of sodium fluoride is greater when the vehicle is milk instead of water.

III. PERIODONTAL DISEASES

Periodontal diseases are chronic infectious disorders characterized by inflammation and progressive loss of soft tissues supporting the teeth, as well as resorption of alveolar bone.[70] Actually, periodontal diseases include several diseases of hard and soft tissues surrounding the teeth: gingivitis (inflammatory gum changes without loss of bone) and periodontitis (inflammatory and destructive changes in the soft tissues and in the bone supporting the teeth). Most Americans will develop gingivitis in which there is mild periodontal disease. Only rarely does this condition progress to severe periodontitis with risk of tooth loss.[70] Because of the potential for severe consequences in terms of tooth loss and treatment costs, as well as ensuing nutritional problems, prevention of periodontal diseases is emphasized.[2,5,70]

Periodontal diseases are initiated by a bacterial infection, but are modified by host response factors including those that affect bone remodeling.[70] Certain individuals are at high risk of periodontal diseases because of a genetic predisposition, diseases such as autoimmune diseases, diabetes, alcoholism, and endocrine disorders; use of certain drugs (e.g., antiepileptic, cancer therapy, corticosteroids); and lifestyle choices such as cigarette smoking, chewing tobacco, and consumption of a nutritionally inadequate diet.[2,70]

Unlike dental caries for which a strong role for diet is suggested, the role of diet, specific foods, or single nutrients in the development of periodontal diseases is unclear. Theoretically, diet may modulate the progression of periodontal diseases in several ways. The composition of the diet can affect accumulation of plaque. Diet may also affect host defense mechanisms important in oral health. Periodontal diseases are infectious disorders and it is well known that dietary imbalances alter inflammatory and immunologic responses and thus resistance to infection.[2]

The role of specific foods such as dairy foods on immune processes and periodontal diseases is unknown. In one study, cheese intake was associated with reduced bone loss (root-surface exposure) in experimental animals receiving a cariogenic diet, leading the authors to suggest that cheese may be important in the prevention of periodontal disease.[16]

Diet may influence the pathogenesis of periodontal diseases by its effect on the metabolism of collagen and alveolar bone. Calcium deficiency has been speculated to be a major factor in periodontitis, and periodontal disease has been hypothesized to be a forerunner of osteoporosis.[71-76] However, studies in experimental animals carried out in the early 1980s to examine the relationship between calcium intake, alveolar bone health, and periodontal diseases provided inconsistent findings.[71] As reviewed by Jeffcoat et al.,[70] findings of studies examining the association between oral bone loss and osteoporosis are conflicting. Although the two conditions share several of the same risk factors (e.g., advancing age, cigarette smoking), and common mechanisms for bone loss may be involved, few controlled clinical trials have examined whether oral bone loss is related to osteoporosis. Nor has it been established whether osteoporosis-related bone loss increases the risk of alveolar bone resorption.[77] A six-year longitudinal trial with a subset of participants in the Women's Health Initiative is currently underway to help determine the relationship between oral bone loss and osteoporosis, including the role of calcium in oral bone loss.[76]

Prevention of the progression of periodontal diseases involves removal of soft and hard deposits and keeping teeth free of bacterial plaque. Consuming a nutritionally adequate diet also may help reduce the risk of periodontal diseases, although further research is necessary to explain the role of diet and specific foods in this oral health disease.

IV. SUMMARY

Given the number of factors, genetic and environmental (diet), that contribute to oral health, how a particular food (e.g., single dairy food), consumed as part of a complex diet, influences dental caries and periodontal diseases is difficult to establish. There is substantial evidence (i.e., from animal testing, human plaque pH measurements, *in vitro* caries models) supporting the protective effect of a variety of cheeses against dental caries. Consuming cheese before, during, or after a meal may reduce the risk of dental caries.

Evidence indicates that milk (whole, lowfat, chocolate), consumed as usual or as part of a diet, does not contribute to dental caries. Further, research findings indicate that milk may be a good saliva substitute for individuals with hyposalivation such as may occur in older people receiving certain medications.

Given the growing population of older adults in the U.S., many of whom are at risk of periodontal diseases and root caries, more research on the role of dairy foods in these conditions seems warranted. Also, the relationship, if any, between oral bone density, periodontal diseases, and osteoporosis needs to be clarified.

The findings reviewed in this chapter regarding the protective effect of milk and other dairy foods in dental health are consistent with those of another review.[12] This latter review concluded that milk and yogurt without added sugar are safe for teeth and that cheese protects against dental caries. The beneficial effect of milk and milk products on oral health is yet another reason to encourage intake of recommended daily servings of foods from the Milk Group. Also, research supporting the caries-protective effects of dairy products should be incorporated into dietary recommendations to help reduce the risk of dental caries.

REFERENCES

1. National Institute of Dental Research, *Oral Health of United States Children, The National Survey of Dental Caries in U.S. School Children: 1986–1987, National and Regional Findings*, NIH # 89-2247, September 1989.
2. DePaola, D.P., Faine, M.P., and Vogel, R.I., Nutrition in relation to dental medicine, In, *Modern Nutrition in Health and Disease*, 8th ed., Shils, M.E., Olson, J.A., and Shike, M. (Eds.), Lea & Febiger, Philadelphia, PA, 1994, 1007.
3. U.S. Department of Health and Human Services, Public Health Service, *Healthy People 2000 1995–96*. DHHS Publ. No. (PHS) 96-1256, Hyattsville, MD, November 1996.
4. Health Care Financing Administration, Office of the Actuary, National Health Statistics Group, U.S. Department of Health and Human Services, Health care spending rise at record low. January 13, 1998, www.HCFA.Gov (5 Feb. 1998).
5. Palmer, C. A. and Papas, A. S., Nutrition and the oral health of the elderly, *World Rev. Nutr. Diet.*, 59, 71, 1989.
6. Navia, J. M., A new perspective for nutrition: the health connection, *Am. J. Clin. Nutr.*, 61(Suppl.), 407s, 1995.

7. Alvarez, J. O., Nutrition, tooth development, and dental caries, *Am. J. Clin. Nutr.*, 61(s), 410s, 1995.

8. Burt, B. A. and Ismail, A. I., Diet, nutrition, and food cariogenicity, *J. Dent. Res.*, 65(spec. issue), 1475, 1986.

9. White, C. H., Milk, milk products, and dental health, *J. Dairy Sci.*, 70, 392, 1987.

10. Bowen, W. H. and Tabak, L. A. Eds., *Cariology for the Nineties*, University of Rochester Press, Rochester, NY, 1993.

11. Herod, E. L., The effect of cheese on dental caries: a review of the literature, *Aust. Dent. J.*, 36(2), 120, 1991.

12. Moynihan, P., The effects of milk and milk products on dental health. A critical update, *Nutrition Monitor* (National Dairy Council, London, UK), April 1997.

13. Tanzer, J. M., Testing food cariogenicity with experimental animals, *J. Dent. Res.*, 65(spec. issue), 1491, 1986.

14. Edgar, W. M., Bowen, W. H., Amsbaugh, S., Monell-Torrens, E., and Brunelle, J., Effects of different eating patterns on dental caries in the rat, *Caries Res.*, 16, 384, 1982.

15. Harper, D. S., Osborn, J. C., Hefferren, J. J., and Clayton, R., Cariostatic evaluation of cheeses with diverse physical and compositional characteristics, *Caries Res.*, 20, 123, 1986.

16. Krobicka, A., Bowen, W. H., Pearson, S., and Young, D. A., The effects of cheese snacks on caries in desalivated rats, *J. Dent. Res.*, 66(6), 1116, 1987.

17. Dreizen, S., Dreizen, J. G., and Stone, R. E., The effect of cow's milk on dental caries in the rat, *J. Dent. Res.*, Sept.–Oct., 1025, 1961.

18. Stephan, R. M., Effects of different types of human foods on dental health in experimental animals, *J. Dent. Res.*, 45(5), 1551, 1966.

19. Navia, M. and Lopez, H., Rat caries assay of reference foods and sugar-containing snacks, *J. Dent. Res.*, 62(8), 893, 1983.

20. Reynolds, E. C. and Johnson, I. H., Effect of milk on caries incidence and bacterial composition of dental plaque in the rat, *Archs. Oral Biol.*, 26, 445, 1981.

21. Harper, D. S., Osborn, J. C., Clayton, R., and Hefferren, J. J., Modification of food cariogenicity in rats by mineral-rich concentrates from milk, *J. Dent. Res.*, 66(1), 42, 1987.

22. Bowen, W. H., Pearson, S. K., Van Wuyckhuyse, B. C., and Tabak, L. A., Influence of milk, lactose-reduced milk, and lactose on caries in desalivated rats, *Caries Res.*, 25(4), 283, 1991.

23. Bowen, W. H. and Pearson, S. K., Effect of milk on cariogenesis, *Caries Res.*, 27, 461, 1993.

24. Bowen, W. H., Pearson, S. K., Rosalen, P. L., Miguel, J. C., and Shih, A. Y., Assessing the cariogenic potential of some infant formulas, milk and sugar solutions, *J. Am. Dent. Assoc.*, 128, 865, 1997.

25. Herod, E. L., The use of milk as a saliva substitute, *J. Publ. Health Dent.*, 3, 184, 1994.

26. Mundorff, S. A., Featherstone, J. D. B., Bibby, B. G., Curzon, M. E. J., Eisenberg, A. D., and Espeland, M.A., Cariogenic potential of foods, *Caries Res.*, 24, 344, 1990.

27. Bibby, B. J., Huang, C. T., Zero, D., Mundorff, S. A., and Little, M. F., Protective effect of milk against *in vitro* caries, *J. Dent. Res.*, 59(10), 1565, 1980.

28. Edgar, W. M. and Geddes, D. A. M., Plaque acidity models for cariogenicity testing - some theoretical and practical observations, *J. Dent. Res.*, 65(spec. issue), 1498, 1986.

29. Jensen, M. E., Harlander, S. K., Schachtele, C. F., Halambeck, S. M., and Morris, H. A., Evaluation of the acidogenic and antacid properties of cheeses by telemetric monitoring of human dental plaque pH, In *Foods, Nutrition and Dental Health.*, Vol. 4. Hefferren, J. J., Ayer, W. A., Koehler, H. M., and McEnery, C. T. Eds., American Dental Assoc., Chicago, IL., 1984, 31–47.

30. Schachtele, C. F. and Harlander, S. K., Will the diets of the future be less cariogenic? *J. Canad. Dent. Assoc.*, 3, 213, 1984.

31. Jensen, M. E. and Schachtele, C. F., The acidogenic potential of reference foods and snacks at interproximal sites in the human dentition, *J. Dent. Res.*, 62(8), 889, 1983.

32. Higham, S. M. and Edgar, W. M., Effects of parafilm and cheese chewing on human dental plaque pH and metabolism, *Caries Res.*, 23, 42, 1989.

33. Jensen, M. E. and Wefel, J.S., Effects of processed cheese on human plaque pH and demineralization and remineralization, *Am. J. Dent.*, 3(5), 217, 1990.

34. Dodds, M. W. J. and Edgar, W. M., The relationship between plaque pH, plaque acid anion profiles, and oral carbohydrate retention after ingestion of several "reference foods" by human subjects, *J. Dent. Res.*, 67(5), 861, 1988.

35. Silva, M. F. de A., Jenkins, G. N., Burgess, R. C., and Sandham, H. J., Effects of cheese on experimental caries in human subjects, *Caries Res.*, 20, 263, 1986.

36. Thomson, M. E., Effects of cheese, breadcrumbs, and a breadcrumb and cheese mixture on microhardness of bovine dental enamel intraoral experiments, *Caries Res.*, 22, 246, 1988.

37. Thomson, M. E., Effect of fruit juice, with or without 1% added whey mineral, on bovine dental enamel in intraoral experiments, *Caries Res.*, 24(5), 334, 1990.

38. Gedalia, I., Ionat-Bendat, D., Ben-Mosheh, S., and Shapira, L., Tooth enamel softening with a cola type drink and rehardening with hard cheese or stimulated saliva *in situ*, *J. Oral Rehabil.*, 18(6), 501, 1991.

39. Featherstone, J. D. B. and Zero, D. T., An *in situ* model for simultaneous assessment of inhibition of demineralization and enhancement of remineralization, *J. Dent. Res.*, 71(spec. 55), 804, 1992.

40. Reynolds, E. C., Riley, P. F., and Storey, E., Phosphoprotein inhibition of hydroxyapatite dissolution, *Calcif. Tissue Int.*, 34(Suppl. 2), 52, 1982.

41. Reynolds, E. C., The prevention of sub-surface demineralization of bovine enamel and change in plaque composition by casein in an intra-oral model, *J. Dent. Res.*, 66(6), 1120, 1987.

42. McDougall, W. A., Effect of milk on enamel demineralization and remineralization *in vitro*, *Caries Res.*, 11, 166, 1977.

43. Gedalia, I., Dukuar, A., Shapira, L., Lewinstein, I., Goultschin, J., and Rahamin, E., Enamel softening with Coca-Cola and rehardening with milk or saliva, *Am. J. Dent.*, 4(3), 120, 1991.

44. Papas, A. S., Joshi, A., Palmer, C. A., Giunta, J. L., and Dwyer, J. T., Relationship of diet to root caries, *Am. J. Clin. Nutr.*, 61(Suppl.), 423, 1995.

45. Rugg-Gunn, A. J., Hackett, A. F., Appleton, D. R., Jenkins, G. N., and Eastoe, J. E., Relationship between dietary habits and caries increment assessed over two years in 405 English adolescent school children, *Archs. Oral Biol.*, 29, 983, 1984.

46. Holund, U., Relationship between diet-related behavior and caries in a group of 14-year-old Danish children, *Community Dent. Oral Epidemiol.*, 15, 184, 1987.

47. Freeman, L., Martin, S., Rutenberg, G., Shirejian, P., and Skarie, M., Relationships between DEF, demographic and behavioral variables among multiracial preschool children, *ASDC J. Dent. Child*, 56(3), 205, 1989.

48. Petti, S., Simonetti, R., and Simonetti D'Arca, A., The effect of milk and sucrose consumption on caries in 6- to 11-year old Italian schoolchildren, *Eur. J. Epidemiol.*, 13, 659, 1997.

49. Papas, A. S., Joshi, A., Belanger, A. J., Kent, Jr., R. L., Palmer, C. A., and DePaola, P. F., Dietary models for root caries, *Am. J. Clin. Nutr.*, 61(Suppl.), 417, 1995.

50. Gedalia, I., Ben-Mosheh, S., Biton, J., and Kogan, D., Dental caries protection with hard cheese consumption, *Am. J. Dentistry*, 7, 331, 1994.

51. Silva, M. F., de A., Burgess, R. C., Sandham, H. J., and Jenkins, G. N., Effects of water-soluble components of cheese on experimental caries in humans, *J. Dent. Res.*, 66(1), 38, 1987.

52. Jenkins, G. N. and Hargreaves, J. A., Effect of eating cheese on Ca and P concentrations of whole mouth saliva and plaque, *Caries Res.*, 23, 159, 1989.

53. Brudevold, F., Tehrani, A., Attarzadeh, F., Goulet, D., and van Houte, J., Effects of some salts of calcium, sodium, potassium, and strontium on intra-oral enamel demineralization, *J. Dent. Res.*, 64(1), 24, 1985.

54. Reynolds, E.-C., Cain, C. J., Webber, F. L., Black, C. L., Riley, P. F., Johnson, I. H., and Perich, J. W., Anticarcinogenicity of calcium phosphate complexes of tryptic casein phosphopeptides in the rat, *J. Dent. Res.*, 74, 1272, 1995.

55. Vacca-Smith, A. M., Van Wuyckhuyse, B. C., Tabak, L. A., and Bowen, W. H., The effect of milk and casein proteins on the adherence of *Streptococcus Mutans* to saliva-coated hydroxyapatite, *Archs. Oral. Biol.*, 39, 1063, 1994.

56. Nesser, J. R., Golliard, M., Woltz, A., Rouvet, M., Dillmann, M. L., and Guggenheim, B., In vitro modulation of oral bacterial adherence to saliva-coated hydroxyapatite beads by milk casein-derivatives, *Oral. Microbiol. Immunol.*, 9, 193, 1994.

57. Vacca-Smith, A. M. and Bowen, W. H., The effect of milk and kappa casein on Streptococcal glucosyltransferase, *Caries Res.*, 29, 498, 1995.

58. Marques, A. P. F. and Messer, L. B., Nutrient intake and dental caries in the primary dentition, *Pediatr. Dent.*, 14, 314, 1992.

59. Stralfors, A., Inhibition of hamster caries by cocoa, The effect of whole and defatted cocoa, and the absence of activity in cocoa fat, *Arch. Oral Biol.*, 11, 149, 1966.

60. Paolino, V. J. and Kashket, S., Inhibition of cocoa extracts of biosynthesis of extracellular polysaccharide by human oral bacteria, *Arch. Oral Biol.*, 30(4), 359, 1985.

61. Glinsmann, W., Irausquin, H., and Park, Y. K., Evaluation of health aspects of sugars contained in carbohydrate sweeteners, *J. Nutr.*, 116(Suppl.), 1, 1986.

62. Bowen, W. H., Response to Seow: biological mechanisms of early childhood caries, *Community Dent. Oral Epidemiol.*, 26(s), 28, 1998.

63. Johnsen, D. and Nowjack-Raymer, R., Baby bottle tooth decay (BBTD): Issues, assessment, and an opportunity for the nutritionist, *J. Am. Diet. Assoc.*, 89, 1112, 1989.

64. The American Dietetic Association, Position of The American Dietetic Association: the impact of fluoride on dental health, *J. Am. Diet. Assoc.*, 94, 1428, 1994.

65. Marino, R., Should we use milk fluoridation? A review, *Bull. PAHO*, 29(4), 287, 1995.

66. Pakhomov, G. N., Ivanova, K., Moller, I. J., and Vrabcheva, M., Dental caries-reducing effects of milk fluoridation project in Bulgaria, *J. Public Health Dent.*, 55(4), 234, 1995.

67. Banoczy, J., Ritlop, B., Solymosi, G., Gombik, A., and Adatia, A., Anticariogenic effect of fluoridated milk and water in rats, *Acta Physiol. Hungarica*, 76(4), 341, 1990.

68. Stosser, L., Kneist, S., and Grosser, W., The effects of non-fluoridated and fluoridated milk on experimental caries in rats, *Adv. Dent. Res.*, 9(2), 122, 1995.

69. Toth, Z., Gintner, Z., Banoczy, J., and Phillips, P. C., The effect of fluoridated milk on human dental enamel in an in vitro demineralization model, *Caries Res.*, 31, 212, 1997.

70. Jeffcoat, M. K., Reddy, M. S., and DeCarlo, A. A., Oral bone loss and systemic osteopenia, In, *Osteoporosis*, Academic Press, New York, 1996, 969–990.

71. Rogoff, G. S., Galburt, R. B., and Nizel, A. E., Role of dietary calcium and vitamin D in alveolar bone health, In, *Calcium in Biological Systems*, Plenum Publ. Co., New York, 1984, 591–595.

72. Paganini-Hill, A., The benefits of estrogen replacement therapy on oral health, The Leisure World cohort, *Arch. Intern. Med.*, 155, 2325, 1995.

73. Kribbs, P. J., Comparison of mandibular bone in normal and osteoporotic women, *J. Prosthet. Dent.*, 63, 218, 1990.

74. Krall, E. A., Dawson-Hughes, B., Papas, A., and Garcia, R. I., Tooth loss and skeletal bone density in healthy postmenopausal women, *Osteoporosis Int.*, 4, 104, 1994.

75. Houki, K., DiMuzio, M. T., and Fattore, L., Mandibular bone density and systemic osteoporosis in elderly edentulous women, *J. Bone Miner. Res.*, 9 (Suppl. 1), 211s, 1994.

76. Jeffcoat, M. K. and Reddy, M. S., Alveolar bone loss and osteoporosis: evidence for a common mode of therapy using the biophosphonate alendronate. In, *Biological Mechanisms of Tooth Movement and Craniofacial Adaptation*. Davidovitch, Z. and Norton, L. A. Eds., Boston, MA, Harvard Society for the Advancement of Orthodontics, 1996, 365–373.

77. Jeffcoat, M. K., and Chestnut, C. H., Systemic osteoporosis and oral bone loss: evidence shows increased risk factors, *J. Am. Dent. Assoc.*, 124, 49, 1993.

CHAPTER 8

Lactose Intolerance

I. INTRODUCTION

Dairy products are an important source of many nutrients including calcium, high-quality protein, potassium, phosphorus, and riboflavin. Dairy foods are an important part of the diets of children and adults in the United States, Canada, and Europe, as well as in other countries. It has been estimated that up to 75% of the world's adult population (approximately 25% of American adults), however, have a genetically controlled limited ability to digest lactose, the principle carbohydrate in milk and other diary foods.[1] This condition is called lactase non-persistence. Limited digestion of lactose can lead to unpleasant gastrointestinal symptoms of varying severity, termed lactose intolerance. However, limited digestion of lactose does not necessarily produce the symptoms of intolerance. Incidence figures greatly overestimate the percentage of those who are lactose intolerant. The estimates are based on studies that employed a 50 gram test dose of lactose, the amount contained in a quart of milk, rather than on an amount usually consumed (12 grams).

All young mammals and human infants (except those with a congenital defect) are born with high levels of the enzyme "lactase" which enables them to digest lactose. Lactase activity declines after weaning in most racial/ethnic groups except most Caucasian North Americans and northern Europeans, so that by approximately 3 to 5 years of age, when the child is consuming a variety of foods, lactase levels are low.[2]

Some have attempted to explain this phenomenon in terms of genetics and evolution. In this culture-historical hypothesis, the selection of a genetic trait (lactase persistence) is influenced by the cultural environment (dairying).[3] A recent analysis supports the hypothesis that lactase persistence is an adaptation to dairying.[4]

The pediatricians Czerny, Finkelstein, and Jacobi who noticed the association between diarrhea and carbohydrate ingestion first described intolerance to milk in 1901.[5] In 1901, the famed biochemist Lafayettte B. Mendel published a series of nine papers demonstrating that in most mammals the lactase enzyme reached maximal activity soon after birth; lactase activity then decreased gradually, reaching a low level after weaning. In 1921, John Howland, in his address to the American Pediatric Society, proposed that milk intolerance in infants and children was due to the lack of the enzyme necessary to hydrolyze lactose. It was not until the mid 1960s that lactose intolerance again attracted the interest of researchers. It was reported that 70% of Black adults, but only 6 to 12% of Caucasian adults studied in Baltimore, were intolerant to the amount of lactose in a quart of milk.[6] As studies were conducted in many populations around the world, it soon became apparent that a marked reduction of lactase activity in early childhood was not uncommon.

Investigators studying lactose intolerance, however, used a large amount of lactose dissolved in water as the test dose. The intolerance symptoms experienced under these experimental conditions has often mistakenly been equated with intolerance to milk in the diet. As a result, the incidence and practical significance of intolerance to milk has been grossly overestimated. Many studies have failed to recognize that cultural and psychosomatic factors as well as biologic mechanisms affect milk intolerance.[2] Researchers investigating lactose intolerance have used a variety of terms to describe the processes involved, making interpretation difficult. Therefore, it is important to carefully define the terms used when comparing the results of research or discussing the topic of lactose indigestion and tolerance. For this reason, a glossary is included at the end of the chapter.

Scientific investigations from many different disciplines, including biochemistry, cultural anthropology, and nutrition have added to our knowledge about lactose digestion. As a result of these studies, we have learned that the ability to digest lactose in adults is most common in northern Europeans and white American ethnic groups; that the trait is genetically transmitted; that the activity of the enzyme cannot be "induced" by continued exposure to lactose, but that adaptation in the colon may improve tolerance to continued milk intake.

Persons who consume less milk and other diary foods as a result of lactose intolerance generally have lower intakes of calcium and other nutrients supplied by milk, such as vitamin D, riboflavin, potassium, phosphorus, and magnesium. An inadequate calcium intake increases the risk of osteoporosis, hypertension, and perhaps colon cancer (see Section VI on long-term consequences of lactose intolerance). Much is now known about the maldigestion of lactose. Research into the factors involved in lactose digestion has fostered the development of strategies that allow those with low lactase activity to consume dairy products without experiencing unpleasant symptoms.

In this chapter, we will review the current literature on the subject to provide a clear understanding of the biologic mechanisms involved in lactose maldigestion and how individuals can best avoid the unpleasant symptoms which often accompany this condition. Since lactose maldigestion in a majority of non-Caucasian children in this country and developing countries has implications for public health and nutrition policy, we will also review recommendations for including milk in food aid programs and for the treatment of diarrheal disease and malnutrition in children.

II. PHYSIOLOGY OF LACTOSE DIGESTION

Lactose, or milk sugar, is the principle carbohydrate in human and animal milk. Human milk contains an average of 7% lactose, while whole cow's milk contains 4.8%. Lactose is a disaccharide made up of equal portions of two monosaccharides, glucose and galactose (Figure 8.1). A unique intestinal enzyme, lactase, a beta-galactosidase, is needed to hydrolyze lactose. It breaks the chemical bond between glucose and galactose, freeing them for absorption.[7] Lactase is one of five disaccharidases located on the brush border of the intestinal epithelium. Activity of the lactase enzyme is highest in the proximal ileum and very low in the first portion of the duodenum and in the terminal ileum.[8]

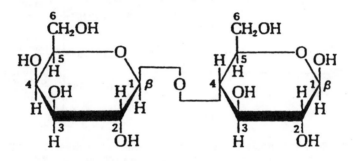

Figure 8 .1 Chemical structure of lactose (βform). O-β-D-galactopyranosyl-(1→4)-βD-glucopy-ranose. (From Lehninger, A. L., *Lehninger: Principles of Biochemistry,* Worth Publishers, New York, 1982, 285. With permission.)

Of all the dietary sugars, lactose is hydrolyzed the most slowly.[7] The hydrolysis of lactose occurs at only half the rate of sucrose hydrolysis. The rate at which lactose is assimilated is dependent on the rate of the hydrolysis. The relative slowness with which lactose is broken down, accompanied by a lack of reserve of the enzyme, helps explain why many people are vulnerable to lactose maldigestion (Figure 8.2).[7] It has been suggested that a faster-than-normal rate of gastric emptying in persons with low lactase activity may also contribute to symptoms of intolerance after milk ingestion.[9] It is thought that when lactose is not hydrolyzed, the osmoreceptors, which lie deeper in the intestinal mucosa than the lactase enzyme, are not stimulated to inhibit gastric emptying.[9]

A. Course of Development of Lactase

In contrast to the other disaccharidases, lactase appears very late in fetal development. It is estimated that at 35 to 38 weeks of gestation lactase levels are approximately 70% of their full-term level.[10] Most studies of lactase development have been conducted in stillborn infants. Because premature infants who survive even for a short time have lactase levels above those of stillborn infants of the same gestational age, it is speculated that feeding might influence the infant's lactase level after birth.[7]

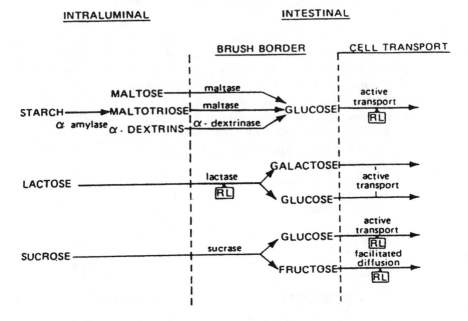

Figure 8.2 Schematic diagram of absorption of dietary carbohydrate at the level of the intestinal brush border. RL indicates the rate-limiting step in the overall digestion and absorption of the sugar. (Reproduced with permission from Saavedra, J. M. and Perman, J. A, *Ann. Rev. Nutr.*, 9, 475, 1989. From the *Ann. Rev. Nutr.*, 9, ©1989, Annual Reviews, Inc. 1989. With permission.)

It is interesting to note that both preterm and term infants in the first few months of life do not completely hydrolyze the lactose in their mother's milk, as indicated by high breath hydrogen concentrations, though they tolerate and thrive on human milk and formulas that contain lactose.[11,12,13] Klein and colleagues at The Ohio State University measured lactose digestion in 14 preterm infants (26 to 31 weeks of gestation).[11] They found that these infants digested <85% of lactose consumed, and an average of 35% was fermented by the colon. Since previous studies conducted by the same group suggested no negative clinical consequences to feeding lactose-containing formulas, the authors concluded that replacement of lactose with other sugars might not be necessary for routine feeding of preterm infants. Lifshitz et al. evaluated lactose digestion in 17 white, normal, breast-fed infants who were 4 to 5 weeks old. Five of the infants (29%) produced large amounts of hydrogen in their breath, indicating that colonic bacteria were fermenting unabsorbed carbohydrate. Three of these infants stopped producing high levels of hydrogen as they grew older; all of them gained weight and grew normally. No glucose appeared in the stools of the infants tested, which indicates that the bacteria fermented the sugars released from lactose. The authors suggest that the fermentation products of unabsorbed lactose may be absorbed in the colon.[13] There is evidence that colonic adaptation also occurs in adults with low lactase activity. This will be discussed later in Section 7.

B. Decline of Lactase Expression

A post-weaning decline in lactase activity is not dependent on the absence of lactose in the diet. Many studies have documented that continued lactose consumption does not maintain or enhance lactase.[2,14] Instead, researchers have concluded that human adult-onset lactase decline is controlled by a single autosomal recessive gene.[15] Researchers using the sucrase/lactase ratio and the lactase/maltase ratio measured in intestinal biopsies, found a trimodal distribution (low, intermediate, and high) of lactase expression. Subjects with a homozygous recessive inheritance pattern had low levels of lactase expression; those who were heterozygous had intermediate levels; those who had a homozygous dominant pattern had high lactase activity.[15]

C. Molecular Regulation

Studies conducted in the fields of molecular and cell biology have provided insight into the gene structure, gene transcription, localization of expression in the small intestine, and biosynthesis of lactase protein. The lactase gene is located on chromosome 2. Differences in the structure of the gene itself, however, are not responsible for differences in lactase expression. Lactase messenger RNA in humans, rats, and rabbits changes coordinately with the amount of enzyme activity, suggesting control of lactase expression at the level of gene transcription.

Researchers in Italy examined lactase lactivity, biosynthesis, and the levels of messenger RNA (mRNA) in jejunal mucosa of lactase persistent and nonpersistent adults. They concluded that both transcriptional and posttranscriptional factors cause the decline of intestinal lactase.[16] Biosynthesis of prolactase (the precursor of lactase) correlated well with lactase mRNA levels, indicating transcriptional control. A high rate of biosynthesis was the main factor distinguishing those with lactase persistence; the rate was five times higher than in those with non-persistence. These Italian researchers found that posttranscriptional factors (e.g., the routing of prolactase from the endoplasmic reticulum to the brush border membrane, the speed of processing during this routing, or the breakdown of lactase), also influenced lactase levels to some degree. However, they observed wide variability of mRNA level, lactase synthesis, and activity in both lactase persistent and nonpersistent individuals. With such a variety of factors responsible for the decrease in intestinal lactase, it is not surprising, say these researchers, that the time of onset of adult-type hypolactasia can vary widely among various population groups.[16] The Caco-2 cell line derived from a human colon adenocarcinoma, which expresses hydrolases such as lactase and sucrase-isomaltase, have been used to study the regulation of lactase expression. Studies using Caco-2 cells have demonstrated that biosynthesis of lactase is preceded by a large increase in messenger RNA levels, indicating transcriptional control.[17,18]

Studies have shown that the decrease in lactase activity is determined by the age of the tissue, not the age of the host. Therefore the pattern for expression is apparently imprinted in the tissue of intestinal epithelum. Several mechanisms for controlling lactase expression have been hypothesized and are currently under investigation, including regulation by corticoid or thyroid hormones. One promising line of research involves a nuclear factor (NF-LPH1), which binds specifically to the lactose promoter and may be an important regulator of gene transcription.[19]

D. Types of Lactase Deficiency

The absence or decline of intestinal lactase can be described as being *congenital, primary,* or *secondary.* Congential lactase deficiency, or alactasia, is an extremely rare condition in which detectable levels of lactase are absent at birth. An infant with congenital lactase deficiency will have severe diarrheal illness beginning a few days after birth. In addition to measuring breath hydrogen production in these infacts, other more aggressive diagnostic procedures such as an intestinal biopsy to measure lactase activity and/or intestinal perfusion study, may be required to rule out other diagnoses.[20] In congenital lactase deficiency the histology of the small bowel is normal, as is the level of other disaccharidases. Symptoms will resolve if the infant is put on a lactose-free diet. According to recent position paper by the American Academy of Pediatrics, soy protein-based formulas (lactose-free), are appropriate for infants with this form of hereditary lactase deficiency.[21] Persons with this disorder are unable to tolerate even small amounts of lactose, and will need to follow a lactose-free diet for the rest of their lives.[22] It is not known whether colonic adaptation might allow a measure of tolerance in these individuals.

In primary lactase deficiency, decline of lactase activity occurs at variable periods after weaning depending on racial/ethnic background (Figure 8.3). In the United States, some degree of lactose maldigestion occurs in an estimated 15% (6% to 19%) of Caucasians, 53% of Mexican Americans, 62% to 100% of Native Americans, 80% of African Americans, and 90% of Asian Americans.[2,23] Although the standard lactose tolerance test is effective for determining genetic differences in lactase among populations, it tends to overestimate the number of individuals who are intolerant to more physiologic amounts of lactose. Lactase deficiency is seldom total, and whether symptoms of intolerance are experienced depends on the level of lactase activity remaining, the amount of lactose consumed, the adaptation of intestinal flora, and the irritibility of the colon. Primary lactase deficiency or lactase non persistence is genetically determined and is inherited as an autosomal recessive trait. In contrast, lactase persistence is inherited as an autosomal dominant characteristic.[2,7]

It is interesting to note that as those who have the ability to digest lactose intermarry with those from a racial/ethnic group that typically does not digest lactose, the rate of maldigestion falls.[24] For example, though African Americans have an expected rate of lactose maldigestion near 100%, the prevalence has decreased to 70% due to intermixing with white Americans.[24] The ability of Native Americans to digest lactose has also increased over time. These examples demonstrate the dominant inheritance pattern of the ability to digest lactose.

A large number of studies have been conducted around the world to examine the incidence and age of onset of lactase non-persistence.[2] Many studies have included wide age ranges of subjects, spanning from the early teens into the 70s, making it difficult to establish a precise relationship between age and prevalence. It appears that the primary reduction in lactase activity occurs in early childhood and

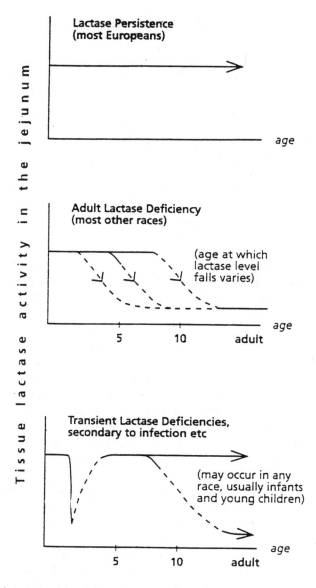

Figure 8.3 Lactase activity, age, race, and deficiencies. (From Ferguson, A., *Allergy,* 50(20 Suppl.), 32, 1995. With permission).

is thought not to progress throughout life.[2,15] A recent study comparing lactose tolerance between adult (20 to 40 years) and elderly (≥65 years) Asian-Americans confirmed this hypothesis.[25] When fed a challenge dose of 0.5 g lactose/kg body weight, there were no significant differences in breath hydrogen production, flatulence, or fecal beta-galactosidase activity between the adult and elderly subjects. Additional studies are needed to confirm these findings in other ethnic populations. Individuals with primary lactase deficiency do not need to avoid all foods containing lactose. By using the management strategies outlined later in this chapter, a variety of dairy foods may be comfortably included in the diet.

Secondary lactase deficiency is a temporary condition, caused by any environmental factors that injure the intestinal mucosa where lactase is expressed. It can occur at any age. The most important causes of secondary lactase deficiency are infectious diarrheal disease, the parasites giardia and ascaria, inflammatory bowel disease such as Crohn's disease, celiac disease, allergy to milk protein, gastrointestinal surgery, radiation treatment, and certain medications such as aspirin, nonsteroidal anti-inflammatory drugs, and antibiotics. Secondary lactase deficiency is reversed upon correction of the causative factor.

When diarrhea is of infectious origin, loss of lactase activity may persist for a long time if the diarrhea is recurrent. In severe protein-calorie malnutrition, such as kwashiorkor, lactase activity is reduced along with all other enzyme activity. Lactose tolerance increases quickly as nutritional status improves. In children who developed a lactase deficiency secondary to cancer chemotherapy treatments, yogurt proved a useful dietary supplement.[26]

Diet therapy for secondary lactose intolerance involves restricting or eliminating lactose-containing foods depending upon the tolerance of the patient. Since tolerance varies between patients, the diet is administered on a trial-and-error basis. Consultation with a nutrition professional will help prevent nutritional deficiencies during treatment of the underlying disease. Patients may need to restrict all lactose-containing foods temporarily or use lactose-hydrolyzed products. A recent commentary on dairy sensitivity in patients with inflammatory bowel disease (IBD), states that patients with either ulcerative colitis or Crohn's disease often avoid dairy products more than they need to because they have incorrect perceptions, and receive arbitrary advice from physicians and authors of popular diet books.[27] Since dairy products are an important source of calcium and other nutrients, the author recommends testing IBD patients for lactose malabsorption using the breath-hydrogen test before recommending the elimination of dairy foods or the use of lactose-reduced products. In a study of 161 IBD patients, those with diagnosed lactose maldigestion (29%) did not have significantly different gastrointestinal symptoms or improvement/worsening of their condition than those who digested lactose. Most of the patients felt, however, that identifying lactose maldigestion helped them to gain awareness of food-symptom relationships.[28]

Manufacturers of candy, confections, and bakery products, such as pancakes, waffles, and toaster pastries use lactose as an ingredient. Its limited sweetness, solubility, crystallization, and browning properties make it ideal for use in these products. Other non-dairy foods that may contain lactose include shakes and instant breakfast mixes, coffee whiteners, commercial breakfast and baby cereals, cake mixes, mayonnaise, salad dressings, luncheon meats, sausage, and frankfurters.[29] If intolerance is severe, patients may need to check ingredient labels and avoid products with the following ingredients: milk, lactose, milk solids, whey, curds, nonfat milk powder, and nonfat milk solids. Medication and vitamin labels should be checked as well, since some contain lactose as a carrier. Some dairy foods, such as Cheddar cheese, have a relatively low lactose content. See the table, Lactose Content of Dairy Products included at the end of this chapter.

E. Lactose Maldigestion

It is estimated that of the lactose that remains unhydrolyzed in the small intestine, approximately 1% is absorbed by passive diffusion into the bloodstream, which is then excreted into the urine unmetabolized. As the remainder of unabsorbed lactose reaches the jejunum, it exerts an osmotic effect, causing water and sodium to be secreted into the intestinal lumen. Transit of the contents of the small bowel accelerates. Significant amounts of lactose may then enter the colon, where it is fermented by colonic bacteria. The majority of the undigested lactose reaching the colon is metabolized to short chain organic acids, and hydrogen, methane, and carbon dioxide gases. Some of the organic acids are absorbed into the bloodstream, while some may be excreted in the feces, resulting in acidic stools (Figure 8.4).[7]

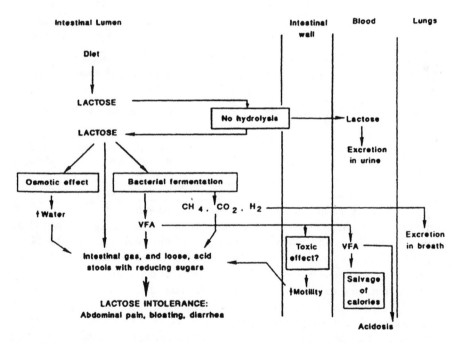

Figure 8.4   Pathophysiologic events following lactose maldigestion. VFA indicates volatile fatty acids. (From Saavedra, J. M. and Perman, J. A., *Ann. Rev. Nutr.*, 9, 475, 1989. Reproduced with permission from the Ann. Rev. Nutr., 9, ©1989, by Annual Reviews Inc.)

III. SYMPTOMS

Lactose intolerance refers to gastrointestinal symptoms associated with the incomplete digestion of lactose. The presence of fermentation products in the colon may produce a variety of symptoms including abdominal discomfort, cramps or distention; nausea; flatulence; or diarrhea.[7,30] Symptoms resulting from lactose maldigestion may be more pronounced in women than in men, according to a study conducted recently in Germany.[31] The women in the study, who were diagnosed as maldigesters by a breath-hydrogen test, had lower breath hydrogen concentrations after ingestion of 50 g of lactose and complained of more abdominal pain, gas, and distension than did their male counterparts. Another recent controlled trial of lactose maldigesters, however, demonstrated no gender differences in lactose digestion or tolerance (unpublished data per personal communication: Dennis Savaiano).

Individuals with an allergy to cow's milk protein may experience symptoms similar to those of lactose intolerance. Therefore it is important to make the distinction between these two very different sensitivities involving the ingestion of milk (Table 8.1).

Table 8.1   Comparison and Contrast of Cow's Milk Allergy and Lactose Intolerance

	Milk Allergy	**Lactose Intolerance**
Cause	Abnormal immune response to ingestion of cow's milk protein	Low intestinal levels of the lactase enzyme that digests lactose (milk sugar)
Age of Onset	Usually in infancy	Early/ late childhood
Symptoms	Abdominal pain, vomiting, diarrhea, nasal congestion, skin rash	Abdominal gas, bloating, cramps, diarrhea
Diagnosis	Food elimination and challenge; RAST blood test	Breath hydrogen test
Dairy Food Use/ Avoidance	Eliminate cow's milk protein from the diet for a time	No need to eliminate dairy foods; experiment with varying amounts/ types of dairy foods to improve tolerance

In milk allergy, gastrointestinal symptoms may predominate, but other symptoms involving the respiratory tract and skin, such as rhinitis and atopic dermatitis, are also common. Cow's milk allergy usually occurs within the first four months of life in bottle-fed infants, though it may in rare instances be first detected in adolescence or adulthood. The incidence of cow's milk allergy as determined by double-blind studies is quite low, in the range of 1 to 3% of infants and children in the first two years of life. Most children with milk allergy outgrow it by age 2-3 years as a result of maturation of the gastrointestinal and immune system.[33] This is the reverse of the time-course of lactose intolerance, which may begin to appear at this age in some individuals.[2]

IV. DIAGNOSIS

Dietary exclusion of lactose is the diagnostic method used by most physicians when they suspect lactose intolerance.[29] There are several reasons why this is an unsatisfactory approach. Most importantly, this approach is highly inaccurate. Several double-blinded studies have shown that many patients who believe they are intolerant to milk and milk products continue to report symptoms when lactose is removed from the diet.[34-39] In addition, exclusion diets usually involve removing only dairy products from the diet and have several drawbacks, whether used by a physician or for self-diagnosis. Excluding dairy foods from the diet for an arbitrary amount of time could result in nutritional shortcomings. If all foods containing lactose are not removed from the diet, symptoms may continue, leading the client to believe lactose was not the cause of the symptoms. Or the reverse could be true; removal of lactose from the diet may happen to coincide with resolution of the symptoms from a totally unrelated cause, thus perpetuating unnecessary dietary restrictions. In addition, self-diagnosis could delay treatment for another more serious gastrointestinal problem. If symptoms are chronic, a physician should be consulted, and an objective test for lactose maldigestion conducted.

Both direct and indirect methods are available to diagnose lactase deficiency. It is possible to directly assay the lactase activity in the small bowel by taking an intestinal biopsy. Researchers have used this method to identify populations with primary lactase deficiency. The procedure is invasive and time-consuming, and may not yield accurate results when intestinal injury is involved. This is because intestinal lesions may affect only a small area that may be missed during the biopsy. Symptoms of intolerance do not correlate as well with mucosal lactase activity as they do with the breath hydrogen test, an indirect measure of lactose maldigestion.[7]

Indirect methods for diagnosing lactose maldigestion include the lactose tolerance test, a stool acidity test, and the breath hydrogen (H_2) test. The lactose tolerance test, which measures the rise in blood glucose after a dose of lactose, is performed in a manner similar to that of the glucose tolerance test used for the diagnosis of diabetes mellitus. A relatively large dose of lactose is required to separate digesters from maldigesters. Typically, an aqueous solution of 50 g of lactose is consumed. In persons who weigh more than 25 kg, a dose of 100 g may be required.[20] Blood is drawn before lactose ingestion, then at intervals of 30, 60, 90, and 120 minutes thereafter.[29] Failure of blood glucose to rise 20 mg/dl from baseline, in the presence of symptoms, indicates lactase deficiency. Even though the lactose tolerance test (actually, a test for lactose maldigestion) is positive, smaller amounts of lactose may be tolerated.[22] This method is mildly invasive, since several blood samplings are involved, and results correlate poorly with actual mucosal lactase levels. Since the rate of gastric emptying slows the rate at which glucose enters the bloodstream, individuals with delayed gastric emptying will have a false-positive test.[20] Results will be questionable if used with diabetic patients or those with malabsorption syndromes.

Testing stool samples for acidity and reducing sugars has been used for years to assess whether infants and young children are absorbing lactose. The test, however, requires the presence of lactose in the diet and availability of fresh stool. The test is not sensitive enough to exclude lactose intolerance, but can be used to confirm the results of another test.[29]

The breath hydrogen (H_2) test has become the "gold standard," or method of choice, for diagnosing lactose maldigestion. The test is noninvasive, inexpensive, and can easily be performed on children and adults. The results of this test are reported to correlate well with lactase activity in mucosal biopsy specimens.[40] When lactose or any other dietary sugar is not completely absorbed, the unabsorbed portion is fermented by colonic bacteria, forming hydrogen (as well as methane in some individuals and CO_2), some of which is absorbed into the portal circulation and exhaled in breath.[7]

Test protocol requires the patient to report after an overnight fast, where a baseline breath sample is taken. Historically, the patients were given a 20% aqueous solution of 2 g of lactose per kg of body weight (10 to 50 g) to drink. Fifty grams of lactose is the amount contained in one quart of milk. The solution may be diluted to 10% in infants younger than 6 months or in adults when severe lactose intolerance is suspected. Breath samples are taken every 30 min for 3 hours; samples are collected in test tubes, and hydrogen in breath is analyzed by gas chromatography. An increase in breath hydrogen of >10 to 20 ppm above the baseline value indicates fermentation of unabsorbed carbohydrate, and is positive for lactose maldigestion.[29]

Even though a rise in breath hydrogen of 10 ppm above baseline indicates the presence of incompletely absorbed lactose in the colon (more than can be accounted for by variability of the technique), many investigators recommend that a rise of 20 ppm be used as the criteria for judging lactose digestion as "abnormal."[20] This criteria is often used because it correlates with less than a 20 mg/dl rise in blood glucose following a 50 g dose of aqueous lactose. However, this rationale has been questioned, because using the >20 ppm criteria unnecessarily limits the sensitivity of the breath hydrogen test to that of the lactose tolerance test, especially when the dose of lactose given is less than 50 g.[41]

Hydrogen production is proportional to the lactose dose. Therefore, when the dose of lactose given is small (10 to 12 g), the criteria of ≥10 ppm above baseline is diagnostic of lactose maldigestion. Patients with a breath hydrogen rise of only 10 ppm are less likely to experience intolerance symptoms than those with a higher rise.[42] The lactose dose used for the test may also be administered in the form of milk, infant formula, or yogurt (not with active cultures). Lactose doses in the range of usual intakes (10 to 12 g) can be used, since the test can determine the maldigestion of as little as 2 g of carbohydrate.[7] When the hydrogen breath test is used for research purposes, many investigators collect samples for 8 hours. This increases the sensitivity of the test when lower doses of lactose are administered. While the breath hydrogen test has the capability of measuring absorption of the amount of lactose in usual milk intakes, the protocol historically used pharmacological doses.

A small percentage of people (2 to 20%) do not have colonic flora which ferment lactose; this can lead to false negative results. This situation is uncommon and may be the result of the use of an antibiotic before the test.[29] Smoking prior to the test may lead to a false-positive result.[7]

The breath hydrogen test is also useful in diagnosing an underlying condition, such as bacterial overgrowth, which can cause secondary lactose intolerance. The bacterial overgrowth in the small bowel can be treated with antibiotic therapy and the secondary lactose maldigestion is managed with a lactose-controlled diet.[29] Lactose maldigestion eventually resolves with the treatment of the underlying condition. In children less than 5 years of age, an abnormal breath hydrogen test indicates an abnormal intestinal mucosa and lactose maldigestion secondary to another problem.[43]

Patients can now easily perform the breath hydrogen test at home using commercially available kits. Breath samples in vacutainers can be mailed to a central laboratory for analysis.[29]

V. RELATIONSHIP BETWEEN LACTOSE MALDIGESTION, INTOLERANCE, AND MILK INTOLERANCE

A. Dose Dependence

Controlled studies have shown that consuming one cup of milk (240 ml) or its lactose equivalent (12 g) at a time produces little or no intolerance symptoms in adults with primary lactase deficiency. The vast majority of those with low lactase levels can tolerate ingestion of 12 g of lactose, particularly if consumed with a meal or other foods.[44,45] Hertzler et al. found that individuals with lactase non-persistence could tolerate up to 6 g of lactose under fasting conditions when consumed in water.[46] When the lactose dose is 50 g vs. 12 g, a much higher percentage of those with hypolactasia experience intolerance symptoms. A group of American Indians studied by Newcomer in 1978 illustrates this phenomenon. Less than 20% of the subjects experienced symptoms when the lactose dose was between 0 and 18 g. However, 88% were symptomatic to a dose of 50 g (Figure 8.5).[47]

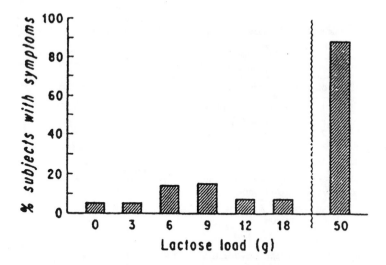

Figure 8.5   Tolerance to various doses of lactose in 59 subjects with lactase deficiency. (From Newcomer, A. D., et al., *Gastroenterology*, 74, 44, 1978. With permission.)

Therefore the term *lactose intolerance* should only be used when referring to the symptomatic response to a defined lactose load. For example, an individual might be tolerant to 12 g of lactose, but be intolerant to 24 g. Determination of the presence and severity of symptoms is somewhat subjective, and may be influenced by factors other than the presence of lactose. Lactose maldigestion, on the other hand, is determined by an objective test, such as the breath hydrogen test. Both the objective determination of maldigestion and the subjective determination of intolerance are needed to develop a dietary strategy. Those with limited lactose digestion may or may not experience intolerance symptoms.

B. Milk Intolerance

Milk intolerance due to lactose is characterized by at least one clinical sign of intolerance experienced a few hours after ingestion of a known quantity of milk or milk-containing products. When the prevalence of milk intolerance is being evaluated rather than lactose maldigestion, several factors, such as the amount and form in which lactose is given, whether it is consumed with a meal, and whether the study is double-blinded, may influence the results.

Johnson et al. evaluated the relationship between maldigestion and intolerance in 164 African American adolescents and adults.[36] Objective testing with the breath hydrogen test revealed that 50% of the subjects maldigested and were intolerant to 25 g of lactose, the amount in 2 cups of milk (480 ml); 86% of this group experienced symptoms of lactose intolerance. Eight percent of the subjects were maldigesters, but tolerant; 15% were digesters but intolerant; and 27% were digesters and tolerant (Table 8.2). This study further confirms what others have observed, that there is a complex relationship between lactose maldigestion, lactose intolerance, and milk intolerance.[7]

Table 8 .2 Outcome of Lactose-Tolerance Breath-Hydrogen Study in 164 Volunteers. All Volunteers Claimed to be Intolerant of a Cup (240 mL) of Milk

Group	Classification	Symptoms*	n (%)
1	Maldigesters, intolerant	+	82 (50)
2	Maldigesters, tolerance	−	13 (8)
3	Digesters, intolerant	+	25 (15)
4	Digesters, tolerant	−	44 (27)
Total			164 (100)

* Symptoms: abdominal fullness, cramps, flatulence, borborygmi, nausea, vomiting, diarrhea.

From Johnson, A. O., et al. *Am. J. Clin. Nutr.*, 57, 399, 1993. With permission.

It is important that studies evaluating lactose tolerance (or other food tolerance) be double blind. This means that neither the subject nor the investigator knows whether the test solution contains lactose or a placebo. Unblinded studies may overestimate intolerance due to expectations of the subjects or the researcher. Lactose is often given in water for tolerance testing, and can be easily distinguished from a solution of glucose and galactose. When different levels of lactose are tested in milk, it is important to give the same volume of milk. When tolerance to milk is compared to that of lactose-hydrolyzed milk, an artificial sweetener should be added to the milk so that subjects cannot distinguish a taste difference between products. Subjects who are aware that the solution they are drinking contains lactose or that the volumes are being increased, sometimes experience symptoms they wouldn't have otherwise. Newcomer states that if all the studies evaluating tolerance were blinded, the percentage of subjects intolerant to 12 g of lactose would be only 10-15%.[48] Results of recent double-blind, randomized, crossover trials indicate that most individuals with primary lactase deficiency can tolerate one cup (240 ml) of milk with a meal or two cups (480 ml) if consumed in divided doses with breakfast and dinner.[34,35] Most recently, the same investigators found that women with limited lactose digestion can eat a dairy-rich diet that includes milk, yogurt, and cheese, supplying about 1500 mg of calcium per day, without major impediment.[49] (Table 8.3).

Table 8.3   Many Individuals Who Describe Themselves as "Lactose Intolerant" (LI) Can Digest Lactose. Most Who are Diagnosed as Lactose Maldigesters Can Tolerate the Amount of Lactose in a Serving or More of Milk and Other Dairy Foods

Study	Subjects	Lactose Dose (g) Breath Hydrogen Test	Lactose Digesters	Lactose Maldigesters	Milk Products Tested	Results
Suarez et al.	30 self-described, LI racially mixed adults	15 g	30%	70%	One cup of milk (12 g lactose) with breakfast	All tolerant
Suarez et al.	49 self-described, LI racially mixed adults	15 g	31%	69%	Two cups of milk/day consumed in divided doses with breakfast and dinner	All tolerant
Suarez et al.	62 female racially mixed adults	15 g	50%	50%	One cup of milk at breakfast, 1 cup of milk, 1 ounce of cheese and 8 ounces of yogurt at lunch, and 1 cup of milk and 1 ounce of cheese at dinner.	All tolerant – increased flatus frequency rated "trivial" in maldigesters

Suarez et al. measured gastrointestinal symptoms in 30 subjects who described themselves as intolerant to very small amounts of milk, such as the amount used on cereal or in coffee.[34] Of the 30 subjects, 21 (70%) were lactose maldigesters based on breath hydrogen concentrations after intake of 15 g of lactose, whereas 9 (30%) were lactose digesters. Both groups then participated in a randomized, double-blind, crossover trial in which they received either one cup of 2% milk (lactose-containing) or lactose-hydrolyzed milk every day with breakfast for one week. Since hydrolysis of the milk increases the sweetness, aspartame was added to the regular milk so that the sensory characteristics of the two milks were indistinguishable. The symptoms reported by both maldigesting and digesting subjects after consumption of one cup of milk (240 ml) were minimal, and were not significantly different than those reported after consumption of lactose-free milk. The researchers concluded that lactose-digestive aids are not necessary when lactose intake is limited to the equivalent of 240 ml of milk or less a day.[34]

The same researchers conducted a similar trial to test tolerance to two cups of milk daily (i.e., the average amount usually consumed).[35] A secondary goal of the study was to determine whether psychological factors play a role in a subjects perception of intolerance (this will be discussed in more detail in the next section). Two groups of lactose maldigesters (confirmed by a breath hydrogen test to 15 g of lactose), participated in the study: those who believed they were markedly intolerant to lactose (symptomatic) and those who believed that lactose did not induce symptoms (asymptomatic). Participants received either one cup of 2% milk (lactose-containing) or one cup of lactose-hydrolyzed milk with breakfast and another at dinner for one week. After a seven-day washout period, study participants switched to the opposite treatment. Both symptomatic and asymptomatic lactose maldigesters reported only minimal symptoms following intake of regular or lactose-free milk. These findings indicate that most self-described lactose intolerant subjects can readily tolerate two cups of milk daily if this milk is ingested in divided doses with breakfast and dinner.[35]

In a subsequent randomized, double-blind, crossover design study, Suarez and colleagues at the University of Minnesota, tested whether lactose maldigesting pre- and postmenopausal women could tolerate a dairy-rich diet providing approximately 1500 mg of calcium/day, the amount recommended by an Expert Panel of the National Institutes of Health to prevent osteoporosis.[49] The intake of dairy products was spread out over the day, and a variety of dairy products were used. The participants (50% maldigesters and 50% digesters per the breath hydrogen test) were randomly assigned to one of two dietary regimens for one week, then switched to the other (1) 240ml of 1% fat milk with breakfast and dinner, plus one serving (30 g) of a hard cheese at lunch and dinner, and 8 ounces of low fat, strawberry flavored yogurt at lunch; or (2) a similar regimen using lactose-hydrolyzed milk and yogurt. The dairy products provided about 1300 mg of calcium per day; it was assumed that the remainder of the diet would provide about 200 mg of calcium daily. Lactose maldigesters who consumed the dairy-rich diet experienced a significantly greater frequency of small flatus, but no differences in bloating, abdominal pain, nausea, fullness, or diarrhea, than when they consumed lactose-hydrolyzed products.

The above findings indicate that primary lactase deficiency need not be an obstacle to meeting calcium needs with milk and milk products. It has been confirmed with double-blind trials that lactose maldigesters can tolerate the amount of lactose in approximately 3 to 4 servings of milk and milk products, which provides the amount of calcium recommended by the expert panel of the National Institutes of Health (i.e., 1000 to 1500 mg) or the National Academy of Sciences for American adults (i.e., 1000 to 1200 mg).[50]

C. Subjective Factors Affecting Milk Tolerance

Some individuals, whether or not they are able to digest lactose, experience intolerance symptoms to whatever placebo is used in double-blind studies. This phenomenon complicates the diagnostic process, making it difficult for clinicians to accurately assess their patient's condition. Tolerance to milk is sometimes affected by factors unrelated to its lactose content, such as psychological factors or cultural attitudes toward milk.

A discussion of studies observing this phenomenon may help illustrate the complexity of the problem. Haverberg et al., in a double-blind trial, evaluated tolerance to 240 ml and 480 ml of a lactose-free and lactose-containing chocolate dairy drink in a group of 110 healthy Boston teenagers, 14 to 19 years of age.[37] Theoretically, symptoms due to lactose should occur only in those with limited lactose digestion in response to a lactose-containing beverage. However, 40% of those identified as lactose digesters per a breath-hydrogen test, and 31% of maldigesters reported symptoms after consuming the lactose-free beverage or after both the lactose-containing and the lactose-free beverage. Suspecting that perhaps the large number of false-positive results were because too much emphasis had been placed on reporting symptoms, the researchers conducted a follow-up study in a similar population of high school students using a simplified questionnaire that placed less emphasis on possible symptoms.[38] This time, 29% of the lactose digesters reported symptoms that apparently were due to an unidentified cause other than lactose. One criticism of these studies is that since chocolate has been shown to improve tolerance to lactose, the addition of chocolate to the dairy drinks (used to make the drinks similar in taste) may have affected the level of symptoms reported. Healthy elderly lactose digesters and maldigesters following a similar protocol to that of Haverberg, reported symptoms with the same degree of frequency to a lactose-containing drink as to a lactose-free drink.[39] The authors concluded that the symptoms were either psychosomatic or were the result of other physiologic causes.

Johnson et al. tested for milk tolerance a subgroup of 45 African American subjects who had confirmed lactose maldigestion and intolerance to 25 g of aqueous lactose.[36] Subjects were given either 315 ml of lactose-containing milk or lactose-hydrolyzed milk alternately on three different days in a double-blind test. One third of the subjects experienced symptoms of intolerance to both types of milk, indicating that their symptoms were not due to lactose. The authors conclude that social and cultural habits and attitudes also affect tolerance to milk drinking.

Two recent studies by Suarez et al. discussed earlier also illustrate this phenomenon.[34,35] In a study testing tolerance to one cup of milk served with breakfast, the researchers recruited subjects who reported severe lactose intolerance and who said they consistently experienced symptoms after consuming less than 240 ml of milk. Surprisingly, approximately one third (9 out of 30) of the subjects who claimed intolerance were able to digest lactose per the breath-hydrogen test. The authors concluded that people who identify themselves as severely lactose intolerant may mistakenly attribute a variety of abdominal symptoms to lactose intolerance.[34]

Similarly, in a second study designed to test tolerance to two cups of milk, approximately a third (31%) of recruited subjects (of mixed ethnic background) who claimed severe intolerance, were able to digest lactose as measured by the breath-hydrogen test. This group was not included in the subsequent milk trial, but was included with the other subjects in a psychological assessment, using the Minnesota Multiphasic Personality Inventory. The lactase deficient subjects who complained of symptoms, demonstrated a high level of psychasthenia (incapacity to resist irrational phobias, obsessions, and compulsions), but no correlations with any clinical psychological conditions (e.g., depression, hypochondriasis, paranoia) in response to the personality inventory. However, since these individuals also failed to respond candidly to the test (they tended to exaggerate, minimize, or conceal information), the researchers question the validity of these findings.

These studies further emphasize the need for objective testing for those complaining of gastrointestinal symptoms after drinking milk, since it appears that a significant portion of the population mistakenly attribute their symptoms to lactose.

D. Lactose Tolerance During Pregnancy

Pregnant women need to consume at least three servings of Milk Group foods to obtain the 1000 mg of calcium/day recommended by the National Academy of Sciences.[50] Women with limited lactose digestion may be encouraged to discover that their tolerance to lactose-containing milk and milk products may improve during pregnancy.

For example, Villar and colleagues demonstrated that 44% of women who maldigested 360 ml of milk (18 g of lactose) before the 15th week of gestation, were able to digest that amount of lactose by the end of their pregnancy.[51] Average breath hydrogen (an indication that undigested lactose is being metabolized by colonic bacteria) decreased by more than half over this time period.

Some researchers hypothesize that slower intestinal transit time during pregnancy improves tolerance to lactose.[52,53] For example, investigators compared lactose maldigestion and symptoms of intolerance between pregnant African American women and nonpregnant controls.[53] The pregnant women reported fewer symptoms than the nonpregnant women after drinking 8 ounces of 1% milk, although their ability to digest lactose did not change. The authors suggest that the improved tolerance was most likely due to slower intestinal transit time. They explain that because the rise in breath hydrogen in response to ingested lactose occurs approximately an hour later in pregnant versus nonpregnant women, breath hydrogen should be measured over a longer time period. This may be why earlier studies showed improved digestion. Whether actual digestion improves or not, it is clear from these studies that women may enjoy improved tolerance to milk and milk products while they are pregnant.

VI. LONG-TERM CONSEQUENCES OF LACTOSE INTOLERANCE

A. Lactose Digestion and Calcium/Nutrient Absorption

Studies conducted in the 1970s and 1980s in both animals and humans failed to provide any evidence that the maldigestion of lactose impaired the absorption of any other nutrient.[2] Nutrients studied include protein, fat, vitamins A and C, calcium, magnesium, copper, manganese, and zinc. In a review of this information, Leichter concluded that "if the unabsorbed lactose has some effect on the absorption of other nutrients it is doubtful whether this effect has significant nutritional consequences in healthy lactose intolerant adults who consume milk and milk products in moderate amounts."[54]

Because some portion of the lactose consumed passes undigested into the colon, those with limited lactose digestion obtain slightly less energy from milk and milk products than do lactose digesters. Part of the unabsorbed lactose is converted by fermentation into volatile fatty acids which are a source of energy and may help maintain the health of intestinal cells.[2] The small amount of energy lost seems to be of no practical significance.

While the presence of lactose stimulates the intestinal absorption of calcium in laboratory animals[55] and in human infants,[56] there is no evidence that it improves calcium absorption in adults.[57] Conversely, limited digestion and absorption of lactose does not appear to decrease calcium absorption. A review of research in this area concludes "the bulk of the evidence indicates a favorable or neutral effect of lactose on Calcium absorption in both lactose digesters and maldigesters."[2]

Tremaine and colleagues investigated how lactose might influence the absorption of calcium from milk in adults with and without lactase deficiency.[58] Using a double-isotope method, the researchers compared calcium absorption between lactose-containing milk and hydrolyzed milk in both lactase-deficient and -sufficient adults. The subjects with lactase deficiency absorbed calcium equally well from lactose-containing or lactose-hydrolyzed milk. Mean calcium absorption was greater in lactase-deficient subjects, presumably due to a lower calcium intake. Decreased calcium intake is known to cause an increase in calcium absorption, although calcium intake was not verified by diet history in this study. Horowitz et al. found no relationship between lactose and calcium absorption when an oral dose of 5 µ Ci of radioactive calcium chloride (20 mg of calcium) was measured in serum an hour later in 46 postmenopausal women with osteoporosis.[59] Roughly half of all subjects, whether or not they were lactose maldigesters, had below normal absorption of calcium. Griessen and colleagues also studied what influence lactase deficiency might have on calcium absorption.[60] Using a double-isotope technique, they compared calcium absorption in young adult lactase-deficient and -sufficient males from two commercial milks, one containing lactose and the other containing glucose. They then compared absorption between lactose-containing milk and water. Results demonstrated that all subjects absorbed calcium equally well from milk and from water. Glucose, when substituted for lactose in milk, did not improve calcium absorption. Lactase-deficient subjects absorbed calcium from the lactose-containing milk better than did the lactase-sufficient subjects. The authors did not attribute the increase to lower calcium status of the lactase-deficient group, since calcium intake of all subjects was normalized prior to the beginning of the study. The authors conclude that avoidance of dairy foods, rather than calcium malabsorption, is most likely the cause of increased risk of osteoporosis in lactase-deficient individuals.

B. Effect on Milk Consumption and Nutritional Status

Lactose intolerance is one factor that may influence milk consumption. Data from most studies, but not all,[61] suggest that individuals with primary lactose deficiency consume less milk than those who digest lactose normally.[39,54,62] For example, in a study conducted at the University of Connecticut, subjects with a history of milk intolerance consumed significantly less milk than the control subjects. The adult subjects consumed an 8-ounce serving (240 ml) of milk less than 1 to 3 times per month, while the lactose tolerant control group consumed an average of 1 to 2 servings of milk per day.[62] Finkenstedt et al. observed that lactose maldigestion affected milk intake in middle aged women. The daily intake of calcium from milk was significantly lower in those women with osteoporosis (125 mg/d) vs. controls (252 mg/d), more of whom were lactose maldigesters. Because of this finding, the investigators suggest that lactose maldigestion be considered a risk factor for osteoporosis.[63]

Interestingly, decreased milk intake as a result of lactose intolerance is not always a deliberate or conscious decision. Horowitz et al. found that even though only 5% of the lactose maldigesters he studied reported a history of milk intolerance, they drank significantly less milk (<1 cup/day) than those who digested milk normally (2 cups/day).[59] Newcomer observed a similar phenomenon.[64] Subjects diagnosed as lactose maldigesters by the breath-hydrogen test were not aware of milk intolerance, yet their intake of milk and calcium was significantly lower than that of lactose digesting subjects. He suggested that perhaps these subjects had decreased their milk intake during childhood as a result of lactose intolerance, but had forgotten that they had done so.[64]

Recent studies demonstrate that a low calcium intake and/or low milk intake results in a low intake of other milk-related nutrients both in adults and teenagers.[65,66,67] Young adult women who had low calcium intakes also had low intakes of protein and 9 other vitamins and minerals.[65] A majority of those nutrients found low in the diets of these women, vitamin A, riboflavin, folate, vitamin B_{12}, vitamin B_6, phosphorus, and magnesium, are provided by milk. Similarly, a recent study revealed that teenagers (13 to 18 years) who drank milk had higher intakes of vitamin A, riboflavin, folate, vitamin B_{12}, vitamin B_6, calcium, magnesium, and potassium than those who did not drink milk.[66] In another study, adults were asked to increase their calcium intake to 1500 mg/day primarily by increasing dairy food intake. Those who increased their dairy food intake also increased their intake of other milk-related nutrients when compared to those who received a calcium supplement (1000 mg/day) or a placebo.[67] During the 12-week experimental period, the group consuming extra dairy foods did not experience weight gain or any change in plasma lipid or lipoprotein concentrations. The authors observed that "a diet which consistently excludes or limits dairy foods will not only provide less calcium, but may also limit those nutrients that track with calcium in foods."[67] In an accompanying editorial, Dr. Robert Heaney states that this study reminds us of the value of food sources of calcium and that "recommended calcium intakes can feasibly be achieved from food sources alone."[68]

Therefore, it is important from a nutritional standpoint to encourage those with lactose intolerance to employ the dietary strategies available for including adequate amounts of dairy foods in the diet. Those with limited lactose digestion do not necessarily dislike dairy foods.[69] Populations with a high incidence of lactose maldigestion often have a positive attitude toward milk and consume moderate amounts without complaint.[2] Teens with lactose intolerance should especially be encouraged to maintain calcium and dairy food intake, since it is now believed that maximizing bone mass attained before age 30 is the most effective way to prevent osteoporosis later in life.[70]

C. Risk of Osteoporosis/Chronic Disease

Low calcium intake has been implicated in the etiology of several chronic diseases, such as osteoporosis, hypertension, and possibly some types of cancer.[71-73] As discussed previously, those with limited lactose digestion tend to have lower calcium and dairy food intakes.

Lactose maldigestion when accompanied by low calcium intake has been suggested as a risk factor for osteoporosis.[74] Studies conducted in the 1970s and 1980s reported a higher prevalence of lactose maldigestion among women with osteoporosis than in those without metabolic bone disease.[59,63,64] Recent research links lactose intolerance (report of symptoms) with low dairy food/calcium intake and low bone density in perimenopausal and postmenopausal women,[75,76] and with increased osteoporotic fractures in both women and men.[77,78]

In a study conducted among 57 postmenopausal Italian women, those who maldigested and were symptomatic to 20 g of aqueous lactose had significantly lower calcium intakes and bone mineral density than those who were maldigesters and asymptomatic.[76] Researchers in Finland investigated the relationship between self-reported lactose intolerance, calcium intake, and bone mineral density in 2025 women aged 48 to 59 who participated in the Kuopio Osteoporosis Risk Factor and Prevention (OSTPRE) study.[75] Mean dairy calcium intake was significantly lower (558 vs. 828 mg/d) and mean bone density of the spine and hip were 2.8% lower in women who reported lactose intolerance than in other women. Dairy calcium intake was an independent predictor of bone mineral density of the hip. These results suggest that perimenopausal bone density is reduced in women who report lactose intolerance, and is possibly due to reduced calcium intake. The same researchers studied all 11,619 women age 38 to 57 years, who were enrolled in the OSTPRE trial to test whether long-term low calcium intake in premenopausal women decreases bone strength differentially in weight-bearing bones.[77] Similar to the previous trial, mean dairy calcium intake was significantly lower in women who reported lactose intolerance than in other women (570 vs. 850 mg/d), while the risk of fracture of the tibia and metatarsal was higher (odds ratio of 3.31 and 2.84, respectively). Fractures of the wrist, ankle, and rib, however, were not related to lactose intolerance. The authors conclude that long-term premenopausal calcium deficiency differentially affects bones, with weight bearing non-ankle bones being at the greatest risk of suffering reduced strength.[77]

The Joint National Committee on Detection, Evaluation, and Treatment of High Blood Pressure, National Institutes of Health, National Heart, Lung and Blood Institute (NHLBI), recommends an adequate intake of calcium, potassium, and magnesium along with other lifestyle modifications for the prevention and treatment of hypertension.[79] Milk and milk products are an important source of all three of these minerals, contributing 73% of the calcium, 19% of the potassium, and 16% of the magnesium to the U.S. food supply.[80] These recommendations came after a clinical trial investigating Dietary Approaches to Stop Hypertension (DASH), funded by the NHLBI, found that a diet including 3 servings of lowfat dairy products and 8 to 10 servings of fruits and vegetables lowered blood pressure in people with or without existing hypertension.[81] The eating plan for the DASH diet, which is low in fat, and high in dietary fiber, potassium, calcium, and magnesium, is included in the appendix of the JNC-VI report. For more detailed information on this topic, see Dairy Foods and Hypertension, Chapter 3.

Epidemiological studies, animal studies, and *in vitro* studies using human cancer cells, indicate that several nutrients/components in milk and milk products may be protective against cancer.[82-86] The potentially anticarcinogenic agents include calcium, vitamin D, protein, vitamin A, beta-carotene, lactic acid bacteria, and components of milkfat, such as sphingolipids, conjugated linoleic acid (CLA), butyric acid, and ether lipids. For further information, see Chapter 4 on Dairy Foods and Colon Cancer.

VII. STRATEGIES FOR DIETARY MANAGEMENT OF PRIMARY LACTOSE MALDIGESTION

Several strategies are available for managing primary lactose maldigestion without compromising nutritional status or health.[1,30,87] Total elimination of dairy foods is unnecessary and not recommended.[2,88] Milk and other dairy foods contribute high quality protein to the diet and contribute 73% of the calcium, 33% of the phosphorus, 31% of the riboflavin, 21% of the vitamin B_{12}, 19% of both the potassium and zinc, and 16% of the magnesium available for consumption in the U.S.[80] Therefore, it is important to help those who maldigest lactose understand how they can include dairy foods in their diet.

Several factors influence an individual's tolerance to dairy foods including: the amount of lactose, type of dairy food, whether the lactose-containing food is eaten with a meal, whether the food has been fermented or hydrolyzed with an enzyme preparation, and colonic adaptation.[89] Employing strategies, which have been developed with these factors in mind, will allow most people with primary lactose intolerance to comfortably include dairy foods in their diet.

A. Amount of Lactose

As discussed earlier, most of those with limited lactose digestion can tolerate the amount of lactose contained in an 8-ounce (240 ml) serving of milk. Few individuals may need to consume smaller amounts (i.e., 4 ounces or 120 ml) at a time. Milk is also better tolerated when it is consumed with a meal.[44] Psyllium fiber, when added to aqueous lactose or milk, reduces hydrogen production and symptoms of intolerance.[90] This finding led to further studies that demonstrated similar alterations in breath hydrogen kinetics when lactose was consumed with a meal.[44,91] When lactose-containing foods are consumed with other solid foods, gastric emptying is delayed, both reducing and delaying peak hydrogen production. Martini and Savaiano found that only 3 out of 12 subjects experienced symptoms following a

19 g lactose load (equivalent to 1.6 glasses or 384 ml of milk) consumed with a breakfast meal.[44] This amounted to a three-fold reduction in both severity and incidence of symptoms when compared to aqueous lactose. Delayed gastric emptying allows more time for any endogenous lactase enzyme present to digest dietary lactose. It also reduces the amount of undigested lactose that reaches the colon at any one time.

B. Type of Dairy Food

People with limited lactose digestion tolerate some types of dairy foods better than others. Some studies have shown that whole milk is better tolerated than lower fat milks,[92,93] however not all studies have confirmed this.[94] The fat content of milk influences milk tolerance, presumably by slowing gastric emptying. When 11 lactose-maldigesting and intolerant subjects were given 50 g of lactose as whole milk, they experienced a significantly lower rise in blood glucose and decreased severity of symptoms, than when they were given the same amount of lactose in either skim milk or an aqueous solution.[92] Dehkordi et al. examined digestion (rather than tolerance) of various milks as measured by breath hydrogen production.[95] They found that absolute hydrogen production of maldigesters was lower for 18 g of lactose in whole milk than for skim milk, but the differences were not significant and neither milk completely alleviated lactose malabsorption (breath hydrogen <20 ppm). Only consumption of whole milk (18 g of lactose) with cornflakes significantly improved lactose digestion when compared to whole, fat free, chocolate, or commercial milk containing *L. acidophilus* and *Bifidobacterium*. Limitations of this study include the small number of subjects (5) and the relatively short collection time for breath hydrogen (5 vs. 8 hours). Vesa reported no differences in symptoms among free-living maldigesting subjects who consumed either fat-free or full-fat milk (8% fat). This group then conducted a more comprehensive study to determine whether raising the energy content of milk slows gastric emptying and improves tolerance.[96] Gastric emptying in 11 lactose maldigesting adults was significantly longer after ingestion of the high-energy milk (18 g of lactose) than after the half-skimmed milk, symptoms were not significantly improved, though there was a trend toward improved lactose digestion. The authors conclude that the positive effect was not strong enough to recommend high-energy milk to lactose maldigesters as a way to improve tolerance. The same group also found that increasing the viscosity of high-energy milk formulas with rice starch did not affect the rate of gastric emptying or improve milk tolerance.[97]

Chocolate milk appears to be better tolerated than unflavored milk by lactose maldigesters,[98] which can be explained by reduced breath hydrogen production when compared to fat free milk.[95] The addition of cocoa to 250 ml of milk formula significantly reduced the breath hydrogen response and symptoms of bloating and cramping in 37 lactose maldigesters.[98] While the mechanism for cocoa's affect on lactose tolerance is unclear, the authors propose three possible mechanisms (1) cocoa might stimulate lactase activity; (2) cocoa might reduce the number of gas-producing bacteria in the colon; or (3) cocoa might slow gastric emptying. These possible mechanisms need further study.

Some dairy foods, such as hard cheeses, cottage cheese, ice cream and yogurt, contain a lower amount of lactose per serving relative to milk, and therefore cause fewer symptoms. For example, Cheddar cheese contains a small amount of lactose. During the cheese-making process, the whey is removed from the curds. Since 94% of the lactose remains primarily with the whey portion, the finished cheese has a relatively low lactose content.

C. Fermented Milk Products

Yogurt with active microbial cultures improves the digestion of lactose. Yogurt with up to 20 g of lactose is well tolerated by a majority of lactase deficient individuals.[99] Improved lactose digestion with yogurt appears to be partly the result of its reduced lactose content, but is primarily due to autodigestion within the intestine by the microbial beta-galactosidase enzyme.[100] Three related factors appear to be important to the survival and expression of microbial enzyme activity from yogurt (1) the buffering of stomach acid by yogurt; (2) protection by the intact microbial cell to degradation by stomach acid or enzymes; and (3) action of digestive enzymes and bile acids on the microbial cell which releases beta-galactosidase activity.[99] In yogurt-making, the starter cultures *Lactobacillus bulgaricus* and *Streptococcus thermophilus* are incubated with fresh milk to which milk solids have been added. Both of these organisms synthesize the beta-galactosidase enzyme. The action of the beta-galactosidase present in these two organisms reduces the level of lactose in the concentrated milk. During the fermentation process the pH falls to about 4.6. (Beta-galactosidase is rapidly destroyed at pH ≤ 3.0.). Further lactase activity is inhibited by the combination of low pH and low temperature during storage. When yogurt is eaten, the casein, lactase, and calcium phosphate in the yogurt act as buffers to the stomach acid, allowing the microbes (and the enzyme activity) to reach the duodenum intact.[89] The buffering capacity of yogurt was found to be almost three times that of whole milk, presumably due to the proteins in the added milk solids.[101] Kolars et al. demonstrated that lactase activity in the duodenum after yogurt ingestion is enough to digest 50 to 100% of a 20 g lactose load.[100]

Factors influencing the extent to which the beta-galactosidase enzyme of the yogurt-borne bacteria facilitates lactose digestion in the human body are not completely understood. A number of variables may influence the delivery of beta-galactosidase to the duodenum, including gastric acid secretion, rate of gastric emptying, quantity of yogurt ingested, pancreatic and intestinal digestive enzyme activity, and lipid emulsification by bile acids.[101] There is some evidence that after the intact bacteria reach the intestinal tract they are disrupted by bile acids, releasing the enzyme to digest lactose. Pochart et al. confirmed the earlier finding of Kolars et al. that beta-galactosidase activity in yogurt survives passage through the stomach (Figure 8.6).[102] In addition they found that minimal lactose hydrolysis occurred in the duodenum after yogurt ingestion, indicating that digestion probably occurs further along the intestinal tract as bacterial (yogurt) lactase activity is stimulated by the progressively increasing pH.

Kolars et al. used the breath hydrogen technique to determine whether lactose in yogurt is better absorbed by lactose maldigesters than is lactose in milk.[100] The

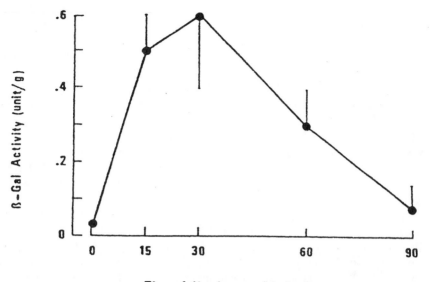

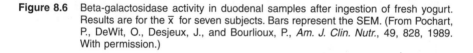

Figure 8.6   Beta-galactosidase activity in duodenal samples after ingestion of fresh yogurt. Results are for the x̄ for seven subjects. Bars represent the SEM. (From Pochart, P., DeWit, O., Desjeux, J., and Bourlioux, P., *Am. J. Clin. Nutr.*, 49, 828, 1989. With permission.)

total area under the breath hydrogen curve was significantly lower for 440 g of yogurt (18 g of lactose) than for milk or a lactose solution containing a similar amount of lactose. Hydrogen production after ingestion of yogurt was only about one third that of milk. A smaller amount of yogurt (270 g) containing 11 g of lactose, an amount closer to that typically consumed, produced only a negligible amount of hydrogen. Symptoms of diarrhea or flatulence were experienced by 80% of the subjects when they consumed 18 g of lactose in milk, but all subjects were symptom-free after consuming the same amount of lactose in yogurt.

Recent studies in adults and children suggest that the semi-solid nature of yogurt, which slows its gastric emptying, may be an important factor in its improved tolerance. Researchers at Johns Hopkins School of Medicine in Boston tested whether yogurt was better tolerated than milk in 14 lactose-malabsorbing children (mean age 9.5 years).[103] The children experienced significantly fewer symptoms after consumption of 8 ounces of yogurt containing active cultures than after consuming milk. Since the children experienced improved tolerance to both yogurt with live active cultures and pasteurized yogurt (which decreased bacterial activity) the authors suggest that yogurt's osmolality, energy density, and delayed transit time played a greater role in improving tolerance than did its ability to "autodigest" lactose. Researchers in France reached a similar conclusion when three yogurts containing different bacterial cultures and lactase activity were equally digested and tolerated by fifteen lactase deficient adults.[104]

Although consuming yogurt (when compared with milk) reduces the occurrence and severity of symptoms associated with lactose maldigestion, lactase activity varies considerably between brands of active-culture yogurt.[105] In addition, if yogurt is pasteurized after the addition of active cultures (which is sometimes done to extend shelf-life of the product), it loses much of its ability to hydrolyze lactose in the gut.[69,106] Furthermore, eating yogurt may not assist the digestion of lactose from other dairy foods eaten with it as part of a meal.[107] Ingestion of yogurt over eight days provided no additional benefit.[106]

Some people find flavored yogurts more acceptable than plain.[69] When lactose digestion was compared between milk, flavored and plain yogurt in 16 lactase deficient subjects, flavored yogurt produced a breath hydrogen level slightly higher than that of plain yogurt, but lower than milk. Although only the hydrogen production from the plain yogurt was statistically significantly lower than that of milk, none of the subjects experienced any symptoms after eating either variety of yogurt, while three reported symptoms after drinking milk.[108] It is unclear how the addition of fruit, sweeteners, and flavorings might reduce the beta-galactosidase activity in flavored yogurts. Frozen yogurt that has been pasteurized prior to freezing (typical commercial practice), lacks beta-galactosidase activity. Lactose maldigestion and tolerance have been found to be similar between frozen yogurt, ice milk, and ice cream. However lactase deficient persons may tolerate significant amounts of these products, presumably due to their slower gastric transit time owing to its high solids and/or fat content.[108]

D. Unfermented Milk with Bacterial Cultures

Whether non-fermented dairy products containing bacterial starter cultures, such as sweet acidophilus milk or yogurt milk, have the potential to improve lactose tolerance is controversial.[109]

Acidophilus milk is a nonfermented beverage made by adding viable L. acidophilus strains to cold milk, then refrigerating to prevent further growth of the organism. It has an advantage over yogurt in that it doesn't have a tart taste. Yogurt milk is prepared in a manner similar to acidophilus milk, except that Streptococcus thermophilus and Lactobacillus bulgaricus are added to the fresh milk.

Several studies conducted in the 1980s found that acidophilus milk or capsules containing high concentrations of mixed lactic acid bacteria or Bifidobacteria bifidum did not improve lactose digestion or alleviate symptoms in lactose maldigesting subjects.[110-113] It has since been learned that certain factors, such as insufficient concentration of the culture, extended storage, use of frozen concentration starter culture, level of lactic acid, and use of inappropriate substrates for culture growth, contribute to the ineffectiveness of these unfermented products.[109,114] The strain of L. acidophillus used in studies of lactose maldigestion is of critical importance, since beta-galactosidase activity, bile sensitivity, and acid tolerance vary considerably among strains.

For example, acidophilus milk (prepared with three different strains of L. acidophilus in two different concentrations) and yogurt milk (prepared with two concentrations of S. thermophilus and L. bulgaricus) were evaluated on the basis of beta-galactosidase activity, bile tolerance, and ability to digest lactose in 10 lactose-maldigesting adults.[115] Only yogurt milk and acidophilus milk prepared with the highest concentration (10^8 cfu/ml) of starter cultures were effective in significantly decreasing breath hydrogen concentrations in the subjects. Only the most bile-sensitive strain of *L. acidophilus* was effective in this regard. This characteristic appears to be important for the release of beta-galactosidase within the intestinal tract. Furthermore, subjects who normally experienced symptoms after ingestion of 20 g of lactose, reported fewer symptoms following consumption of 400 ml of yogurt milk containing 10^8 cfu/ml than with 400 ml of acidophilus milk containing the same cell concentration. The researchers conclude that consumption of non-fermented yogurt milk containing high concentrations of yogurt cultures was able to reduce breath hydrogen concentrations 3-fold. This is similar to the effect of fermented yogurt, which reduces gas production by 3 to 4-fold, when compared to milk.[115] Montes et al. tested digestibility and tolerance of unfermented milks among 20 children with limited lactose digestion.[116] They found that consumption of 250 ml of lowfat milk inoculated with 10^{10} cells of *Lactobacillus acidophilus* improved tolerance, while consumption of the same amount of milk inoculated with a commercial yogurt starter culture containing 10^8 cells of *Lactobacillus lactis* and 10^{10} cells of *Streptococcus thermophilus*, improved both digestion and tolerance, compared to regular milk.

Most recently, researchers at Purdue University tested four strains of *L. acidophilus* with varying degrees of lactose transport, beta-galactosidase activity, and bile acid sensitivity on lactose digestion and tolerance in a group of lactose maldigesting adults.[114] Acidophilus milk prepared with the bacterial strain with the greatest bile and acid tolerance was the most effective in improving lactose digestion and tolerance. Further studies are needed, however, to determine the extent of the importance of these factors.

Bifidobacteria may have potential for use in products designed to improve lactose digestion because they contain a relatively high level of beta-galactosidase activity and are stable under normal storage conditions. A study conducted among 15 lactose-maldigesting adults showed that unfermented milk containing *Bifidobacteria longum* that was grown in a lactose-containing medium, had the greatest beta-galactosidase activity and significantly improved lactose digestion (per breath hydrogen) and symptoms of flatulence compared to other bifido strains or regular lowfat milk.[117]

E. Enzyme Preparations

Lactose-hydrolyzed milk or commercial oral enzyme replacement therapy has proven beneficial in adults and children and is recommended as a strategy for improving lactose tolerance.[2,7,87,118,119] Oral enzyme replacement in tablet form offers the advantage of allowing a more liberal use of lactose-containing dairy foods. This may prove a useful therapy even for young children, making specialized nutritional management unnecessary.[120] Beta-galactosidases extracted from yeast, *Kluyveromyces lactis*; or fungi, *Aspergillus niger* or *Aspergillus oryzae*, have been found effective.[72,121,122] These enzymes as well as the final products of their addition to food have been classified as Generally Recognized as Safe (GRAS) by the Food and Drug

Administration under the broad classification of carbohydrates.[123] Lactose reduced milk is prepared at a processing plant by adding the liquid enzyme to previously pasteurized milk and holding for 24 hours. When the appropriate level of reduction has been reached, usually 70%, the milk is pasteurized again to stop lactose hydrolysis.[124] Milk that has 99.9% of its lactose hydrolyzed, labeled "lactose free," is now available on the market.[125] A milk labeled "lactose reduced" must contain at least 70% less lactose than regular milk.[126] In addition to lactose-reduced milk, other lactose-reduced dairy products are now on the market.

Lactose hydrolyzed milk and an oral enzyme tablet taken with milk were evaluated along with milk, acidophilus milk, and yogurt, for their effectiveness in facilitating lactose digestion and for their acceptability.[112] Acidophilus milk induced the greatest rise in breath hydrogen production, followed by whole milk, whole milk plus a lactase tablet, hydrolyzed lactose milk, and yogurt, respectively. Even though yogurt was the most effective at reducing breath hydrogen production compared to exogenous lactase products, the study subjects did not like it as well as milk. Acceptability of hydrolyzed-lactose milk did not differ significantly from yogurt. While some found yogurt unacceptable because of its tart taste, others gave hydrolyzed lactose milk a lower rating due to its sweetness.[112] When lactose is hydrolyzed into glucose and galactose, the free glucose makes the product taste slightly sweeter. Children have found lactose hydrolyzed milk quite acceptable for this reason.[127] At least a 50% reduction of lactose content in milk is adequate to relieve symptoms of lactose intolerance in a majority of lactose maldigesters.[128] Those more sensitive to lactose (e.g., those with secondary lactose intolerance) may need lactose free milk or additional lactase tablets to relieve symptoms.

Below is a summary of management strategies aimed at improving lactose tolerance while keeping dairy foods and the nutrients they provide in the diet:

Management Strategies for Those with Lactose Intolerance

1. Drink milk in servings of one cup or less.
2. Drink milk with a meal or with other food.
3. Try whole or chocolate milk.
4. Try cheese. Much of the lactose is removed during processing.
5. Try yogurt with active cultures.
6. Use milk and other dairy foods that are lactose-reduced or lactose-free.
7. Prepare lactose-reduced milk at home using an enzyme preparation.
8. Use an oral lactase supplement before consuming dairy foods.

F. Colonic Adaptation

Although continued exposure to lactose does not induce the intestinal synthesis of the lactase enzyme, there is evidence that adaptation to lactose occurs in the colon. This phenomenon was first noted in the 1950s when supplemental milk feeding programs for preschool and school-aged children were initiated as part of global relief efforts. When milk was first introduced, it was sometimes associated with complaints of diarrhea and gastrointestinal discomfort. However, these complaints soon stopped as the program continued. This phenomenon was initially explained as a child's psychological reaction to an unfamiliar food. An early clinical trial, however, demonstrated that continued lactose intake increases the amount of lactose tolerated without symptoms, and without change in intestinal lactase activity.[129]

Recent clinical trials have demonstrated that the colonic flora of persons with limited lactose digestion adapts to continued milk intakes. Twenty-five African American adolescents and young adults, who were confirmed lactose maldigesters and intolerant to the amount of lactose in one glass of milk (12 g), were given gradually increasing amounts of lactose in milk (beginning at 5 g) over a period of time until their maximum level of tolerance was determined.[130] Of the 22 subjects who completed the study, 77% tolerated ≥12 g of lactose (the amount in 8 ounces or 240 ml of milk) without disturbing symptoms. All individuals were able to adapt to ≥7 g of lactose, the amount in 150 ml of milk. Objective testing of breath hydrogen production revealed that a majority of the subjects continued to maldigest the lactose dose they tolerated.

Hertzler and Savaiano conducted a two-part blinded, controlled crossover trial to determine the effect of continued lactose feeding on (1) the ability of fecal bacteria to metabolize lactose, and (2) the symptomatic response to lactose.[131] Results from the first part of the study indicated that lactose feeding altered the ability of fecal bacteria to metabolize lactose. Fecal beta-galactosidase began to rise within 48 hours of beginning lactose feeding, and by 10 days had peaked at 3 times the control value. In part two of the study, subjects were given 0.6 g/kg body weight per day of lactose in water divided between breakfast, lunch, and dinner. This amount was increased by 0.2 g/kg increments every other day, up to a maximum of 1.0 g/kg per day. Subjects increased their intake of lactose over a 10-day period from an average of 42 g to 70 g per day (equivalent to the amount of lactose in 800 to 1500 ml of milk). Symptoms in the lactose group were not significantly different from the control group (fed dextrose), and did not increase from the beginning to the end of the lactose feeding period, even though the lactose dose was nearly doubled. In fact, a breath-hydrogen test, administered at the end of the study, indicated that the subjects had no increase in breath hydrogen. The authors conclude that adaptation of the colonic flora offers a simpler and less expensive solution for subjects who wish to consume large amounts of lactose containing foods on a regular basis.

A double-blind study conducted by researchers in France among severely intolerant (all experienced diarrhea) Asian subjects, also demonstrated metabolic adaptation and reduction of symptoms (except diarrhea) to lactose in water feeding (17 g twice daily) over 13 days.[132] The control group (fed sucrose), also reported fewer symptoms, though they did not demonstrate biochemical adaptation (e.g., increased fecal beta-galactosidase activity, lower pH, and decreased breath hydrogen), as did the group fed lactose. The authors suggest that improved clinical tolerance may sometimes be the result of becoming familiar with the test procedures. They recommend that those with severe symptoms avoid consuming lactose in the fasting state. Instead, they should consume lactose in the form of yogurt or together with other foods.

The mechanism by which adaptation occurs is not completely understood, however, the following mechanisms have been proposed (1) The presence of unhydrolyzed lactose in the colon stimulates organic acid production which lowers the pH inhibiting further fermentation and hydrogen production; (2) undigested lactose may alter the composition of colonic bacteria by reducing the number of gas-forming bacteria in favor of non-gas-producing organisms; or (3) lactose in the colon stimulates colonic bacterial fermentation and the removal of end products.[130]

Theoretically, a reduction in breath hydrogen after continued lactose feeding could be either the result of decreased absolute hydrogen production or increased hydrogen consumption by colonic bacteria. Using a technique that distinguishes production from consumption, Hertzler et al. established that lactose feeding decreased absolute hydrogen production, possibly by stimulating the proliferation of bacterial species such as bifidobacteria, which ferment lactose without producing hydrogen.[133] Jiang and Savaiano, simulating lactose adaptation *in vitro*, found that supplementation of the culture medium with *Lactobacillus acidophilus* enhanced lactose utilization during the first day.[117] They conclude that *L. acidophilus* may enhance lactose fermentation in the colon during the early period of lactose feeding before adaptation is established.

VIII. TREATMENT OF MALNUTRITION/DIARRHEAL DISEASE IN CHILDREN

Infants and children with infectious gastroenteritis and accompanying diarrhea, experience lactase deficiency and intolerance secondary to damage of the intestinal mucosa. Diarrhea caused by most common organisms is self-limiting, and rarely persists for more than 4 to 5 days. Even during acute infectious enteritis, the gut retains a significant capacity to assimilate nutrients.[134] During this phase, the goal of nutritional management is to maintain hydration status and prevent starvation in the malnourished infant; the number and character of stools should not guide management.[134] Current recommendations support continued breast-feeding of infants during diarrhea with concurrent use of a glucose-electrolyte solution to maintain hydration. For bottle-fed infants and those receiving solid foods, usual feedings can be reintroduced after the rehydration phase, but should not be delayed longer than 24 hours.[135]

Whether lactose containing formulas should be used for young children with acute diarrhea has been a matter of frequent debate. No firm recommendations have been developed. This issue has policy implications for feeding programs in developing countries where diarrheal disease in children is a common health problem, and where lactose-reduced products are expensive and unavailable.

Recently a meta-analysis of 29 randomized clinical trials was conducted evaluating the use of non-human milks or formulas in the dietary management of acute diarrhea in children.[136] The studies compared the effectiveness of lactose containing vs. non-lactose containing diets and the effect of using undiluted vs. diluted milk or delayed milk feeding. In general, treatment failure, defined as greater stool frequency, increased duration of symptoms, recurrent dehydration, and weight loss, was increased in those receiving lactose containing diets, but only in patients who initially presented with severe dehydration. The authors conclude, however, that "nondehydrated children can be managed as successfully with lactose containing diets as with lactose-free regimens." They emphasize the importance of rapidly correcting dehydration with an oral electrolyte solution, as recommended in the standardized treatment protocol of the World Health Organization (WHO).[135] Feeding with undiluted milk was a less effective treatment than diluted milk in children with the most severe illness. This small advantage of feeding with diluted milk was offset by poorer weight gains. Thus, there is a trade-off between risking relapsing diarrhea and suboptimal nutritional status. Therefore, when the diarrhea is relatively mild, it is preferable to feed with undiluted milk. The clinical trials taken as a whole indicate that children who continue to receive lactose containing milk diets have a treatment failure rate of about 10%. The authors conclude, "the vast majority of young children with acute diarrhea can safely continue to receive undiluted, nonhuman milk."[136]

Some practitioners recommend that infants younger than 6 months who have persistent diarrhea should be treated with a lactose-free soy-based formula or a low lactose protein hydrolysate formula for the first few days or weeks after acute gastroenteritis.[119] Cow's milk formula may be reintroduced after the diarrhea and intestinal damage which promote lactase deficiency have resolved, usually in about four weeks. Others, however, contend that infants under 6 months with diarrhea should be given full-strength formula as soon as dehydration is corrected.[137] The generally accepted method of treatment for children older than 9 months is full-strength milk or formula immediately following 24 hours of treatment with a glucose-electrolyte solution.[119] Infants or children with secondary lactose intolerance due to gastrointestinal diseases leading to villus atrophy such as Crohn's disease or protein-sensitive enteropathy must be managed by temporarily restricting lactose in the diet,[118] and may benefit from a protein-hydrolyzed formula.[138]

In the case of older children who are eating a variety of solid foods, practitioners should assess the severity of the lactose maldigestion and individualize the diet accordingly. Lower lactose dairy products such as yogurt, aged cheeses, and lactose hydrolyzed milk should be encouraged. Many children will be able to tolerate 4 to 6 ounces of milk with meals. Various types of milks and infant formulas can be treated with a lactase enzyme preparation that is added to milk in the form of drops, then allowed to incubate for 24 hours. As much as 100% of the lactose can be hydrolyzed in this manner for severe cases of lactose intolerance. In severe cases of intolerance it will also be necessary to read labels on non-dairy foods and avoid purchasing products that have ingredients that contain lactose: these include whey powder, casein, casein hydrolysate, sodium caseinate, and lactalbumin.[118]

Children with severe protein energy malnutrition (PEM) commonly have reduced activity of intestinal lactase due to nutritional injury and infection.[87] Milk has been used extensively along with other protein sources in refeeding programs aimed at reversing PEM. A study involving 20 Guatemalan preschool children with PEM demonstrated that lactose-hydrolyzed milk offered no advantages over lactose containing milk in recovery from PEM.[139] The group receiving intact lactose experienced more diarrhea, but recovery was satisfactory in both groups during the 45-day refeeding period, with no differences in rates of growth, body protein repletion, restoration of energy reserves, or intestinal function. A study of malnourished Senegalese children age 6 to 36 months demonstrated that fermented milk may also be useful in the treatment of malnourished children with acute diarrhea and sugar intolerance.[140]

IX. RECOMMENDATIONS FOR FEEDING PROGRAMS

The American Academy of Pediatrics stated the following position in 1978, which was reaffirmed in 1990, "On the basis of present evidence it would be inappropriate to discourage supplemental milk feeding programs targeted at children on the basis of primary lactose intolerance."[88]

A. International

Milk can provide an inexpensive source of carbohydrate, protein, and calcium to children in countries where protein-calorie malnutrition is prevalent. In Gambia West Africa, for example, growth failure and undernutrition is common, as is lactose maldigestion after the second year of life. In a study involving Gambian children, lactose maldigestion was not associated with growth failure. Consumption of cow's milk was common among the children and was rarely associated with any adverse affects.[141] The authors recommend that cow's milk be given to Gambian children after weaning as a means of supplementing their diet.

As discussed in the section on adaptation, children who receive milk as part of a supplemental feeding program usually tolerate it quite well. Powdered fermented milk might also be a viable option for providing supplemental milk to children in countries where there is a high prevalence of lactase deficiency.[142] When 25 Gabonese lactase deficient children consumed 150 ml of powdered fermented milk formula containing 10.5 g lactose, breath hydrogen production was reduced to normal levels and symptoms of intolerance were reduced by one-third, when compared to a regular milk formula. Since this product may be purchased in dry powdered form, it has advantages for use in developing countries where refrigeration may not be available.

B. United States

Supplemental feeding programs in the United States, such as the National School Lunch Program (NSLP), the National School Breakfast Program (NSBP) and the Women, Infants and Children Supplemental Food Program (WIC), serve clients with a variety of ethnic backgrounds. While many schools serve populations where lactose maldigestion is common, milk is not contraindicated, and dairy products are included as part of the standard meal plan. Nearly all children with low lactase activity can tolerate the 8 ounces of milk required in the school meal pattern, especially since it is served with a meal.

However, studies of milk drinking among African American children at school report that some students may reject milk at school or drink only part of the 240 ml provided.[143] There is evidence that children's milk drinking habits may be more influenced by cultural attitudes towards milk as they get older than by lactose tolerance status.[37] This is illustrated by the fact that, regardless of lactose tolerance status, the parents of Black children consume less milk than those of White children.[144]

After the age of eight, milk intake decreases in some student populations, increasing the chance of clinical consequences.[143] Therefore it may be beneficial for schools serving such populations to make available a selection of dairy foods, such as aged cheese, yogurt, whole and chocolate milk. Yogurt is approved for use in school meals as a meat alternate.[145]

High school students have the option of declining milk if they so choose under the offer versus serve guidelines. If a younger child has severe milk intolerance, however, the school is allowed (or required in some states) to make an appropriate substitution. The child must bring a letter from a physician, dietitian, or nurse describing the need for a food substitution and a recommendation of substitute foods.[146]

Fifty-eight percent of those enrolled in the WIC program belong to ethnic groups with a high prevalence of lactose maldigestion, including Black (25.4%), Hispanic (26.1%), Asian (2.6%), and Native American (1.7%).[147] Lactose intolerance is not a major issue for WIC-eligible children, since the prevalence of lactose maldigestion for children under age 5 is low. A review of WIC food packages, conducted by researchers at Pennsylvania State University in cooperation with the Food Nutrition Service, concluded that although many adults in the ethnic minority populations served by WIC are potentially affected by lactose maldigestion, dairy products can be and are consumed by these individuals.[148] They add that dairy foods of some type may be acceptable to most WIC participants, and a number of management strategies are available for improving tolerance to dairy foods. Educational materials that outline these strategies are supplied to WIC participants who need them. In addition to milk and cheese, it has been a long-standing policy of the WIC program to allow lactose-reduced milk to participants with lactose intolerance.

Cultural food values, rather than lactose intolerance, is the main factor affecting acceptance of dairy products among WIC participants.[148] Nevertheless, the panel who reviewed WIC food packages feels there are valid scientific reasons for accommodating food preferences, whether they have a biological or cultural basis. Therefore, several non-dairy foods that would provide alternative sources of calcium and protein are under consideration for inclusion in WIC food packages.[149] Though USDA solicited public comment on this issue in 1994, they have not yet published a final ruling.

X. FUTURE RESEARCH NEEDS

Further work is needed in the areas of genetics, management, and education. Animal studies are continuing to investigate the molecular mechanisms involved in developmental changes in the lactase enzyme. Studies are underway investigating the regulation of lactase gene expression in the human intestine.[19] A further understanding of how the colon adapts to continued milk intakes is important; this will allow development of protocols for encouraging milk intake in those with lactase nonpersistence. More research is needed on the strains of organisms used as bacterial cultures in fermented and nonfermented dairy foods that will aid the hydrolysis of lactose *in vivo* most effectively. This knowledge will lead to the development of new, more effective products. More can be done to educate practitioners and the public about appropriate diagnosis and treatment strategies available for those with lactose intolerance.

XI. CONCLUSION

Lactose intolerance, whether real or perceived, causes individuals to reduce or eliminate milk and milk products from their diet. Tolerance to dairy foods can be improved by following the simple strategies outlined in this chapter. Research has shown that current calcium recommendations can be met through the strategic use of dairy foods by most people who have low lactase levels. While most with limited lactose digestion can tolerate milk in moderate amounts, the loss of intestinal lactase in early childhood does have clinical and nutritional significance. A low intake of milk and milk products has been shown to increase the risk of osteoporosis, hypertension, and some forms of cancer. Future research will further our knowledge in the areas of genetics and the development of new dairy products that will be well tolerated by those with low lactase activity. Nearly all children and most adults should be encouraged to benefit from the nutritional value of milk, even if lactose intolerance limits the quantities they can consume at one time, or the forms in which they may enjoy dairy products.

XII. GLOSSARY OF TERMS

Lactase Beta-galactosidase, an enzyme of the hydrolase class that catalyzes the hydrolysis (digestion) of lactose, a disaccharide, into its monosaccharide components of glucose and galactose. Lactase is present on the brush border of the intestinal mucosa where such digestion takes place.

Lactase nonpersistence Refers to the decrease in lactase activity that occurs after weaning. This characteristic is transmitted as an autosomal-recessive trait.

Lactase persistence Refers to the retention of significant intestinal lactase into adulthood. This characteristic is transmitted as an autosomal-dominant trait.

Low lactase activity or **hypolactasia** Low levels of the intestinal enzyme, lactase, in the brush border membrane. Low lactase activity (lactase deficiency) can be measured directly by small bowel biopsy, or indirectly using the lactose tolerance test or the breath-hydrogen test.

Lactose A disaccharide which yields upon hydrolysis the monosaccharides, glucose and galactose. Since milk is the sole natural source of lactose, it is commonly referred to as *milk sugar.*

Lactose intolerance The clinical signs and symptoms which include bloating, flatulence, abdominal pain, and diarrhea following consumption of a dose of lactose greater than the body's ability to digest and absorb. "Tolerance" and "intolerance" are not synonymous with "digestion" and "maldigestion" and should be used only in reference to a defined dose of lactose delivered in a specific vehicle (i.e., the subject was intolerant to 50 g of lactose in aqueous solution).

Congenital lactase deficiency A rare genetic abnormality in which the enzyme lactase is very low or absent at birth.

Primary lactase deficiency The normal developmental decrease in lactase activity beyond the age of weaning.

Secondary lactase deficiency Temporary low levels of the lactase enzyme due to an underlying disease or medical condition affecting the gastrointestinal tract, such as gastroenteritis, tropical sprue, recovery from gastrointestinal surgery, radiation therapy, or certain drugs.

Lactose maldigestion Reduced digestion of lactose due to low lactase activity.

Milk intolerance due to lactose One or more clinical signs of abdominal pain, bloating, flatulence, or diarrhea experienced a few hours after ingestion of a known quantity of milk or milk-containing products in a person with proven lactose maldigestion.

XIII. LACTOSE CONTENT OF DAIRY PRODUCTS

Product	Lactose (g)
Milk (1 cup)	
Whole	9 – 12
2% reduced fat	9 – 13
1% low fat	12 – 13
Fat free	11 – 14
Chocolate	10 – 12
Buttermilk	9 – 12
Evaporated	24 – 28
Sweetened condensed	31 – 50
*Lactaid (lactose-reduced lowfat milk)	3
Goat's milk	11 – 12
Acidophilus, skim	11
Yogurt, lowfat (1 cup)	4 - 17
Cheese (1 oz.)	
Cottage (1/2 cup)	0.7 – 4
Cheddar, sharp	0.4 – 0.6
Swiss	0.5 – 1
Mozzarella, part skim, low moisture	.08 – .9
American, pasteurized, processed	0.5 – 4
Ricotta (1/2 cup)	0.3 – 6
Cream	0.1 – .8
Butter (1 pat)	0.04 – 0.05
Cream (1 tbsp.)	
Light	0.6
Whipping	0.4 – 0.5
Sour	0.4 – 0.5
Ice Cream (1/2 cup)	2 – 6
Ice Milk (1/2 cup)	5
Sherbet (1/2 cup)	0.6 – 2

Sources: Scrimshaw, N.S. and Murray, E.B., *Amer. J. Clin. Nutr.*, Supplement 48(4), 1988.
* Bowes & Church's *Food Values of Portions Commonly Used*, Jean A. Pennington, 1989.

Studies have shown that yogurt with live active cultures is significantly better tolerated than milk because of its high lactase activity.[100]

REFERENCES

1. National Digestive Diseases Information Clearinghouse, *Lactose Intolerance*, NIH Publication No. 91-2751, 1991.
2. Scrimshaw, N. S. and Murray, E. B., The acceptability of milk and milk products in populations with a high prevalence of lactose intolerance, *Am. J. Clin. Nutr.*, 48 (Suppl. 4), 1988.
3. Johnson, J. D., Kretchmer, N., and Simoons, F. J., Lactose malabsorption: its biology and history, in *Advances in Pediatrics*, Vol. 21, Schulman, I., Ed., Yearbook Medical Publishers, Chicago, 1974, 197.
4. Holden, C. and R. Mace, Phylogenetic analysis of the evolution of lactose digestion in adults, *Human Biology*, 69(5), 605, 1997.
5. Kretchmer, N., The significance of lactose intolerance: an overview, in *Lactose Digestion: Clinical and Nutritional Implications*, Paige, D. M. and Bayless, T. M., Eds., Johns Hopkins University Press, Baltimore and London, 1981, chap. 1.
6. Bayless, T. M. and Rosensweig, N. S., A racial difference in incidence of lactase deficiency, *J. Am. Med. Assoc.*, 197, 968, 1966.
7. Saavedra, J. M. and Perman, J. A., Current concepts in lactose malabsorption and intolerance, *Ann. Rev. Nutr.*, 9, 475, 1989.
8. Torun, B., Solomons, N. W., and Viteri, F. E., Lactose malabsorption and lactose intolerance: implications for general milk consumption, *Archivos Latinoamericanos De Nutricion*, 29(4), 446, 1979.
9. Troncon, L. E., de Oliveira, R. B., Collares, E. F., and Padovan, W., Gastric emptying of lactose and glucose-galactose in patients with low intestinal lactase activity, *Arquivos De Gastroenterologia*, 20(1), 8, 1983.
10. Grand, R. J, Watkins, J. B., and Torti, F. T., Development of the human gastrointestinal tract: a review, *Gastroenterology*, 70, 790, 1976.
11. Kien, C. L., McClead, R. E., and Leandro, C., In vivo lactose digestion in preterm infants, *Am. J. Clin. Nutr.*, 64, 700, 1996.
12. MacLean, Jr., W. C., and Fink, B. B, Lactose malabsorption by premature infants: magnitude and clinical significance, *J. Pediatr.*, 97, 383, 1980.
13. Lifschitz, C. H., Smith, E. O., and Garza, C., Delayed complete functional lactase sufficiency in breast-fed infants, *J. Pediatr. Gastroenterol. Nutr.*, 2(3), 478, 1983.
14. Gilat, T., Russo, S., Gelman-Malachi, E., and Aldor, T. A., Lactase in man: a non-adaptable enzyme, *Gastroenterology*, 62, 1125, 1972.
15. Lee, M-F, and Krasinski, S. D., Human adult-onset lactase decline: an update, *Nutr. Rev.*, 56(1), 1, 1998.
16. Rossi, M., Maiuri, L, Fusco, M. I., Salvati, V. M., Fuccio, A., Auriccio, S., Mantei, N., Zecca, L., Gloor, S. M., and Semenza, G., Lactase persistence versus decline in human adults: multifactorial events are involved in down-regulation after weaning, *Gastroenterology*, 112, 1506, 1997.
17. Hauri, H-P, Sander, B., and Naim, H., Induction of lactase biosynthesis in the human intestinal epithelial cell line Caco-2, *Eur. J. Biochemistry*, 219, 539, 1994.
18. Van Beers, E., Al, R. H., Rings, E. H., Einerhand, W. C., Dekker, J, and Buller, H. A., Lactase and sucrase-isomaltase gene expression during Caco-2 cell differentiation, *J. Biochem.*, 308, 769, 1995.

19. Rings, E. H. H. M., van Beers, E. H., Kransinski, S. D., Verhave, M., Montgomery, R. K., Grand, R. J., Dekker, J., and Buller, H. A., Origin, gene expression, localization, and function, *Nutr. Res.*, 14(5), 775, 1994.

20. Solomons, N. W., Diagnosis and screening techniques for lactose maldigestion: advantages of the hydrogen breath test, in *Lactose Digestion: clinical and nutritional implications*, Paige, D. M. and Bayless, T. M., Eds., Johns Hopkins University Press, Baltimore and London, 1981, 105, Chap. 8.

21. American Academy of Pediatrics, Committee on Nutrition, Soy protein-based formulas: Recommendations for use in infant feeding, *Pediatrics*, 101(1), 148, 1998.

22. Aurisicchio, L. N. and Pitchumoni, C. S., Lactose Intolerance: recognizing the link between diet and discomfort, *Postgraduate Med.*, 95(1), 113, 1994.

23. Sahi, T, Genetics and epidemiology of adult-type hypolactasia, *Scandinavian J. Gastroenterol.*, 29(Suppl. 202), 7, 1994.

24. American Academy of Pediatrics, Practical significance of lactose intolerance in children: supplement, *Pediatrics*, 86(4), 643, 1990.

25. Suarez, F. L. and Savaiano, D. A., Lactose digestion and tolerance in adult and elderly Asian-Americans, *Am. J. Clin. Nutr.*, 59, 1021, 1994.

26. Pettoello-Mantovani, M., Guandalini, S., diMartino, L., Corvino, C., Indolfi, P., Casale, F., Giuliano, M., Dubrovsky, L., and Di Tullio, M., Prospective study of lactose absorption during cancer chemotherapy: Feasibility of a yogurt-supplemented diet in lactose malabsorbers, *J. Pediatric Gastroenterol. Nutr.*, 20, 189, 1995.

27. Mishkin, S., Dairy sensitivity, lactose malabsorption, and elimination diets in inflammatory bowel disease, *Am. J. Clin. Nutr.*, 65, 564, 1997.

28. Tolliver, B. A., Jackson, M. S., Jackson, K. L., Barnett, E. D., Chastang, J. F., and DiPalma, J. A., Does lactose maldigestion really play a role in the irritable bowel?, *J. Clin. Gastroenterol.*, 23(1), 15, 1996.

29. Montes, R. G. and Perman, J. A., Lactose intolerance: pinpointing the sources of nonspecific gastrointestinal symptoms, *Postgraduate Med.*, 89(8), 175, 1991.

30. Martens, R. A. and Martens, S., *The Milk Sugar Dilemma: living with lactose intolerance*, Medi-Ed Press, Lansing, 1987.

31. Krause, J., Kaltbeitzer, I., and Erckenbrecht, J. F., Lactose malabsorption produces more symptoms in women than in men, (Abstr.), *Gastroenterology*, 110(Suppl.), A339, 1996.

32. Husby, S., Halken, S., and Host, A., Food allergy, in *Nutrition and Immunology*, Klurfeld, Ed., Plenum Press, New York, 1993, 25-29.

33. Bock, S. A., Prospective appraisal of complaints of adverse reactions to foods in children during the first 3 years of life, *Pediatrics*, 79, 683, 1987.

34. Suarez, F. L., Savaianno, D. A., and Levitt, M. D., A comparison of symptoms with self-reported severe lactose intolerance after drinking milk or lactose-hydrolyzed milk, *N. Engl. J. Med.*, 333, 1, 1995.

35. Suarez, F. L, Savaiano, D., Arbisi, P., and Levitt, M. D., Tolerance to the daily ingestion of two cups of milk by individuals claiming lactose intolerance, *Am. J. Clin. Nutr.*, 65, 1502, 1997.

36. Johnson, A. O., Semenya, J. G., Buchowski, M. S., Enwonwu, C. O., and Scrimshaw, N. S., Correlation of lactose maldigestion, lactose tolerance, and milk intolerance, *Am. J. Clin. Nutr.*, 57, 399, 1993.

37. Haverberg, L., Kwon, P. H., and Scrimshaw, N. S., Comparative tolerance of adolescents of differing ethnic backgrounds to lactose-containing and lactose-free dairy drinks, I. Initial experience with a double-blind procedure, *Amer. J. Clin. Nutr.*, 33, 17, 1980.

38. Haverberg, L., Kwon, P. H., and Scrimshaw, N. S., Comparative tolerance of adolescents of differing ethnic backgrounds to lactose-containing and lactose-free dairy drinks, I. Initial experience with a double-blind procedure, *Amer. J. Clin. Nutr.*, 33, 17, 1980.

39. Rorick, M. H. and Scrimshaw, N. S., Comparative tolerance of elderly from differing ethnic backgrounds to lactose-containing and lactose-free dairy drinks: a double-blind study, *J. Gerontology*, 34(2), 191, 1979.

40. Barr, R. G., Watkins, R. B., and Perman, J. A., Mucosal function and breath hydrogen excretion: comparative studies in the clinical evaluation of children with nonspecific abdominal complaints, *Pediatrics*, 68(4), 526, 1981.

41. Barr, R. G., Limitations of the hydrogen breath test and other techniques for predicting incomplete lactose absorption, in *Lactose Digestion: clinical and nutritional implications*, Paige, D. M., and Bayless, T. M., Eds., Johns Hopkins University Press, Baltimore and London, 1981, Chap. 9.

42. Bayless, T. M., Lactose malabsorption, milk intolerance, and symptom awareness in adults, in *Lactose Digestion: Clinical and Nutritional Implications*, Paige, D. M., and Bayless, T. M., Eds., The Johns Hopkins University Press, Baltimore and London, 1981, Chap. 10.

43. Buller, H. A. and Grand, R. J., Lactose intolerance, *Ann. Rev. Med.*, 41, 141, 1990.

44. Martini, M. C. and Savaiano, D. A., Reduced intolerance symptoms from lactose consumed during a meal, *Am. J. Clin. Nutr.*, 47, 57, 1988.

45. Villako, K. and Maaroos, H., Clinical picture of hypolactasia and lactose intolerance, *Scand. J. Gastroenterol.*, 29 (Suppl. 202), 36, 1994.

46. Hertzler, F. R., Huynh, B.-C. L., and Savaiano, D. A., How much lactose is low lactose?, *J. Am. Diet. Assoc.*, 96, 243, 1996.

47. Newcomer, A. D., McGill, D. B., Thomas, P. J., and Hoffman, A. F., Tolerance to lactose among lactase-deficient American Indians, *Gastroenterology*, 74, 44, 1978.

48. Newcomer, A., Immediate sympotomatic and long-term nutritional consequences of hypolactasia, in *Lactose Digestion: clinical and nutritional implications*, Paige, D. M. and Bayless, T., M., Eds., The Johns Hopkins University Press, Baltimore and London, 1981, Chap. 11.

49. Suarez, F. L., Adshead, J., Furne, J. K., and Levitt, M. D., Lactose maldigesters tolerate ingestion of a dairy-rich diet containing approximately 1500 mg calcium/day, *Am. J. Clin. Nutr.*, 68, 1118, 1998.

50. Food and Nutrition Board/Institute of Medicine, *Dietary reference intakes for calcium, phosphorus, magnesium, vitamin D, and fluoride*, uncorrected proofs, National Academy Press, Washington, D.C., 1997.

51. Villar, J., Kestler, E., Castillo, P., Juarez, A., Mendndez, R., and Solomons, N. W., Improved lactose digestion during pregnancy: A case of physiologic adaptation?, *Obstet. Gynecol.*, 71(5), 697, 1988.

52. Szilagyi, A., Salomon, R., Martin, M., Fokeeff, KI., and Seidman, E., Lactose handling by women with lactose malabsorption is improved during pregnancy, *Clin. Invest. Med.*, 19(6), 416, 1996.

53. Paige, D., M., Witter, E., R., Kessler, L. A., Bronner, Y., and Perman, J. A., Lactose intolerance in pregnant African-American women, *J. Am. Coll. Nutr.*, 16, 5 (Abstr. 69), 488, 1997.

54. Leichter, J., Effects of lactose on the absorption of other nutrients: implications in lactose-intolerant adults, in *Lactose Digestion: clinical and nutritional implications*, Paige, D. M. and Bayless, T. M., Eds., John Hopkins University Press, Baltimore and London, 1981, Chap. 13.

55. Buchowski, M. S. and Miller, D. D., Lactose, calcium source, and age affect calcium bioavailability in rats, *J. Nutr.*, 121, 1746, 1991.

56. Ziegler, E. E. and Foman, S. J., Lactose enhances mineral absorption in infancy, *J. Pediatr. Gastroenterol. Nut.*, 2, 288, 1983.

57. Miller, D. D., Calcium in the diet: food sources, recommended intakes, and nutritional bioavailability, *Adv. Food Nutr. Res.*, 33, 103, 1989.

58. Tremaine, W. J., Newcomer, A. D., Riggs, B. L., and McGill, D. B., Calcium absorption from milk in lactase-deficient and lactase-sufficient adults, *Dig. Dis. Sciences*, 31(4), 376, 1986.

59. Horowitz, M., Wishart, J., Mundy, L., and Nordin, B. E. C., Lactose and calcium absorption in postmenopausal osteoporosis, *Arch. Inter. Med.*, 147, 534, 1987.

60. Griessen, M., Cochet, B., Infante, F., Jung, A., Bartholdi, P., Donath, A., Loizeau, E., and Courvoisier, B., Calcium absorption from milk in lactase-deficient subjects, *Am. J. Clin. Nutr.*, 49, 377, 1989.

61. Garza, C. and Scrimshaw, N. S., Relationship of lactose intolerance to milk intolerance in young children, *Am. J. Clin. Nutr.*, 29, 192, 1976.

62. Rosado, J. L., Allen, L. H., and Solomons, N. W., Milk consumption, symptom response, and lactose digestion in milk intolerance, *Am. J. Clin. Nutr.*, 45, 1457, 1987.

63. Finkenstedt, G., Skrabal, F., Gasser, R. W., and Braunsteiner, H., Lactose absorption, milk consumption, and fasting blood glucose concentrations in women with idiopathic osteoporosis, *Br. Med. J.*, 292(6514), 161, 1986.

64. Newcomer, A. D., Hodgson, S. F., and McGill, D. B., Lactase deficiency: prevalence in osteoporosis, *Ann. Inter. Med.*, 89, 218, 1978.

65. Barger-Lux, M. J., Heaney, R. P., Packard, P. T., Lappe, J. M., and Recker, R. R., Nutritional correlates of low calcium intake, *Clin. Appl. Nutr.*, 2(4), 39, 1992.

66. Fleming, K. and Heimbach, J. R., Consumption of calcium in the U.S.: food sources and intake levels, *J. Nutr.*, 124, 1426s, 1994.

67. Karanja, N., Morris, C. D., Rufolo, P., Snyder, G., Illingworth, D. R., and McCarron, D. A., Impact of increasing calcium in the diet on nutrient consumption, plasma lipids, and lipoproteins in humans, *Am. J. Clin. Nutr.*, 59, 900, 1994.

68. Heaney, R. P., Food: what a surprise!, *Am. J. Clin. Nutr.*, 64, 791, 1996.

69. Varela-Moreairas, G., Antoine, J. M., Ruiz-Roso, B., and Varela, G., Effects of yogurt and fermented-then-pasteurized milk on lactose absorption in an institutionalized elderly group, *J. Am. Coll. Nutr.*, 11(2), 168, 1992.

70. Recker, R. R., Prevention of osteoporosis: calcium nutrition, *Osteoporosis Int.*, Suppl. 1, S163, 1993.

71. Heaney, R. P., Nutritional factors in osteoporosis, *Ann. Rev. Nutr.*, 13, 287, 1993.

72. Barger-Lux, M. J. and Heaney, R. P., The role of calcium intake in preventing bone fragility, hypertension, and certain cancers, *J. Nutr.*, 124, 1406s, 1994.

73. U.S. Department of Health and Human Services, National Institutes of Health, *Consenus Development Conference, Optimal Calcium Intake*, Washington, D.C., June 6-8, 1994.

74. Wheadon, M., Goulding, A., Barbezat, G. O., and Campbell, A. J., Lactose malabsorption and calcium intake as a risk factor for osteoporosis in elderly New Zealand women, *New Zealand Med. J.*, 104(921), 417, 1991.

75. Honkanen, R., Pulkkinen, P., Jarvinen, R., Kroger, H, Lindstedt, K., Tuppurainen, M., and Uusitupa, M., Does lactose intolerance predispose to low bone density? A population-based study of perimenopausal Finnish women, *Bone*, 19(1), 23, 1996.

76. Corazza, G. R., Benati, G., Di Sario, A., Tarozzi, C., Strocchi, A., Passeri, M., and Gasbarrini, G., Lactose intolerance and bone mass in postmenopausal Italian women, *Br. J. Nutr.*, 73, 479, 1995.

77. Honkanen, R., Kroger, H., Alhava, E., Turpeinen, P., Tuppurainen, M., and Saarikoski, S., Lactose intolerance associated with fractures of weight-bearing bones in Finnish women aged 38-57 years, *Bone*, 21(6), 473, 1997.

78. Laroche, M., Bon, E., Moulinier, L., Cantagrel, A., and Mazieres, B., Lactose intolerance and osteoporosis in men, *Expansion Scientifique Francaise*, 62(11), 766, 1995.

79. The Sixth Report of the Joint National Committee on Detection, Evaluation, and Treatment of High Blood Pressure (JNC-VI), *Arch. Intern. Med.*, 157, 2413, 1997.

80. USDA, *Nutrient Content of the U.S. Food Supply*, 1909-1994, Report no. 53.

81. Appel, I. J., Moore T. J., Obarzanek, E.,Vollmer, W. M., Svetkey, L. P., Sacks, F. M., Bray, G. A., Vogt, T. M., Cutler, J. A., Windhauser, M. M., Lin, P-H., and Karanja, N., A clinical trial of the effects of dietary patterns on blood pressure, *N. Engl. J. Med.*, 336, 1117, 1997.

82. Parodi, P. W., Cow's milk fat components as potential anticarcinogenic agents, *J. Nutr.*, 127, 1055, 1997.

83. Risio, M., Lipkin, M., Newmark, H., Yang, K., Rossini, F. P., Steele, V. E., Boone, C. W., and Kelloff, G. J., Apoptosis, cell replication, and Western-style diet-induced tumorigenesis in mouse colon, *Cancer Res.*, 56, 4910, 1996.

84. Knekt, P., Jarvinen, R., Seppanen, R., Pukkala, E., and Aromaa, A., Intake of dairy products and the risk of breast cancer, *Br. J. Cancer*, 73, 687, 1996.

85. Chiu, B., Cerhan, C.-H., Folsom, A. R., Sellers, T. A., Kushi, L. H., Wallace R. B., Zheng, W., and Potter, J. D., Diet and risk of non-Hodgkin lymphoma in older women, *JAMA*, 275(17), 1315, 1996.

86. Lupton, J. R., Steinbach, G., Chang, W. C., OíBrien, B. C., Wiese, S., Stoltzfus, C. L., Glober, G. A., Wargovich, M. J., McPherson, R. S., and Winn, R. J., Calcium supplementation modifies the relative amounts of bile acids in bile and affects key aspects of human colon physiology, *J. Nutr.*, 126, 1421, 1996.

87. Dobler, M. L., *Lactose Intolerance–Revised Edition*, The American Dietetic Association, Chicago, 1991.

88. The American Academy of Pediatrics, Committee on Nutrition, Practical significance of lactose intolerance in children: supplement, *Pediatrics*, 86(4), 643, 1978.

89. Savaiano, D. A. and Kotz, C., Recent advances in the management of lactose intolerance, *Contemporary Nutr.*, 13(9,10), 1988.

90. Nguyen, K. N., Welsh, J. D., Manion, C. V., and Ficken, V. J., Effect of fiber on breath hydrogen response and symptoms after oral lactose in lactose malabsorbers, *Am. J. Clin. Nutr.*, 35, 1347, 1982.

91. Solomons, N. W., Guerrero, A., and Torun, R., Dietary manipulation of postprandial colonic lactose fermentation: I. effect of solid foods in a meal, *Am. J. Clin. Nutr.*, 41, 199, 1985.

92. Leichter, J., Comparison of whole milk and skim milk with aqueous lactose solution in lactose tolerance testing, *Am. J. Clin. Nutr.*, 26, 393, 1973.

93. Dehkordi, N., Rao, D. R., Warren, A. P., and Chawan, C. B., Lactose malabsorption as influenced by chocolate milk, skim milk, sucrose, whole milk, and lactic cultures, *J. Am. Diet. Assoc.*, 95, 484, 1995.

94. Vesa, T. H., Lember, M., and Korpela, R., Milk fat does not affect the symptoms of lactose intolerance, *Eur. J. Clin. Nutr.*, 51, 633, 1997.

95. Dehkordi, N., Warren, A. P., and Chawan, C. B., Lactose malabsorption as influenced by chocolate milk, skim milk, sucrose, whole milk, and lactic cultures, *J. Am. Diet. Assoc.*, 95(4), 484, 1995.

96. Vesa, T. H., Marteau, P. R., Briet, F. B., Boutron-Ruault, M.-C., and Rambaud, J.-C., Raising milk energy content retards gastric emptying of lactose in lactose-intolerant humans with little effect on lactose digestion, *J. Nutr.*, 127, 2316, 1997.

97. Vesa, T. H. Marteau, P. R., Briet, F. B., Flourie, B., Briend, A., and Rambaud, J.-C., Effects of milk viscosity on gastric emptying and lactose intolerance in lactose maldigesters, *Am. J. Clin. Nutr.*, 66,123, 1997.

98. Chong, M. L. and Hardy, C. M., Cocoa feeding and human lactose intolerance, *Am. J. Clin. Nutr.*, 49, 840, 1989.

99. Savaiano, D. A. and Levitt, M. D., Milk intolerance and microbe-containing dairy foods, *J. Dairy Sci.*, 70, 397, 1987.

100. Kolars, J. C., Levitt, M. D., Aouji, M., and Savaiano, D., Yogurt, — an autodigesting source of lactose, *N. Engl. J. Med.*, 310, 1, 1984.

101. Martini, M. C., Bollweg, G. L., Levitt, M. D., and Savaiano, D. A., Lactose digestion by yogurt beta-galactosidase: influence of pH and microbial cell integrity, *Am. J. Clin. Nutr.*, 45, 432, 1987.

102. Pochart, P., DeWit, O., Desjeux, J., and Bourlioux, P., Viable starter culture, beta-galactosidase activity, and lactose in duodenum after yogurt ingestion in lactase-deficient humans, *Amer. J. Clin. Nutr.*, 49, 828, 1989.

103. Shermack, M. A, Saavedra, J. M., Jackson, T. L., Huang, S. S., Bayless, T. M., and Perman, J. A., Effect of yogurt on symptoms and kinetics of hydrogen production in lactose-malabsorbing children, *Am. J. Clin. Nutr.*, 62, 1003, 1995.

104. Vesa, T. H., Marteau, P., Zidi, S., Briet, F, Pochart, P., and Rambaud, J. C., Digestion and tolerance of lactose from yogurt and different semi-solid fermented dairy products containing *Lactobacillus acidophilus* and bifidobacteria in lactose maldigesters — Is bacterial lactase important?, *Eur. J. Clin. Nutr.*, 50, 730, 1996.

105. Wytock, D. H. and DiPalma, J. A., All yogurts are not created equal, *Am. J. Clin. Nutr.*, 47, 454, 1988.

106. Lerebours, E., Ndam, C., Lavoine, A., Hellot, M. F., Antoine, J. M., and Colin, R., Yogurt and fermented-then-pasteurized milk: effects of short-term and long-term ingestion on lactose absorption and mucosal lactase activity in lactase-deficient subjects, *Am. J. Clin. Nutr.*, 49, 823, 1989.

107. Martini, M. S., Kukeilka, D., and Savaiano, D. A., Lactose digestion from yogurt: influence of a meal and additional lactose, *Am. J. Clin. Nutr.*, 53, 1253, 1991.

108. Martini, M. C., Smith, D. E., and Savaiano, D. A., Lactose digestion from flavored and frozen yogurts, ice milk, and ice cream by lactase-deficient persons, *Am. J. Clin. Nutr.*, 46, 636, 1987.

109. Gilliland, S. E., Acidophilus milk products: a review of potential benefits to consumers, *J. Dairy Science*, 72, 2483, 1989.

110. Payne, D. L., Welsh, J. D., Manion, C. V., Tsegaye, A., and Herd, L. D., Effectiveness of milk products in dietary management of lactose malabsorption, *Am. J. Clin. Nutr.*, 34, 2711, 1981.

111. Savaiano, D. A., AbouElAnouar, A., Smith, D. E., and Levitt, M. D., Lactose malabsorption from yogurt, pasteurized yogurt, sweet acidophilus milk, and cultured milk in lactase-deficient individuals, *Am. J. Clin. Nutr.*, 40, 1219, 1984.

112. Onwulata, C. I., Rao, D. R., and Vankineni, P., Relative efficiency of yogurt, sweet acidophilus milk, hydrolyzed-lactose milk, and a commercial lactase tablet in alleviating lactose maldigestion, *Am. J. Clin. Nutr.*, 49, 1233, 1989.

113. Hove, H., Nordgaard-Andersen, I., and Mortensen, P. B., Effect of lactic acid bacteria on the intestinal production of lactase and short-chain fatty acids, and the absorption of lactose, *Am. J. Clin. Nutr.*, 59, 74, 1994.

114. Mustapha, A., Jiang, T, and Savaiano, D. A., Improvement of lactose digestion by humans following ingestion of unfermented acidophilus milk: Influence of bile sensitivity, lactose transport, and acid tolerance of *lactobacillus acidophilus, J. Dairy Sci.*, 80, 1537, 1997.

115. Lin, M., Savaiano, D., and Harlander, S., Influence of nonfermented dairy products containing bacterial starter cultures on lactose maldigestion in humans, *J. Dairy Sci.*, 74, 87, 1991.

116. Montes, R. G., Bayless, T. M., Saavedra, J. M., and Perman, J. A., Effect of milks inoculated with *Lactobacillus acidophilus* or a yogurt starter culture in lactose-maldigesting children, *J. Dairy Science,* 78, 1657, 1995.

117. Jiang, T., Mustapha, A., and Savaiano, D. A., Improvement of lactose digestion in humans by ingestion of unfermented milk containing *Bifidobacterium longum, J. Dairy Sci.*, 79, 750, 1996.

118. Solomons, N. W., Guerrero, A., and Torun, B., Dietary manipulation of postprandial colonic lactose fermentation: II. addition of exogenous, microbial beta-galactosidases at mealtime, *Am. J. Clin. Nutr.*, 41, 209, 1985.

119. Sinden, A. A., and Sutphen, J. L., Dietary treatment of lactose intolerance in infants and children, *J. Am. Diet. Assoc.*, 91, 1567, 1991.

120. Medow, M. S., Kerry, D. T., Newman, L. J., Berezin, S., Glassman, M. S., and Schwarz, S. M., Beta-galactosidase tablets in the treatment of lactose intolerance in pediatrics, *Am. J. Diseases of Childhood,* 144, 1261, 1990.

121. Corazza, G. R., Benati, G., Sorge, M., Strocchi, A., Calza, G., and Gasbarrini, G., Beta-galactosidase from aspergillus niger in adult lactose malabsorption: a double-blind crossover study, *Aliment. Pharmacol. Ther.*, 6(1), 61, 1992.

122. DiPalma, J. A. and Collins, M. S., Enzyme replacement for lactose malabsorption using a beta-d-galactosidase, *J. Clin. Gastroenterol.*, 11(3), 290, 1989.

123. Food and Drug Administration/HHS, Direct food substances generally recognized as safe, 21 CFR, 184.1, 1992.

124. Holsinger, V. H. and Kligerman, A. E., Applications of lactase in dairy foods and other foods containing lactose, *Food Technol.*, 45(1), 92, 1991.

125. Gannett News Service, Missing enzyme means body can't handle lactose: alternative products lack lactose, *St. Cloud Times*, Dec. 5, 1993.

126. Food and Drug Administration, HHS, Code of Federal Regulations, 21 CFR, 184.1388, April 1, 1993.

127. Nielson, O. H., Schiotz, P. O., Rasmussen, S. N., and Krasilnikoff, P. A., Calcium absorption and acceptance of low-lactose milk among children with primary lactase deficiency, *J. Pediatr. Gastroenterol. Nutr.*, 3(2), 219, 1984.

128. Brand, J. C. and Holt, S., Relative effectiveness of milks with reduced amounts of lactose in alleviating milk intolerance, *Am. J. Clin. Nutr.*, 54, 148, 1991.

129. Reddy, V. and Pershad, J., Lactase deficiency in Indians, *Am. J. Clin. Nutr.*, 25, 114, 1972.

130. Johnson, A. O., Semenya, J. G., Buchowski, M. S., Enowonwu, C. O., and Scrimshaw, N. S., Adaptation of lactose maldigesters to continued milk intakes, *Am. J. Clin. Nutr.*, 58, 879, 1993.

131. Hertzler, S. R. and Savaiano, D. A., Colonic adaptation to daily lactose feeding in lactose maldigesters reduces lactose intolerance, *Am. J. Clin. Nutr.*, 64, 232, 1996.

132. Briet, R., Pochart, P., Marteau, P., Flourie, B., Arrigoni, E., and Rambaud, J. C., Improved clinical tolerance to chronic lactose ingestion in subjects with lactose intolerance: a placebo efffect?, *Gut*, 41, 632, 1997.

133. Hertzler, S. R., Savaiano, D. A., and Levitt, M. D., Fecal hydrogen production and consumption measurements, *Dig. Dis. Sciences*, 42(2), 348, 1997.

134. Heird, W. C. and Cooper, A., Nutrition in infants and children, in *Modern Nutrition in Health and Disease*, Shils, M. E. and Young, V. R., Eds., Lea and Febiger, Philadelphia, 1988, 958.

135. Committee on Nutrition, American Academy of Pediatrics, Oral fluid therapy and posttreatment feeding after enteritis, *Pediatric Nutrition Handbook, Third Edition*, Barness, L. A., Ed., The American Academy of Pediatrics, Elk Grove Village, 1993, Chap. 23.

136. Brown, K. H., Peerson, J. M., and Fontaine, O., Use of nonhuman milks in the dietary management of young children with acute diarrhea: a meta-analysis of clinical trials, *Pediatrics*, 93(1), 17, 1994.

137. Chew, F., Penna, F. J., Filho, L. A., Quan, C., Lopes, M. C., Mota, J. A. C., and Fontaine, O., Is dilution of cow's milk formula necessary for dietary management of acute diarrhea in infants aged less than 6 months?, *The Lancet*, 341, 194, 1993.

138. Lifschitz, F., Fagundes-Neto, U., Ferreira, V. C., Cordano, A., and da Costa Ribeiro, H., The response to dietary treatment of patients with chronic post-infectious diarrhea and lactose intolerance, *J. Am. Coll. Nutr.*, 9(3), 231, 1990.

139. Solomons, N. W., Torun, B., Caballero, B., Flores-Huerta, S., and Orozco, G., The effect of dietary lactose on the early recovery from protein-energy malnutrition, *Am. J. Clin. Nutr.*, 40(3), 591, 1984.

140. Beau, J.P., Fontaine, O., and Garenne, M., Management of malnourished children with acute diarrhea and sugar intolerance, *J. Tropical Pediatr.*, 35(6), 281, 1989.

141. Erinoso, H. O., Hoare, S., Spencer, S., Lunn, G., and Weaver, L. T., Is cow's milk suitable for the dietary supplementation of rural Gambian children? 1. prevalence of lactose maldigestion, *Ann. Tropical Pediatr.*, 12, 359, 1992.

142. Gendrel, D., Dupont, C., Richard-Lenoble, D., Gendrel, C., and Chaussain, M., Feeding lactose-intolerant children with a powdered fermented milk, *J. Pediatr. Gastroenterol. Nutr.*, 10(1), 44, 1990.

143. Paige, D. M., Lactose malabsorption in children: prevalence, symptoms and nutritional considerations, in *Lactose Digestion: clinical and nutritional implications*, Paige, D. M. and Bayless, T. M., Eds., Johns Hopkins University Press, Baltimore, 1981, Chap. 14.

144. Garza, C. and Scrimshaw, N., Relationship of lactose intolerance to milk intolerance in young children, *Am. J. Clin. Nutr.*, 29, 192, 1976.

145. Department of Agriculture/Food and Consumer Service, National School Lunch Program, School Breakfast Program, Summer Food Service Program for Children and Child and Adult Care Food Program: Meat Alternates Used in the Child Nutrition Programs, *Federal Register*, 7 CFR Parts 210, 220, 225, and 226, Vol. 62, No. 44, March 6, 1997.

146. Heise, C., Food and Nutrition Service, Child Nutrition Division, Special Nutrition Programs, personal communication, 1994.

147. Food and Nutrition Service, Financial Management Program Information Division, Data Base Monitoring Branch, Special Supplemental Food Program (WIC) For Women, Infants and Children: Racial Participation, January 1993.

148. United States Department of Agriculture/Food and Nutrition Service, *Technical Papers: Review of WIC Food Packages*, 1991.

149. USDA, Food and Nutrition Service, Notice of solicitation of comments, Special supplemental food program for women, infants and children (WIC): accommodation of cultural food preferences in the WIC program, *Federal Register*, 59(120) FR 32406, June 23, 1994.

CHAPTER 9

Contribution of Milk and Milk Products to Health Throughout the Life Cycle

I. INTRODUCTION

Adequate amounts of milk and milk products are needed throughout the life cycle to promote bone health, to help reduce the risk of chronic diseases such as osteoporosis, hypertension, and cancer, and to contribute to overall nutritional status. Age and life stage influence the need for calcium and other nutrients supplied by dairy foods, due to changes in physiological need, hormonal status, the absorption and retention of nutrients, among other factors. However, many population groups in the United States, particularly adolescent and adult females and older Americans, consume significantly less calcium and fewer servings of Milk Group foods than recommended. Psychosocial and environmental factors influence the intake of milk and milk products differently throughout life, so that no one educational approach to improve consumption is relevant to all ages. In this chapter we will discuss the benefits of milk and milk products enjoyed at each stage of the life cycle, as well as important issues and concerns unique to each life stage group from infancy to old age. Although the information in this chapter focuses primarily on the role of dairy foods and health, this information should be viewed in the context of the total diet and life style of the individual.

II. INFANCY

A. Characteristics

The infant period is characterized by rapid growth and development. Infant growth rates are highly variable and are influenced by genetic, hormonal, nutritional, and environmental factors. The average infant generally triples his birth weight and gains about 50% in length, and approximately 30% in head circumference over the first year.[1] The infant grows about an inch in length and adds about 2.2 pounds per month for the first six months. During the second six months, growth velocity slows to about 0.5 inches in length and about one pound per month.[1] As the infant grows, his body composition changes; the percentage of water decreases and the proportions of fat and protein increase. About 3.2% of the infant's body weight is composed of minerals (mostly bone). Between five and nine months the first deciduous teeth erupt, and by one year of age, most infants have four to eight teeth.[1] Occurring simultaneously with physical development is neurological, cognitive, language, and psychosocial development.

B. Recommendations for Feeding

The infant's first food is human milk or iron-fortified infant formula. The American Academy of Pediatrics and the Canadian Paediatric Society strongly recommend human milk as the exclusive nutrient source for feeding full-term infants during the first six months after birth, which should be continued, with the addition of solid foods, at least through the first 12 months.[2,3] This recommendation stems from the acknowledged benefits of human milk to infant nutrition, gastrointestinal function, host defense, and psychological well-being.[4]

Adequate amounts of calcium in the diet of infants is needed for skeletal growth and for the development of teeth. Table 9.1 presents both the 1997 calcium recommendations for infancy from the Food and Nutrition Board of the National Academy of Sciences and those established by an Expert Panel of the National Institutes of Health in 1994.[5,6] The calcium recommendations of these groups differ substantially from each other because these organizations did not use the same approach. The NAS recommendations are Adequate Intakes (AI), and for infancy are based on the amount of calcium supplied by human milk. Recommended intakes for children 6 to 12 months were based on expected intakes from human milk and solid food. The NIH Expert Panel did not take this approach.

Table 9.1 Calcium Recommendations for Infancy

NIH Expert Panel		NAS	
Age	Calcium (mg)	Age	Calcium (mg)
Birth – 6 months	400	Birth – 6 months	210
6–12 months	600	6–12 months	270

From National Institutes of Health Expert Panel, 1994 and Dietary Reference Intakes, National Academy of Sciences, 1997.

1. Standard Cow's Milk-Based Formulas

Standard iron-fortified cow's milk-based formula is the "feeding of choice," when breastfeeding is not used or is stopped before one year of age.[7] Commercial cow's milk-based infant formulas have been tested extensively, and can provide adequate nutrition for the healthy infant. Their nutrient composition, however, can differ substantially from human milk and from each other (Table 9.2). Since calcium is absorbed more efficiently from human milk, cow's milk-based formulas are formulated to contain approximately 40% more calcium. Soy formulas are a nutritionally equivalent alternative to cow's milk formula for infants with hereditary or transient lactase deficiency, or for patients seeking a vegetarian diet for their infant. Protein hydrolysate formulas are also available for preterm infants or for infants who are allergic to cow's milk or soy protein.[7]

2. Cow's Milk

Full-fat cow's milk, goat's milk, fat free milk, 1% to 2% fat milk, and evaporated milk are not recommended for use during the first 12 months of life.[8] There are several reasons for this recommendation. Since cow's milk contains a low concentration and bioavailability of iron when compared to human milk, feeding cow's milk to infants increases the risk of iron deficiency anemia and the possibility of increased intestinal blood loss in infants with milk sensitivity. Cow's milk also increases the risk of deficiency of essential fatty acids, vitamin E, and zinc, since concentrations of these nutrients are lower than in human milk. In addition, fat free, lowfat, and reduced fat milk may cause the infant to consume excessive amounts of protein as the infant consumes an increased volume of milk to satisfy caloric needs. Excessive protein intake increases the renal solute load and risks overtaxing the kidneys, particularly if the infant becomes dehydrated.[7]

3. Cow's Milk Allergy

Cow's milk hypersensitivity involves a reaction by the infant's previously sensitized immune system to milk protein. It develops in 2.2 to 2.8% of infants, of whom 85% outgrow the reactivity by their third birthday.[9] Children who develop a sensitivity after age 3 are less likely to outgrow the problem. Symptoms may involve the gastrointestinal and respiratory systems, and the skin. Infants typically exhibit diarrhea, vomiting, and failure to thrive.

Treatment should be based on a diagnosis using proper diagnostic procedures. Sensitivity to cow's milk can be tested using either a skin prick test or a blood test (Radioallergosorbent Test or RAST), which estimates the amount of antigen-specific IgE antibodies in the serum. Infants who have confirmed cow's milk sensitivity should be fed a substitute hypoallergenic formula (e.g., protein hydrolysate) at least until they are one year of age. Because soy protein-based formulas may be equally as allergenic as cow's milk protein-based formulas, they are not recommended for infants with a documented allergy to cow's milk.[9] Appropriate dietetic counseling will be needed for older infants to assure the elimination of all food sources of the antigen and to assure the nutritional adequacy of the diet. A rechallenge with milk or soy in a controlled setting will determine whether symptoms persist. When cow's milk allergy is diagnosed in infancy, controlled rechallenges are recommended every 6 to 12 months, to avoid prolonging a milk free diet unnecessarily.[10]

Experts agree that eliminating allergenic foods from the maternal diet during pregnancy is unlikely to prevent food allergies in the infant. The following recommendations from the American Academy of Pediatrics may help delay or prevent

Table 9.2 Composition of Human Milk and Standard Infant Formulas (per Liter)

	Mature Human Milk (Estimate)	Enfamil[†] (Mead Johnson, Evansville, IN)	Gerber[‡] (Gerber, Fremont, MI)	Good Start[*] (Carnation, Glendale, CA)	Similac[*†] (Ross, Columbus, OH)	SMA[*†‡] (Wyeth, Philadelphia, PA)
Energy, kcal	680	680	680	676	676	676
Protein, g	10.5	14.2	15	16.2	14.5	15
Casein, % of total protein	30	40	82	0	82	40
Whey, % of total protein	70	60	18	100[§]	18	60
Fat, g	39	35.8	37	34.5	36.5	36
Polyunsaturated, %	14.2	29	36	32	37	15
Monounsaturated, %	41.6	16	18	26	17	41
Saturated, %	44.2	55	46	43	46	44
Predominant oil	Human milk fat	Palm olein soy coconut, high-oleic sunflower	Palm olein soy coconut, high-oleic sunflower	Palm olein soy coconut, high-oleic safflower	Soy, coconut	Oleo, coconut, oleic soy
Carbohydrate (lactose), g	72	73.7	73	74[a]	72.3	72
Mineral						
Calcium, mg	280	528	510	433	492	426
Phosphorus, mg	140	358	390	243	380	284
Magnesium, mg	35	54	41	45.3	41	47.3
Iron, mg	0.3	12.2	12.2	10.1	12.2	12.2
Zinc, mg	1.2	6.8	5.1	5.1	5.1	5.4
Manganese, µg	6	101	34	47	34	101
Copper, µg	252	507	610	541	610	473
Iodine, µg	110	68	54	54	95	61
Sodium, mEq	7.8	8	9.6	7	8	6.5
Potassium, mEq	13.5	18.7	18.7	17	18.1	14.3
Chloride, mEq	11.9	12.1	13.5	11.3	12	10.6

Vitamin						
A, µg	675	630	600	676	676	667
D, µg	0.5	10.8	10.3	10	10	10
E, IU	4	13.6	13.6	8	20	9.5
K, µg	2.1	54	54	55	54	54
Thiamin (B$_1$), µg	210	541	680	406	680	676
Riboflavin (B$_2$), µg	350	947	1020	913	1010	1014
Pyridoxine, µg	205	406	410	507	410	423
B$_{12}$, µg	0.5	2	1.7	1.5	1.7	1.4
Niacin, mg	1.5	6.8	7.1	5.1	7.1	5.1
Folic acid, µg	50	108	102	61	100	51
Pantothenic acid, mg	1.8	3.4	3.1	3	3	2.1
Biotin, µg	4	20.3	30	14.9	30	14.9
C(ascorbic acid), mg	40	81.2	61	54.1	60	57.5
Choline, mg	92	81	109	81	108	101
Inositol, mg	149	115	32	122	32	29

* Liquid and powder.
† High iron level.
‡ No longer available in the United States
§ Enzymatically hydrolyzed.
a Lactose and maltodextrin.

From American Academy of Pediatrics, *Pediatric Nutrition Handbook, Fourth Edition*, Appendix E, American Academy of Pediatrics, Elk Grove Village, IL, 1998. With permission.

some food allergy in infants at high risk of atopic disease (e.g., parents or siblings have allergies):

1. breastfeed exclusively for the first 4 to 6 months of life or use a protein hydrolyzed formula
2. delay introduction of solid foods until after 4 to 6 months of age
3. delay introduction of cow's milk until 1 year of age (eggs until 2 years; peanuts, nuts, and fish until 3 years).[9]

Soy formulas should not be considered hypoallergenic or be used to prevent food allergy in infants.[9,11] Recent studies indicate that feeding a partially hydrolyzed whey formula (or exclusive breast feeding) decreases the risk of food allergy in high risk infants for up to five years.[12,13] A study in laboratory rats found that feeding a partially hydrolyzed whey formula suppressed an immune response to cow's milk protein.[14] The authors suggest that selected peptides in cow's milk protein may induce oral tolerance.

Whether eliminating allergenic foods from the diet of the mother during lactation will help prevent milk (or other food) allergy remains controversial, since study results conflict.[15] In a recent review, Zeiger states, "More definitive randomized studies with both food challenges and immunologic confirmation are mandatory before maternal lactation diets can be recommended as effective in the prevention of atopic disease."[11]

C. Vitamin D and Rickets

Vitamin D is essential to a healthy skeleton throughout life. Vitamin D promotes the intestinal absorption of calcium as well as acting directly on bone mineralization. The vitamin D deficiency disease, rickets, results in soft and deformed bones. Vitamin D is synthesized in the skin when exposed to sunlight and is also obtained from foods. Only a few foods, such as egg yolks, butter, fatty fish (e.g. salmon), and liver contain vitamin D. Human milk contains very little vitamin D (0.5 µg).[16] One liter of standard infant formula contains 10 µg (400 IU) of vitamin D. According to the Dietary Reference Intake Report (DRI) from the National Academy of Sciences, breast- or formula-fed infants do not need supplementary vitamin D if they are exposed to habitual small doses of sunshine. However, they recommend at least 5 µg (200 IU) of vitamin D daily for infants 0 to 12 months not exposed to sunlight; they do not deem the amount of vitamin D contained in standard infant formulas as excessive.[5] The same level of vitamin D is recommended for infants, children, and adults through age 50. After age 1, the recommended amount of vitamin D may be supplied by 2 eight-ounce servings of vitamin D fortified cow's milk, which is voluntarily fortified to a level of 400 IU per quart.

D. Introduction of Solid Foods

By 4 to 6 months of age the infant is developmentally ready for the introduction of solid foods to complement the liquid diet. By this time the extrusion reflex (tongue pushes food out of the mouth) has disappeared, pureed solids can be swallowed, and the infant can sit with support.[17] Solid single foods, such as infant cereals, strained fruits and vegetables, and then meats (by about 7 to 8 mos.), should be introduced one at a time for 3 to 5 days, before trying a different food, so that allergic reactions can be identified. In all cases, single foods should be introduced before mixtures.

As the infant's eye-hand coordination develops, he can begin to feed himself. By 7 months he will begin to finger-feed soft foods.[18] Although human milk or infant formula is still the mainstay of the infant's diet, milk products, such as yogurt and cheese may be introduced, which contribute calcium and other vitamins and minerals. Cheese cubes/slices and cottage cheese are among the foods appropriate for self-feeding (Table 9.3). Yogurt can be introduced at 8 to 10 months of age.[19] The ingestion of lactic acid bacteria found in yogurt may have a beneficial effect on an infant's intestinal microflora. In a recent study conducted among 39 healthy infants aged 10 to 18 months, the daily ingestion of 125 g of yogurt or milk fermented with yogurt cultures (*Lactobacillus casei*), significantly reduced the activity of harmful intestinal enzymes.[20] The authors state that feeding of these foods may prove useful in the prevention of infectious disease, stimulation of the immune system, and in protection against some carcinogens.

Table 9.3 Some Appropriate Foods for Infant Self-Feeding

Fruits	Soft, fresh or canned, unsweetened, such as bananas, peeled apples, apricots, peaches, or pears
Vegetables	Tender pieces of cooked vegetables, such as carrots, potatoes, green beans, summer squash, yellow squash, sweet potatoes
Dairy	Cubes or slices of milk cheese, cottage cheese
Meat, Poultry, Fish	Small, tender pieces of cooked chicken, turkey, or white flaky fish without bones; ground meat, such as meat balls, pieces of hamburger patty, or meatloaf
Bread/Cereals	Toast, plain unsalted crackers, teething biscuits, individual cereal pieces
Other	Plain wafer cookies

From Mitchell, M. K., Nutrition during infancy, In: *Nutrition Across the Life Span*, W. B. Saunders Co, 1997. With permission.

III. PRESCHOOL YEARS

A. Characteristics

During the preschool years, the rate of growth gradually decelerates from the rapid growth in height and weight seen in infancy. During the second and third year of life, height increases about 12 cm (5 inches) and weight increases about 2.5 kg (5 to 6 pounds) per year. From 3 to 5 years of age, the child gains about 2 kg (4.5 pounds) and grows about 6 to 8 cm (2.5 to 3.5 inches) in height per year. Appetite decreases proportionately to decreases in growth rates, and at times the child's food intake is erratic and unpredictable. Motor skills are becoming fine-tuned. At 12 months (or before), a toddler is able to pick up and release a piece of food and hand feed himself, and by age 2 he is able to handle a spoon and fork.[21] At 15 months, the child can drink from a cup, though not without spilling.[22]

Social, intellectual and emotional growth is rapid. Speech develops, so that by the time a child is 3 years of age he can use short sentences and hold a brief conversation. During the second year, the child begins to imitate parents, siblings, and playmates. As the child becomes increasingly aware that he will become a larger child and eventually an adult, he begins to emulate role models.

B. Recommendations for Milk Group Foods

Milk and milk products provide the majority of calcium in the diets of toddlers and preschoolers. Calcium is needed throughout childhood to maintain existing bone and for bone growth. In children 1 to 2 years of age, milk and milk products contribute 83% of the calcium in their diet; milk used as an ingredient contributes 10% of that amount.[23] Data are not available for older preschoolers. In addition to calcium, milk is either a good or an excellent source of eight other essential nutrients needed for good health (i.e., protein, phosphorus, potassium, vitamins A, B_{12}, and D, riboflavin, and niacin). Vitamin D plays an important role in calcium absorption and metabolism; however, dietary sources are limited. Vitamin D fortified milk is the primary food source of vitamin D in the U.S. For example, 2 eight-ounce glasses of vitamin D fortified milk provide the amount of vitamin D currently recommended for this age group (200 IU). Other milk products are not fortified with vitamin D, so a child who consumes only yogurt and cheese may not be getting enough, particularly if exposure to sunlight is limited.

The portion sizes recommended for young children are $^2/_3$ the size of adult servings. Three smaller servings of Milk Group foods are recommended for children ages 1 to 2. As the child grows, larger servings are recommended. Children ages 3 to 5 should consume 3 servings from the Milk Group; a serving is 8 ounces of milk or yogurt and $1^1/_2$ ounces of cheese (Table 9.4).

C. Calcium Recommendations and Consumption

Milk and milk products provide calcium, protein, phosphorus, and vitamin D needed for maximum skeletal growth. Few studies have measured the accretion of calcium into bone in this age group. However, it is estimated that about 100 mg of calcium per day is retained in the skeleton of children 2 to 3 years old.[5] The National Institutes of Health Expert Panel recommends 800 mg of calcium per day for children ages 1 to 5.[6] The National Academy of Sciences recommends 500 mg of calcium (expressed as Adequate Intakes) per day for children ages 1 to 3 and 800 mg per day for children ages 4 to 8 (Table 9.5).[5] The NAS chose to develop separate recommendations for children ages 1 to 3. Although calcium balance data was not available for this age group, the committee chose an estimate of net calcium retention to establish what they felt was a reasonable recommendation. They acknowledge the need for more information to more precisely estimate calcium needs.[5] Approximately 81% of children ages 1 to 2 meet the NAS calcium recommendations, but only about 56% of children

Table 9.4 Food Guide for Children and Adults

SERVING GUIDELINES FOR ALL AGES

FOOD GROUP	SERVINGS					FOODS	SERVING SIZE
	CHILDREN				ADULTS		
	1–3	4–5	6–8*	9–18*	19+		
MILK GROUP	3†	3†	3	4	3–4	▲ milk ▲ yogurt ▲ cheese ▲ cottage cheese ▲ pudding ▲ ice cream, frozen yogurt	1 cup 1 cup 1½–2 oz ½ cup ½ cup ½ cup
MEAT GROUP	2†	2	2	2	2–3	▲ cooked lean meat, fish or poultry ▲ egg ▲ peanut butter ▲ cooked dried peas ▲ cooked dried beans ▲ nuts, seeds	2–3 oz 1 2 tbsp ½ cup ½ cup ⅓ cup
VEGETABLE GROUP	3†	3	3	3	3–5	▲ cooked vegetables ▲ chopped, raw vegetables ▲ raw, leafy vegetables ▲ vegetable juice	½ cup ½ cup 1 cup ¾ cup
FRUIT GROUP	2†	2	2	2	2–4	▲ apple, banana, orange, pear ▲ grapefruit ▲ cantaloupe ▲ raw, canned, or cooked fruit ▲ raisins, dried fruit ▲ fruit juice	1 medium ½ ¼ ½ cup ¼ cup ¾ cup
GRAIN GROUP	6†	6†	6	6	6–11	▲ bread ▲ tortilla, roll, muffin ▲ bagel, English muffin, hamburger bun ▲ rice, pasta, cooked cereal, grits ▲ ready-to-eat cereal	1 slice 1 ½ ½ cup 1 oz
"OTHERS" CATEGORY	Eat in moderation					▲ fats, oils, and spreads ▲ candy ▲ cookies ▲ chips and other salty snacks ▲ soft drinks	1 tsp/1 tbsp 1 oz 2 small 1 oz 12 oz

†For children 1-3, serving sizes are about 2/3rds of typical serving sizes.

‡For children 4-5, serving sizes depend on the appetite of the child. If you offer smaller-sized servings, you should increase the number of servings so that children 4-5 eat the equivalent of 3 cups of milk, 4 oz. of meat, 6 slices of bread, etc. daily.

*These represent the *minimum* number of servings recommended each day for children and teens ages 6–18. Some children and teens may need more servings—depending on their size, activity level, and growth.

Table 9.5   Calcium Recommendations for Preschool
            Children

NIH Expert Panel		NAS	
Age	Calcium (mg)	Age	Calcium (mg)
1–5 years	800	1–3 years	500

From National Institutes of Health Expert Panel, 1994 and
Dietary Reference Intakes, National Academy of Sciences,
1997.

ages 3 to 5 do so.[24] This low intake is reflective of a dietary pattern that is already
becoming low in milk and milk products.

D. Strategies to Improve Intake

1. Snacks

Because children in this age group have a small stomach capacity, they do best
when fed four to six times a day. Snacks should be treated as mini-meals that are
planned to contribute to the daily nutrient intake.[22] Foods chosen for snacks should
come mainly from the Five Food Groups. Milk, yogurt, and cheese are excellent snack
choices, and will help young children meet daily calcium requirements. Offer a variety
of foods from each Food Group. If a child dislikes white milk, offer a flavored milk,
such as chocolate milk, to encourage milk consumption. Flavored milk has a similar
sugar content to orange juice, and contains all the same nutrients as white milk.

2. Parental Role Modeling

Children begin to acquire their adult food preferences during the preschool years.
Parental role models can have a profound impact on a child's food preferences and
eating patterns. Young children will not choose a well-balanced diet unassisted.
Parents must provide the child with a variety of nutritious foods and model patterns
of food acceptance.[22] A child will become more positive toward a food the more
often it is presented. A parent may need to offer a food 8 or 10 times before the
child will accept it.[25] Parents can encourage adequate intake of Milk Group foods
both by serving milk, yogurt, and cheese at meal and snack time, and by consuming
these foods themselves. Since the child begins to emulate role models at this stage
of life, it is important for the preschooler to see her parents, preschool teachers, and
other children enjoying these foods.

E. Nutritional Concerns

1. Low fat diets

Fat modified foods, including fat free and lowfat milks, are not recommended
for children between the ages of 1 and 2.[22] Children of this age need foods with

high caloric density for growth. Failure to thrive has been reported in preschool children whose overzealous parents have offered their children very low fat, restrictive diets in the misguided hope of preventing adult obesity and/or cardiovascular disease.[25] After the age of two years, the 1995 Dietary Guidelines recommends that children "gradually adopt a diet that, by about five years of age, contains no more than 30% of calories from fat."[27] Canada revised its recommendations for fat intake in children after a Working Group concluded that there was "no evidence that any reduction of blood cholesterol levels in childhood persists into adulthood."[28] They determined that there was no scientific evidence that a fat-restricted diet during childhood had any demonstrated value either while the child was a child or later in adulthood. Therefore, Health Canada recommends that complete adherence to adult fat recommendations not occur until linear growth has ceased.[29]

Because of a growing recognition in the health professional community that kids are not little adults, the American Dietetic Association advises that the U. S. consider separate dietary guidelines for children, and states that individual foods should not be restricted because of calorie, fat, or sugar content.[30] Instead of focusing on fat restriction, parents and caregivers of young children should emphasize foods that will provide the energy and variety of nutrients needed for growth and development which is the top priority for children's nutrition.

2. Excessive Fruit Juice Consumption

Natural fruit juice is nutritious, and an appropriate food for preschoolers, but when fruit juice replaces milk in the diet, it can have a negative nutritional impact.[22] Smith and Lifshitz reported that toddlers (14 to 27 months) with growth failure consumed large amounts of fruit juice, primarily apple juice.[31] The fruit juice displaced other calorie- and nutrient-dense foods from the diet, such as milk, starches, and fruits and vegetables. The result was an inadequate intake of calories, protein, fat, calcium, vitamin D, iron, and zinc. All of the parents perceived fruit juice as being a healthy food choice because it was "natural," and it was readily accepted by the children because of the sweet taste. One mother gave her child fat free milk after weaning because she felt she was getting too heavy. When the child refused the fat free milk, she offered juice as a "healthy" substitute. When juice consumption was replaced by whole milk and increased amounts of solid foods (three meals and two or three snacks), the dietary intakes of calcium, vitamin D, iron, and zinc increased to recommended levels in these children. More recently, it was reported that excess fruit juice consumption is associated with short stature and obesity in preschool children,[32] though these results have been challenged.[33] These studies highlight the importance of encouraging a balanced intake of a variety of foods for children.

3. Lead Toxicity

Lead toxicity, from exposure to high levels of lead in the environment (lead-based paint, newspaper ink dust, automobile emissions), is the number one environmental health threat to infants and children.[21] It can impair growth and result in lowered IQ and learning disabilities. Blood lead levels in the general population have decreased dramatically since the 1970s due to regulatory and voluntary bans on the use of lead in gasoline, household paint, food and drink cans, and plumbing. The Centers for Disease Control (CDC) reports that 4.4% of children ages 1 to 5 have blood lead levels in the toxic range (≥10 mg/dl).[34] The prevalence in this age group decreased about 4% between 1991 and 1994. Even so, blood lead levels in children 1 to 5 years are more likely to be higher among lower income minorities living in older urban housing.

Some nutrients, including calcium and iron, influence the handling of lead, and protect against toxicity by decreasing lead's absorption into the bloodstream.[21,35] Deficiencies of calcium, phosphorus, iron, and zinc make children more susceptible to lead intoxication. Also, lead is absorbed more rapidly in the fasting state. All children with blood lead levels between 15 and 19 µg/dl should receive nutritional and environmental counseling.[36] The Centers for Disease Control recommends that all children from 6 to 36 months of age have a blood test for lead.[37] They recommend more frequent screening for children who live in environments with higher exposure to lead (e.g., old houses). Dietary recommendations to prevent and treat lead toxicity are (1) evaluate and treat iron deficiency; (2) eat three meals and a midmorning and midafternoon snack daily; and (3) give 4 to 6 ounces of milk or yogurt with meals and snacks. The molar excess of calcium in milk is high enough to inhibit lead absorption. Milk also contains phosphorus, which further decreases lead absorption.[38] A balanced diet that includes a variety of foods, including adequate amounts of meat and dairy foods, will help decrease the risk of lead toxicity in young children.

IV. SCHOOL-AGED CHILD

A. Characteristics

Children between 7 and 12 years of age enjoy slow, but steady growth, with an increase in appetite and food intake. Since they spend much of their day in school, they eat fewer times a day, but after-school snacks are almost universal. Elementary school children often take responsibility for preparing their own breakfast, packing their own lunch, and finding snacks after school. Less frequently they assume responsibility for grocery shopping and preparing the evening meal. Although children at this age make their own eating decisions, parents still influence family food habits, attitudes, and expectations. Peers and the media begin to have a stronger influence on food attitudes and choices.[21,22]

B. Importance of Milk Group Foods

1. Bone Growth and Fracture Prevention

Bone growth begins to accelerate in the mid-grade school years, making this an important time for building optimal bone mass (Figure 9.1). Achieving an optimal genetically-determined peak bone mass by as early as late adolescence is considered

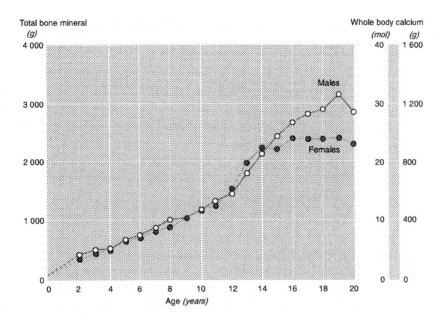

Figure 9.1 Accumulation of total bone mineral and whole body calcium in boys and girls as a function of age. (From FAO Food, Nutrition and Agriculture Division, *Food, Nutrition, and Agriculture: Calcium Throughout Life*, 20, 14, 1997. With permission.)

the best way to prevent osteoporosis later in life. Osteoporosis prevention should ideally begin in childhood. An adequate intake of dietary calcium throughout the growing years will help maximize calcium retention and bone density.

Numerous studies showing that increasing calcium intake during childhood (and puberty) increases bone mass led a National Institutes of Health (NIH) Expert Panel in 1994, then the National Academy of Sciences (NAS) in 1997, to increase calcium recommendations for this age group. (For more information about these studies, see Chapter 5, Dairy Foods and Osteoporosis). The NIH Expert Panel recommends 800 to 1200 mg of calcium per day for children ages 6 to 10, and NAS recommends 800 mg of calcium for children ages 4 to 8 and 1300 mg of calcium for pre-adolescents and adolescents ages 9 to 18 (Table 9.6).[6,5] This translates into a daily consumption of 3 or 4 servings of Milk Group foods (Table 9.4). Calcium absorption efficiency is about 28% in prepubertal children and increases to 34% in early puberty,

Table 9.6 Calcium Recommendations for School-Age Children

NIH Expert Panel		NAS	
Age	Calcium (mg)	Age	Calcium (mg)
6–10	800–1,200	4–8 years	800
		9–13 years	1,300

From National Institutes of Health Expert Panel, 1994 and Dietary Reference Intakes, National Academy of Sciences, 1997.

giving this age group the greatest potential for bone mass development.[39] Several retrospective studies have associated higher milk intake in early life with higher bone density and/or osteoporosis risk in later years. For more details on these studies, see Chapter 5.

Low bone density may contribute to fracture risk during childhood. The incidence of forearm fractures in children peaks during the growth spurt, leading some experts to suggest that the cause is low bone density due to the rapid increase in linear growth. To test this hypothesis, researchers in New Zealand measured the bone density at several sites in 100 girls ages 3 to 15 who had a recent forearm fracture with 100 girls who had not.[40] Osteopenia (a Z score below −1) of the forearm, spine, and hip was significantly more common among the fracture patients than in girls who had never broken a bone. In fact, one third of the fracture cases had low bone density. The older girls with forearm fracture reported lower current and past calcium intakes than controls.

2. Prevention of Dental Caries

Although the prevalence of dental caries in children is declining, 45% of school-aged children have dental caries in their permanent teeth, and this exceeds the goal for the year 2000.[41]

Dental caries in children can be prevented by increasing tooth resistance (e.g., fluoride), changing the oral environment (e.g., dietary intervention), and by reducing oral microorganisms with proper oral hygiene. Diet plays an important role in dental caries risk. Fermentable carbohydrates (e.g., sugar, starches) in a food are cariogenic, while cheese and milk may protect against tooth decay.[42,43] Components in cheese or milk such as protein (casein and whey), lipids, calcium, and phosphorus may be responsible for the caries protective effects of these foods. Milk, particularly casein, has been demonstrated to decrease the adherence of cavity causing bacteria to the teeth.[44] Although it is not known exactly how cheese protects against tooth decay, water soluble components of cheese, such as calcium and possibly phosphorus, may inhibit demineralization and promote the remineralization of teeth. Researchers have demonstrated an anticariogenic effect of aged Cheddar, Swiss, Monterey Jack, Edam, Gouda, Muenster, mozzarella, Port Salut, Roquefort, Roman, Stilton, Tilsit, and American processed cheeses.[42]

Although the cariogenicity of chocolate milk has not been determined, it is less likely to contribute to dental caries than sucrose alone or snack foods such as potato chips, cookies, and raisins. There is evidence that its cocoa milk fat, calcium, and phosphorus content may contribute to this favorable effect.[45] In addition, since chocolate milk is a liquid that clears the mouth rapidly, it is less likely to cause dental caries than sticky carbohydrate foods.

To prevent dental caries, children should limit their intake of sugar containing foods to mealtimes, should eat plenty of noncariogenic foods, such as cheese, fresh fruits or vegetables, and practice good oral hygiene. Since eating frequency increases caries risk, the American Academy of Pediatrics suggests that parents should not feed their children more than three meals and three snacks per day.[46]

C. Strategies to Improve Milk Consumption

Many children fail to consume the recommended amount of calcium and servings of Milk Group foods. Data from the USDA Continuing Food Intakes of Individuals, 1994–96, indicates that U. S. males and females ages 6 to 11 consume an average of 970 mg and 857 mg of calcium daily.[24] Approximately 62% of boys and 70% of girls ages 6 to 11 are not meeting their current recommendation for calcium. Milk intake is correspondingly low, with males in this age group consuming about one and one third cups of milk and females consuming about one cup.[24]

In addition to calcium, milk and milk products provide a number of nutrients to children's diets that contribute to overall health. A recent analysis of dietary sources of nutrients in the diets of U.S. children reported that milk was the number one source of calcium, magnesium, and protein, and a major source of zinc, vitamin A, and folate.[47] The authors found that milk and milk products (milk, cheese, and ice cream/sherbet/frozen yogurt) supplied 69.7% of the calcium in the diets of children ages 6 to 11 (Table 9.7).

Table 9.7 Contribution of Milk Group Foods to Children's Diets (Ages 2-5 and 6-11)

Milk Group Foods	Ages 2–5				Ages 6–11			
	Milk %	Cheese %	Ice Cream %	Total %	Milk %	Cheese %	Ice Cream %	Total %
Energy	15.4	3.3	2.6	21.3	12.4	3.4	2.8	18.6
Fat	19.0	7.1	3.3	29.4	15.0	7.0	3.1	25.1
Carbohydrate	10.2	—*	2.8	13.0	8.2	—*	3.3	11.5
Protein	25.0	5.8	1.1	31.9	20.5	6.3	1.2	28.0
Calcium	58.9	10.8	2.5	72.2	53.6	13.2	2.9	69.7
Magnesium	27.8	1.7	1.3	30.8	24.2	2.0	1.6	27.8
Vitamin A	22.4	4.3	2.0	28.7	19.9	4.9	2.2	27.0
Zinc	21.1	5.3	1.5	27.9	16.7	5.5	1.6	23.8
Folate	9.4	—*	—*	9.4	8.1	—*	—*	8.1
Carotene	3.9	1.4	—*	5.3	3.0	1.3	—*	4.3

* Not a significant source in this age group.

From Subar, A. F. et. al., *Pediatrics*, 102(4), 913, 1999. With permission.

Following are some important ways parents, teachers, and health professionals can encourage children to consume the recommended amounts of milk and milk products.

1. Encourage Consumption of All Milk Types

There has been a steady decline in milk consumption among U.S. children since the 1970s.[48] Since milk and milk products are the most important source of calcium in children's diets, low milk consumption makes it difficult for children to meet their calcium needs.[49] There is evidence that the public health message to "eat less fat," has been mistranslated by consumers and pediatric health practitioners into "drink less milk," since whole and 2% milk are sources of fat in children's diets. Johnson and Wang analyzed nutrient intake data in school-aged children (ages 5 to 17) and found that calcium and fat intakes were closely related.[50] The lowest fat intake group (27% of calories) had the lowest percent of recommended amounts of calcium when compared to the other four fat intake groups. The authors state that "Recommendations to lower fat in the diets of school-aged children must be counterbalanced by guidance that promotes optimal calcium intakes." Since calcium qualifies as a "problem nutrient" (30% or more of the sample have intakes below 77% of recommended levels) for grade-school children, children should not necessarily be counseled to drink only lowfat and fat free milk. The authors suggest that those who do not like the taste of lower fat milks should instead be encouraged to switch to lower fat versions of less nutrient dense, non-dairy sources of fat (e.g., salad dressings, snack foods, desserts).

2. School Meals

In 1997, schools served nearly 7 million breakfasts and 26 million lunches daily in 94,000 schools.[51] Milk is required to be offered to every student at every school meal, although children are not required to select it as one of their food choices.[52] The milk children receive at school, through the National School Lunch Program and/or the School Breakfast Program, accounts for roughly 12 to 14% of all milk drinking occasions for children 6 to 11 years of age.[53,54]

Consuming milk or milk products at breakfast (whether at home or at school) is an important way for school children to meet their daily calcium needs. In a study conducted among school children (ages 9 to 13) in Spain, children with the greatest intakes of milk products and/or calcium at breakfast also showed greater intakes over the rest of the day.[55] An accompanying editorial states that children in the U.S. who eat breakfast enjoy higher intakes of calcium and other nutrients than those who skip breakfast.[56] Recognizing the benefits of a nutritious breakfast for children, the U.S. government established the School Breakfast Program in 1975. An evaluation of the School Breakfast Program in the 1980s revealed that breakfast participants had superior intakes of milk related nutrients, such as calcium, phosphorus, riboflavin, and protein, and had higher overall nutrient intakes over 24 hours than breakfast skippers.[57] Expansion of this program into more schools, and greater student participation within schools would likely improve school children's calcium and nutritional status.

School lunch also contributes significantly to a child's intake of calcium and milk products. The U.S. Department of Agriculture's School Nutrition Dietary Assessment Study found that children who participated in the National School Lunch Program consumed nearly two times the amount of milk and milk products as nonparticipants.[58] In a nationwide sample of over two thousand children ages 5 to 17, only those who drank milk at the noon meal met or exceeded 33% of the 1989 RDA for calcium for that meal or the recommended amount of calcium over the whole day.[59] Those who drank other beverages at lunch, such as soft drinks, juice, tea, or fruit drinks failed to meet their calcium recommendations. When milk was included in the noon meal, diet quality improved. The authors identified four "problem" nutrients (vitamin A, vitamin E, calcium, and zinc) for which 30% or more of the sample children had three-day average intakes that fell below 77%

of the Recommended Dietary Allowance (1989). When children consumed milk at lunch, that meal, as well as the total daily diet, contained some of the highest amounts of these "problem" nutrients. The authors conclude that "noon meals that include milk are associated with improved vitamin and mineral intakes."[59]

Children need to select and consume milk at breakfast and lunch in order to meet the current recommendations for calcium for 9 to 18 year olds (1300 mg/d). An informal analysis of one week's worth of sample school lunch and breakfast menus indicates that a child must consume an 8 ounce serving of milk at breakfast to meet the required 1/4 of the current recommendation for calcium (325 mg) required of this meal. However, even if children consume 8 ounces of milk with lunch, this meal may fall short of the 1/3 of the current recommendation for calcium (433 mg) required for this meal.[60] Since calcium recommendations were increased for this age group, it may be beneficial to provide school children with larger servings of milk at school. In a recent survey of 600 children ages 8 to 13, 45% said they "would drink more school milk if the cartons/containers were bigger."[54] This was especially true for older boys (58%).

The growing presence of soft drink marketers in the schools encourages students to drink beverages other than milk with their meals. Leading soft drink manufacturers in the U.S. are offering monetary incentives to school districts in return for exclusive contracts to provide products and advertising within schools. Forty-five percent of school foodservice directors surveyed recently agree that "competing drinks sold a la carte threaten milk consumption at school."[54] When children choose a beverage other than milk with their meal, this further erodes already low calcium intakes during the years when skeletal demand for bone-building nutrients is the highest.

Other barriers to milk consumption at school include (1) lack of parental support for milk consumption; (2) temperature problems (milk not cold enough); (3) lack of colorful, eye-catching packaging; and (4) taste. The dairy industry is working with government, industry, nutrition/health partners to help overcome these barriers and encourage greater milk consumption at school. For example, in 1998 National Dairy Council® initiated a national effort to improve milk quality in schools. State and regional offices distributed a *Totally Cool Milk Temperature* survey kit, including a thermometer, to schools to increase awareness among school foodservice personnel of the importance of keeping milk cold.

3. Flavored Milk

Most children and adults like the taste of chocolate milk, though most parents said in a recent survey they do not buy chocolate milk or keep chocolate milk (or the necessary syrups/powders) on hand at home.[61] However, in the same survey, 4 out of 10 children said they would rather drink chocolate milk if it were available, especially 10 to 11 year old boys (46%). In restaurants, almost as many children drink chocolate milk as white milk; it is especially popular with girls ages 8 to 9 and with boys ages 10 to 11. Children prefer to drink chocolate milk with lunch or with foods such as sandwiches, cake, and other dry foods. More children view chocolate milk as "best with lunch" (46%) than soft drinks (33%). At school, chocolate and white milk are equally popular. About half the children consume either white or chocolate milk weekly.

Providing a choice of milks at school is an effective way to encourage milk consumption. Although milk's image ("cool people drink milk") declines during the grade-school years, boys between the ages of 8 and 11 increasingly say "I would drink more milk if milk at school came in more flavors."[62] Most schools (91%) currently offer chocolate milk or other flavored milks daily. Although most foodservice directors are positive about its nutritional contribution to the diet, chocolate milk still suffers from a "bad boy" image. In 1998, National Dairy Council® developed a program (*Choc' it Up!*™) targeting food service directors, parents, and children with information to dispel any negative notions about offering chocolate milk in schools. Messages delivered through the program assure parents/teachers/foodservice personnel that chocolate milk is just as nutritious as white milk (Figure 9.2), that the sweeteners do not cause hyperactivity[63] or tooth decay,[64] and that the calcium is just as well absorbed as from white milk.[65] In addition, chocolate milk may be better tolerated than white milk for people with lactose intolerance,[66] and it is nutritionally superior to soft drinks and fruit drinks.

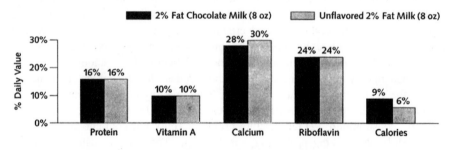

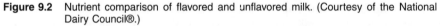

Figure 9.2   Nutrient comparison of flavored and unflavored milk. (Courtesy of the National Dairy Council®.)

A recent study compared the nutritional contribution of flavored milks to that of other beverages children frequently consume.[67] The children who consumed flavored milk had higher intakes of key nutrients such as calcium, protein, and vitamin A than did consumers of alternative beverages such as soft drinks, fruit juices, fruit drinks, and tea. However, soft drinks were the most popular beverage among 6 to 11 year olds (over 50% consumed them)—and less than 20% of this age group consumed flavored milk.

4. Parental Role Modeling

Children's eating patterns are strongly influenced by adults as well as by the marketplace.[47] Parents serve as role models for their children's eating behavior and in this age group a parent's persistence in encouraging milk consumption has a positive influence on their children's milk intake. In a recent analysis of USDA 1994–95 CSFII data, researchers found that the amount of milk consumed by the mothers of children ages 5 to 17 was the strongest predictor of the children's milk intake.[68] Children's milk intake increased by one gram for every 0.64 grams of milk consumed by their mothers. The authors suggest that the influence of parental role modeling should be considered when designing nutrition intervention programs designed to increase children's milk intake.

A nationally representative survey of children and their parents revealed that most parents of boys ages 5 to 8 increasingly agreed that, "milk is absolutely essential to a child's growth," and "I try to make sure everyone in my household has milk every day."[62] These parental attitudes corresponded with an 8% yearly increase in milk consumption in this age group. However, fewer parents of boys 9 to 12 years felt that milk was "absolutely essential" to their child's growth, and they increasingly agreed that, "It's less important for older children to drink milk," and that, "It's hard to get my older children to drink milk." Consequently, boys of this age felt less compelled to drink milk, and their consumption decreased by 6% yearly. Other factors, such as problems with away from home portability and school milk quality also influenced this decline.

The pattern is similar for girls. Although girls' milk consumption remains fairly steady between the ages of 6 and 11, the stage is being set for a dramatic decline in consumption during their teenage years. Fewer parents say that they "Encourage my kids to drink milk at school," and "Insist kids drink at least one glass of milk at mealtime" as their girls get older. Unfortunately, parents set the stage for girls' weight concerns. As girls approach age 11, more and more parents say "I'm concerned about the calories in milk for members of my household." This is matched by girls who say increasingly more frequently as they age that "Drinking milk will make me fat."[62] This belief is a barrier preventing many young girls from consuming the milk they need to reach their bone mass potential and is not supported by research. In a study conducted in Utah, 9 to 13 year old girls who increased their calcium intake to recommended levels by eating more milk, yogurt, and cheese (no fat level specified) had an increased rate of bone mineralization, but did not gain weight or increase body fatness compared to girls who followed their normal diet.[69] Similarly, 12 year old girls who consumed an additional two cups of either whole or lowfat milk per day, gained bone mineral density, but not weight or fat mass compared to the control group.[70]

Parents of girls in particular need to be very careful not to criticize their children about their weight or communicate through their own actions that outward appearance is of greater importance than health. Doing so increases the likelihood that children will restrict their dietary intake and develop nutritional deficiencies.

V. ADOLESCENCE

A. Characteristics

The adolescent period is characterized by rapid physical growth as well as maturational changes. The adolescent "growth spurt" which begins at the onset of puberty, contributes 15% to adult height, 50% to adult weight, and 45% to adult skeletal mass.[71] It typically occurs between the ages of 10 and 13 in girls and two years later in boys. A nutritionally adequate diet is needed for growth, but the rate of growth is influenced by a number of factors including genetics, physical activity, age, gender, and endocrine balance.[72] Socially, the adolescent moves from a state of dependence upon parents and family to become more independent and self-directing. The peer group becomes more important as a source of support, self-esteem, and behavioral standards.[71]

Various aspects of teen culture, life style, and environment influence food selection and nutritional status. Teens receive most of their nutrition information from television and magazines. Their growing independence means they eat fewer meals with the family and eat more meals in fast food restaurants and at concession stands at sporting events.

B. Importance of Adequate Calcium/Dairy Food Intake

1. Peak Bone Mass

Calcium is important for building bone mass and strength. Optimizing the amount of bone laid down during the adolescent period appears to be the most effective strategy for reducing the risk of osteoporosis (porous bones) later in life.[73] The most opportune time to initiate efforts to increase calcium intake is during the five year period from 11 to 16 years of age, since this is when a substantial part of bone accretion takes place.[74] However, efforts to improve calcium intake may need to begin even earlier to be successful. Although the data are not conclusive, there is considerable evidence supporting the importance of physical activity, especially activity initiated before puberty, on the bone status of youth.[75]

2. Nutritional Status

Milk supplies calcium, as well as eight other essential nutrients that contribute to the nutritional status of teens. In an analysis of calcium consumption and food sources of calcium in the U.S., Fleming and Heimbach compared the nutrient profiles of teenage girls (13 to 18 years) who drank milk with those who did not (Table 9.8).[23] Milk-drinkers consumed 80% more calcium, 59% more vitamin B_{12}, 56% more riboflavin, 38% more folate, 35% more vitamin A, 24% more of each vitamin B_6 and potassium, and 22% more magnesium than did non-milk drinking teenagers. The authors urge placing emphasis on changing current consumption patterns of milk, since milk and milk products are the source of more than three-fourths (77%) of the calcium in the diets of teenage girls. Encouraging adolescent girls to consume more milk and dairy foods will likely help improve their overall nutrient profile as well.

Table 9.8 Nutrient Density of Diets of Teenage Girls 13–18 Years Who Use and Do Not Use Milk*

Nutrient	Mean intake (d-1000 kcal) per day per 1,000 kcal		(Users – Nonusers)/ Nonusers %
	Users of Fluid Milk	Nonusers of Fluid Milk	
Fat, g	41	42	
Protein, g	38	36	
Vitamin A, RE	475	351	35
Folate, μg	121	88	38
Riboflavin, mg	1.03	0.66	56
Vitamin B6, mg	0.78	0.63	24
Vitamin B-12, μg	2.57	1.62	59
Calcium, mg	495	275	80
Magnesium, mg	117	96	22
Potassium, mg	1232	994	24

* 1987–88 Nationwide Food Consumption Survey weighted data.

From Fleming, K. H. and Heimbach, J. T., *J. Nutr.*, 124, 1426S, 1994. With permission.

C. Calcium/Dairy Food Recommendations and Consumption

An Expert Panel convened by the National Institutes of Health recommends that adolescents and young adults ages 11 to 24 consume 1200 to 1500 mg of calcium daily for the prevention of osteoporosis.[6] This amount of calcium is the equivalent of 4 to 5 servings of milk, yogurt, or cheese. These recommendations were subsequently endorsed by the American Medical Association. In order to help pediatricians screen adolescents for nutritional problems and provide dietary guidance, the American Academy of Pediatrics adapted the Food Guide Pyramid to meet the nutritional needs of teenagers (Figure 9.3).[76] This guide recommends five servings of Milk Group foods to meet the highest calcium needs of this age group. Although other foods, such as green vegetables, nuts, and dried beans, may supply up to 300 mg of calcium in the overall diet of the average American, these foods are not routinely eaten by teenagers. Therefore, AAP's recommendations are not dependent on foods other than dairy foods to supply calcium in the teen diet. In 1997 the National Academy of Sciences released new recommendations for calcium and other bone-related nutrients that were more in line with the recommendations of the NIH Expert Panel. They increased the recommendation for calcium to 1300 mg per day for children and teens ages 9 to 18 (Table 9.9).[5]

Unfortunately, many teens do not consume enough calcium, and the increased recommendations only widened the gap. According to USDA's Continuing Survey of Food Intakes by Individuals (CSFII), nine out of ten (88%) adolescent girls and

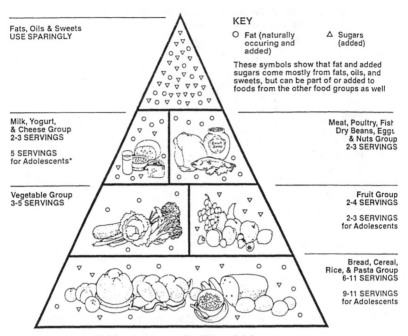

*5 dairy servings provide 1500mg Calcium

Modified from the "Food Guide Pyramid," USDA, DHHS, 1992. Modifications for adolescents are based upon "Basic Concepts in Identifying the Health Needs of Adolescents," Center for Continuing Education in Adolescent Health, Division of Adolescent Medicine, University of Cincinnati, 1994. The increase to 1500 mg calcium per day is based upon recommendations of the National Health Consensus Conference, 1994.

Figure 9.3   How to adapt the Food Guide Pyramid to meet nutritional needs in adolescence. (AAP, *Adolescent Health Update: A Clinical Guide for Pediatricians*, 9, 2, February 1997. With permission.)

Table 9.9   Calcium Recommendations for Adolescents

NIH Expert Panel		NAS	
Age	Calcium (mg)	Age	Calcium (mg)
11–24 years	1,200–1,500	9–18	1,300
Pregnancy/lactation	1,200–1,500	Pregnancy/lactation ≤ 18 years	1,300

From National Institutes of Health Expert Panel and Dietary Reference Intakes, National Academy of Sciences.

seven out of ten (68%) adolescent boys fail to meet calcium recommendations.[24] An evaluation of food sources of calcium for adolescent females reports that calcium intakes in girls ages 11 to 18 have "declined over time, with age, and appear to be related to a decline in fluid milk consumption."[77] According to 1994-96 CSFII, boys ages 12 to 19 consume an average of about $1\frac{1}{4}$ glasses of milk per day, while girls consume only about $\frac{3}{4}$ of a cup.[24]

D. Factors Contributing to Low Milk Intake

1. Lack of Knowledge

A recent study conducted in over 1000 ninth grade students found that most are aware that dietary calcium "is healthy" (98%), it "strengthens bones" (92%), and it "prevents osteoporosis" (51%).[78] However, only 19% knew how much calcium was recommended for their age group, and only 10% knew the calcium content of various dairy products. The authors conclude that this lack of information may contribute to adolescents' suboptimal intake of calcium. Parents, teachers, and health care providers need to disseminate information about calcium recommendations and food sources to teens and motivate them to consume more Milk Group foods.

2. Eating Away from Home

Fully 72% of teenage boys (12 to 19 years) and 64% of teenage girls eat away from home on any given day, according to a USDA survey.[24] However, milk is most often consumed at home, rather than away from home. Only about a third of milk drinkers report away-from-home usage.[79] More than half of young teens surveyed said they would rather not drink milk in a restaurant.[80] Thus, the trend to away from home eating has likely contributed to the low calcium and milk intake of adolescents. In addition, how milk is viewed in teen culture may also affect consumption. Researchers in Toronto found that adolescent girls categorized milk as a "healthy food" which was associated in their minds with home and family, while "junk foods" were associated with peers and independence.[81] Consequently, teens may leave milk at home as they seek independence and peer acceptance. Therefore, it is important for any nutrition intervention to identify and address the functional meaning of foods in the teen culture in order to bring about more healthful food choices.

3. Soft Drinks Substituted for Milk

There is evidence that adolescents may be substituting fruit juice and soft drinks for milk, putting them at greater risk for deficiencies of bone-building nutrients such as calcium, magnesium, and zinc. Soft drink consumption has risen steadily among teens over the last 20 years.[82] As teens have doubled or even tripled their consumption of soft drinks, their consumption of milk has decreased by more than 40% (Figure 9.4).[82] Twenty years ago, boys consumed more than twice as much milk as soft drinks, and girls consumed 50% more milk than soft drinks. By 1994 to 1996, the tables were turned. Both boys and girls consumed twice as much soda pop as milk. Compared to teens who do not consume soft drinks, heavy drinkers (26 ounces or more per day) are almost four times more likely to drink less than one glass of milk a day. Currently, the average teenage boy (12 to 19 years) who consumes soft drinks consumes about 2.3 cans (12 ounce) per day and girls drink about 1.7 cans.[24]

Teens who substitute soft drinks for milk or milk products will likely have low calcium intakes, putting them at risk for low peak bone mass and osteoporosis later

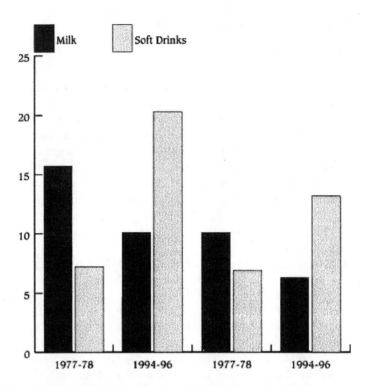

Figure 9.4 Teens (ages 12-19) consumption of milk and soft drinks (ounces per day). (From Jacobson, M. F., *Liquid Candy: How Soft Drinks Are Harming Americans' Health*, Center for Science in the Public Interest, October 1998. With permission.)

in life. Research has shown that trading soft drinks for milk can have short-term consequences as well. Researchers found a strong association between carbonated beverage consumption (particularly colas containing phosphoric acid) and the occurrence of bone fractures in 14 year old girls.[83] They found, however, that a high intake of dietary calcium was protective.

Parents should consider how many soft drinks they and their children are consuming and return to using them as an occasional treat, instead of a routine meal beverage. Soft drinks should not routinely replace milk as a beverage even when eating away from home.

4. Body Image/Weight Concerns

Milk consumption dramatically declines by 12% per year in girls 12 to 17 years of age.[62] Weight concerns that were beginning to surface in late childhood now take center stage, and play a large part in this decline. One third of older teen girls surveyed in 1997 said they were currently on a diet and two thirds said they would like to lose weight. Weight concerns increase with age, so by the age of 16 and 17, almost 60% of girls said they "pay more attention to beverages I drink than before," and almost a third said they "cut back on dairy when I'm dieting."[62]

Fear of obesity which leads to excessive dieting may adversely affect an adolescent's growth and development.[84] Dieting teenage girls tend to have poor eating habits (i.e., skip meals) and low intakes of nutrients, particularly calcium and iron. In spite of all the dieting by adolescents, rates of obesity continue to rise. Studies conducted among restrained and unrestrained eaters indicate that on and off dieting produces little if any weight loss. On the contrary, an expert in eating behavior warns that dieting frequently results in feelings of psychological deprivation that result in binge eating.[85] By willfully training oneself not to eat in response to internal hunger signals, the dieter becomes susceptible to other signals to eat. Since dietary restraint is often counterproductive, the author recommends that individuals who are of normal weight (up to a BMI of 25-27) avoid food restrictions. Instead, they should be advised to establish a healthful life style that incorporates moderate exercise, and a balanced diet without restrictions of any particular food. Even those who are obese should be taught to incorporate their favorite foods into more moderate levels of intake, while increasing energy expenditure with physical activity.[86]

The prevention of chronic dieting and other eating disorders could be included as part of a comprehensive health education program in schools. Programs to change dieting and eating behaviors need to address both psychological (body image) and cognitive issues (nutrition knowledge/attitudes). Health professionals can help encourage teens to consume more Milk Group foods by explaining that teens who increase their dairy food intake to meet calcium recommendations do not necessarily experience weight gain.[69,70]

E. Groups at Risk for Low Consumption

1. Vegetarians

Adolescents are increasingly expressing interest in following a vegetarian diet and life style for a variety of reasons, including an increased sensitivity about animals. According to a 1995 Roper poll, more teens ages 13 to 17 than adults say they "do not ever eat" meat (8% vs. 6%), poultry (6% vs. 3%), fish (17% vs. 4%), and eggs (8% vs. 4%).[87] In addition, 3% of teen girls avoid all dairy products, sparking concern among health professionals that these girls are at risk for low peak bone density and osteoporosis.[88] (See Chapter 6 for more information on the bone health of vegetarians.) The American Academy of Pediatrics emphasizes that lacto-vegetarian teens who have a high intake of milk and milk products decrease their risk of inadequate calcium nutrition.[89]

2. Pregnant Teens

Adequate calcium intake to maximize peak bone mass is particularly important for pregnant teens since their bone mass is still increasing.[90] The NIH Expert Panel recommends that pregnant teens consume 1200 to 1500 mg of calcium daily, and lactating teens consume 1500 mg.[6] The NAS recommends 1300 mg of calcium daily for both pregnant and lactating teens, or the equivalent of four servings of milk, yogurt, or cheese (Table 9.9).[5]

Adequate dairy food intake during pregnancy can help pregnant teens preserve bone mass and achieve an adequate nutrient intake. Chan and colleagues compared bone mineral content after 16 weeks of lactation between adolescents who consumed at least 1600 mg of calcium per day (primarily as dairy foods) and those who consumed their usual 900 mg of calcium daily.[91] The group who consumed their usual diet experienced a 10% decrease in bone mineral content, while those consuming the high calcium diet maintained bone mineral. By increasing milk and dairy food intake, those in the experimental group also increased their intake of other nutrients including calcium and protein.

F. Strategies to Improve Consumption

In response to the critically low calcium intakes among adolescents, the National Institute of Child Health Development (NICHD) is sponsoring a publicly funded calcium awareness campaign, "Milk Matters." The campaign will educate pediatricians, other health care professionals, children, adolescents, and their parents about the importance of calcium for building strong bones and a healthy body. The campaign is designed to help prevent the next generation from suffering the devastating effects of osteoporosis.

While the campaign encourages children and teens to consume a variety of calcium-rich foods, the emphasis is on drinking more milk. The NICHD believes that milk is the best source of calcium because it is already a part of most American diets, the calcium from milk is easily absorbed by the body, and along with calcium, it provides several other essential nutrients, including vitamin D, potassium, and magnesium, essential for bone growth. In addition, the 1994 NIH Consensus Conference on Optimal Calcium Intake designated milk and milk products as the preferred source of calcium.

The materials available in the "Milk Matters" campaign include:

1. *Why Milk Matters for Children and Teens*, a fact sheet for parents and kids explaining the role of calcium for good health
2. *Why Milk Matters: Questions and Answers for Professionals*, a research fact sheet for health care professionals
3. *Count Your Calcium*, an erasable board/refrigerator magnet that lists sources of calcium and allows kids to fill in how much calcium they have had each day
4. *Milk Matters for Your Child's Health*, an educational brochure for parents
5. Print public service announcements for newspapers and magazines. (The materials are available free from the NICHD/Milk Matters Clearinghouse, 1-800-370-2943).

Choosing to eat a healthful diet is a behavior influenced by a complex interaction between environmental factors, personality factors, and behavioral factors of an individual. To be successful, nutrition education programs to increase consumption of Milk Group foods need to recognize and address these factors. Adolescents can understand abstract nutrition concepts, such as causality. Therefore, evaluation of their own diet and eating behavior patterns is very useful at this age.[92] Other components of nutrition interventions that may encourage behavioral change include

(1) teaching adolescents how to respond to the media and social pressures; (2) helping students make the connection between food and health; and (3) letting students identify potential problem areas and set goals for more healthful behavior.[92]

VI. ADULTS

A. Characteristics

The main physiologic characteristic of adulthood is stability. In general, the cells of most tissues are catabolized and replaced at about the same rate. Over time, however, catabolism slightly exceeds anabolism, and there are small changes in structure and function. The adult reaches maximum strength, endurance, and agility about five years after maximum height is attained.[93] Although the bone mass of the hip and vertebrae peaks in late adolescence, the long bones continue to slowly increase in mass well into the third decade.[94] After bone mass has peaked, the bones grow wider. This process is called consolidation. Physical activity, particularly resistance training, may help prevent both bone and muscle loss associated with aging.[93]

B. Calcium/Dairy Food Recommendations and Consumption

Adequate calcium intake throughout the adult years is important for maintaining bone mass between the time peak bone mass has been reached and menopause in women or about age 50 in men. (See Chapter 5 for more details on research in this area.) Although the age cut-offs are different, both the NIH Expert Panel and the NAS currently recommend that adult men and women age 25 and above consume 1000 mg of calcium per day (Table 9.10).[6,5] This is the equivalent of about three servings of milk, yogurt, or cheese.

Table 9.10 Calcium Recommendations for Adults

NIH Expert Panel		NAS	
Age	Calcium (mg)	Age	Calcium (mg)
11–24 years	1,200–1,500	19–30 years	1,000
25–65 years (men)	1,000	31–50 years	1,000
25–50 years (women)	1,000	Pregnancy/lactation (19–50 years)	1,000
Pregnancy/lactation	1,200–1,500		

From National Institutes of Health Expert Panel, 1994 and Dietary Reference Intakes, National Academy of Sciences, 1997.

A majority of American adults are neither meeting current calcium recommendations nor recommendations for consumption of Milk Group foods. Roughly two thirds of males ages 20 to 29 (64%), 30 to 39 (65%), and 40 to 49 (68%) are not meeting 100% of their current calcium recommendations.[24] Even more women underconsume calcium. Roughly nine out of ten females ages 20 to 29 (85%), 30 to 39 (86%), and

40 to 49 (89%) are not meeting 100% of their calcium recommendations, putting them at greater risk for low bone density and osteoporosis.[24]

Consumption of milk and milk products tends to be higher in males than females, and higher in Whites than Blacks. For example, White adult males ages 20 to 39 and 40 to 59 consume an average of 1.8 and 1.5 servings of Milk Group foods, while women consume an average of only 1.3 (ages 20 to 39) and 1.1 (ages 40 to 59) servings.[24] Black males consume an average of 1.5 (ages 20 to 39) and 0.9 (ages 40 to 59) servings of Milk Group foods, while Black females the same ages consume less than one serving (0.8 and 0.7, respectively).[24]

USDA's 1994–96 Diet and Health Knowledge Survey (which accompanies the Continuing Survey of Food Intakes by Individuals), reveals that many adults perceive their calcium intake to be better than it actually is. When asked "Compared to what is healthy, do you think your diet is too low, too high, or about right in calcium?," only 26% of adult males and 43% of adult females thought their calcium intake was too low.[24] However, consumption data show that about two out of three men and eight out of ten women have diets low in calcium. Most adults believe it is either "very important," (28% of males and 43% of females) or "somewhat important," (38% of males and 32% of females) to eat at least two servings of dairy products daily. However, there is also a substantial proportion who believe it is "not too important" (26% of males and 20% of females).[24] Some may not be motivated to increase their calcium intake until they learn how many servings of Milk Group foods are needed to meet calcium requirements, then have the opportunity to assess their own intake.

C. Milk Group Foods and the Reduction of Chronic Disease Risk

A prolonged low calcium intake has been linked to the development of several chronic diseases, including osteoporosis, hypertension, and cancer.[95,96] Experts have proposed that disease occurs either when the body's adaptation to low intakes is inadequate to maintain the calcium regulatory system or when the constant, forced adaptive response itself produces adverse consequences.[96]

1. Osteoporosis

Although reduced bone mass leading to osteoporosis has many contributing causes (i.e., genetic predisposition, inactivity, excessive alcohol use, cigarette smoking), a low calcium/dairy food intake throughout life can substantially increase the risk of osteoporosis and fracture. A state of calcium deficiency exists when calcium intakes are so low that the body can no longer conserve enough calcium (by increasing absorption and/or decreasing excretion) to maintain serum ionized calcium levels. Calcium stored in bone is the most vulnerable to the effects of calcium deficiency. Calcium deficiency leads to parathyroid hormone mediated release of calcium from bone to maintain the serum level of ionized calcium, a higher physiological priority. This deficiency state, over time, leads to bone fragility and risk of fracture.[96] Chapter 5 reviews the scientific evidence illustrating the positive influence of lifelong adequate calcium or milk consumption on adult bone density.

2. Hypertension

In 1980, McCarron and colleagues hypothesized that chronic calcium deficiency may lead to hypertension.[97] In subsequent intervention trials, calcium supplementation successfully reduced blood pressure in participants who had low serum ionized calcium, and elevated parathyroid hormone and 1, 25-dihydroxy vitamin D levels.[98] These conditions are consequences of and adaptations to restricted calcium intake. Parathyroid hormone and 1, 25-dihydroxy vitamin D are thought to increase blood pressure through increases in intracellular free calcium and in muscle tone.[98] These observations serve to confirm the hypothesis that at least some cases of hypertension are secondary to the adaptive response to conserve calcium in a calcium deficient state.[96] Other studies showed that potassium and magnesium, nutrients abundantly supplied by fruits, vegetables, and dairy foods, may also be effective in reducing hypertension. Two meta-analyses found calcium to be significantly effective in reducing blood pressure in normotensive and hypertensive individuals, and in preventing pregnancy-induced hypertension and preeclampsia.[99,100]

The NHLBI funded DASH (Dietary Approaches to Stop Hypertension) Trial, studied the effects of dietary patterns on blood pressure, both in hypertensive and normotensive populations. The results published in the April 1997 issue of *The New England Journal of Medicine*, demonstrated that a combination diet, low in fat, and rich in fruits, vegetables, and lowfat dairy products, can substantially lower blood pressure.[101] This dietary pattern was found to be especially effective for African Americans. Among other life style modifications, the Sixth Report of the Joint National Committee on Prevention, Detection, Evaluation, and Treatment of High Blood Pressure, published in November 1997, now recommends a diet adequate in calcium, potassium, and magnesium for hypertension prevention and management.[102] The report endorses the DASH diet as used in the clinical trial, and provides the DASH eating plan and sample menu in Appendix A of the report.

The DASH diet is an attractive option for individuals seeking to control blood pressure. The DASH diet may replace or reduce the need for drug treatment for some patients. In addition, the DASH diet was effective without sodium restriction. DASH participants consumed an average of 3 grams of sodium daily.

3. Cancer

Colon cancer in susceptible persons may also be the unfortunate result of adaptation to a low calcium intake.[96] On a high calcium diet, much of the unabsorbed calcium (75 to 85%) remains in the intestinal lumen, where it forms insoluble complexes with bile acids and unabsorbed fatty acids, and protects the mucosal lining of the colon from their toxic effects. Conversely, on a low calcium diet, the body adapts by increasing calcium absorption, leaving less unabsorbed calcium reaching the colon to complex with irritant acids. This increases the likelihood that the cells lining the colon will be damaged, proliferate, and progress toward cancer.

Epidemiologic research as well as studies in animals and humans indicates that dairy foods and/or their components have a protective effect against cancer. The potential anticancer agents identified so far in dairy foods include conjugated linoleic acid (CLA), calcium, vitamin D, sphingomyelin, butyric acid, ether lipids, protein, and lactic acid bacteria.[103] Most recently, Holt et al. conducted a randomized controlled trial to evaluate whether increasing the intake of lowfat dairy foods in patients at high risk of colon cancer would normalize changes in the colon believed to be precancerous.[104] Seventy adults (average age 66 to 67 years), who had previously had an adenomatous polyp removed from their colon, were randomly assigned to either increase their intake of calcium with lowfat dairy foods to approximately 1500 mg/day or consume their normal daily diet containing about 600 to 700 mg of calcium (control group). At six and twelve months, those who consumed additional dairy foods, when compared to controls, had significantly reduced cell proliferation of the colonic mucosa; cell differentiation and maturation was significantly returned toward normal. Since dairy foods were used in the intervention, the authors do not attribute these results to calcium alone. Calcium, or any of the components of dairy foods mentioned above, could have produced the positive effect. Most recently, in a study of individuals who had had at least one adenomatous polyp removed, supplementation with 1200 mg of calcium reduced the risk of recurrent colorectal adenomas by 19% and the number of polyps by 24%.[105]

It is interesting to note that similar amounts of calcium or its equivalent in servings of Milk Group foods are being recommended for the prevention of osteoporosis (1000 to 1500 mg of calcium or 3 to 5 servings of dairy foods), and hypertension (at least 3 servings of dairy foods). Science emerging in the area of chemoprevention of cancer suggests that similar amounts of calcium/dairy foods may be protective for cancer as well. Since the sequelae of calcium deficiency appear to increase the risk of several chronic diseases, and several components of dairy foods are potentially protective, it makes sense for health practitioners to encourage a lifelong adequate intake of milk and milk products.

D. Special Needs of Women

1. Pregnancy and Lactation

During pregnancy a woman's requirement for calcium increases by approximately 33%.[106] Adequate calcium is needed to maintain maternal bone density, to mineralize infant bone, to regulate blood pressure, and to supply a readily available source of calcium in breast milk during lactation. Over the course of pregnancy, a remarkable series of physiological adjustments occur to preserve maternal bone mass, while providing for the skeletal growth of the fetus. Thus, under normal conditions and adequate calcium intake, pregnancy exerts little influence on net bone mineral content, even when calcium intake is not increased.[107] Both biochemical and clinical data suggest that increased calcium needs during pregnancy are met primarily by an increase in calcium absorption (by 50% or more), and by increased bone turnover. Although the hormones responsible for triggering these changes are still under investigation, production of 1,25-dihydroxyvitamin D may almost double, stimulating the synthesis of calcium binding protein and an increased intestinal absorption of calcium.[108]

The demand for calcium during lactation can be twice that of pregnancy. Lactating women secrete 240 to 320 mg of calcium daily in breast milk.[108] The major source of calcium for milk secretion appears to be maternal bone. Studies have shown, however, that increased intestinal absorption and renal retention of calcium in the postweaning period facilitate the recovery of bone lost during pregnancy and/or lactation.[109,110] A recent study indicates that calcium supplementation during this time may be beneficial. Kalkwarf et al. found that lactating women who received a calcium supplement of 1000 mg/day post-weaning (12 months after delivery) had a 5.9% increase in spinal bone density, which was significantly greater than the 4.4% increase in those who received a placebo.[111]

The National Academy of Sciences 1997 Dietary Reference Intake report concluded that "the maternal skeleton is not used as a reserve for fetal calcium needs . . . provided that dietary calcium intake is sufficient for maximizing bone accretion rates in the nonpregnant state."[5] Therefore, they recommend a calcium intake during pregnancy and lactation no higher than for nonpregnant women of the same age (Table 9.10). Data on the calcium intake of pregnant and lactating women, presented in the NAS report on Dietary Reference Intakes, shows that while half (median intake) are meeting the recommended intake of 1000 mg/day, many are not (Table 9.11). According to the report, roughly two thirds of pregnant adolescents and one third of pregnant adults are not meeting their AI for calcium.[5] It should be noted that although the data was statistically adjusted to account for day-to-day variation of the small number of women sampled, it is less reliable than the data for females in general.

Table 9.11 Current Calcium Intake of Females

	Calcium (mg) Percentiles		
	5th	50th	95th
9–13 years (200)	486	889	1,452
14–18 years (169)	348	413	1,293
19–30 years (302)	300	612	1,116
31–50 years (590)	297	606	1,082
51–70 years (510)	294	571	1,001
>70 years (221)	277	517	860
Pregnancy (33)	656	1,154	1,729
Lactation (16)	794	1,050	1,324

Source: CSFII, 1994

It seems unlikely that the Healthy People 2000 goal that "at least 50% of pregnant and lactating women will consume at least 3 or more servings daily of calcium-rich foods" will be met. According to USDA data (CSFII 1985-86) that was submitted to provide a baseline for the HP 2000 goal, only 24% of pregnant and/or lactating women met the goal.[112] Rather than improving over time, the 1995 to 96 Healthy People 2000 Review reported that only 22% of pregnant and/or lactating women were meeting the goal.[113]

A low intake of calcium during pregnancy and lactation (defined by NAS as 600 mg/day or less) has been associated with biochemical indices of bone resorption in the mother,[114] low bone density in the infant,[115] reduced calcium in breastmilk,[116] and increased exposure of the fetus and breast-fed infant to lead mobilized from bone.[117] The effects of maternal calcium intake on breast milk calcium and infant bone are not fully understood and require further study.[118] There is substantial evidence that adequate calcium intake is important for maintaining normal blood pressure during pregnancy and in preventing preeclampsia.[119,100] A meta-analysis of fourteen randomized trials found that calcium supplementation during pregnancy reduced the incidence of pregnancy-induced hypertension by 70% and preeclampsia by 62%.[100] However, the results of the Calcium for Preeclampsia Prevention (CPEP) trial, conducted among over 4500 pregnant women at five U.S. medical centers, found only a slight, but nonsignificant beneficial effect of 2000 mg of supplemental calcium on preeclampsia, pregnancy-associated hypertension, or other adverse outcomes of pregnancy.[120] It is difficult to reconcile these conflicting results. It may be that increasing calcium intake may be most important when baseline calcium intake is low (CPEP participants had an average calcium intake of 1000 mg/d), or for those at the highest risk for preeclampsia, such as women with diabetes or who are pregnant with twins.

Mothers who model a healthy eating pattern that includes at least 3 servings of milk and milk products both during pregnancy and afterward, can have a profound effect on a family's dietary patterns and nutrient status. A recent review reported that children's food acceptance patterns are well established by age 5 or 6, and familiarity with food plays a large role in a child's food preferences.[25] In general, children tend to prefer those foods which are served most often and therefore are the most familiar. A study conducted among urban high school students revealed that calcium intake, even in these older children, is positively related to taste enjoyment of dairy foods and whether friends and family modeled milk-drinking behavior.[121]

2. Premenstrual Syndrome (PMS)

Although there is no scientific agreement as yet that nutritional factors cause or alleviate PMS, there is some evidence suggesting that increasing dietary calcium intake may reduce PMS symptoms. For example, a double-blind cross-over trial among 33 women with PMS showed that increasing calcium intake by 1000 mg/day for three months significantly reduced PMS related symptoms.[122] In a recent multicenter trial, researchers found that women ages 18-45 who received 1200 mg of calcium/day reported a 48% decrease in premenstrual symptoms (cramping, bloating, food cravings, irritability) when compared to those who received a placebo.[123] Women suffering from PMS should be encouraged to consume a diet adequate in calcium from foods.

E. Strategies to Improve Intake

Reversing the decline in intake of calcium-rich foods, especially milk consumption, is one of the two major challenges dietitians and other health professionals face as they work as agents for behavior change, concluded participants at a multi-disciplinary seminar, "Changing Behaviors to Optimize Women's Health."[124] The other major challenge highlighted by this seminar (sponsored by the Center of Nutrition Education at the University of Wisconsin and The American Dietetic Association's Nutrition and Health Campaign for Women), was helping women of all ages change their attitudes about their bodies. This second challenge influences the first, since concerns about body weight can influence milk and dairy food intake. At this seminar, nutrition professionals were encouraged to build partnerships with patients, understand the patient, start where the patient is, and concentrate on small changes for success.[124]

Knowledge of personal characteristics associated with either meeting or not meeting calcium/dairy food recommendations is useful for developing nutrition education programs. A survey of factors influencing milk and milk product consumption among both young and elderly New Zealand women with low calcium intakes, found that among the younger women (ages 19 to 23), the main reasons given for low consumption of dairy foods were a "change in lifestyle" (i.e., leaving the family home) and "health reasons," primarily weight reduction and lowering fat intake.[125] Nearly a third of the younger women reported that the reason they did not consume dairy foods other than milk (e.g., yogurt or cheese) was their concern for calorie/fat intake and body weight. The authors conclude, that education for younger women should emphasize the availability of lowfat versions of dairy foods and that weight control does not require the exclusion of Milk Group foods from the diet. A randomized, placebo-controlled intervention study conducted among adults (ages 18 to 70) in Oregon demonstrated that calcium intake can be increased to 1500 mg/d with dairy foods without causing weight gain or increasing blood lipid levels.[126]

All but one of the young women in the above-mentioned study said they would be willing to make changes in their diets if it would improve their health. Eighty-six percent said they would drink more milk, 55 and 64% said they would eat more cheese or lowfat cheese, respectively, and 91% said they would eat more yogurt, if it would improve their health.

A study of 2261 women (not pregnant or lactating) who participated in USDA's 1990–91 Continuing Survey of Food Intakes by Individuals — Diet and Health Knowledge Survey, identified several factors positively associated with meeting the RDA for calcium from food sources.[127] According to this study, women who met or exceeded the RDA for calcium were more likely to be working part time, taking vitamin-mineral supplements, reporting avoidance of whole milk only, aware of a relationship between calcium intake and health, and to report a higher number of Milk Group servings as being recommended daily. Women who met calcium recommendations also met recommendations for magnesium, vitamin E, vitamin B_6, iron, and vitamin A, but the other women did not. This confirms earlier research that showed that women who had low intakes of calcium, also had low intakes of several other vitamins and minerals.[128] This data should encourage health professionals to continue to communicate the benefits of dairy foods for bone health, blood pressure maintenance, reduction of cancer risk, and nutrient adequacy of the diet, particularly to adult women.

A nationally representative consumer survey conducted in 1997 found that adult milk drinkers fall into three categories, those who drink milk at several meal occasions, those who drink milk at only one meal, and those who are "light" milk drinkers or use it only on cereal.[62] People in all three of these groups have common motivations for drinking milk. They like the taste of milk, they believe that milk is needed for strong bones at every stage of life, and they believe milk to be compatible with food. However, they have barriers to drinking milk in certain situations. For example, they may feel that milk is incompatible with certain foods, they may prefer another beverage with a particular meal, and they note that milk is not readily available when they are eating away from home. Health professionals can help their clients increase their intake of milk and milk products by identifying the behavioral routines and attitudes of their clients, and suggesting new ways to include these foods with their meals. For example, a person who only consumes milk with a sandwich at lunch, may be encouraged to add a café latte at breakfast, or a carton of yogurt as a between-meal snack.

As mentioned previously, men and women may believe their calcium and dairy food intake is adequate, when it actually needs improvement. Nutrition education, conducted either in a group or private counseling session, or communicated through articles in consumer publications, may help bring the consumer's perceptions closer to reality. First and foremost, communicating the many health benefits of Milk Group foods will help motivate consumers to increase their intake. Information should also focus on what constitutes a serving of dairy foods, and how many servings are needed to meet calcium recommendations. Tools that allow the client to assess their own calcium/dairy food intake may also be effective. In addition, it is important for health practitioners to assess and help remove a client's individual barriers to meeting their calcium and dairy food requirements.

VII. OLDER ADULTS

A. Characteristics

As adults age they experience a gradual functional decline in many physiological processes and changes in body composition. A majority of older adults enjoy good health, and overall, less than 17% require assistance with day-to-day activities. Aging is associated with slow declines in weight, bone mass (Figure 9.5), lean body mass, and gains in adipose tissue. For example, muscle mass declines approximately 2 to 3% per decade, contributing to a reduced basal metabolic rate. Resistance training can help preserve fat free mass and increase muscular strength in the elderly. Likewise, adequate calcium and vitamin D intakes can help slow age-related bone loss.[129]

Several of the physiological changes of aging influence the intake and metabolism of bone-related nutrients, increasing the older adult's need for these nutrients and the susceptibility to bone loss. For example, as physical activity and lean body mass decline with age, so do energy needs and food intake. Reduced food intake in the elderly contributes to low intakes of bone-related nutrients, including calcium,

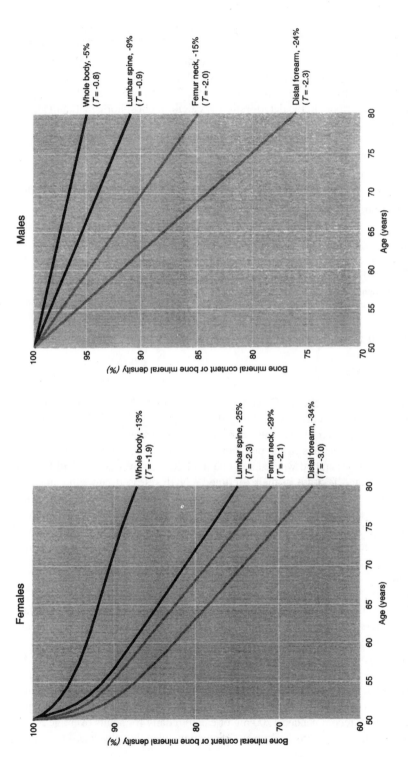

Figure 9.5 Percentage loss of bone at four different sites as a function of age in men and women. (From FAO Food, Nutrition, and Agriculture Division, *Food, Nutrition, and Agriculture: Calcium Throughout Life*, 20, 15, 1997. With permission.)

vitamin D, phosphorus, and protein.[130] Calcium absorption and the renal conservation of calcium decreases with aging, increasing its requirement. Reduced sun exposure, impaired renal conversion of the circulating form of vitamin D [25(OH)D] to the active form [1, 25(OH)$_2$D], and partial intestinal resistance to the active form of vitamin D, increases the requirement of vitamin D with age (Table 9.12). All of these changes contribute to the deterioration of calcium, phosphorus, vitamin D, and protein nutriture often seen in older adults.[130]

Table 9.12 Calcium and Vitamin D Recommendations for Older Adults

NIH (Expert Panel)		NAS		
Age	Calcium (mg)	Age	Calcium (mg)	Vitamin D (IU)
Men up to 65 years				
Women over 50 years on estrogen	1,000	51–70 years	1,200	400
		> 70 years	1,200	600
Men and women over 65 years and women over 50 years not on estrogen	1,500			

From National Institutes of Health Expert Panel and Dietary Reference Intakes, 1994; National Academy of Sciences, 1997.

B. Milk Group Foods and the Reduction of Chronic Disease Risk

1. Osteoporosis

According to the National Osteoporosis Foundation (NOF), "osteoporosis is reaching epidemic proportions in the elderly population."[131] The incidence of osteoporosis is expected to rise with increasing life expectancy and the increasing number of older Americans in the population. Eighty percent of those affected are women, however one in two women and one in eight men over age 50 will have an osteoporosis related fracture in their lifetime.[132] NOF released new guidelines for the physician in the prevention and treatment of osteoporosis. The guidelines included universal recommendations for adequate intake of calcium and vitamin D, regular weight-bearing exercise, and the avoidance of tobacco use and alcohol abuse.[131] Chapter 5 has additional information on osteoporosis risk in this age group.

a. Calcium

Both the National Institutes of Health (NIH) Expert Panel and the National Academy of Sciences (NAS) recognize that the calcium requirement increases with age (Table 9.12). In 1994, an NIH Expert Panel recommended optimal calcium intakes for the prevention of osteoporosis.[6] They recommended 1000 mg of calcium daily for postmenopausal women over age 50 on estrogen replacement therapy and for men up to 65 years. They recommended 1500 mg of calcium daily for all men and women over age 65 years, and for postmenopausal women over age 50 years not on estrogen. In 1997, the NAS recommended 1200 mg of calcium daily for adults over age 50.[5] In 1998, the National Osteoporosis Foundation recommended that physicians encourage a calcium intake of at least 1200 mg daily for all their patients, both to prevent and treat osteoporosis.[131] They state, as does the NIH Expert Panel, that calcium-rich foods should be the primary source of calcium, and that calcium supplements be used only when "an adequate dietary intake cannot be achieved."[131]

Calcium intakes for older adults age 50 and above are critically low, and decrease slightly with age. Older men's mean calcium intakes are close to 800 mg/day, while women's are roughly 600 mg/day. To correct the calcium deficit, older men would need to consume roughly one additional serving of milk, yogurt, or cheese, and women would need to consume about two additional servings. According to USDA data, 85% of males ages 50 to 59 and 87% of men over age 60 are not meeting current calcium recommendations. These intakes are comparable to the critically low intakes of teenage girls. Calcium intakes of older women are even worse; few women meet recommendations. Ninety five percent of women ages 50 to 59 and 96% of women over age 60 are not meeting current calcium recommendations.

Since nutritional status clearly influences the rate of physiological and functional declines with age,[133] such a large calcium deficit in the elderly population is likely to accelerate rates of bone loss and increase the risk of fracture and disability. Conversely, clinical trials in which older adults were given calcium and/or vitamin D supplements (1000 to 1700 mg of calcium per day) have demonstrated a significant reduction in age-related bone loss, and incidence of fractures.[134,135,136] According to Heaney, "many of the features of the calcium economy in the older adult which we had once attributed to age, turn out to be manifestations of calcium privation."[130]

a. Vitamin D

Because of the vital role vitamin D plays in calcium absorption, poor vitamin D status profoundly affects bone and mineral metabolism, increasing the risk of osteomalacia and fracture.[133] Many older adults are deficient in vitamin D as indicated by low blood levels of the circulating form, 25-hydroxyvitamin D, especially those who are homebound or institutionalized.[137] Deficiency is a result of a lack of exposure to sunlight, the age-related decrease in both cutaneous and endogenous synthesis of vitamin D, and a low dietary intake of vitamin D. Fortified milk is one of the few dietary sources of vitamin D; it is voluntarily fortified to a level of 400 IU per quart. However, older adults consume little milk. Men and women over age 50 consume little more than a half cup of milk daily (120 to 187 grams).[24] A number of studies indicate that increasing the vitamin D intake of older adults (either alone or with calcium) reduces bone loss and risk of fractures.[134,136,138]

The latest recommendations for vitamin D intake for older adults is two to three times higher than that for younger adults and children, and higher than the previous RDAs set in 1989. Currently, 400 IU/day is recommended for adults ages 51 to 70, and 600 IU is recommended for adults over age 70 (Table 9.12).[5] Older adults who drink more milk will increase both their calcium and vitamin D intake and improve their bone health, though vitamin D supplementation may be needed to meet recommendations. Vitamin D expert, Dr. Michael Holick, says that older adults can satisfy their vitamin D needs by exposing their hands, arms, and face briefly to sunlight two or three times a week.[139] Those who choose to get a little more sunlight by walking outdoors, should apply sunscreen after the initial exposure. Walking outdoors will maintain muscle tone and increase bone strength as well as improve vitamin D status.

b. Protein

Although protein intake in the adult is usually more than sufficient, in the older adult it is often low.[130] In fact protein malnutrition is prevalent in hip fracture patients. Heaney sites two clinical trials in which hip fracture patients who were supplemented with protein, averted some of the bad outcomes associated with hip fracture, namely death and institutionalization.[130] In a recent randomized, double-blind, placebo-controlled trial, elderly persons with hip fracture who were given a protein supplement supplying 250 kcals and 20 g of protein (90% milk proteins) had less bone loss, improved muscle strength, and reduced length of stay in a rehabilitation hospital.[140] In addition, intake of dietary protein, especially from animal sources, was associated with reduced incidence of hip fracture in a group of postmenopausal women in the Iowa Women's Health Study.[141]

It is unclear whether preventing protein malnutrition will prevent fracture. Some have suggested that older adults utilize protein less efficiently, so need more protein per kilogram of body weight than younger adults. For example, Campbell et al. recommends that older adults consume 1.0 to 1.25 g/kg/day of high quality protein, rather than the RDA of 0.8 g/kg/day.[142] Dairy foods, meat, and eggs provide high quality protein, as well as many other essential nutrients needed by older adults.

2. Hypertension

Hypertension is very common among older Americans. As in younger patients, hypertension therapy, as outlined in the Sixth Report of the Joint National Committee on Prevention, Detection, Evaluation, and Treatment of High Blood Pressure, should begin with life style modifications that include consuming adequate amounts of calcium, magnesium, and potassium in a diet rich in lowfat dairy foods, fruits, and vegetables.[102] See complete discussion in the adult section of this chapter.

3. Cancer

The risk of developing cancer increases with age, as does the risk of all chronic diseases. Emerging research in this area is showing a protective benefit for dairy foods and/or their components in reducing the risk of some cancers. See complete discussion in adult section.

C. Strategies to Improve Intake

Many older Americans would benefit by increasing their intake of milk and milk products to recommended levels. Eating more dairy foods would not only help reduce the risk of developing chronic diseases such as osteoporosis, hypertension, and possibly cancer, but will help improve nutritional status. Also of interest to older adults are the preliminary results from a study in Georgia showing that age-related hearing loss may be associated with poor bone health and low intakes of calcium.[143] Adequate intakes of calcium, protein, vitamin D, and vitamin B_{12} are of concern in the elderly population. Dairy foods are an abundant source of these and other nutrients (vitamin D in fortified milk only), so are an important way to help older adults meet their requirements.

Attention to diet and nutrition tends to increase steadily with age. A recent survey found that by 65 years of age, 39% agree with the statement "I am very careful about the foods I eat."[79] This is a decline from 45% reported in 1994, but is still higher than the number of younger adults who agree. Therefore, older adults may be the most receptive to information geared to improving their calcium intake. Even a brief educational intervention resulted in a significantly increased calcium intake in persons over age 60.[144]

Adults over age 65 may be the biggest challenge for the nutrition professional who wants to encourage clients to meet calcium recommendations with food. Adults over age 65 have higher calcium requirements, but lower energy needs compared to younger adults. Therefore, nutrition education for the elderly should focus on the value of high quality, nutrient-dense foods.[133] Due to reduced physical activity, the prevalence of obesity among older persons is growing, but their food and nutrient intake may be declining.[145] The overweight elderly should be encouraged to increase their physical activity and be taught how to eat a high calcium, but low calorie diet.

A recent study emphasized the need for caution when educating older Americans about decreasing their fat intake. After receiving advice and education materials on dietary fat reduction, adults 45 to 59 years of age increased their fruit and vegetable intake, but adults 60 to 75 years of age significantly *decreased* their intake of fruits and vegetables.[146] More than half of the 60 to 75 year olds also consumed less than two thirds of their recommended intake for calcium and 45% exhibited low vitamin D intakes. The authors concluded that educational materials for dietary fat reduction should contain balanced eating messages, to prevent the restriction of nutrient-dense foods such as dairy foods. As discussed earlier, a diet rich in fruits, vegetables, and lowfat dairy products is recommended for the prevention of hypertension.[102]

A study involving 100 postmenopausal women over age 50, recruited from three midwestern churches, evaluated how attitudes toward health promotion affect osteoporosis preventive behaviors, such as calcium intake and exercise.[147] They found that women who perceived greater benefits and fewer barriers to calcium intake tended to consume a greater amount of milk. Women who consumed the most calcium-rich foods perceived themselves as more self-efficacious (believed their actions could influence their health), believed health was internally controlled or influenced by significant others (such as physicians), perceived themselves to be in good health, and perceived fewer barriers to calcium intake. The authors conclude that, "Effective education about osteoporosis prevention needs to emphasize the required daily calcium amount for postmenopausal women, provide examples of the calcium content of calcium-rich foods, educate women about supplements, assess and address individual barriers, explain benefits, and use research findings to support information provided."[147]

A telephone survey of 495 of older adults, ages 60 to 94 years found that nutrition knowledge was positively associated with drinking fat free and 1% milk and with drinking milk more often.[148] Total milk consumption was positively influenced by consumption of milk during youth and negatively influenced by a perception of milk intolerance. The authors state that a self-report of milk intolerance is not a clinical diagnosis of lactase non-persistence. Research has shown that most of those who perceive themselves intolerant to milk can tolerate up to four servings of dairy foods (milk, yogurt with active cultures, and aged cheese) per day with minimal symptoms, and can meet even the highest calcium requirement for older adults (1500 mg/d) with dairy foods.[149] In this study, 1300 mg of the total 1500 mg of calcium in the diet was provided by dairy foods. Education about strategies for including dairy foods in the diet of those with perceived milk intolerance is important to assure adequate calcium and dairy food intake among both older and younger adults. (See Chapter 8 for more information about lactose intolerance.)

In a study of New Zealand women with low calcium intakes, a major barrier to improving calcium/dairy food intake in elderly women was the common misperception that increasing the intake of milk or milk products will have either no effect or an adverse effect on health.[125] The health reasons mentioned by the older women included lowering fat and cholesterol intake, kidney stones, asthma, and pancreatic problems. Thirteen percent of all participants (young and older) reported they had been advised by their doctors not to consume milk or milk products. The elderly women said their doctors advised against consuming dairy foods to reduce cholesterol intake or mucus production, to ameliorate kidney or pancreatic problems, or for the management of bronchitis, diabetes, or a heart condition. The authors conclude that "there is a need to actively counter misconceptions concerning the adverse effects of milk or milk products on medical conditions, particularly amongst elderly women."[125] Several studies, discussed in the concluding section of Chapter 5, highlight calcium's effectiveness at reducing the risk of kidney stones.

Older Americans should be encouraged to use food first, rather than supplements to meet their calcium needs because older adults often have low intakes of several nutrients that milk and milk products can supply. For those who are not able to consistently obtain enough calcium from dairy foods, a judicious use of calcium-fortified foods or a calcium supplement is preferable to neglecting the difference. A four-year longitudinal study among 64 postmenopausal women in Australia demonstrated the value of fat free milk at improving diet quality.[150] When compared to the women who took a calcium supplement (1000 mg/day in addition to diet), those who increased their calcium intake to 1600 mg/day with fat free milk also significantly increased their intakes of protein, potassium, magnesium, phosphorus, riboflavin, thiamin, and zinc. They did so without increasing their total fat or saturated fat intake. In an accompanying editorial, Robert Heaney, MD, world-renowned calcium researcher from Creighton University in Omaha, Nebraska, emphasizes that "Diets low in calcium are typically low in other nutrients, too.[151] When you drink milk, you're getting an entire nutrient package." He chastised nutrition practitioners for having a "defeatist attitude toward encouraging increased milk consumption and a too easy acceptance of supplements."[151]

Based on the documented concerns of older adults, nutrition initiatives to increase the consumption of calcium-rich foods might contain the following elements:

- Design educational materials to appeal to both men and women. A survey of over 400 older Americans (ages 55 to 89) found no gender-related differences in health concerns or behaviors. Eighty-five percent of older married men shopped for food and 84% cooked at least part of the time.[152]
- Present information about the benefits of milk and milk products for reducing the risk of several chronic diseases, including osteoporosis, hypertension, and possibly cancer, and improving the quality of their latter years. Actively counter any misinformation they may have received about adverse health effects of milk.
- Compare the calcium, fat, and calorie content of various calcium-rich foods. Weight control ranked second among the diet concerns of the elderly.[152] Provide clients with sample high calcium, low calorie menus; help them customize the menus to their own taste preferences.
- Discuss how Milk Group foods can improve the nutrient adequacy of the total diet. In a screening initiative designed to identify older adults at nutritional risk, over one third said they ate few fruits and vegetables, and drank little milk.[153] A majority of those surveyed had inadequate (<75% of the RDA) calcium intakes and 40% had inadequate intakes of vitamin A – both nutrients provided by dairy foods.
- Discuss the client's attitudes toward health promotion in general and perceptions of barriers to milk intake. Strategize with the client to overcome these barriers.

VIII. CONCLUSION

An adequate intake of milk and milk products as part of a healthy, balanced diet, is needed throughout the lifespan to promote health. Milk and milk products contain a high calcium content, substantial amounts of other essential nutrients, and health-promoting components. Because of their unique nutritional package, dairy foods contribute significantly to the nutritional adequacy of the diets of children and adults. Research has established the benefit of dairy foods for reducing the risk of chronic diseases, such as osteoporosis, hypertension, and possibly some cancers. Results from human clinical trials suggest that dairy foods, with their unique nutritional profile, may be more effective than a single nutrient (i.e. calcium, potassium, magnesium, vitamin D) for reducing the risk of hypertension and colon cancer.

Unfortunately, the consumption of dairy foods by many Americans is grossly inadequate – particularly among females and the elderly. As this century is coming to a close, we are moving away, rather than toward, the Healthy People 2000 goal for at least 50% of people ages 11 to 24 and pregnant and lactating women to consume at least three servings of calcium-rich foods daily, and for those 25 years of age and older to consume two or more servings. Although educational efforts are important for all age groups, children in particular deserve special attention. Increasing dairy food consumption to recommended levels in children and adolescents, and physical activity, appears to be the most effective strategy for reducing the risk of osteoporosis later in life. It affords the best chance to influence peak bone mass and to establish eating habits that will continue throughout life. To turn this tide, we will need a concerted effort of governmental agencies, industry sponsors, individual health professionals, and the media, to educate consumers about the important health benefits of milk and milk products and to address personal and social barriers to their consumption.

REFERENCES

1. Mitchell, M. K., Nutrition during infancy, In: *Nutrition Across the Lifespan*, Philadelphia, W.B. Saunders, 1997, 76.
2. American Academy of Pediatrics, Work Group on Breastfeeding, Breastfeeding and the use of human milk, *Pediatrics*, 100, 1035, 1997.
3. Nutrition Committee of the Canadian Paediatric Society and the Committee on Nutrition of the American Academy of Pediatrics, Breastfeeding: a commentary in celebration of the International Year of the Child, 1979, *Pediatrics*, 65, 591-601, 1978.
4. Committee on Nutrition, American Academy of Pediatrics, Breastfeeding, in, *Pediatric Nutrition Handbook, Fourth Edition*, Kleinman, R. E., Ed., American Academy of Pediatrics, Elk Grove Village, IL, 1998, 3.
5. Food and Nutrition Board/Institute of Medicine, Dietary Reference Intakes, Calcium, phosphorus, magnesium, vitamin D, and fluoride, National Academy Press, Washington, D.C., 1997.
6. NIH Consensus Conference, Optimal Calcium Intake, *JAMA*, 272(24), 1942, 1994.
7. Committee on Nutrition, American Academy of Pediatrics, Formula feeding of term infants, In, *Pediatric Nutrition Handbook, Fourth Edition*, Kleinman, R. E., Ed., American Academy of Pediatrics, Elk Grove Village, IL, 1998, 31.
8. American Academy of Pediatrics, Committee on Nutrition, The use of whole cow's milk in infancy, *Pediatrics*, 89, 1105, 1992.
9. Committee on Nutrition, American Academy of Pediatrics, Food sensitivity, In, *Pediatric Nutrition Handbook, Fourth Edition*, Kleinman, R. E., Ed., American Academy of Pediatrics, Elk Grove Village, IL, 1998, 469.
10. Host, A., Cow's Milk Allergy, *J. Royal Society of Med.*, 90 (Suppl. 30), 34, 1997.
11. Zeiger, R. S., Dietary manipulations in infants and their mothers and the natural course of atopic disease, *Pediat. Allerg. Immunol.*, 5 (Suppl. 1), 33, 1994.
12. Baumgartner, M., Brown, C. A., Secretin, M-C, van't Hof, M., and Haschke, F., Controlled trials investigating the use of one partially hydrolyzed whey formula for dietary prevention of atopic manifestations until 60 months of age: an overview using meta-analytical methods, *Nutr. Res.*, 18(8), 1425, 1998.
13. Chandra, R. K., Five-year follow up of high risk infants with family history of allergy exclusively breast-fed or fed partial whey hydrolysate, soy and conventional cow's milk formulas, *Nutr. Res.*, 18(8), 1395, 1998.
14. Fritsche, R., Induction of oral tolerance to cow's milk proteins in rats fed with a whey protein hydrolysate, *Nutr. Res.*, 18(8), 1335, 1998.
15. Halken, S. and Host, A., Prevention of allergic disease: Exposure to food allergens and dietetic intervention, *Pediatr. Allerg. Immunol.*, 7 (Suppl. 9), 102, 1996.
16. Committee on Nutrition, American Academy of Pediatrics, Human milk and standard milk-based infant formulas, In, *Pediatric Nutrition Handbook, Fourth Edition*, Kleinman, R. E., Ed., American Academy of Pediatrics, Elk Grove Village, IL, American Academy of Pediatrics, 1998, Appendix E.

17. Committee on Nutrition, American Academy of Pediatrics, Supplemental foods for infants, In, *Pediatric Nutrition Handbook, Fourth Edition*, Kleinman, R. E., Ed., American Academy of Pediatrics, Elk Grove Village, IL, 1998, 43.

18. Mitchell, M. K., Nutrition during infancy, In, *Nutrition Across the Lifespan*, W. B. Saunders, Philadelphia, 1997, 98.

19. Personal communication with Ray Coteras, Director of the Committee on Nutrition, the American Academy of Pediatrics, June 1998.

20. Guerin-Danan, C., Chabanet, C., Pedone, C., Popot, F., Vaissade, P., Bouley, C., Szylit, O., and Andrieux, C., Milk fermented with yogurt cultures and Lactobacillus casei compared with yogurt and gelled milk: influence on intestinal microflora in healthy infants, *Am. J. Clin. Nutr.*, 67, 111, 1998.

21. Mitchell, M. K., Nutrition during growth: preschool and school years, In, *Nutrition Across the Lifespan*, Philadelphia, W. B. Saunders, 1997, Chapter 6.

22. Committee on Nutrition, American Academy of Pediatrics, Feeding from age 1 to adolescence, In, *Pediatric Nutrition Handbook, Fourth Edition*, Kleinman, R. E., Ed., W. B. Saunders, Elk Grove Village, IL, 1998, Chapter 8.

23. Fleming, K. H. and Heimbach, J. T., Consumption of calcium in the U.S.: food sources and intake levels, *J. Nutr.*, 124, 1426S, 1994.

24. Agricultural Research Service/U. S. Department of Agriculture, *Continuing Survey of Food Intakes of Individuals and Diet and Health Knowledge Survey*, Food Surveys Research Group, Beltsville Human Nutrition Research Center, 1994-96.

25. Birch, L. L., Children's food acceptance patterns, *J. Nutr.*, 31(6), 234, 1997.

26. Pugliese, M. T., Weyman-Daum, M., Moses, N., Lifshitz, F., Parental health beliefs as a cause on nonorganic failure to thrive, *Pediatrics*, 80, 175, 1987.

27. U. S. Department of Agriculture/Department of Health and Human Services, *Nutrition and Your Health: Dietary Guidelines for Americans, 4th Edition*, Home and Garden Bulletin No. 232, U. S. Government Printing Office, Washington, D.C., December 1995.

28. Joint Working Group of the Canadian Paediatric Society and Health Canada, Nutrition recommendations update: dietary fats and children, *Nutr. Rev.*, 53(12), 367, 1995.

29. Zlotkin, S. H., A review of the Canadian "Nutrition Recommendations Update: Dietary Fat and Children," *J. Nutr.*, 126(Suppl.), 1022, 1996.

30. Timely Statement of the American Dietetic Association: Dietary guidance for healthy children, *J. Am. Diet. Assoc.*, 95(3), 370, 1995.

31. Smith, M. M. and Lifshitz, F., Excess fruit juice consumption as a contributing factor in nonorganic failure to thrive, *Pediatrics*, 93(3), 438, 1994.

32. Dennison, B. A., Rockwell, H. L., Baker, S. L., Excess fruit juice consumption by preschool-aged children is associated with short stature and obesity, *Pediatrics*, 88(1), 15, 1997.

33. Skinner, J. D., Carruth, B. R., Moran III, J., JHouck, K., and Coletta, F., Fruit juice intake is not related to children's growth, *Pediatrics*, 103(1), 58, 1999.

34. Centers for Disease Control, Update: Blood lead levels – United States, 1991–1994, *JAMA*, 277(13), 1031, 1997.

35. Miller, G. D. and Groziak, S., Essential and nonessential mineral interactions, In, *Handbook of Human Toxicology*, Massaro, E. J., Miller, G. D., Kang, Y. J., Morgan, D. L., Rodgers, K. E., and Schardein, J. L., Eds., CRC Press, Boca Raton, FL, July 1997.

36. Haan, M. N., Gerson, M., and Zishka, B. A., Identification of children at risk for lead poisoning: An evaluation of routine pediatric blood lead screening in an HMO-insured population, *Pediatrics*, 97(1), 79, 1996.

37. Centers for Disease Control, Preventing lead poisoning in young children, Atlanta: U.S. Department of Health and Human Services, October 1991.

38. Sargent, J. D., The role of nutrition in the prevention of lead poisoning in children, *Pediatr. Ann.*, 23(11), 636, 1994.

39. Abrams, S.A. and Stuff, J. E., Calcium metabolism in girls: current dietary intakes lead to low rates of calcium absorption and retention during puberty, *Am. J. Clin. Nutr.*, 60, 739, 1994.

40. Goulding, A., Cannan, R., Williams, S. M., Gold, E. J., Taylor, R. W., and Lewis-Barned, N. J., Bone mineral density in girls with forearm fractures, *J. Bone Miner. Res.*, 13(1), 143, 1998.

41. U.S. Department of Health and Human Services, Public Health Service, *Healthy People 2000, 1995–96,* DHHS Publ. No. (PHS) 96-1256, Hyattsville, MD, November 1996.

42. Jenkins, G. N., Cheese as a protection against dental caries, *Nutr. Q.*, 13, 33, 1990.

43. Bowen, W. H. and Pearson, S. K., Effect of milk on cariogenesis, *Caries Res.*, 27, 461, 1993.

44. Vacca-Smith, A. M., Van Wuyckhuyse, B. C., Tabak, L. A., and Bowen, W. H., The effect of milk and casein proteins on the adherence of *Streptococcus mutans* to saliva-coated hydroxyapatite, *Arch. Oral Biology*, 39(12), 1063, 1994.

45. Paolino, V. J. and Kashket, S., Inhibition of cocoa extracts of biosynthesis of extra-cellular polysaccharide by human oral bacteria, *Arch. Oral Biology*, 30(4), 359, 1985.

46. American Academy of Pediatrics, Nutrition and oral health, In, *Pediatric Nutrition Handbook, Fourth Edition*, Kleinman, R. E., Ed., American Academy of Pediatrics, Elk Grove Village, IL, 1998, Chapter 35.

47. Subar, A. F., Krebs-Smith, S. M., Cook, A., and Kahle, L. L., Dietary sources of nutrients among US children, 1989–91, *Pediatrics*, 102(4), 913, 1998.

48. Borrud, L., Enns, C. W., and Mickle, S., What we eat: USDA surveys food consumption changes, *Nutrition Week, Community Nutrition Institute*, 4, April 18, 1997.

49. Margarey, A., Seal, L., and Boulton, J., Calcium, fat, and the p. s. ratio in children's diets: a mixed public health message?, *Austr. J. Nutr. Diet.*, 48, 58, 1991.

50. Johnson, R. K. and Wang, M. Q., Decrease fat, increase calcium, a mixed nutrition message for school-aged children?, *Am. J. Health Studies,* 13(4), 174, 1997.

51. Katz, F., New sophistication marks school lunch and breakfast programs, *Food Technol.*, 52(9), 60, 1998.

52. United States Government, National School Lunch Act, P.L. 103-448 as amended, 11, 1994.

53. DMI, Milk Consumption Tracking Studies, 1990. 1991, 1996.

54. DMI, Milk Consumption Tracking Benchmark Study, Oct-Dec, 1997.

55. Ortega, R. M, Requejo, A. M., Lopez-Sobaler, A. M., Andres, P., Quintas, M. E., Navia, B., Izquierdo, M., and Rivas, T., The importance of breakfast in meeting daily recommended calcium intake in a group of school children, *J. Am. Coll. Nutr.*, 17(1), 19, 1998.

56. Miller, G. D., Forgac, T., Cline, T., and McBean, L., Breakfast benefits children in the U.S. and abroad, *J. Am. Coll. Nutr.*, 17(1), 4, 1998

57. Hanes, S., Vermeersch, J., Gale, S., The national evaluation of school nutrition programs: program impact on dietary intake, *Am. J. Clin. Nutr.*, 40, 390, 1984.

58. Mathematica Policy Research, Inc., The School Nutrition Dietary Assessment Study, Princeton, NJ, Food and Nutrition Service, U.S. Department of Agriculture, 1993.

59. Johnson, R. K., Panely, C., and Wang, M. Q., The association between noon beverage consumption and diet quality of school-age children, *J. Child Nutr. Manage.t*, 22(2), 95, 1998.

60. Groziak, S. M., Boning up on calcium, *School Foodservice and Nutrition*, 23, November 1998.

61. DMI Children's Chocolate Milk Survey, conducted by McDonald Research, May 1998.

62. DMI, Consumer Segmentation Study, 1997.

63. Wolraich, M. L., Wilson, D. B., White, J. W., The effect of sugar on behavior or cognition in children: a meta-analysis, *JAMA*, 274(20), 1617, 1995.

64. Bowen, W. J. and Pearson, S. K., Effect of milk on cariogenesis, *Caries Res.*, 27, 461, 1993.

65. Recker, R. R., Bammi, A., Barger-Lux, M. J., and Heaney, R. P., Calcium absorbability from milk products, an imitation milk, and calcium carbonate, *Am. J. Clin. Nutr.*, 47, 93, 1988.

66. Lee, C. M. and Hardy, C. M., Cocoa feeding and human lactose intolerance, *Am. J. Clin. Nutr.*, 49(5), 840, 1989.

67. Grove, T. M., Heimbach, J. T., Douglass, J. S., Doyle, E., DiRienzo, D. B., and Miller, G. D., Nutritional contribution of flavored milks and alternative beverages in the diets of children, *FASEB J.*, 12(4), A225, abstract #1316, 1998.

68. Panley, C. V., Johnson, R. K., Wang, M. Q., Predictors of milk consumption in U.S. school-aged children: Evidence from the 1994-95 USDA Continuing Survey of Food Intakes by Individuals, *J. Am. Diet. Assoc.*, 98(9), A-52, 1998.

69. Chan, G. M., Hoffman, K., and McMurry, M., Effects of dairy products on bone and body composition in pubertal girls, *J. Pediatr.*, 126, 551, 1995.

70. Cadogan, J., Eastell, R., Jones, N., and Barker, M. E., Milk intake and bone mineral acquisition in adolescent girls: randomized, controlled intervention trial, *Br. Med. J.*, 315, 1255, 1997.

71. Gong, E.J. and Heald, F. P., Diet, nutrition, and adolescence, In, *Modern Nutrition in Health and Disease*, 8th edition, Shils, M. E., Olsen, J. A., and Shike, M., Eds., Lea & Febiger, Philadelphia, 1994, 759-69.

72. Wotecki, C. E. and Filer, L. J., dietary issues and nutritional status of American children, In, *Child, Health, Nutrition, and Physical Activity*, Ceung, L. W. Y., and Richmond, J. B., Eds., Human Kinetics, 1995, 3-40.

73. Weaver, C. M., Peacock, M., Martin, B. R., Plawecki, K. L., and McCabe, G. P., Calcium retention estimated from indicators of skeletal status in adolescent girls and young women, *Am. J. Clin. Nutr.*, 64, 67, 1996.

74. Gunnes, M., Bone mineral density in the cortical and trabecular distal forearm in healthy children and adolescents, *Acta Paediatrics*, 83, 463, 1994.

75. Barr, S. I. and McKay, H. A., Nutrition, exercise, and bone status in youth, *Int. J. Sport Nutr.*, 8, 124, 1998.

76. Skiba, A., Loghmani, E., and Orr, D. P., Nutritional screening and guidance for adolescents, *Adolescent Health Update*, 9(2), 3, 1997.

77. Albertson, A. M., Tobelmann, R. C., Marquart, L., Estimated dietary calcium intake and food sources for adolescent females: 1980-92, *J. Adolescent Health*, 20, 20, 1997.

78. Harel, Z., Riggs, S., Vaz, R., White, L, and Menzies, G., Adolescents and calcium: what they do and do not know and how much they consume, *J. Adolescent Health*, 22, 225, 1998.

79. Dairy Management, Inc., Attitude and Usage Trends Study, 1998.

80. Teenage Research Unlimited, National Teen Nutrition Quantitative Research Final Report, June 1996.

81. Chapman, G. and Maclean, H., "Junk food" and "healthy food": meanings of food in adolescent women's culture, *J. Nutr. Educ.*, 25(3), 108, 1993.

82. Jacobson, M. F., Liquid candy: How soft drinks are harming Americans' health, www.cspinet.org/sodapop/liquid-candy.htm, October 22, 1998.

83. Wyshak, G. and Frisch, R. E., Carbonated beverages, dietary calcium, the dietary calcium/phosphorus ratio and bone fractures in girls and boys, *J. Adolescent Health*, 15, 210, 1994.

84. Pugliese, M.T., Lifshitz, F., Grad, G., Fort, P., and Marks-Katz, M., Fear of obesity: a cause of short stature and delayed puberty, *New England J. Med.*, 309, 513, 1983.

85. Polivy, J., Psychological consequences of food restriction, *J. Am. Diet. Assoc.*, 96, 589, 1996.

86. Epstein, L. H., Coleman, K. J., and Myers, M. D., Exercise in treating obesity in children and adolescents, *Med. Sci. Sports Exer.*, 28(4), 428, 1996.

87. "Notes from the Scientific Department – Special Report: Vegetarian Resource Group conducts Roper poll on eating habits of youths," *Vegetarian Journal*, November/December, 1995.

88. Tatiana , R., More teenagers forsaking meat: diet's shortcomings draw concern, advice on healthy nutrition, *Boston Globe*, December 7, 1997.

89. The American Academy of Pediatrics, Nutritional aspects of vegetarian diets, In, *Pediatric Nutrition Handbook, Fourth edition*, Kleinman, R. E., Ed., American Academy of Pediatrics, Elk Grove Village, IL, 1998, Chapter 40.

90. Story, M. and Alton, I., Nutrition issues and adolescent pregnancy, *Nutr. Today*, 30(4), 142, 1995.

91. Chan, G. M., McMurry, M., Westover, K., Engelbert-Fenton, K., and Thomas, M. R., Effects on increased dietary calcium intake upon the calcium and bone mineral status of lactating adolescent and adult women, *Am. J. Clin. Nutr.*, 46, 319, 1987.

92. Lytle, L., Nutrition education for school-aged children: a review of research, prepared for: U.S. Department of Agriculture, Food and Consumer Service, Office of Analysis and Evaluation, September 1994.

93. Mitchell, M. K., Adult years, In, *Nutrition Across the Lifespan*, W. B. Saunders, Philadelphia, 1997, Chapter 11.

94. Haapasalo, H., Kannus, P., Sievanen, H. Pasanen, M., Uusi-Rasi, K., Heinonen, A., Oja, P., and Vuori, I., Development of mass, density, and estimated mechanical characteristics of bones in Caucasian females, *J. Bone Min. Res.*, 11, 1751, 1996.

95. Heaney, R. P. and Barger-Lux, J., Low calcium intake: the culprit in many chronic diseases, *J. Dairy Sci.*, 77, 1155, 1994.

96. McCarron, D. A., Lipkin, M., Rivlin, R. S., and Heaney, R.P., Dietary calcium and chronic diseases, *Med. Hypoth.*, 31, 265, 1990.

97. McCarron, D. A., Pingree, P. A., Rubin, R. J., Gaucher, S. M., Molitch, M., and Krutzik, S., Enhanced parathyroid function in essential hypertension: a homeostatic response to a urinary calcium leak, *Hypertension*, 2, 162, 1980.

98. Sowers, J. R., Zemel, M. B., Zemel, P. C., and Standley, R. P., Calcium metabolism and dietary calcium in salt sensitive hypertension, *Am. J. Hypertension*, 4, 557, 1991.

99. Bucher, H. C., Cook, R. J., Guyatt, G. H., Lang, J. D., Cook, D. J., Hatala, R., and Hunt, D. L., Effects of dietary calcium supplementation on blood pressure, *JAMA*, 275(13), 1016, 1996.

100. Bucher, H. C., Cook, R. J., Guyatt, G. H., Lang, J. D., Cook, D. J., Hatala, R., and Hunt, D. L., Effects of dietary calcium supplementation on blood pressure, *JAMA*, 275(14), 1113, 1996.

101. Appel, L. J., Moore, T. J., Obarzanek, E., Vollmer, W. M., Svetkey, L. P., Sacks, F. M., Bray, G. A., Vogt, T. M., Cutler, J. A., Windauser, M. M., Lin, P-H., and Karanja, N., A clinical trial of the effects of dietary patterns on blood pressure, *N. Engl. J. Med.*, 336, 1117, 1997.

102. National Institutes of Health, National Heart, Lung, and Blood Institute, *The Sixth report of the Joint National Committee on Prevention, Detection, Evaluation, and Treatment of High Blood Pressure*, NIH Publication No. 98-4080, November 1997.

103. National Dairy Council, New perspectives on diet and cancer, *Dairy Council Digest*, September/October 1997.

104. Holt, P. R., Atillasoy, E. O., Gilman, J., Guss, J., Moss, S. F., Newmark, H., Fan, K., Yang, K., and Lipkin, M., Modulation of abnormal colonic epithelial cell proliferation and differentiation by low-fat dairy foods, *JAMA*, 280(12), 1074, 1998.

105. Baron, J. A., Beach, M., Mandel, J. S., VanStolk, R. U., Haile, R. W., Sandler, R. S., Rothstein, R., Summers, R. W., Snover, D. C., Back, G. J., Bond, J. H., and Greenberg, E. R., Calcium supplements for the prevention of colorectal adenomas, *N. Engl. J. Med.*, 340(2), 101, 1999.

106. Repke, J. T., Calcium homeostasis in pregnancy, *Clin. Obstetr. and Gynecology*, 37(1), 59, 1994.

107. Pitkin, R. M., Calcium metabolism in pregnancy and the perinatal period: A review, *Am. J. Obstetr. Gynecology*, 151, 99, 1985.

108. King, J. C., Halloran, B. P., Huq, N., Diamond, T., and Buckendahl, P. E., Calcium metabolism during pregnancy and lactation, In, *Mechanisms Regulating Lactation and Infant Nutrient Utilization,* Wiley-Liss, New York, 1992, 129-146.

109. Kalkwarf, H. J. and Specker, B. L., Bone mineral loss during lactation and recovery after weaning, *Obstet. and Gynecol.*, 86, 26, 1995.

110. Cross, N. A., Hillman, L. S., Allen, S. H., Krause, G. F., and Vierira, N. E., Calcium homeostasis and bone metabolism during pregnancy, lactation, and postweaning: a longitudinal study, *Am. J. Clin. Nutr.*, 61, 514, 1995.

111. Kalkwarf, H. J., Specker, B. L., Bianchi, D. C., Ranz, J., and Ho, M., The effect of calcium supplementation on bone density during lactation and after weaning, *N. Engl. J. Med.*, 337(8), 523, 1997.

112. U. S. Department of Health and Human Services, Public Health Service, *Healthy People 2000 National Health Promotion and Disease Prevention Objectives*, DHHS Publication No. (PHS) 91-50212, September 1990.

113. U. S. Department of Health and Human Services, Public Health Service, *Healthy People 2000 Review 1995-96*, Hyattsville, Maryland: Public Health Service, 1996.

114. Donangelo, C. M., Trugo, N. M. F., Melo, G. J. O., Gomes, D. D., and Henriques, C., Calcium homeostasis during pregnancy and lactation in primiparous and multi-parous women with sub-adequate calcium intakes, *Nutr. Res.*, 16(10), 1631, 1996.

115. Raman, L., Rajalskshmi, K., Krishnamachari, K. A. V. R., and Sastry, J. C., Effect of calcium supplementation to undernourished mothers during pregnancy on the bone density of the neonates, *Am. J. Clin. Nutr.*, 31, 466, 1978.

116. Ortega, R. M., Martinez, R. M., Quintas, M. E., Lopez-Sobaler, A. M., and Andres, P., Calcium levels in maternal milk: Relationships with calcium intake during the third trimester of pregnancy, *Br. J. Nutr.*, 79, 501, 1998.

117. Gulson, B. L., Mahaffey, K. R., Jameson, C. W., Mizon, K. J., Korsch, M. J., Cameron, M. A., Eisman, J. A., Mobilization of lead from the skeleton during the postnatal period is larger than during pregnancy, *J. Lab. Clin. Med.*, 131, 324, 1998.

118. Prentice, A., Maternal calcium requirements during pregnancy and lactation, *Am. J. Clin. Nutr.*, 59(Suppl.), 477S, 1994.

119. Repke, J. T., and Villar, J., Pregnancy-induced hypertension and low birth weight: the role of calcium, *Am. J. Clin. Nutr.*, 54, 237S, 1991.

120. Levine, R. J., Hauthy, J. C., Curet, L. B., Sibai, V. M., Catalano, P. M., Morris, C. D., DerSimonian, R., Esterlitz, J. R., Raymond, E. G., Bild, D. E., Clemens, J. C., and Cutler, J. A., Trial of calcium for prevention of preeclampsia, *N. Engl. J. Med.*, 337(2), 69, 1997.

121. Barr, S. I., Associations of social and demographic variables with calcium intakes of high school students, *J. Am. Diet. Assoc.*, 94, 260, 1994.

122. Thy-Jacobs, S., Ceccarelli, S., Bierman, A., Weisman, H., Cohen, M.-A., and Alvir, J., Calcium supplementation in premenstrual syndrome: a randomized crossover trial, *J. Gen. Intern. Med.*, 4, 183, 1989.

123. Thy-Jacobs, S., Starkey, P., Bernstein, D., Tian, J., and the Premenstrual Syndrome Study Group, Calcium carbonate and the premenstrual syndrome: Effects on premenstrual and menstrual symptoms, *Am. J. Obstetr. Gynecol.*, 179, 444, 1998.

124. Fahm, E. G. and Jocelyn, J., Changing behaviors to optimize women's health: A multidisciplinary seminar, *J. Am. Diet. Assoc.*, 98(7), 818, 1998.

125. Horwath, C. C., Govan, C. H., Campbell, A. J., Busby, W., and Scott, V., Factors influencing milk and milk product consumption in young and elderly women with low calcium intakes, *Nutr. Res.*, 15(12), 1735, 1995.

126. Karanja, N., Morris, C., Rufolo, P., Snyder, G., Illingworth, D. R., and McCarron, D. A., Impact of increasing calcium in the diet on nutrient consumption, plasma lipids, and lipoproteins in humans, *Am. J. Clin. Nutr.*, 59, 900, 1994.

127. Guthrie, J. F., Dietary patterns and personal characteristics of women consuming recommended amounts of calcium, *Family Econ. Nutr. Rev.*, 9(3), 1996.

128. Barger-Lux, M. J., Heaney, R. P., Packard, P. T., Lappe, J. M., and Recker, R. R., Nutritional correlates of low calcium intake, *Clin. Appl. Nutr.*, 2(4) 39, 1992.

129. Mitchell, M. K., Aging and older adults, In, *Nutrition Across the Lifespan*, W. B. Saunders, Philadelphia, 1997, 309.

130. Heaney, R. P., Age considerations in nutrient needs for bone health: older adults, *J. Am. Coll. Nutr.*, 15(6), 575, 1996.

131. National Osteoporosis Foundation, *Physician's Guide to Prevention and Treatment of Osteoporosis*, National Osteoporosis Foundation, Washington, D.C., 1998.

132. Fast facts on osteoporosis, National Osteoporosis Foundation, 1998.

133. Blumberg, J., Nutritional needs of seniors, *J. Am. Coll. Nutr.*, 16(6), 517, 1997.

134. Chapuy, M. C., Arlot, M. E., Duboeu, F., Brun, J., Crouzet, B., Arnaud, S., Delmas, P. D., Meunier, P. J., Vitamin D3 and calcium to prevent hp fractures in elderly women, *N. Engl. J. Med.*, 327, 1637, 1992.

135. Aloia, J. F., Vaswani, A., Yeh, J. K., Ross, P., Flaster, E., Dilmanian, A., Calcium supplementation with and without hormone replacement therapy to prevent postmenopausal bone loss, *Ann. Intern. Med.*, 120, 97, 1994.

136. Dawson-Hughes, B., Harris, S. S., Krall, E. A., Dallal, G. E., Effect of calcium and vitamin D supplementation on bone density in men and women 65 years of age or older, *N. Engl. J. Med.*, 337(10), 670, 1997.

137. Dawson-Hughes, B., Harris, S. S., and Dallal, G. E., Plasma calcidiol, season, and serum parathyroid hormone concentrations in healthy elderly men and women, *Am. J. Clin. Nutr.*, 65(1), 67, 1997.

138. Dawson-Hughes, B., Harris, S. S., Krall, E. A., Dallal, G. E., Falconer, G., and Green, C. L., Rates of bone loss in postmenopausal women randomly assigned to one of two dosages of vitamin D, *Am. J. Clin. Nutr.*, 61(5), 1140, 1995.

139. Holick, M. F., McCollum Award Lecture, 1994: Vitamin D – new horizons for the 21st century, *Am. J. Clin. Nutr.*, 60, 619, 1994.

140. Schurch, M-A., Rizzoli, R., Slosman, D., Vadas, L., Vergnaud, P., and Bonjour, J-P., Protein supplements increase serum insulin-like growth factor-I levels and attenuate proximal femur bone loss in patients with recent hip fracture, *Ann. Intern. Med.*, 128, 801, 1998.

141. Munger, R. G., Cerhan, J. R., and Chiu, B. C-H., Prospective study of dietary protein intake and risk of hip fracture in postmenopausal women, *Am. J. Clin. Nutr.*, 69, 147, 1999.

142. Campbell, W. W., Crim, M. C., Dallal, G. E., Young, V. R., Evans, W. J., Increased protein requirements in the elderly: new data and retrospective reassessments, *Am. J. Clin. Nutr.*, 60, 501, 1994.

143. Johnson, M. A., Houston, D. K., Edmonds, J., Nozza, R. J., Shea, K., Cutler, M., Lewis, R. D., Modlesky, C., and Gunter, E. W., Age-related hearing loss is associated with poor bone health and low calcium intake in women, *FASEB J.*, 12(5), A878, 1998.

144. Constans, T., Delarue, J., Rival, M., Theret, V., and Lamisse, F., Effects of nutrition education on calcium intake in the elderly, *J. Am. Diet. Assoc.*, 94(4), 447, 1994.

145. Jensen, G. L. and Rogers, J., Obesity in older persons, *J. Am. Diet. Assoc.*, 98(11), 1308, 1998.

146. Greene, G. W., The relationship between dietary change over 18 months and the aging process, *J. Am. Diet. Assoc.*, 98(9), A-69, 1998.

147. Ali, N. S. and Twibell, R. K., Health promotion and osteoporosis prevention among postmenopausal women, *Preventive Med.*, 24, 528, 1995.

148. Elbon, S. M., Johnson, M. A., and Fischer, J. G., Milk consumption in older Americans, *Am. J. Public Health*, 88(5), 1221, 1998.

149. Suarez, F. L., Adshead, J., Furne, J. K., and Levitt, M. D., Lactose maldigestion is not an impediment to the intake of 1500 mg calcium daily as dairy products, *Am. J. Clin. Nutr.*, 68(5), 1118, 1998.

150. Devine, A., Prince, R. L., and Roma, B., Nutritional effect of calcium supplementation by skim milk powder or calcium tablets on total nutrient intake in postmenopausal women, *Am. J. Clin. Nutr.*, 64, 731, 1996.

151. Heaney, R. P., Food: What a surprise!, *Am. J. Clin. Nutr.*, 64, 791, 1996.

152. Goldberg, J. P., Gershoff, S., N., and McGandy, R. B., Appropriate topics for nutrition education for the elderly, *J. Nutr. Educ.*, 22, 303, 1990.

153. Posner, B. M., Jette, A. M., Smith, K. W., and Miller, D. R., Nutrition and health risks in the elderly: The nutrition screening initiative, *Am. J. Public Health*, 83, 972, 1993.

Index